Differential Diagnosis in **PEDIATRICS**
(Including Color Atlas)

Differential Diagnosis in PEDIATRICS
(Including Color Atlas)

Sixth Edition

Suraj Gupte MD FIAP FSAMS (Sweden) FRSTMH (London)
Professor and Head (Emeritus)
Postgraduate Department of Pediatrics
Mamata Medical College and Mamata General and
Superspecialty Hospitals
Khammam, Telangana, India
drsurajgupte@gmail.com
www.drsurajgupte.com

Editor: The Short Textbook of Pediatrics; Recent Advances in Pediatrics (Series), Textbook of Pediatric Emergencies, Neonatal Emergencies, Pediatric Nutrition, and Pediatric Gastroenterology, Hepatology and Nutrition; Pediatric Infectious Diseases; Influenza: Complete Spectrum; Case-based Reviews in Pediatric Emergencies, Clinical Problem Solving in Neonatal Emergencies and Intensive Care, etc.
Author: Pediatric Drug Directory, Instructive Case Studies in Pediatrics, Influenza, Perspectives in Influenza, Nutrition in Neonatal ICU, Speaking of Child Care, etc. *Chief Editor* (Gastroenterology Section): International Journal of Gastroenterology, Hepatology, Transplant and Nutrition.
Co-editor: Asian Journal of Maternity and Child Health (Manila, Philippines). *Section and Guest Editor:* Pediatric Today (New Delhi).
Editorial Advisor: Asian Journal of Pediatric Practice (New Delhi). Editorial Advisory Board
Member/Reviewer: Indian Journal of Pediatrics (New Delhi), Indian Pediatrics (New Delhi), Indian Journal Child Health (Gwalior), Synopsis (Detroit, USA), Maternal and Child Nutrition (Preston, UK), Journal of Infectious Diseases (Turkey), EC Pediatrics (London), Journal of Clinical Pediatrics (Patna), etc.
Examiner: Several Universities, including National Board of Examinations (NBE) for DNB, New Delhi; All India Institute of Medical Sciences (AIIMS), New Delhi; Postgraduate Institute of Medical Education and Research (PGIMER), Chandigarh; Sher-I-Kashmir Institute of Medical Sciences (SKIMS), Srinagar; Indira Gandhi National Open University (IGNOU), New Delhi
Pediatric Faculty Selection Expert: All India Institute of Medical Sciences (AIIMS), Punjab Public Service Commission, J&K Public Service Commission, Union Public Service Commission, etc.

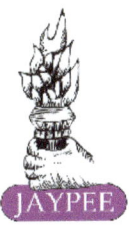

JAYPEE BROTHERS MEDICAL PUBLISHERS
The Health Sciences Publisher

New Delhi | London

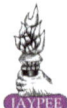 **Jaypee Brothers Medical Publishers (P) Ltd**

Headquarters

Jaypee Brothers Medical Publishers (P) Ltd
4838/24, Ansari Road, Daryaganj
New Delhi 110 002, india
Phone: +91-11-43574357
Fax: +91-11-43574314
Email: jaypee@jaypeebrothers.com

Overseas Office

J.P. Medical Ltd
83 Victoria Street, London
SW1H 0HW (UK)
Phone: +44 20 3170 8910
Fax: +44 (0)20 3008 6180
Email: info@jpmedpub.com

Website: www.jaypeebrothers.com
Website: www.jaypeedigital.com

© 2020, Manu Gupte, Executive Editor

The views and opinions expressed in this book are solely those of the original contributor(s)/author(s) and do not necessarily represent those of editor(s) of the book.

All rights reserved. No part of this publication may be reproduced, stored or transmitted in any form or by any means, electronic, mechanical, photocopying, recording or otherwise, without the prior permission in writing of the publishers/editors.

All brand names and product names used in this book are trade names, service marks, trademarks or registered trademarks of their respective owners. the publisher is not associated with any product or vendor mentioned in this book.

Medical knowledge and practice change constantly. This book is designed to provide accurate, authoritative information about the subject matter in question. However, readers are advised to check the most current information available on procedures included and check information from the manufacturer of each product to be administered, to verify the recommended dose, formula, method and duration of administration, adverse effects and contraindications. It is the responsibility of the practitioner to take all appropriate safety precautions. Neither the publisher nor the author(s)/editor(s) assume any liability for any injury and/or damage to persons or property arising from or related to use of material in this book.

This book is sold on the understanding that the publisher is not engaged in providing professional medical services. If such advice or services are required, the services of a competent medical professional should be sought.

Every effort has been made where necessary to contact holders of copyright to obtain permission to reproduce copyright material. If any have been inadvertently overlooked, the publisher will be pleased to make the necessary arrangements at the first opportunity. the **CD/DVD-ROM** (if any) provided in the sealed envelope with this book is complimentary and free of cost. **Not meant for sale.**

Inquiries for bulk sales may be solicited at: jaypee@jaypeebrothers.com

Differential Diagnosis in Pediatrics (Including Color Atlas)

First Edition: 1986

Sixth Edition: **2020**

ISBN 978-93-5270-247-3

Dedicated to

*My Parents
Who always gave my efforts
the necessary blessings
Their inspiration has been a
tower of strength in
bringing out
this book and other books*

Foreword

At the very outset, I wish to record my indebtedness to Prof Suraj Gupte, India's outstanding pediatric educationist, researcher and innovator with a multitude of high-quality books and other publications to his credit. He is gracious enough in asking me to again write a Foreword to the sixth edition of his noted book, *Differential Diagnosis in Pediatrics*.

Having carefully gone through the drafts of the new edition, I have no doubt that this already popular book has considerably improved its excellence and utility for the intended readership. The first section, i.e. Color Atlas, has many more high-quality photographs added to it. **The contents of the 62 topics** included in the second section are significantly improved and updated with fresh matter plus illustrations, tables and boxes. Additionally, incorporation of "investigative component" has further strengthened the usefulness of the book. Notably, each chapter in this section is provided with key references for further reading. The remaining three sections deal with differential diagnosis of select clinical signs, laboratory findings and radiologic signs. Prof Gupte has done well to complement these too with illustrative photographs.

Furthermore, all through this fine book, the presentation is simple, lucid, straightforward and easy-to-understand. Over and above the richness of the contents, Prof Gupte's well-known style of driving home the important points to the readers is not just profusely evident but also a very strong points of the title.

In my considered opinion, the sixth edition of Prof Suraj Gupte's *Differential Diagnosis in Pediatrics* is a strongly recommended treatise for the target audience (undergraduate and postgraduate medical students, residents, and practitioners of child health). By virtue of its several unique qualities, it has attained the powerful potentials to sharpen the readers' skill in effectively dealing with signs and symptoms and quickly formulating the differential diagnoses in a given situation.

EA Robert MD PhD
Professor Emeritus
Department of Pediatrics
University School of Medicine
Formerly, WHO Regional Adviser
New York, United States

Preface to the Sixth Edition

The sixth edition of the *Differential Diagnosis in Pediatrics,* the pioneer and the solo textbook in the field from the Indian subcontinent stands thoroughly revised, updated, enlarged and further rendered state-of-the-art to meet the requirements of the medical students, residents, teachers and practitioner.

Section 1 exclusively presents *Color Atlas* comprising over 300 instructive clinical photographs with explanatory legends.

Section 2 presents chapters dealing with differential diagnosis of as many as 62 common presenting clinical manifestations such as abdominal distention, abdominal pain, chronic diarrhea, headache, short stature, jaundice, ambiguous genitalia, wheezing, etc. Each and every chapter is now complemented with key information about the investigative part over and above the clinical details.

Section 3 deals with the differential diagnosis of select clinical signs. Addition of clinical photographs has further enhanced its utility.

Section 4 is an illustrated spotlight on select laboratory findings and their significance.

Section 5 focuses on select radiologic signs. To enhance the impact, a multitude images are provided as illustrations.

Hopefully, the new revised, updated and enlarged edition of the *Differential Diagnosis in Pediatrics* shall receive yet warmer welcome and prove yet more beneficial to the target readership.

Preface to the First Edition

The vital importance of differential diagnosis, the backbone of deductive reasoning process and professional skill in clinical medicine, is widely recognized. Yet, for one or the other reason, the pediatric textbooks are not able to deal with this important aspect in a reasonably comprehensive way. A couple of books devoted exclusively to differential diagnosis are written by the European authors. These provide only very little information on problems relevant to the children of the developing countries and are, therefore, only of limited value in our settings.

The sustained and overwhelming demand from various quarters to fill this glaring "vacuum" has given birth to this new textbook, the first and the only one of its kind. I have designed it to provide a comprehensive up-to-date discussion on topics of day-to-day practical importance with special emphasis on problems encountered in the pediatric population in India and rest of the Third World.

As many as 48 topics ranging from *abdominal distention, abdominal pain or anemias* through *diarrhea, failure to thrive* or *hepatomegaly* to *splenomegaly, vomiting* or *wheezing,* are covered. Each topic organized alphabetically as a separate Section, starts off with an introductory note and sets out to highlight salient points in the history and physical examination having bearing on the differential diagnosis. Finally, I have discussed the various conditions that fall in the differential diagnosis, laying special stress on clinical features of particular diagnostic value. As and when indicated, a suitable reference is made to the investigative aspect.

All through this problem-oriented work, I have tried to be simple, straight-forward and lucid as also comprehensive and yet-to-the point. Hopefully, the volume would fulfill its aims and objectives and provide stimulating and informative reading for clinical diagnosis to the readers.

The book is addressed primarily to the medical students (both undergraduates and postgraduates), pediatric residents, junior pediatricians, family doctors and general practitioners whose clientage includes infants and children.

The eminent pediatric teacher, Dr N Sundaravalli, President, Indian Academy of Pediatrics, has done me great honor in writing the *Foreword* to this textbook at a time when she is extremely busy and preoccupied with, among the other things, affairs of the Academy. My salutation to her for recommending the volume so warmly!

The preparation of this textbook has needed cooperation of many people, including colleagues in and outside the country. I acknowledge my gratitudes to each one of them.

I record my sincere gratitudes to my parents and other family folks for providing generous help and encouragement while I was working on the manuscript. My wife, Shamma; daughter; Novy, and son, Manu; were gracious enough to make available to me the "time" that indeed needed to be spent with them. Their forbearance and understanding have contributed considerably to the entire endeavour taking the present solid shape.

Thanks are also due to the publishers, M/s Jaypee Brothers and their staff, for the excellent production qualities of the book.

Last, but in no way the least, any *feedback* for enhancing the practical utility of this textbook will be most welcome.

November 1986
"Gupte House"
60 Lower Gumat
Jammu 180001

Suraj Gupte MD

Special Acknowledgments

Grateful acknowledgments are hereby made to:
- Professor EA Robert, Professor Emeritus (Pediatrics), University School of Medicine, and Former WHO Regional Advisor, New York, for writing the Foreword and warmly recommending the book.
- World Health Organization, UNICEF, Recent Advances in Pediatrics, The Short Textbook of Pediatrics, Instructive Case Studies in Pediatrics, Dr EW Warner, Dr Sheffali Kapoor, Dr Arnold Bake, etc. for allowing access to some color images.
- Dr Gagan Hans, Dr Novy Gupte, Shamma-Bakshi Gupte and Shivanu Mahendru for voluntarily helping us in various ways in taking the project to its logical conclusion.
- Various journals and periodicals for critical reviews of previous editions of the book and for permission to use their references in the state-of-the-art chapters
- The readers who provided us the feedback to maintain and enhance the excellence of the book.
- M/s Jaypee Brothers Medical Publishers (P) Ltd, New Delhi, India, and their dedicated staff deserve our appreciation for the skilful and commendable production qualities of the book.

Finally, though all attempts have been made to acknowledge the source of information correctly here or in the text per se, error, if any, is unintentional and regretted.

Contents

SECTION 1: Color Atlas

SECTION 2: Differential Diagnosis of Common Pediatric Presentations

1. Abdominal Distension — 55
2. Abdominal Pain — 58
3. Ambiguous Genitalia (Intersex) — 65
4. Anemia — 68
5. Ataxia — 72
6. Blood in Stools — 74
7. Chest Pain — 77
8. Child Abuse and Neglect — 79
9. Clubbing — 82
10. Coma — 85
11. Constipation — 89
12. Seizures — 93
13. Cough — 100
14. Cyanosis — 103
15. Deafness — 106
16. Delayed Puberty — 109
17. Diarrhea — 111
18. Dyspnea — 117
19. Dysuria — 130
20. Edema — 132
21. Encopresis — 138
22. Enuresis — 140
23. Epistaxis — 142
24. Floppy Baby Syndrome — 144
25. Failure to Thrive — 148
26. Frequency of Micturition — 153
27. Feeding Problems — 155
28. Gingivostomatitis — 159
29. Halitosis — 161
30. Headache — 163
31. Heart Murmurs — 166
32. Hematemesis — 170
33. Hematuria — 173
34. Hemoptysis — 177
35. Hepatomegaly — 179
36. Hoarseness — 188
37. Involuntary Movements — 190
38. Irritability — 193
39. Jaundice — 195
40. Joint Pain — 203
41. Large Head — 209
42. Limping — 213
43. Lethargy — 218
44. Lymphadenopathy — 220
45. Mass in Abdomen — 225
46. Mouth Breathing — 233
47. Nystagmus — 235
48. Obesity — 237
49. Precocious Puberty — 239
50. Purpura — 242
51. Fever of Unknown Origin — 246
52. Rash — 254
53. Short Stature — 259
54. Small Head — 265
55. Splenomegaly — 267
56. Stiff Neck — 272
57. Stridor — 275
58. Sudden Infant Death Syndrome — 278
59. Tall Stature — 280
60. Vertigo — 283
61. Vomiting — 285
62. Wheezing — 289

SECTION 3: Differential Diagnosis of Selected Clinical Signs

63. Differential Diagnosis of Selected Clinical Signs — 295
    - Micrognathia 295
    - Stridor in First Few Days of Life 295
    - Macrocephaly 295
    - Microcephaly 295
    - Sparse and Light-colored Scalp Hair 296
    - Frontal/Parietal/Occipital Bossing 296

- Large Anterior Fontanel 296
- Craniotabes 296
- Rickets with Mental Retardation 296
- Bulging Anterior Fontanel 296
- Low-Set Ears 297
- Short Neck 297
- Depressed Bridge of Nose 297
- Hypertelorism 297
- Hypotelorism 297
- Periorbital Edema 297
- Mongoloid (Upward and Lateral) Slant of Eyes 297
- Epicanthal Folds 298
- Antimongoloid (Downward and Lateral) Slant of Eyes 298
- "Sunset" Sign 298
- Ptosis 298
- Proptosis (Exophthalmos) 299
- Blue Sclera 299
- Subconjunctival Hemorrhage 299
- White Reflex (Cat's Eye) 299
- Cataract 299
- Discoloration of Teeth 299
- Macroglossia 299
- Gingival Hyperplasia 300
- Blindness 300
- Pinpoint Pupil 300
- Iris Coloboma 300
- Acute Uveitis 300
- Deafness (Hearing Loss) 300
- Parotid Swelling 300
- Preauricular Tags/Pits 301
- Retarded (Delayed) Speech 301
- Pectus Carinatum (Pigeon Chest) 301
- Pectus Excavatum (Funnel Chest) 301
- Harrison Sulcus 301
- Costochondral Beading 301
- Senile Appearance 302
- Congenital Limb Hypertrophy 302
- Clinodactyly 302
- Polydactyly 302
- Knock-Knee Deformity (Genu Valgum) 302
- Bowleg Deformity (Genu Varus) 302
- Painful Swelling of Thigh 302
- Dry, Scaly, Hyperkeratotic Skin 303
- Skin Tuberculosis 303
- Scrofuloderma 303
- Sinus Bradycardia 303
- Sinus Tachycardia 303
- Paroxysmal Supraventricular Tachycardia 303
- Innocent Cardiac Murmur 304
- Cardiomegaly without Murmur 304
- Atrial Flutter or Fibrillation 304
- Umbilical Hernia 304
- Scoliosis 304
- Flat Foot 304
- Talipes Equinovarus (Club Foot) 304
- Congenital Goiter 304
- Gynecomastia 305
- Simian Crease 305
- Cafe-au-lait Spots 305
- Drug-induced Lupus 305
- Butterfly Rash 305
- Recurrence of Fever in Meningitis (on Treatment) 305
- Recurring Meningitis 305
- Opisthotonos 305
- Neck Rigidity (Stiffness) 305
- Acute Ataxia 305
- Chronic Ataxia (Static) 306
- Chronic Ataxia (Progressive) 306
- Calf Hypertrophy 306
- Painful/Tender Hepatic Enlargement 306
- Dull Percussion Note (Chest) 306
- Pigeon Chest Deformity 306
- Hemihypertrophy 306
- Microorchidism 306
- Macroorchidism 306
- Micropenis 306
- Vaginal Bleeding 306
- Syndrome of Inappropriate Secretion of ADH 306
- Ascites 306
- Gastroenteritis with Arthritis 307
- Gastrointestinal Bleeding 307
- Ulcerative Colitis-like Manifestations 307
- Soft Neurologic Signs 307
- Premature Graying of Hair 307
- Potter Facies and Syndrome 307

SECTION 4: Differential Diagnosis of Salient Laboratory Findings

64. **Differential Diagnosis of Salient Laboratory Findings**   311
    - Normocytic Anemia 311
    - Increased Mean Corpuscular Volume (Macrocytic Anemia) 311
    - Hypochronic Anemia 311
    - Decreased Mean Corpuscular Volume (Microcytic Anemia) 311
    - Increased Mean Corpuscular Hemoglobin Concentration 311
    - Target Cells 311
    - Basophilic Stippling 311
    - Howell–Jolly Bodies 311
    - Tear Drop Cells 312
    - Elliptocytosis 312
    - Acanthocytosis 312
    - Rouleaux Formation 312
    - Stomatocytes 313
    - Neutrophilia (Neutrophil Leukocytosis) 313
    - Neutropenia (Neutrophil Leukopenia) 313
    - Eosinophilia 313
    - Eosinopenia 314

- Lymphocytosis 314
- Lymphopenia 314
- Monocytosis 314
- Leukemoid Reaction 315
- Thrombocytopenia 315
- Poor Thrombocytopoiesis 315
- Poor Platelet Survival 315
- Sequestration of Platelets 315
- Thrombocytosis 315
- Hypocellular Bone Marrow 315
- Hypercellular Bone Marrow 315
- Megakaryocytic Hyperplasia 316
- Megakaryocytic Hypoplasia (Depression) 316
- Erythroid Hyperplasia 316
- Erythroid Hypoplasia 316
- Low-Serum Proteins (Total) 316
- High-Serum Proteins (Total) 316
- Low-Serum Albumin 316
- High-Serum Albumin 316
- Low Alpha-1 Globulin 316
- High Alpha-1 Globulin 316
- Low Alpha-2 Globulin 316
- High Alpha-2 Globulin 316
- High Beta Globulin 317
- Low Gamma Globulin 317
- High Gamma Globulin 317
- High Immunoglobulin G 317
- Low Immunoglobulin G 317
- Low Immunoglobulin A 317
- High Immunoglobulin A 317
- Low Immunoglobulin M 317
- High Immunoglobulin M 317
- High Immunoglobulin E 317
- Low Complement (C3, C4) 317
- High C-reactive Protein 317
- High Alpha-1-Fetoprotein 317
- High Creatine Phosphokinase 317
- High Serum Glutamic Oxaloacetic Transaminase or Aspartate Aminotransferase 318
- High Serum Glutamic-Pyruvic Transaminase or Alanine Aminotransferase 318
- High Alkaline Phosphatase 318
- Low Alkaline Phosphatase 318
- High Serum Amylase 318
- High Serum Lactate Dehydrogenase 318
- High Serum Calcium 318
- Low Serum Calcium 318
- High Serum Phosphate 318
- Low Serum Phosphate 318
- High Serum Magnesium 319
- Low Serum Magnesium 319
- High Serum Urea (Azotemia) 319
- Low Serum Urea 319
- High Serum Urea–Creatinine Ratio 319
- Low Serum Urea–Creatinine Ratio 319
- Aminoaciduria 319
- Phosphaturia 319
- Smell and Taste as Clues to Diagnosis 319
- Simple Observation on Urine as a Clue to Diagnosis 319
- Frothy: Albuminuria 319
- Hyaline: Normal 319
- Pathognomonic Jejunal Biopsy Findings 319
- High Sweat Chloride 320
- False Negative Sweat Chloride 320
- False Negative Tuberculin (Mantoux) Test 320
- Xanthochromic Cerebrospinal Fluid 320
- Albuminocytological Dissociation 320

SECTION 5: Differential Diagnosis of Selected Radiologic Signs

65. **Differential Diagnosis of Selected Radiologic Signs**   323
    - Mediastinal Shift 323
    - Hilar Enlargement 323
    - Enlargement of Anterior Mediastinum 323
    - Enlargement of the Superior Mediastinum 324
    - Enlargement of the Middle Mediastinum 324
    - Enlargement of the Posterior Mediastinum 324
    - Multiple Finely Granular Shadows (Miliary Mottling) in the Lungs 324
    - Solitary Lung Densities 325
    - Multiple Lung Densities 325
    - Large Lung Density 326
    - Overwhelming Interstitial Changes in Lung Field 326
    - Unilateral Increase in Lung Radiolucency 326
    - Pulmonary Edema (Unilateral) 326
    - Pulmonary Metastases 327
    - Middle Lobe Consolidation 327
    - Enlarged Cardiac Shadow 327
    - Air Bronchogram 327
    - Opaque Hemithorax 327
    - Kerley Lines in Chest X-ray 328
    - Nodular Opacities in Chest X-ray 328
    - Calcification in Chest X-ray 328
    - Reticular Granular Pattern in Chest X-ray 328
    - Soap Bubble Appearance in Abdomen Film of Neonates 328
    - Left Ventricular Enlargement 328
    - Left Atrial Enlargement 328
    - Right-sided Heart 328
    - Abnormal Intra-abdominal Air Collection 328
    - Bowel Showing Opaque Material (Calcification/Opacities) in Abdominal Film 329
    - Intra-abdominal Cyst 329

- Unilateral Small Kidney   329
- Bilateral Small Kidney   329
- Unilateral Large Kidney   329
- Bilateral Large Kidney   329
- Double Bubble Appearance   329
- Multiple Air-Fluid Levels   330
- Absent Radii   330
- Wormian Bones   330
- Hair-on-end Appearance (Skull)   330
- Abnormal Skull Shape   330
- Craniosynostosis   331
- J-shaped Sella Turcica   331
- Intracranial Calcification   331
- Sutural Diastasis   331
- Silver/Copper-beaten Appearance   332
- Increased Bone Density   332
- Enhancing Lesions (Neuroimaging)   332
- Nonenhancing Lesions (Neuroimaging)   332
- Calcification (Neuroimaging)   333
- Metacarpal Sign   333
- Pathologic Fractures   333

Index   *335*

SECTION 1

Color Atlas

Color Atlas 3

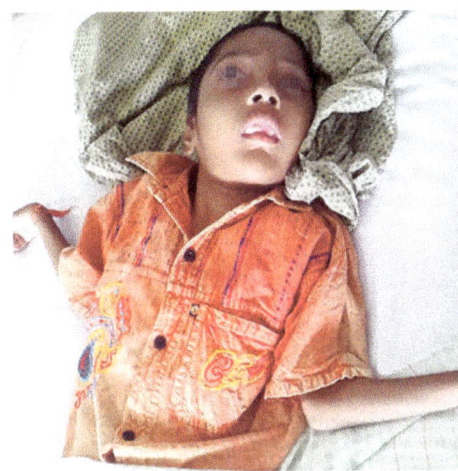

Fig. 1: *Tuberculous meningitis*—Note the features of third stage, especially flexion posturing as a result of decorticate rigidity.

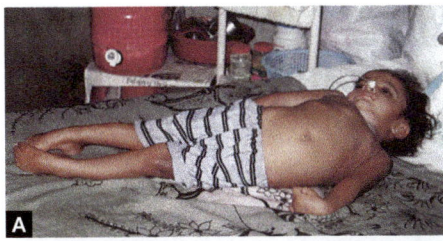
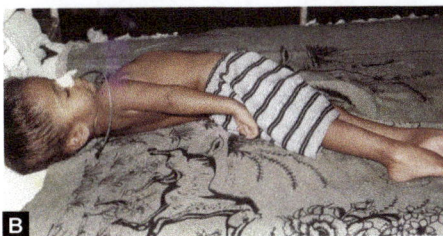

Figs. 2A and B: *Tuberculous meningitis*—Note the features of third stage, including coma and motor (neurologic) deficit in the form of extensor posturing from decerebrate rigidity.

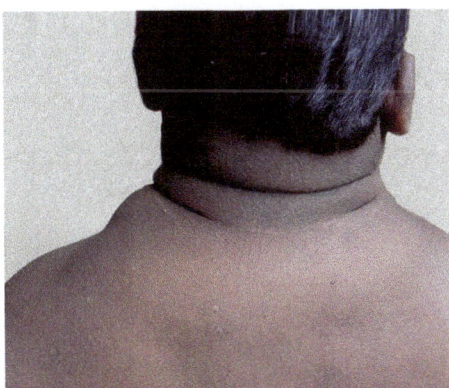

Fig. 3: *Buffalo hump*—Note the huge extra fat around the neck and upper part of the back. Typically, it is a feature of Cushing syndrome.

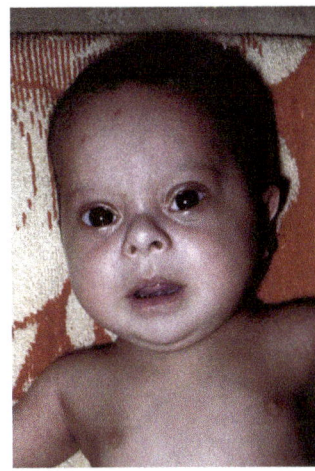

Fig. 4: *Down syndrome*—Note the characteristic facial and dysmorphic features—flat face, epicanthal folds, upward slant of eyes, and microcephaly with cheerful look and short neck. Flat nasal bridge and epicanthal fold give the impression of widely placed eyes, the so-called "pseudohypertelorism". In "true hypertelorism", the inter-pupillary distance between the eyes is actually increased due to overgrowth of the lesser wing and hypoplasia of greater wing of the sphenoid.

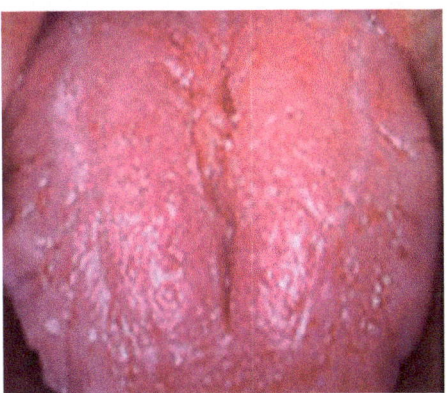

Fig. 5: *Down syndrome*—Note the typical scrotal tongue with fissures and wrinkles.

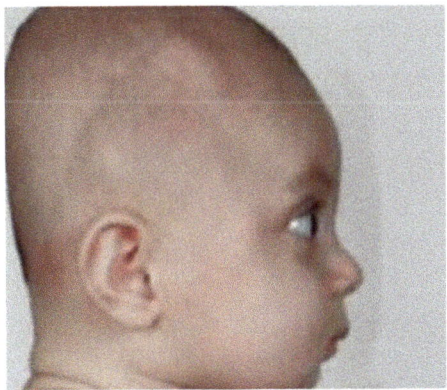

Fig. 6: **Downs syndrome*—Note the brachicephaly characterized by reduced anteroposterior diameter with flattened occiput.
*After the British physician, John Down, who first described it in 1886 as "mongolism".

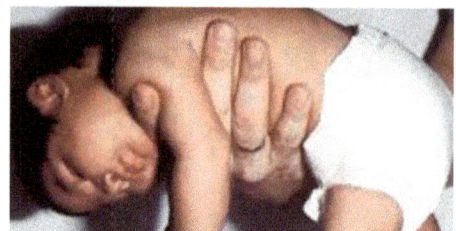

Fig. 7: *Down syndrome*—Note hypotonia over and above the facial features.

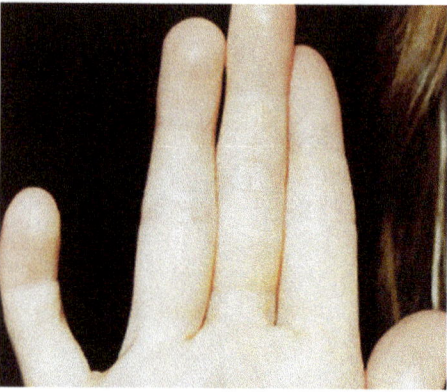

Fig. 10: *Down syndrome*—Note the bend (incurving) of the little finger towards the ring finger (clinodactyly). It may occur in other syndromes such as Turner syndrome, Russell–Silver syndrome.

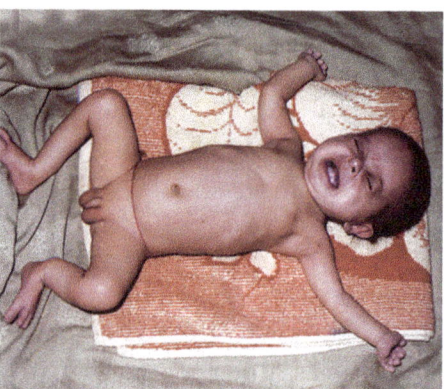

Fig. 8: *Down syndrome*—Note the hypotonia.

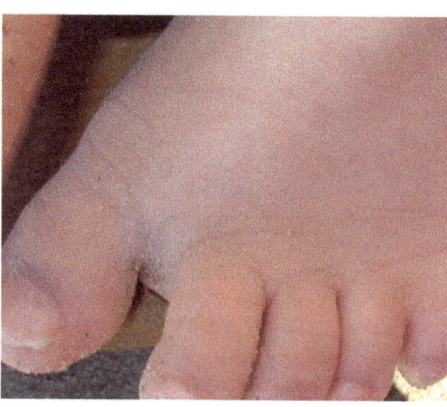

Fig. 11: *Down syndrome*—Note the unusual large gap between big toe and second toe.

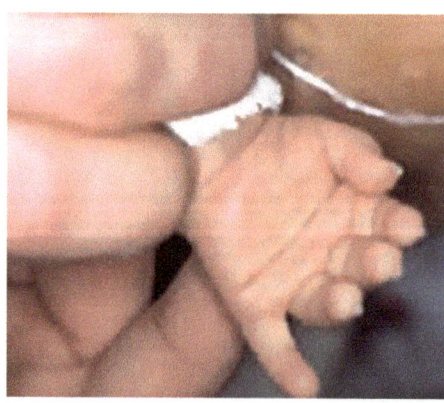

Fig. 9: *Down syndrome:* Note the single palmar (simian) crease.

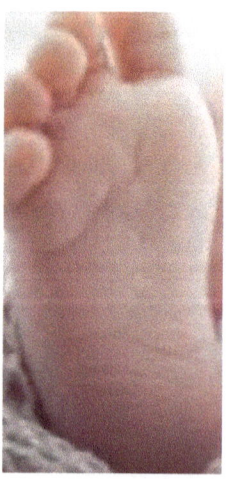

Fig. 12: *Down syndrome*—Note the unusual sole creases.

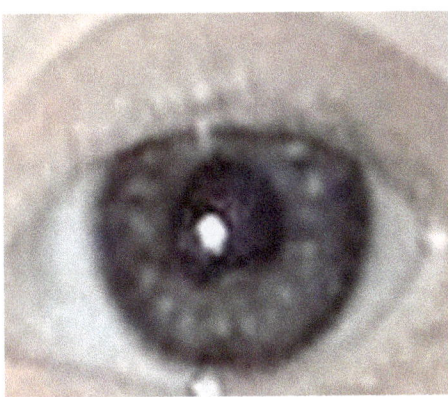

Fig. 13: *Down syndrome*—Note the whitish spots in the periphery of the iris (Brushfield spots).

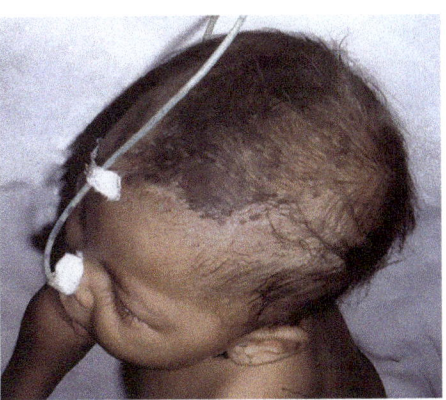

Fig. 14: *Infantile seborrheic dermatitis (cradle cap)*—Note the scaling and crusting of the scalp. The greasy erythematous papular lesions involving the face, neck, retroauricular areas, axillae, and diaper area, which are initially mild, become quite pronounced—virtually resembling psoriasis. Differential diagnosis includes, besides psoriasis, atopic dermatitis, candidiasis, and dermatophytosis.

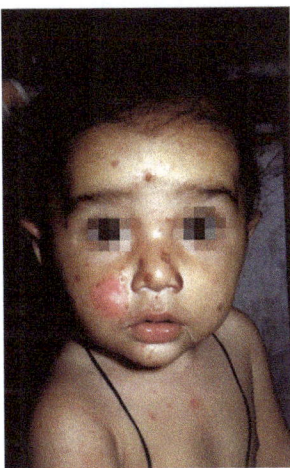

Fig. 15: *Atopic dermatitis (eczema)*—Note the characteristic highly pruritic erythematous papules over the face of the 8-month-old infant. Supportive features for this diagnosis include chronic remitting behavior of the eczema with positive family history of atopy, say asthma, immediate skin test reactivity, hay fever, or high immunoglobulin E (IgE). Differential diagnosis includes inflammatory skin diseases, infectious diseases, infestations, genetic disorders, immunodeficiency, and skin malignancy.

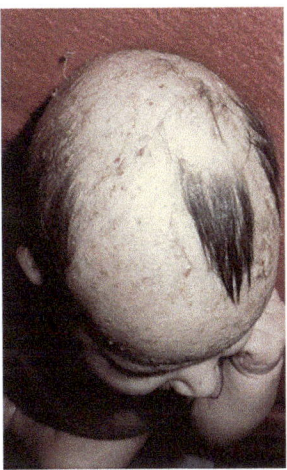

Fig. 16: *Atopic dermatitis (partially treated)*—In addition to the erythematous papules over the scalp and face, intense pruritus is a dominant feature. It may coexist with infantile seborrhea. Both parents and an elder sibling of this infant were asthmatic.

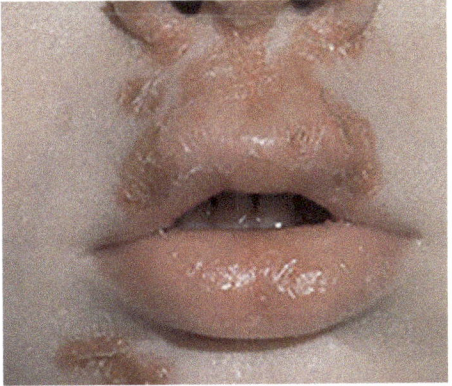

Fig. 17: *Impetigo*—Usually, *Streptococcus* and, less frequently, *Staphylococcus* are the etiologic agents.

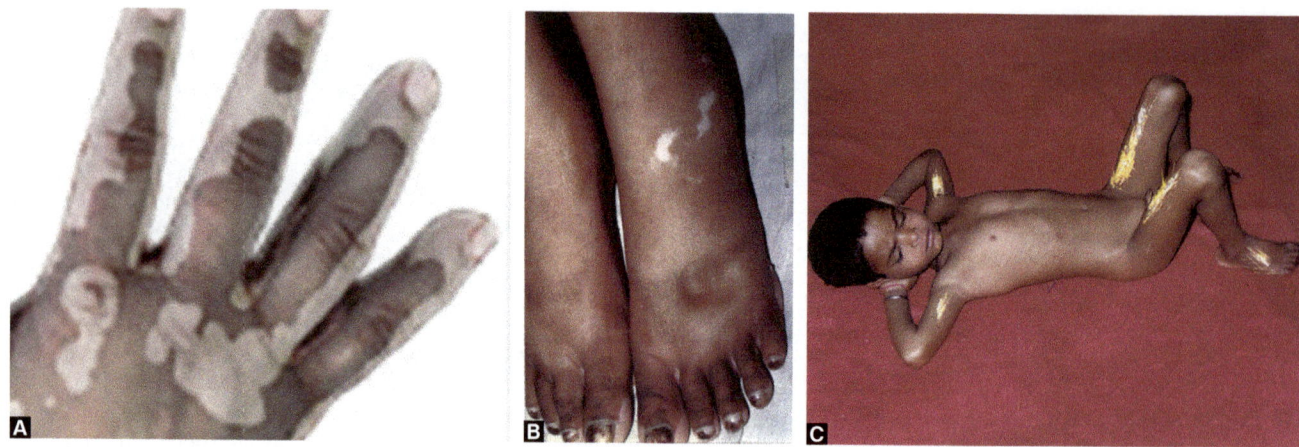

Figs. 18A to C: *Vitiligo*—Note the sharply circumscribed completely depigmented macules of varying size and shape (more or less symmetrical), due to absence of melanocytes and melanin in the epidermis. Uveitis and premature graying of hair may also be present. The disorder is more prevalent in subjects with immunologic disorders, e.g. thyroid disease (both hypothyroidism and hyperthyroidism), adrenal insufficiency, pernicious anemia, diabetes mellitus, etc. Note that depigmentation of the macules is complete. In case of pityriasis, depigmentation is only partial.

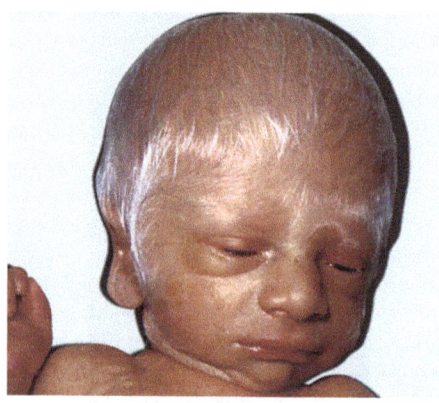

Fig. 19: *Generalized (oculocutaneous) albinism*—Note the remarkable hypopigmentation of hair and skin. Irides were translucent and pink and there was marked photophobia. When seen last, the patient was 11-month-old child and had developed strabismus and the irides had become light blue.

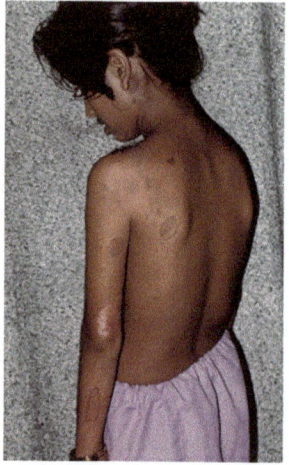

Fig. 20: *Café-au-lait spots*—Note the several dark macules. More than six spots measuring 5–15 mm in preadolescents and more than 15 mm later are considered pathologic (as was the case in this girl with neurofibromatosis). Differential diagnosis includes neurofibromatosis, ataxia telangiectasia, Fanconi anemia, Gaucher's disease, and McCune–Albright syndrome.

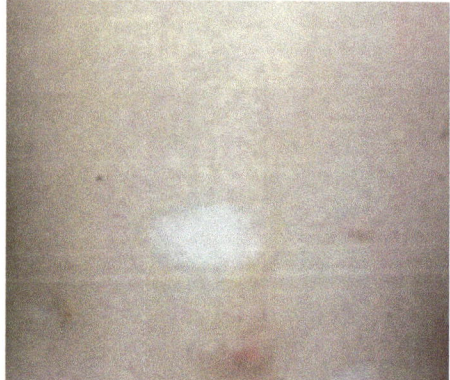

Fig. 21: *Ash-leaf spot*—Note the white, hypopigmented leaf-like patch in tuberous sclerosis.

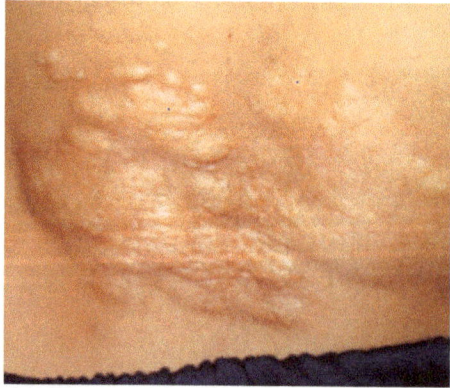

Fig. 22: *Shagreen patch*—Note areas of thick leathery skin that are dimpled like an orange peel, and pigmented in tuberous sclerosis. Lower back, nape of the neck, trunk, and thighs are the common sites.

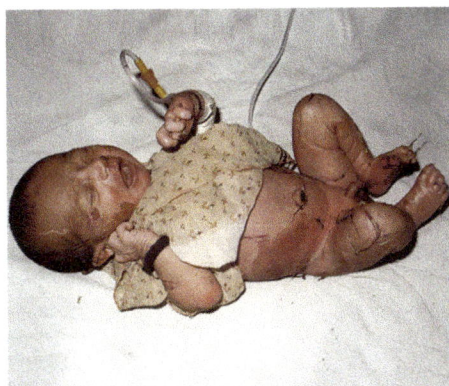

Fig. 23: *Ritter's disease*—Note the conjunctivitis, circumoral lesions, and areas of epidermis showing separation in response to gentle pressure (Nikolsky sign). An extensive sheet of epidermis may peel off, leaving behind raw and glistening areas. Risk of super added sepsis and fluid and electrolyte balance is considerable.

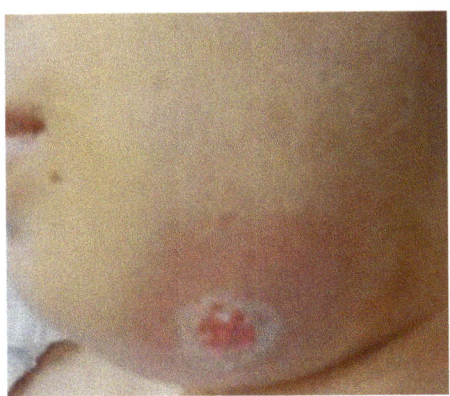

Fig. 26: Abscess.

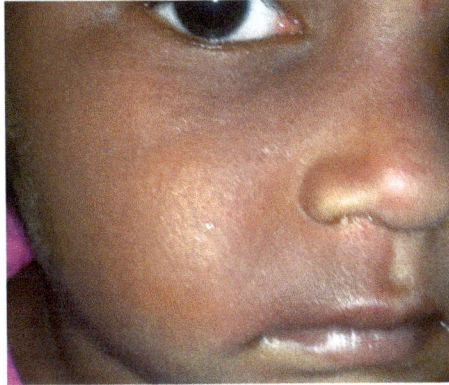

Fig. 24: *Erysipelas (Holy fire, St Anthony's fire)*—Note the erythema from superficial infection of skin (involving upper dermis) and lymphatics. Beta hemolytic group A *Streptococcus* (GAS) is the usual causative bacteria.

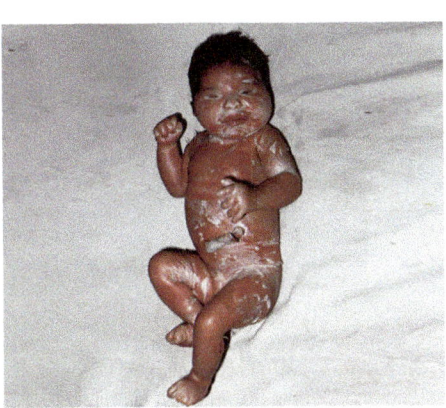

Fig. 27: *Collodion baby*—Note the remnants of the thick taut membrane, flat nose and ears, and ectropion. Now over 12 years of age, the child has ichthyosis.

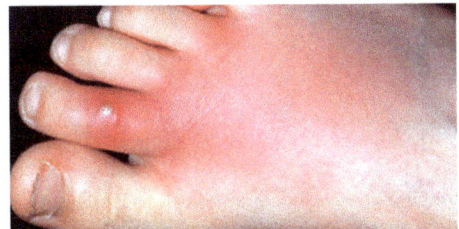

Fig. 25: *Cellulitis*—Note that, compared to erysipelas, the skin involvement is deeper.

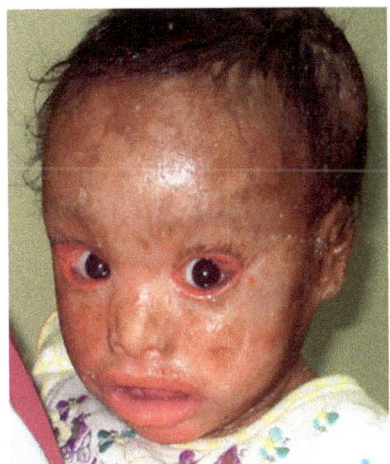

Fig. 28: *Congenital ichthyosis*—Note the skin lesions and upper and lower lid ectropion in both eyes.

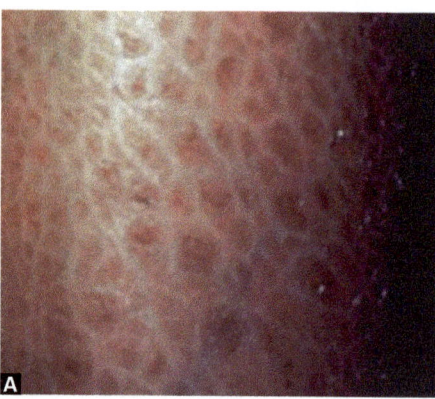
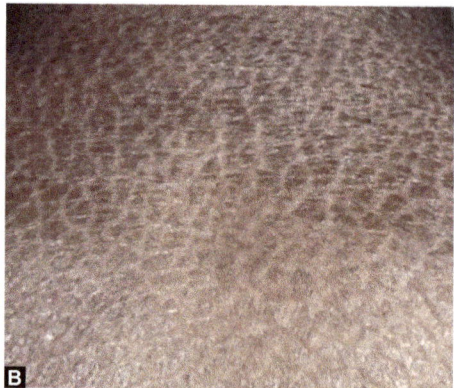

Figs. 29A and B: *Ichthyosis vulgaris*—Note the roughening and scaling over extensor aspects of legs in an 8-month-old child. The flexural surfaces were unaffected. Involvement of upper limbs and palms and soles was mild whereas face, neck, and abdomen were spared. The lesion showed worsening in winter and improvement in summer. This is the most common among the hereditary causes of keratinization.

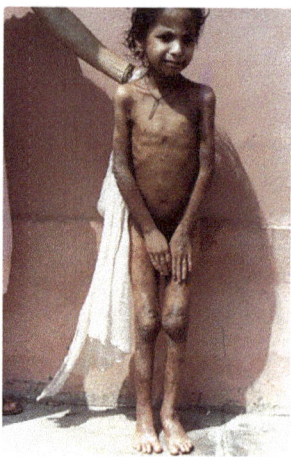

Fig. 30: *Psoriasis*—Note the erythematous papules that, at places, coalesce to form plaques with irregular sharp borders. The valuable diagnostic signs of psoriasis are—pitting of nail plate, Auspitz sign, removal of yellowish-white scale causing pinpoint bleeding, and Koebner/isomorphic response, appearance of new lesions at sites of trauma.

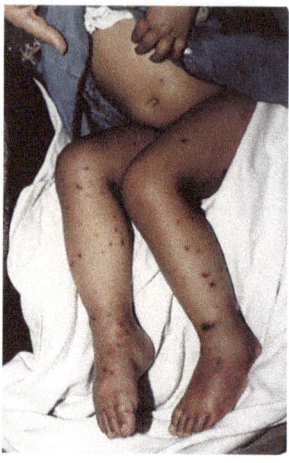

Fig. 31: *Scabies*—Note the eczematous dermatitis, papules, and nodules. In infants, involvement of palms and soles, face and scalp is more common than that of interdigital spaces. The classical thread-like burrows may not be seen in infants.

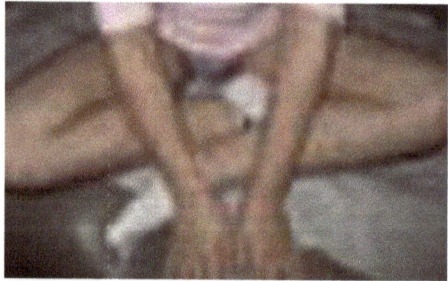

Fig. 32: *Scabies*—Note the characteristic itchy lesions with burrows in the skin involving particularly the hands (especially interdigital space and sides of fingers), wrists, elbows, feet, buttocks, axillae, and external genitalia. The child developed superimposed infection (presumably with group A beta-hemolytic streptococcal followed by acute glomerulonephritis).

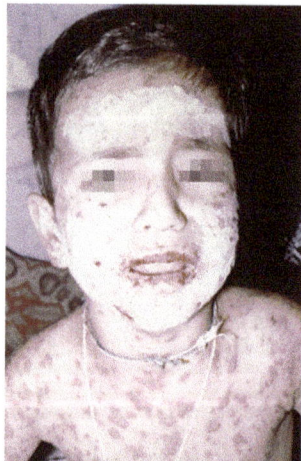

Fig. 33: *Stevens–Johnson syndrome*—Note the extensive lesions involving both skin and mucous membrane. The offending agent was phenobarbital.

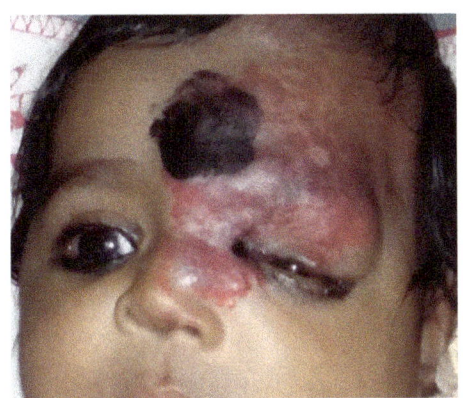

Fig. 34: *Capillary hemangioma*—Note the hemangioma on child's left side involving upper eyelid and nose.

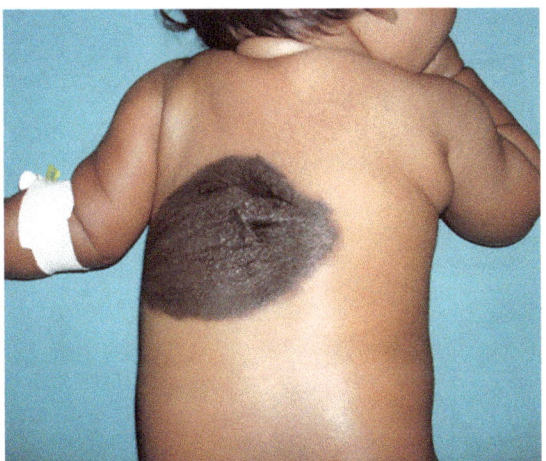

Fig. 35: *Congenital cutaneous nevus*—Note its intermediate size.

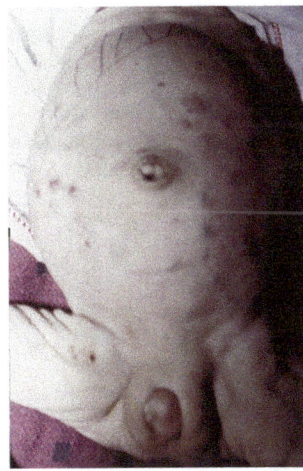

Fig. 36: *Purpura complicating—Gram-negative sepsis*—Note the widespread petechia and purpuric spots.

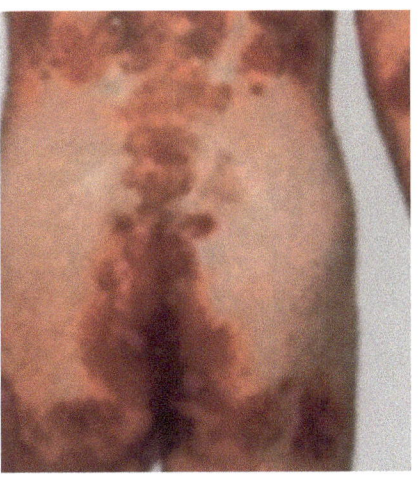

Fig. 37: *Pemphigus vulgaris.*

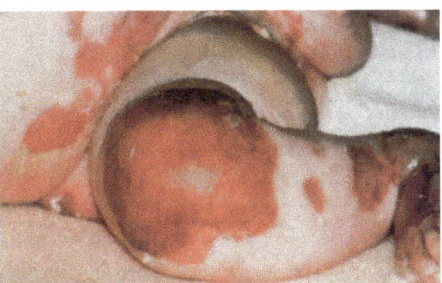

Fig. 38: *Epidermolysis bullosa simplex*—Note the extensive hemorrhagic blisters with erosions (which are vulnerable to super-added infection) in a neonate.

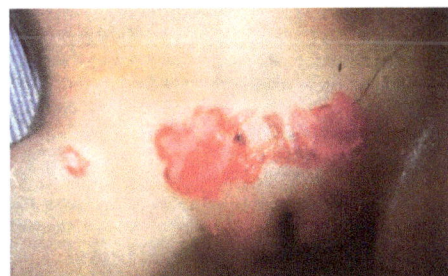

Fig. 39: *Chronic bullous dermatosis*—Note the cluster of jewels with new bullae over older lesions.

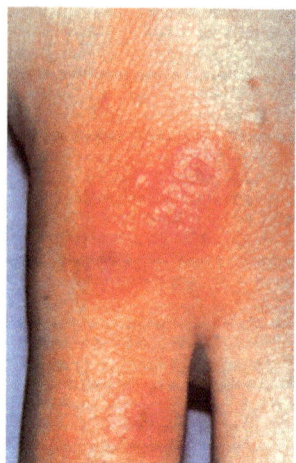

Fig. 40: *Erythema multiforme*—Note the typical target lesions over the knuckles (series of concentric circles). Etiologic factors include viruses, bacteria, fungi, vaccination, and drugs (especially sulfas, penicillins, and anticonvulsants).

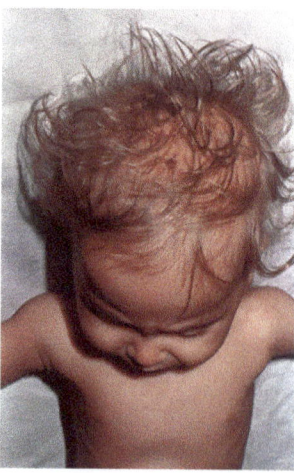

Fig. 41: *Sparse, light-colored hair*—Differential diagnosis includes kwashiorkor, infantile tremor syndrome (ITS), acrodermatitis enteropathica, zinc deficiency, and acrodynia.

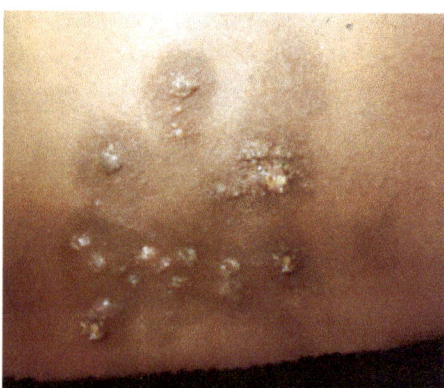

Fig. 42: *Herpes zoster (HZ)*—Note the vesicular lesions clustering within a dermatome. Unlike the disease in adults, in children the neurologic manifestations (pain, hyperesthesia, etc.) are minimal and full recovery usually occurs. In immunocompromised children, however, severe disease may occur. Varicella in the mother in third trimester or in the child in the first year is particularly a risk factor for HZ.

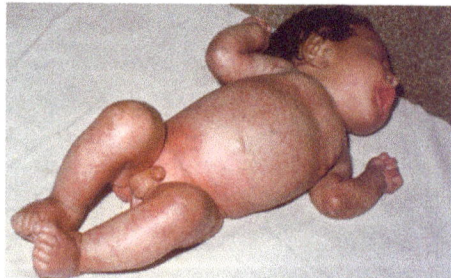

Fig. 43: *Acrodermatitis enteropathica (AE)*—Note the vesicobullous and eczematous skin and perioral lesions (symmetrically distributed), blepharitis, some alopecia, growth failure, and paronychia in an artificially fed infant with chronic diarrhea. Response to oral zinc was excellent. In some cases, psoriasiform skin lesions may be encountered. Skin lesions of AE may be seen in maple syrup urine disease, organic aciduria, essential fatty acid deficiency, cystic fibrosis, and kwashiorkor.

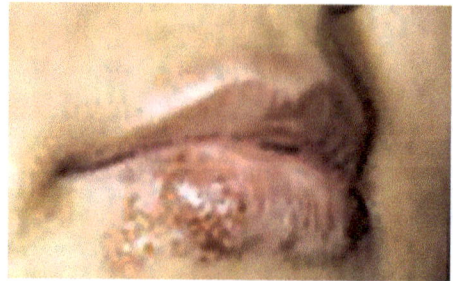

Fig. 44: *Herpes labialis*—Note the painful lesions (vesicles) over lips together with erythema and edema preceded by a prodrome of fever. Accompanying these lesions, the child had gingivostomatitis and cervical lymphadenitis. Healing occurred by ulceration and crust formation in the following 3 weeks. Caused by herpes simplex virus, the disease has a tendency for recurrences.

Color Atlas

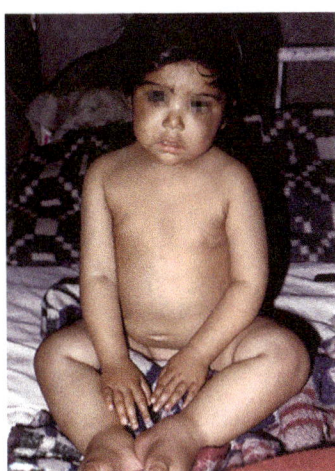

Fig. 45: *Nephrotic syndrome*—Note the generalized edema. The 24-hour urine protein was 10 g, serum cholesterol 310 mg/dL, serum albumin 1.8 g/dL. Response to steroids was excellent.

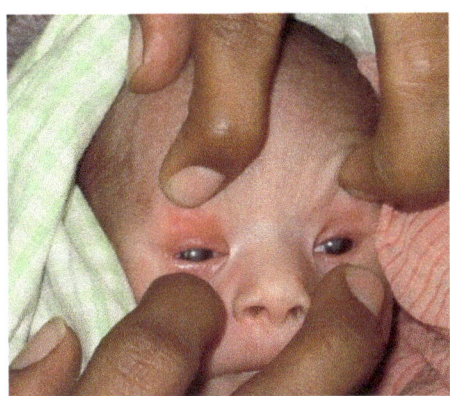

Fig. 48: *Congenital rubella syndrome*—Note the microphthalmia plus bilateral cataract.

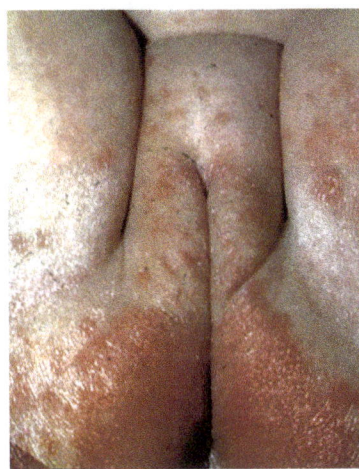

Fig. 46: *Nappy (diaper) rash*—Note that erythema is apparent on convexities with sparing of the inguinal folds, giving it the W-shape.

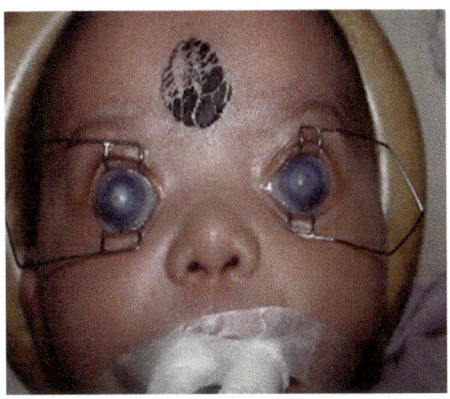

Fig. 49: *Congenital rubella syndrome*—Note bilateral cataract.

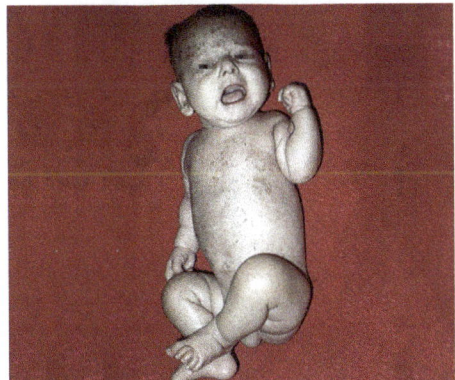

Fig. 47: *Seborrheic dermatitis*—Note the cradle cap and poorly circumscribed erythematous rash extending downward to involve forehead, ears, eyebrows, nose, and trunk.

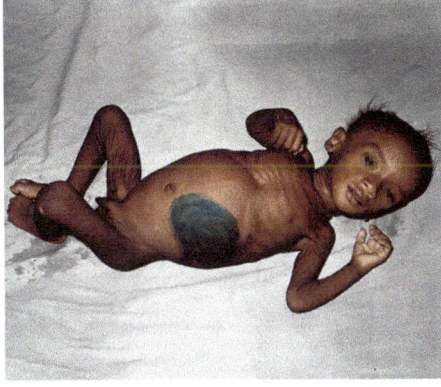

Fig. 50: *Wilms' tumor (nephroblastoma)*—Note the large mass (not crossing the midline) in the child brought for increasing abdominal distention, failure to thrive (FTT), and hematuria. X-ray and imaging studies confirmed the diagnosis. Differential diagnosis includes neuroblastoma, non-Hodgkin's lymphoma, hepatoblastoma, hepatoma, etc.

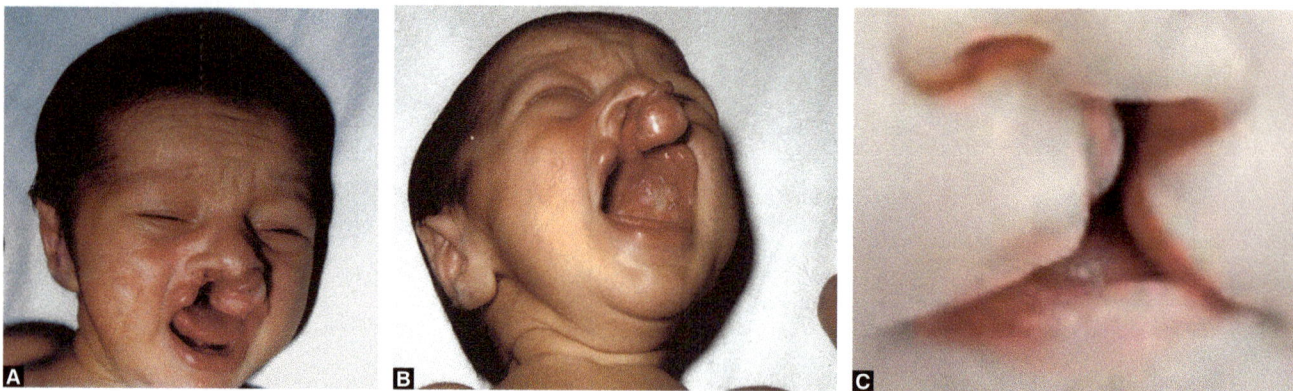

Figs. 51A to C: *Cleft lip*—Note the complete separation (bilateral) involving skin, muscle, mucosa, and alveolar border. Associated cleft palate should carefully be excluded. Surgical closure (modification of Millard rotation advancement technique) should be done by 3 months when a reasonable weight gain has occurred and the infant is infection free.

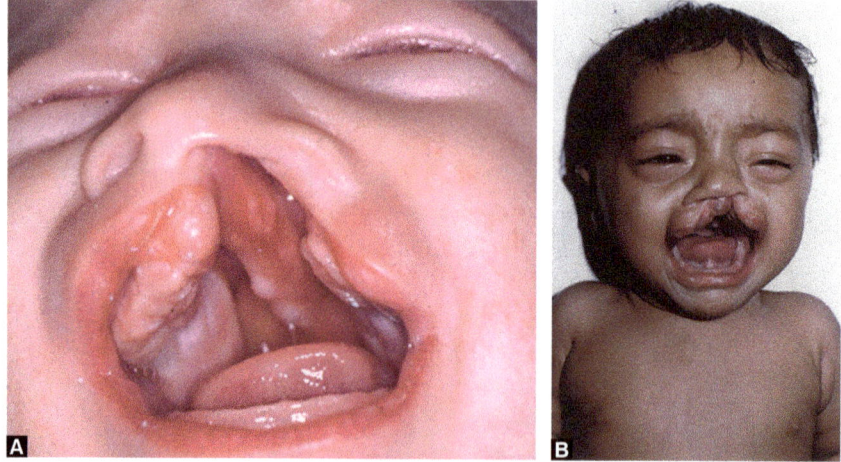

Figs. 52A and B: *Cleft lip and palate*—Note complete separation of lip involving all layers, including alveolar ridge (bilateral) plus defect involving the midline of the soft palate and extending into the hard palate. Surgical closure is recommended by 12 months of age to ensure normal speech development. Besides speech defects, sequelae may include recurrent otitis media and hearing loss.

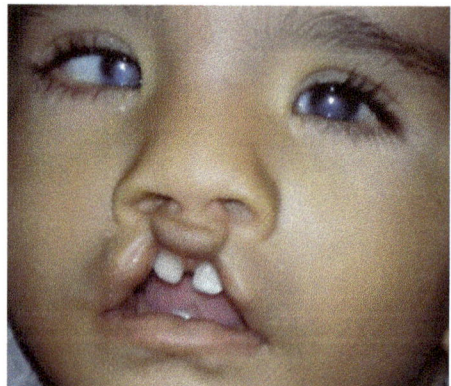

Fig. 53: *Peter's anomaly*—Note bilateral corneal opacity, depressed nasal bridge, and cleft lip with cleft palate in an infant born premature. Peter's plus syndrome includes disproportionate short stature, developmental delay, dysmorphic facial features, cardiac, genitourinary, and central nervous system malformations.

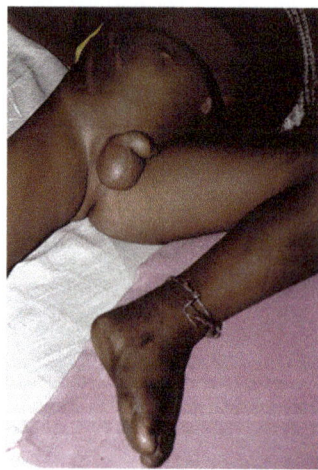

Fig. 54: *Snakebite*—Note the inflammation all around and spreading to the leg.

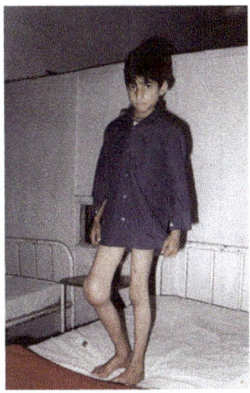
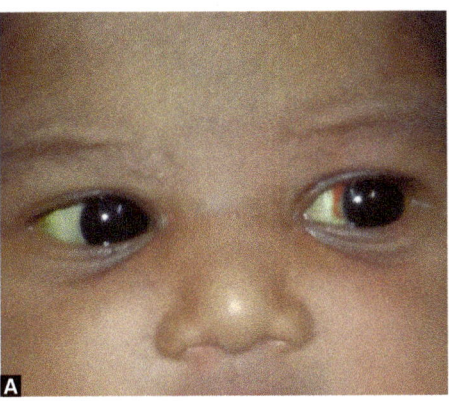

Fig. 55: *Hemophiliac arthropathy*—Note the chronic arthropathy involving the right knee joint, following cyclic recurrent bleeds.

Figs. 56A and B: *Subconjunctival hemorrhage*—Note the bright hemorrhage in bulbar conjunctiva. The causes include violent coughing (pertussis), violent sneezing, bleeding diathesis [scurvy, idiopathic thrombocytopenic purpura (ITP), leukemia] or inflammation (conjunctivitis).

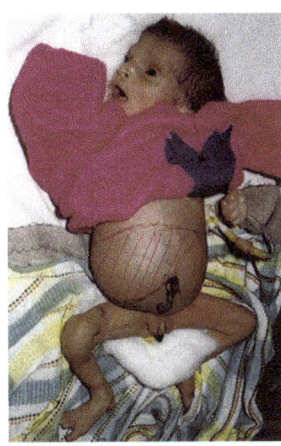
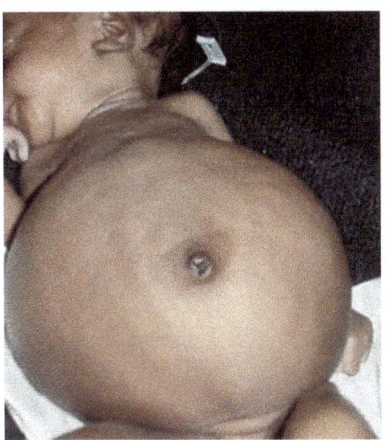

Fig. 57: *Alpha1-antitrypsin deficiency*—Note the icterus with massive hepatomegaly. Stools were alcoholic. The infant eventually died of cirrhosis at 6 months of age. Diagnosis stool established by determination of an alpha1-antitrypsin (Pi) phenotype and liver biopsy. The sole curative treatment is liver transplantation.

Fig. 58: Massive ascites secondary to biliary cirrhosis.

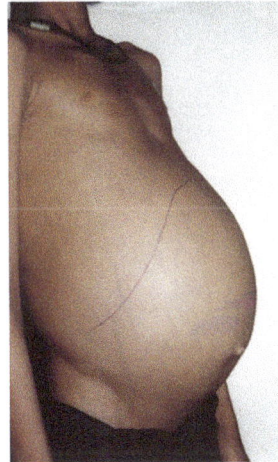
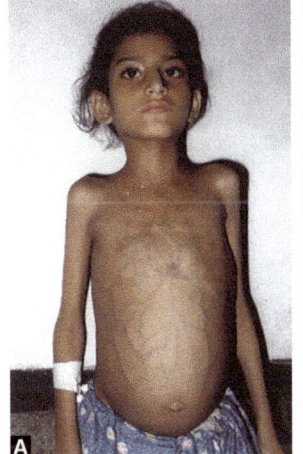
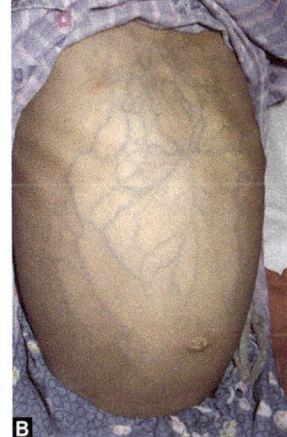

Fig. 59: *Massive tense ascites*—Note the massive abdominal distention with hepatomegaly, engorged superficial abdominal wall veins and positive fluid thrill in a known case of hepatitis B. Serum-ascites albumin gradient (SAAG) was high (71.1 g/dL). Liver biopsy confirmed clinical diagnosis of cirrhosis.

Figs. 60A and B: *Extrahepatic portal hypertension*—Note the tortuous veins over anterior abdominal wall and splenomegaly in a girl who presented with recurrent bouts of hematemesis and endoscopy showed both esophageal and gastric varices. Portal pressure turned out to be 16 mm Hg; (normal 7 mm Hg; upper limit 10–12 mm Hg).

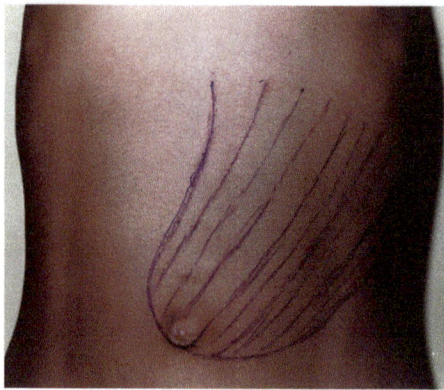

Fig. 61: *Tropical splenomegaly*—Note the massive splenomegaly in a 10-year-old child with moderate anemia and growth retardation. The boy came from a hyperendemic area for malaria.

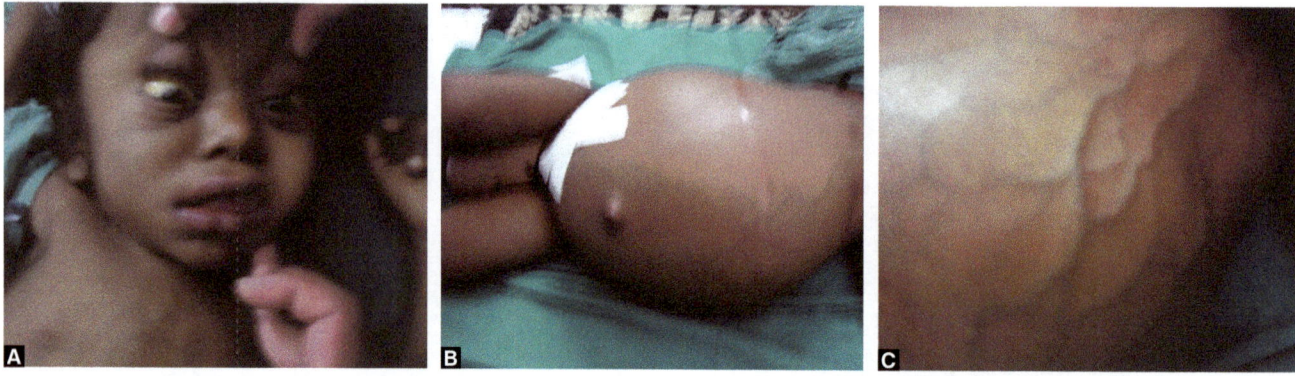

Figs. 62A to C: *Extrahepatic biliary atresia ending up as cirrhosis*—Note the (A) icterus; (B and C) ascites recently undergone tapping, and engorged superficial abdominal venous network. Surgical intervention well in time when the infant had presented with cholestatic jaundice in first few weeks of life could prevent progression to cirrhosis.

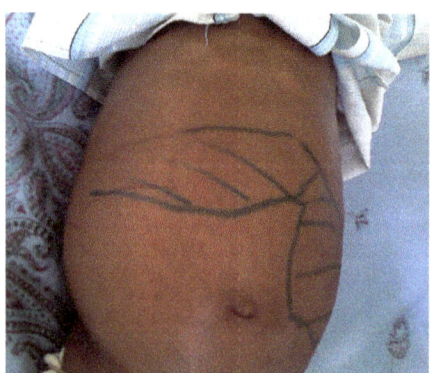

Fig. 63: *Hepatosplenomegaly in a case of suspected chronic liver disease*—The child suffered from viral hepatitis approximately 6 months back with only partial recovery.

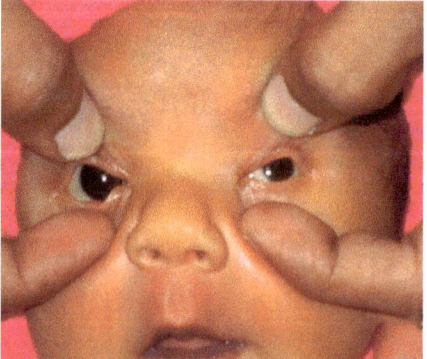

Fig. 64: *Microphthalmia*—Note remarkably small left eye. It may be a part of fetal alcohol syndrome, intrauterine infections (herpes simplex virus, rubella, cytomegalovirus, etc.), chromosomal abnormalities such as trisomy 13 (Patau syndrome).

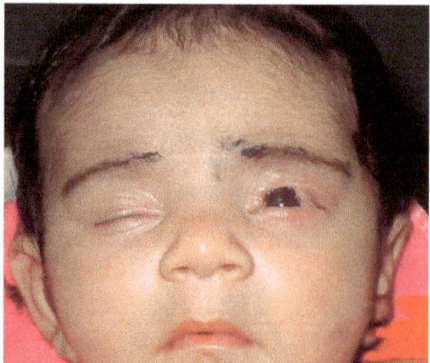

Fig. 65: *Coloboma*—Note the lesion involving the left upper eyelid.

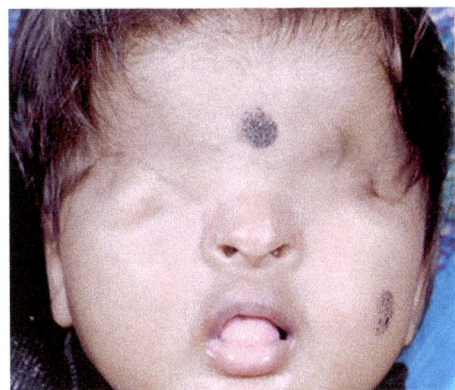

Fig. 66: Bilateral cryptophthalmos.

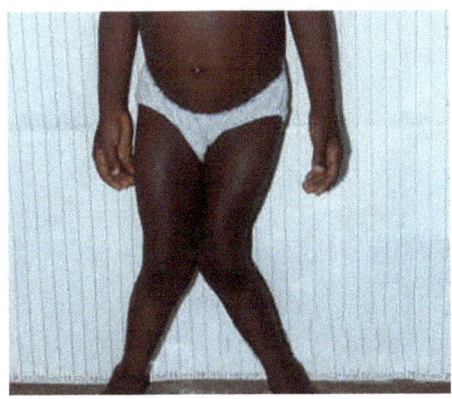

Fig. 69: *Genu valgus*—Note the severe knock knee deformity in a 6-year-old child. Vitamin D deficiency is likely to cause rickets in them.

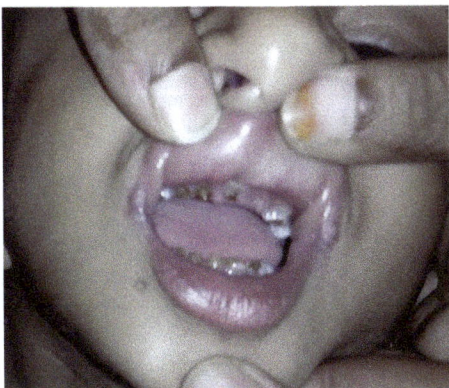

Fig. 67: *Dental caries*—Note the severe caries in a bottle-fed child.

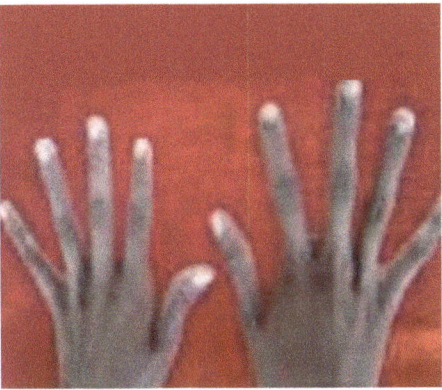

Fig. 70: *Arachnodactyly*—Note the unusually long fingers. Most common organic cause is Marfan's syndrome.

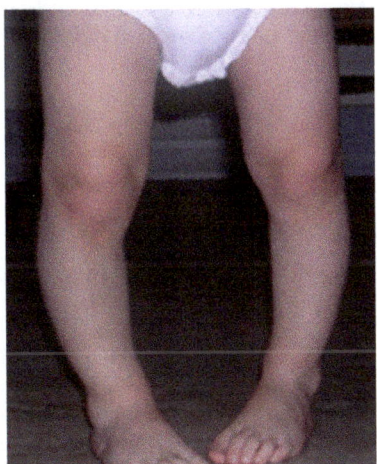

Fig. 68: *Genu varum*—Note the bowlegs. Often, it is a physiological finding in first 2 years of life after which it slowly recedes, often giving way to knock knee (genu valgus) which may persist up to 5 years or so.

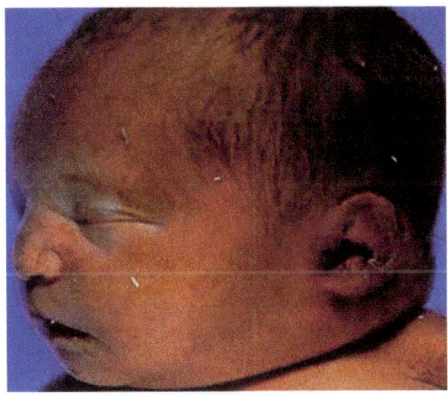

Fig. 71: *Potter facies*—Note flat facial profile, beaked nose, small chin, and low-set deformed ears.

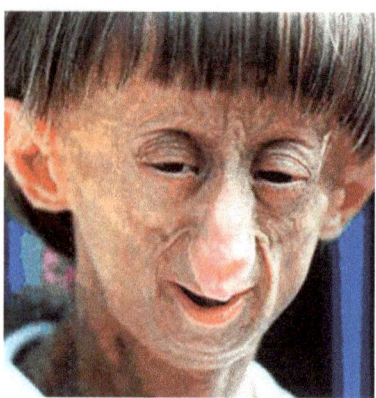

Fig. 72: *Progeria*—Note the features of premature senility.

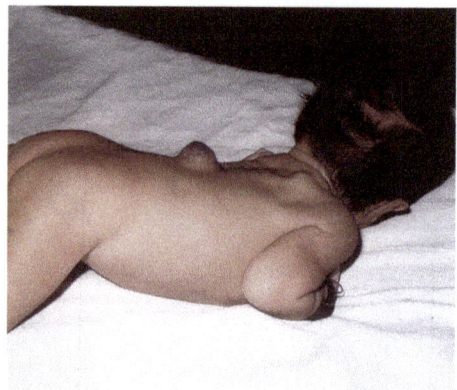

Fig. 75: *Dorsal meningocele*—Note the well-covered midline mass. Transillumination was positive, indicating lack of any neurologic tissues. The child was asymptomatic. Investigative workup, including magnetic resonance imaging (MRI), showed neither any neural tissue involvement nor associated anomalies like tethered spinal cord, lipoma or diastematomyelia.

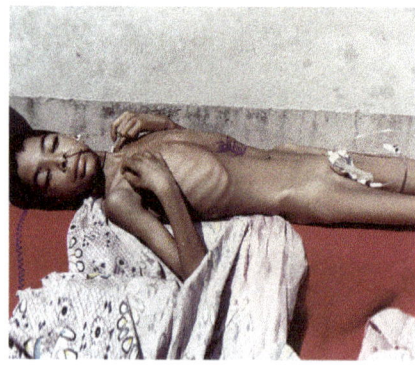

Fig. 73: *Salmonella (enteric) encephalopathy in a 9-year-old child with sickle-cell disease*—Complications such as encephalopathy, meningitis, fecal brown abscess, osteomyelitis, etc. are more common in subjects with immunocompromised status [human immunodeficiency virus (HIV), leukemias, chronic granulomatous disease], sickle-cell disease, chronic malaria, and schistosoma mansoni infection.

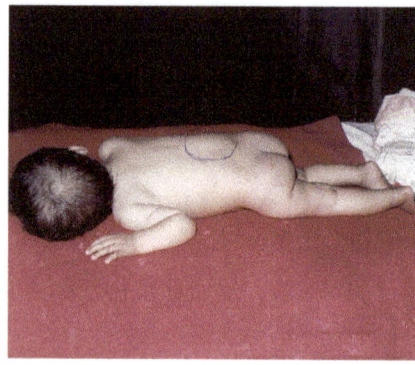

Fig. 76: *Lumbodorsal abscess*—Note that the swelling is towards the right of the spine rather than midline. This was a part of the multiple pyemic abscesses.

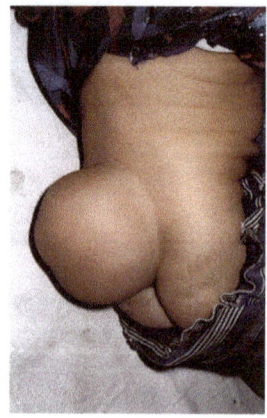

Fig. 74: *Sacral lipoma*—Classically the swelling is soft, compressible, lobulated, and subcutaneous. It is important to exclude occult spinal dysraphism (say, involvement of the conus) by magnetic resonance imaging (MRI) studies.

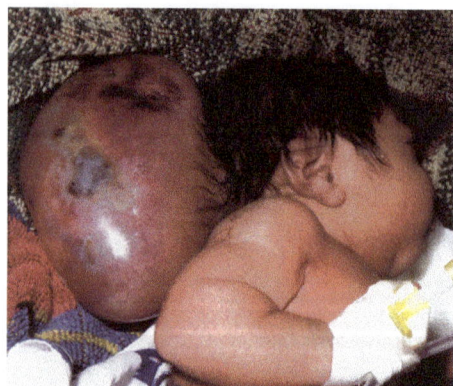

Fig. 77: *Cranial (occipital) encephalocele*—Note the very large sac covered with skin (denuded at places) and containing neural tissue. The infant also had cleft lip and cleft palate, microcephaly microphthalmia, ambiguous genitalia, and polydactyly (Meckel–Gruber syndrome).

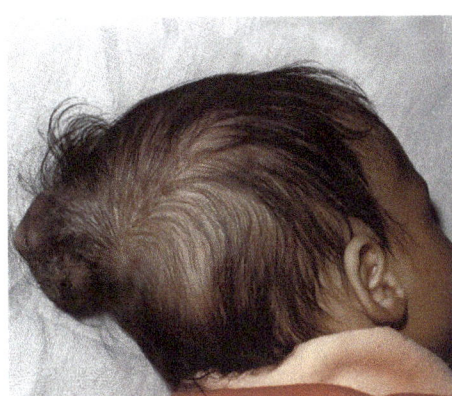

Fig. 78: *Cranial (occipital) meningocele*—The transillumination of the sac showed that it was a sheer cerebrospinal-fluid-filled sac protruding through a midline defect in the skull.

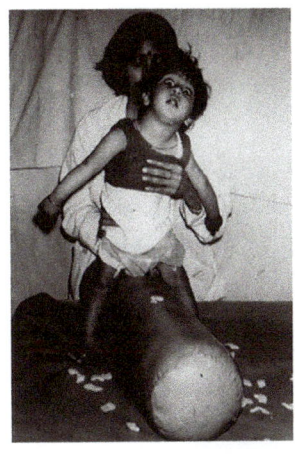

Fig. 81: *Spastic cerebral palsy*—Note the spasticity of all the four limbs (quadriplegia) in the child with speech, visual, and feeding difficulties, delayed milestones, mental retardation, and seizures.

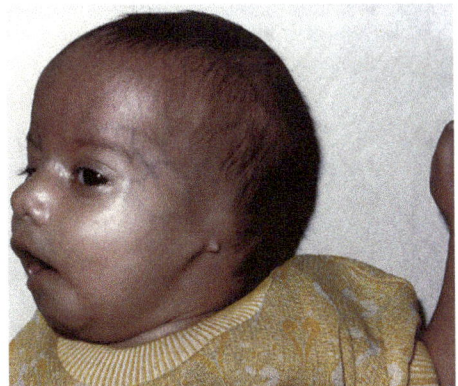

Fig. 79: *Anotia*—Note almost complete absence of the pinna and ear canal together with facial paralysis and micrognathia. The infant also had ventricular septal defect (VSD).

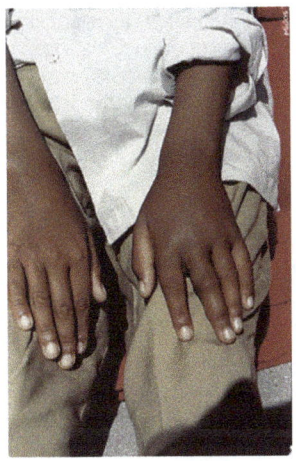

Fig. 82: *Juvenile idiopathic polyarticular arthritis*—Note the symmetrical inflammatory swellings of metacarpophalangeal joints, proximal interphalangeal joints, and distal interphalangeal joints together with involvements of wrists. In pauciarticular juvenile rheumatoid arthritis (JRA), permanent involvement is of knee and ankle (lower limbs). Large joints of the upper limbs are usually spared.

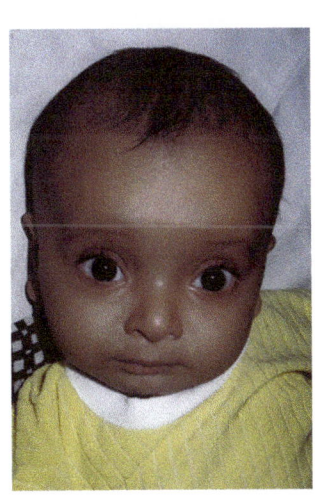

Fig. 80: *Hypertelorism*—Note the wide separation of the eyes secondary to increased inter pupillary distance. The depressed bridge of nose is also apparent. It may occur as a morphogenic variant or as a secondary phenomenon in association with developmental anomalies.

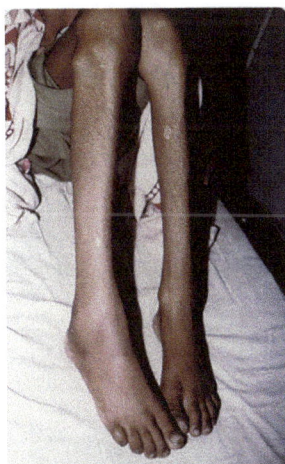

Fig. 83: *Pauciarticular juvenile idiopathic arthritis*—Note the involvement of the right knee and ankle. Large joints of the upper limb remain unaffected.

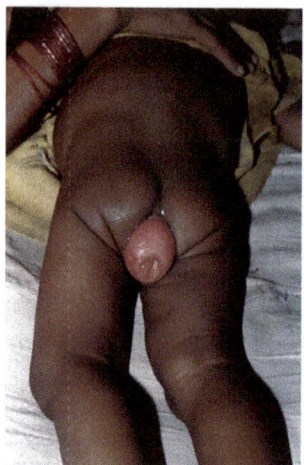

Fig. 84: *Rectal prolapse*—Note the exteriorization of mucosa and other layers of the rectal wall through the anus. Predisposing conditions include protein-energy malnutrition (PEM), heavy intestinal parasitosis, whooping cough, cystic fibrosis, chronic constipation, chronic diarrhea, meningocele, and Ehler–Danlos syndrome. Occasionally, true rectal prolapse may need differentiation from polyps or intussusception.

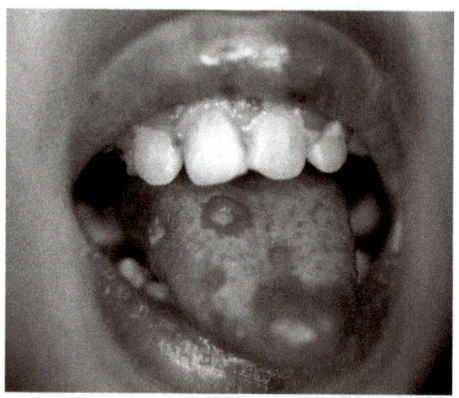

Fig. 86: *Aphthous stomatitis/ulcers*—Note the distinct, well-circumscribed ulcerative lesions having a white necrotic base surrounded by red halos. Such infections like *Helicobacter pylori*, herpes simplex virus, and measles may have a causative role. Healing occurs in 10–14 days, leaving no scarring, treatment is purely palliative and mainly in the form of local analgesic anesthetic agent.

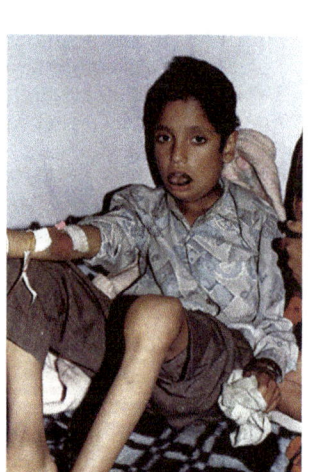

Fig. 85: *Hemophilia*—Note swelling of the knee and ankle as a result of bleeding into joints, the so-called "hemarthrosis" which is considered the hallmark of the disease. Also note bleeding from oral mucosa. Also had pain in the groin and difficulty to extend the hip. These were ascribed to probable bleeding into the iliopsoas muscle. Ultrasonography confirmed this impression. Laboratory diagnosis of hemophilia was established by activated partial thromboplastin time (APTT) and factor VIII.

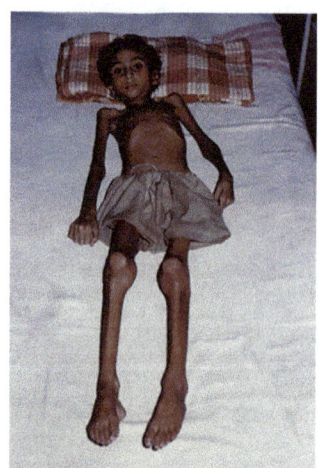

Fig. 87: *Celiac disease*—Note the severe malnutrition (weight 15 kg, height 120 cm, and mid-arm circumference 13 cm) with remarkable wasting of muscles and subcutaneous fat in the 10-year-old girl. A known case of chronic diarrhea since late infancy the diagnosis of celiac disease was confirmed on investigations (stool fat: 25 g/24 hours, D-xylose absorption: grossly impaired, jejunal biopsy: subtotal villous atrophy) and response to gluten-free diet (GFD) and gluten challenge.

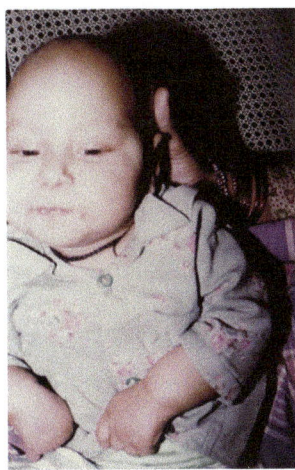

Fig. 88: *Microcephaly with mental retardation*—The head circumference of this 5-month-old baby was 38 cm. Note the stunted forehead. History was suggestive of hypoxic encephalopathy as the cause of microcephaly and mental retardation.

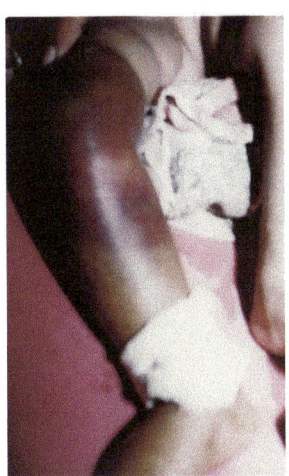

Fig. 90: *Thrombophlebitis*—The cause was infected intravenous needle.

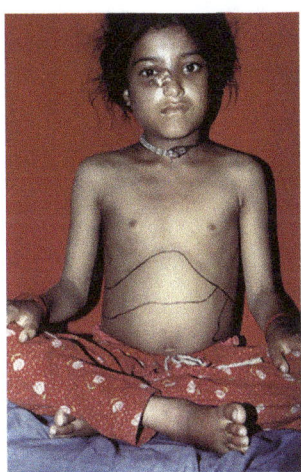

Fig. 89: *Systemic lupus erythematosus (SLE)*—Note the hepatosplenomegaly, butterfly rash over bridge of nose and cheeks (with superadded infection on right side) in this 12-year-old girl who presented with prolonged, irregular fever with remissions, weight loss, and joints pains of 3 months duration. Diagnosis of SLE was established by LE preparation and anti-nuclear antibody (ANA).

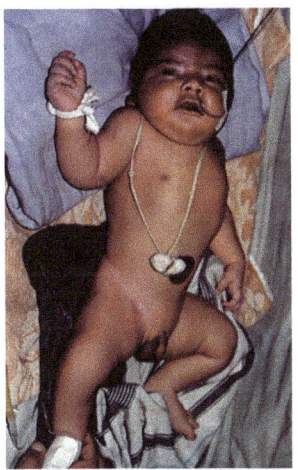

Fig. 91: *Overgrown (large-for-dates) baby*—The infant, weighing 4.6 kg, was born to a tall and heavy mother with diabetes. Overgrowth of the fetus appears to be secondary to islet-cell hyperplasia and increase in the growth hormone-like substance (human placental lactogen). Differential diagnosis includes constitutional overgrowth, cerebral gigantism (Sotos syndrome), transposition of the great vessels (TGVs), hydrops fetalis, congenital hypothyroidism, and overgrowth with advanced bone age (congenital adrenal hyperplasia, thyrotoxicosis, maternal intake of progestins, etc.).

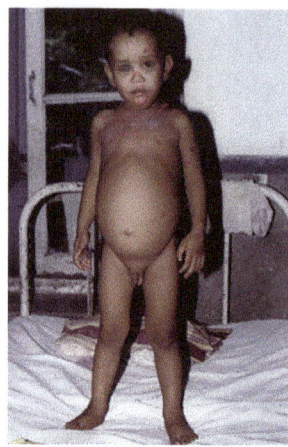

Fig. 92: *Abdominal distention secondary to massive ascariasis*—Note growth failure and rickets in this 3-year-old boy despite voracious appetite. He was hospitalized for acute on recurrent abdominal pain of over a year's duration.

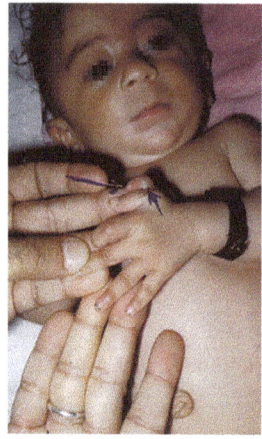

Fig. 93: *Polydactyly*—Note the extra finger lateral to thumb. Though frequently a familial trait, it may be associated with several syndromes, e.g. Laurence Moon–Biedl, trisomy 13, Carpenter, Ellis-van Creveld, Rubinstein–Taybi, Meckel–Gruber, polysyndactyly, orofaciodigital, etc.

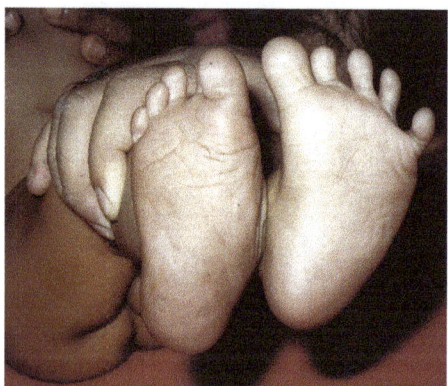

Fig. 94: *Flexible flat feet*—A common finding in neonates and toddlers due to the laxity of bone ligament complexes of foot and fat in the region of medial longitudinal arch. By 6 years, most children demonstrate considerable improvement. Conditions causing rigid flat feet include cerebral palsy, tarsal coalitions, Achilles tendon contracture. It may well be a familial trait.

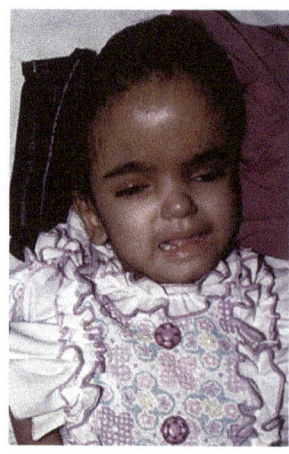

Fig. 95: *Craniosynostosis*—Note the left-sided frontal plagiocephaly due to premature fusion of the ipsilateral coronal suture together with the sphenofrontal suture. Surgical intervention is important from cosmetic angle.

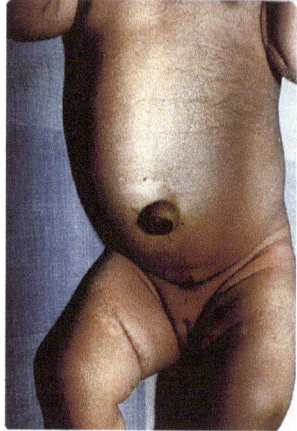

Fig. 96: *Umbilical granuloma*—Note the persistence of granulation tissue, which is soft, vascular, granular, and dual red or pink with mucoid, mucopurulent or seropurulent discharge. Differential diagnosis is umbilical polyp, which is bright red, firm, and resistant.

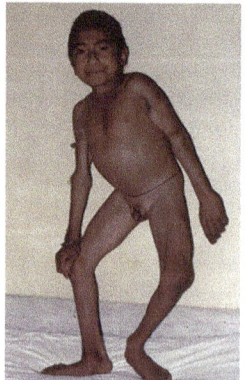

Fig. 97: *Pseudohypoparathyroidism*—Note the short stature with round face, mental retardation, and brachydactyly. The child suffered from recurrent attacks of tetany. The condition is also termed as Albright hereditary osteodystrophy.

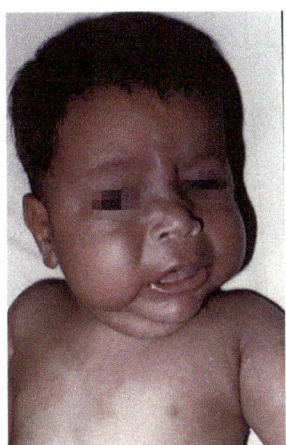

Fig. 98: *Glycogen storage disease (Von Gierke disease)*—Note the doll-like faces with prominent fat cheeks. The infant also had protuberant abdomen with massive hepatomegaly and palpable kidneys. Hypoglycemia, lactic acidosis, hyperlipemia, and hyperuricemia are the hallmarks of the disease which is caused by the absence or deficiency of G-6-P activity in the liver, kidneys, and gut mucosa.

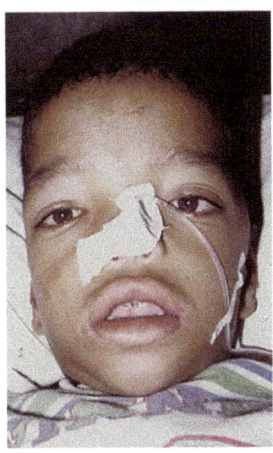

Fig. 101: *Cerebral gigantism (Sotos syndrome)*—Note the large head (circumference 56 cm), hypertelorism, antimongoloid slant, prominent jaw in this 5-year-old boy who had large hands and feet and somewhat thickened subcutaneous tissue. His accelerated growth was reflected in his height (123 cm) and weight (25 kg). Thus, the height and weight age was 8 years.

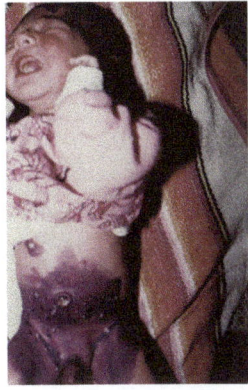

Fig. 99: *Neonatal sepsis*—Note the pustules, septic umbilicus (omphalitis), and abdominal wall cellulitis.

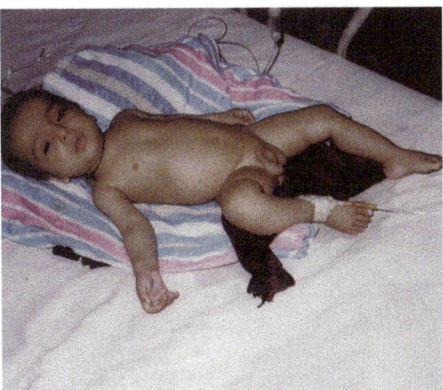

Fig. 102: *Poliomyelitis*—Note the patchy and asymmetrical paralysis of extremities (of lower motor neuron type) with no sensory loss. Differential diagnosis includes Guillain–Barré syndrome (GBS) and other entities under the shield of acute flaccid paralysis (AFP).

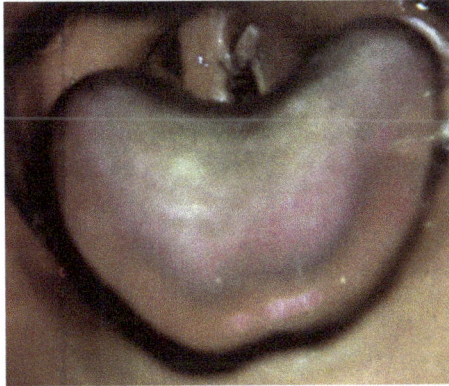

Fig. 100: *Tonsillar diphtheria*—Note the grayish membrane formation over tonsils with extension to involve the uvula, soft palate, posterior oropharynx, and hypopharynx. Underlying soft tissue edema together with lymphadenopathy may cause "bull-neck" appearance.

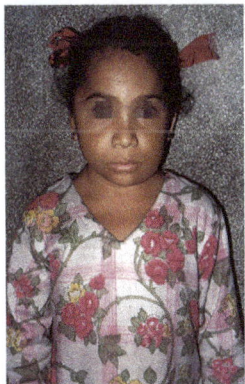

Fig. 103: *Goitrogenous hypothyroidism*—Hypothyroidism in this 12-year-old girl was secondary to endemic iodine deficiency. Iodine deficiency causes deficient thyroid hormone production, thyroid stimulating hormone (TSH) hypersecretion, increased iodine trapping with goiter and high T3:T4 ratio.

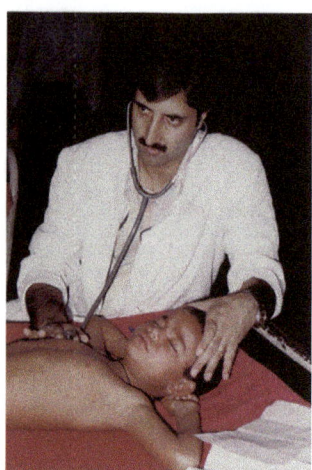

Fig. 104: *Measles encephalitis*—Note the fading rash and progressive drowsiness. The child presented with recurrence of fever (after a 5-day afebrile period since appearance of rash), severe cough, severe headache, vomiting, and worsening sensorium. There was doubtful history of atypical febrile seizures (thrice over the preceding 12 hours). Usually, recovery occurs but chances of permanent cerebral damage are high in measles encephalitis or postmeasles encephalomyelitis.

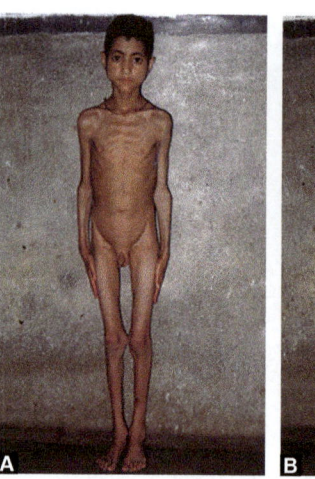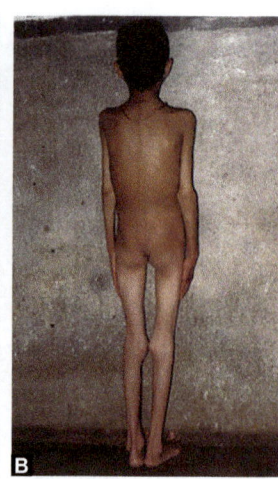

Figs. 106A and B: *Acute on chronic malnutrition*—Note the wasting of muscles and subcutaneous adiposity in this 10-year-old boy whose height was 120 cm and weight 26 kg. He, therefore, had not only stunting (as a result of chronic malnutrition) but also superadded wasting (as a result of a recent attack of enteric fever which further reduced his dietary intake).

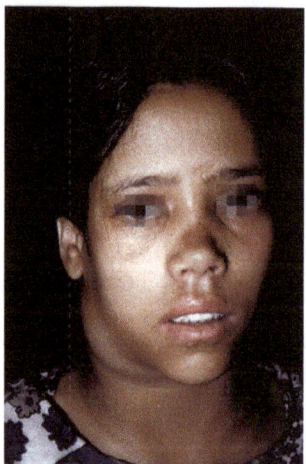

Fig. 105: *Hodgkin's lymphoma*—Note the characteristic unilateral cervical lymphadenopathy, the involved lymph nodes are being matted, firm, nontender, and mobile. Over and above cervical lymphadenopathy, the presenting complaints were fever, anorexia, pruritus, weight loss, and night sweats. The diagnosis of Hodgkin's lymphoma was confirmed by histopathologic study of the biopsy material from the involved nodes.

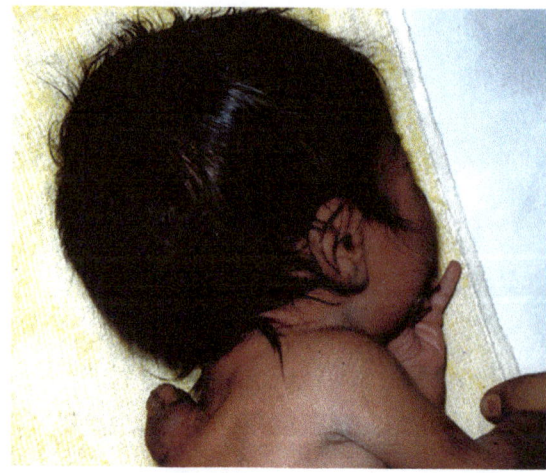

Fig. 107: *Congenital hydrocephalus with meningocele*—Note the large head (circumference 43 cm) with a cystic mass at the upper back (cervical). The mass is covered with thick skin and does not contain the myelodysplasia or spinal cord. As a rule, there is no neurologic deficit (unlike meningomyelocele).

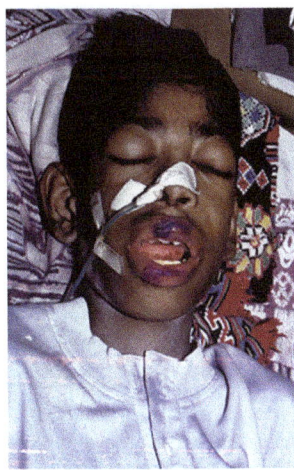

Fig. 108: *Peutz–Jeghers syndrome*—Note the characteristic mucosal pigmentation of the lips. The boy, with history of recurrent abdominal pain and blood in stools over several years, was hospitalized for intestinal obstruction. Investigations revealed multiple polyps (pathologically hamartomas). This is a rare autosomal dominant syndrome. Vulnerability to cancer (colorectal, breast, gynecological, etc.) is as high as up to 50%.

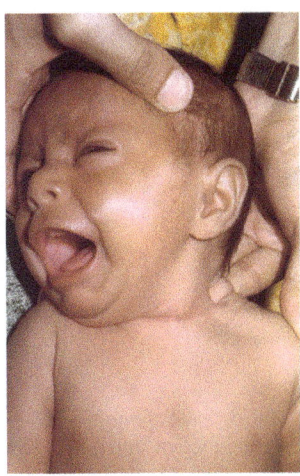

Fig. 110: *Sternomastoid tumor*—Note the hard, immobile, fusiform, and well-defined mass in the middle of the sternomastoid muscle. *Cause:* Birth trauma from difficult breech delivery.

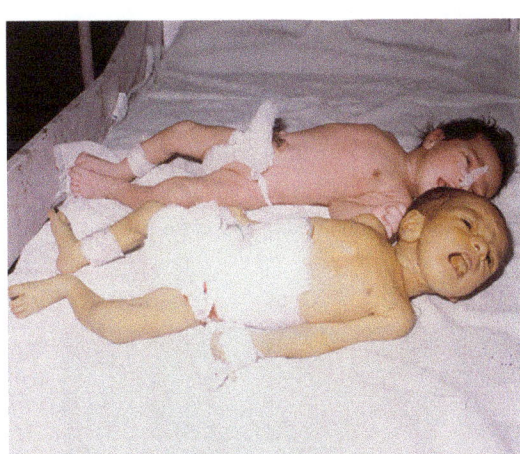

Fig. 109: *Rhesus (Rh) isoimmunization*—Note the severe icterus (in the neonate on left) which appeared in the first 24 hours and showed rapid progression to 22 mg/dL.

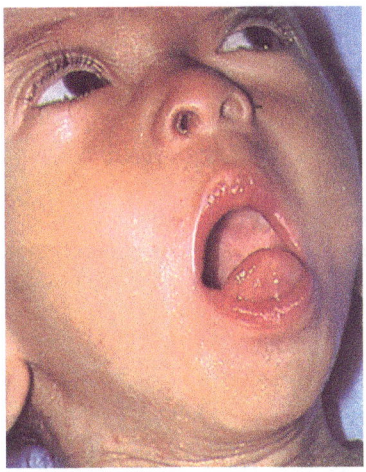

Fig. 111: *Pertussis (paroxysmal stage)*—Note the hallmark of the stage, lasting 2–6 weeks after the catarrhal stage (1–2 weeks). As the child struggles to cough, his face gets congested, tongue protrudes, eyes bulge, and chin and neck are held forward. After a machine-gun burst of uninterrupted coughs, coughing stops. At this point, a loud "whoop" results as the inspired air passes the still partially closed airway. The child usually vomits after the whoop. Invariably, he becomes exhausted. More than one such attack per hour may occur at the peak of the paroxysmal stage.

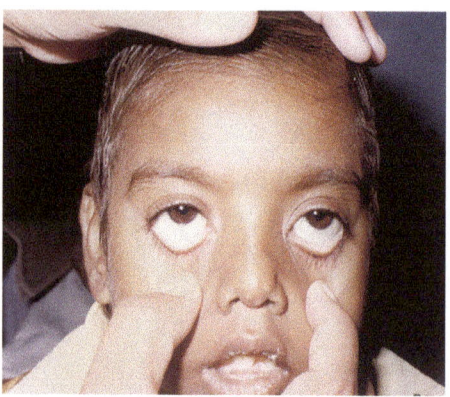

Fig. 112: *Chronic iron deficiency anemia (IDA)*—Note the severe pallor of palpebral conjunctiva and skin. The child presented with progressive pallor, easy fatigability, anorexia, and pica with recurrent abdominal pain. Stool was positive for occult blood. Stool microscopy showed *Ancylostoma duodenale*.

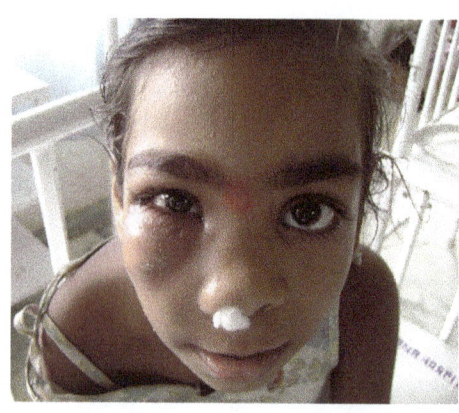

Fig. 114: *Periorbital cellulitis*—Note the periorbital inflammation with involvement of the lids and nose as a result of direct extension of the paranasal sinusitis. It may progress to true orbital cellulitis with proptosis and limitation of eye movements.

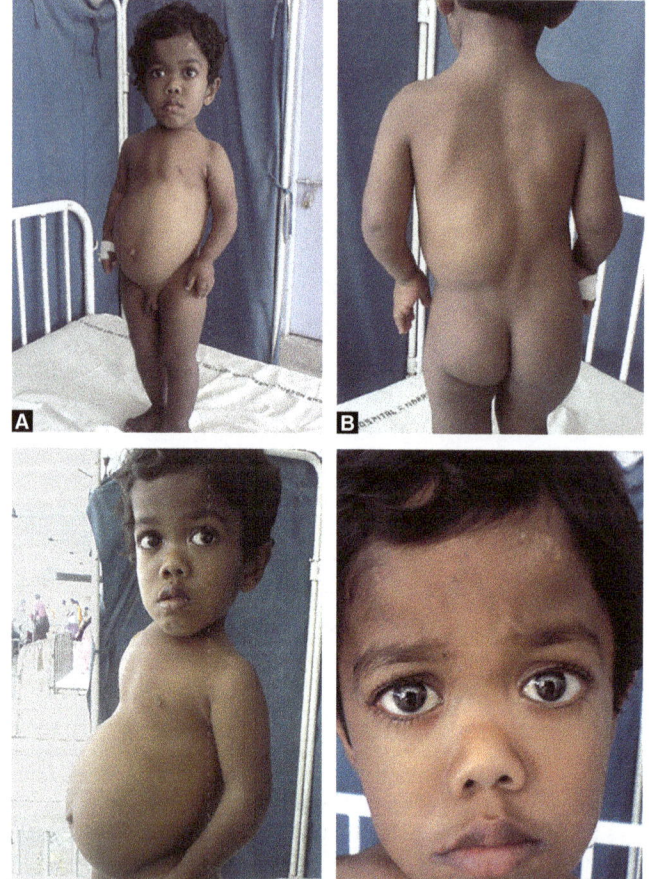

Figs. 113A to D: *Achondroplasia*—Note the disproportionate short stature of short-limbed variety—(A to C) arms barely reaching the inguinal level; U/L segment ratio 1.6:1, small chest compared to a large protuberant abdomen, exaggerated lumbar lordosis and (D) large head with prominent forehead and flat nasal bridge. Hypochondroplasia is a milder form resulting from different mutations in Figure 75 gene. Major differential diagnosis includes pituitary dwarfism, congenital hypothyroidism and Turner syndrome.

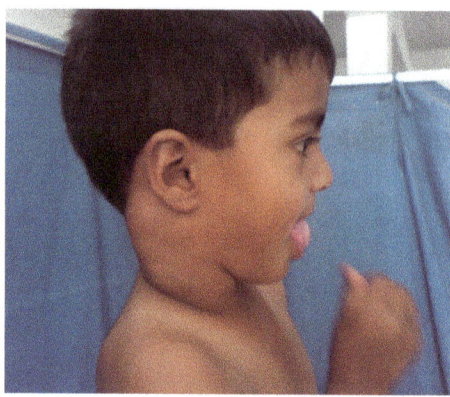

Fig. 115: *Tumor-bearing cervical lymphadenitis*—The nodes are firm or matted and nontender and often fixed to the skin or underlying structures.

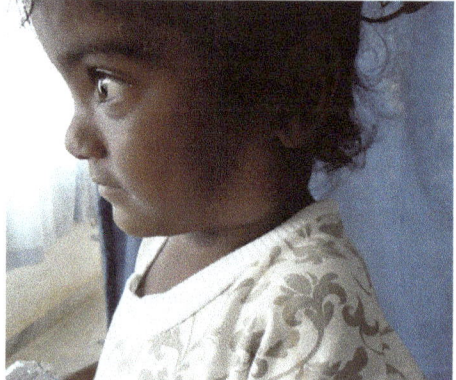

Fig. 116: *Tuberculous cervical lymphadenopathy*—The nodes are typically matted. Note the hydrocephalus in this child recovering from tuberculous meningitis.

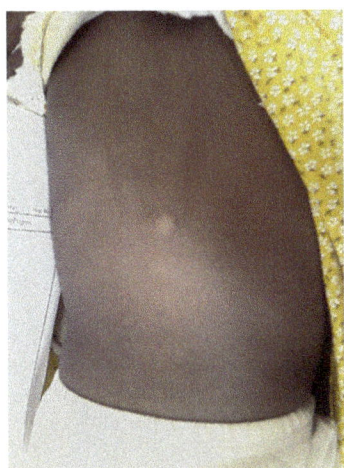

Fig.117: *Tuberous sclerosis*—Note the shagreen patch and hypopigmented spot. The child also had pink telangiectatic papules (adenoma sebaceum) in nasolabial folds. She was on carbamazepine for epilepsy. Computed tomography (CT) and magnetic resonance imaging (MRI) revealed a few tubers in cortex and subcortex.

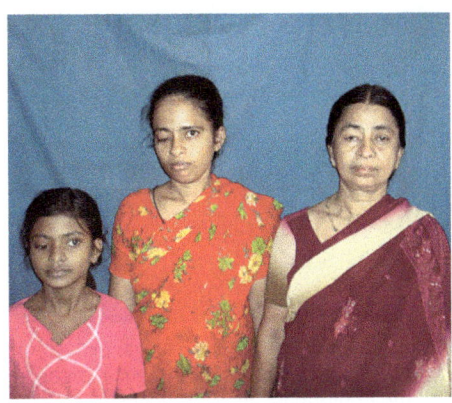

Fig. 118: *Familial ptosis*—Note the presence of ptosis in the sister and the mother of the child as well.

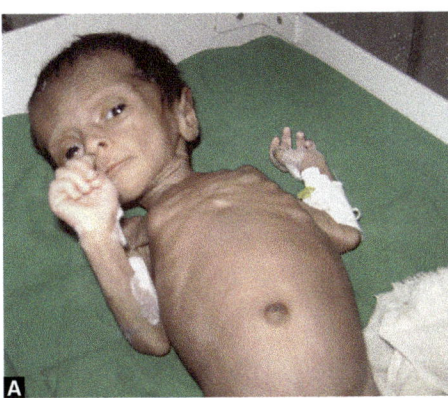
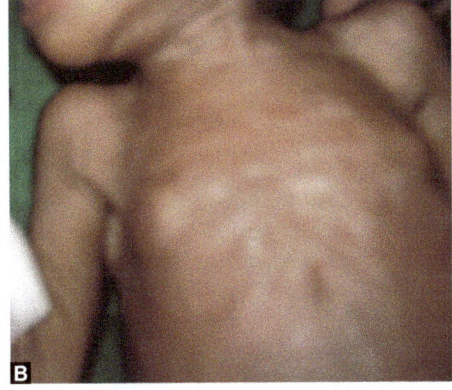

Figs. 119A and B: *Bottle-baby disease*—Note the remarkable wasting in this infant on bottle-feeding employing highly diluted, contaminated, and dirty formula.

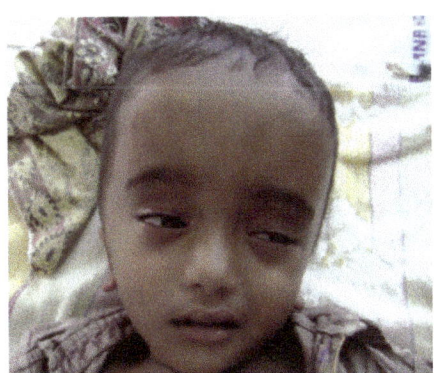

Fig. 120: *Acquired hydrocephalus*—Note the large head (52 cm) in this 3-year-old child convalescing from tuberculous meningitis.

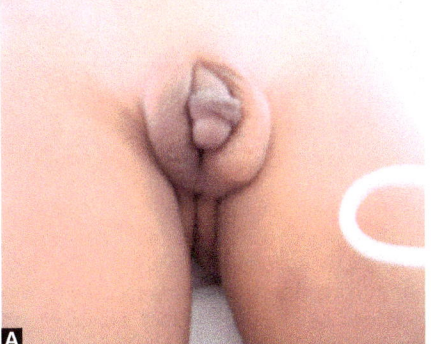
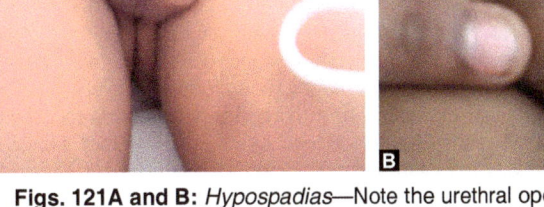

Figs. 121A and B: *Hypospadias*—Note the urethral opening at the ventral surface of the penis.

26 Section 1: Color Atlas

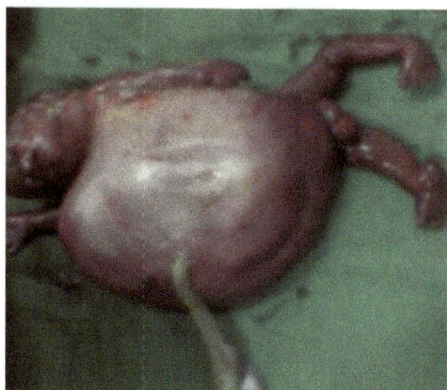

Fig. 122: *Hydrops fetalis*—Note the clinical picture of excessive abnormal fluid in different fetal compartment such as skin, pleura, pericardium, and peritoneum, causing death in utero or soon after birth.

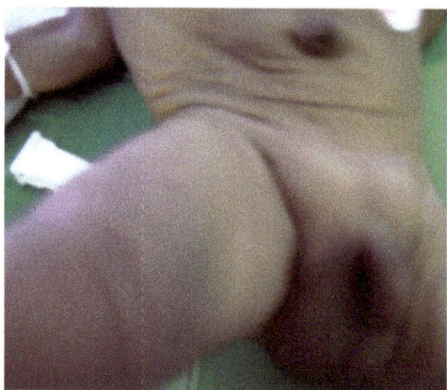

Fig. 123: *Congenital inguinal hernia*—Note the obvious bilateral inguinal swelling which showed impulse on crying.

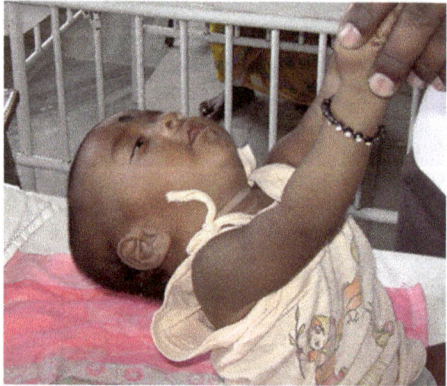

Fig. 124: *Floppy infant*—Note the head lag. It may well be physiological in a premature infant and an incidental nonspecific finding in an acutely sick infant. Differential diagnosis includes neuromuscular [hereditary spinal muscular atrophy, congenital myopathies, metabolic diseases, Guillain–Barré syndrome (GBS), neonatal myasthenia], CNS (cerebral palsy), endocrinal (hypothyroidism), metabolic (rickets, renal tubular acidosis, etc.), nutritional [protein-energy malnutrition (PEM)], and chromosomal (Down syndrome) disorders. Benign congenital hypotonia should also be borne in mind.

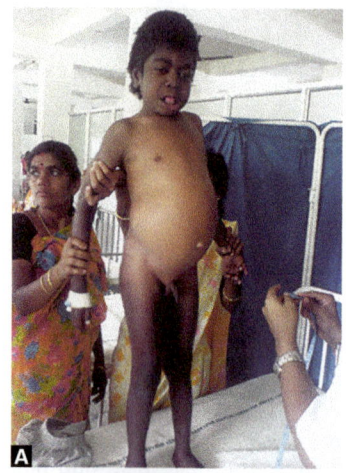

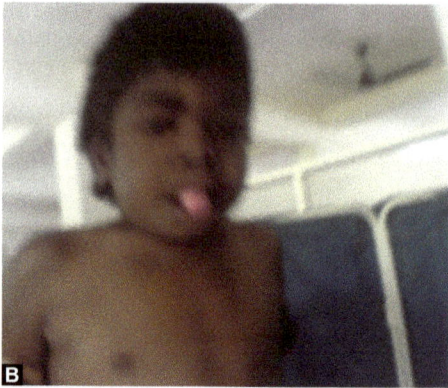

Figs. 125A and B: *Hurler's disease*—Note mental retardation and grotesque facial features with hepatosplenomegaly (not highlighted in the photos).

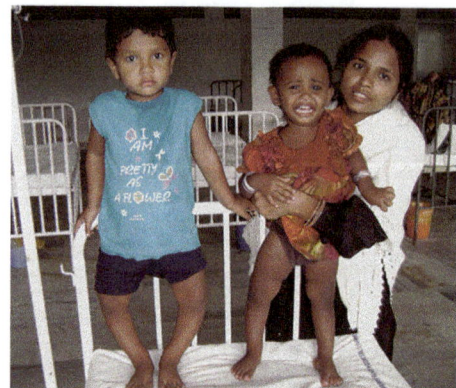

Fig. 126: *Vitamin D deficiency rickets*—Note that both children are suffering from bowleg deformity (genu varus) as a result of nutritional rickets. The diagnosis was supported by classical changes in X-ray of wrist and biochemical findings. The poor nutritional environment in the family is known to affect the siblings with similar nutritional disorders.

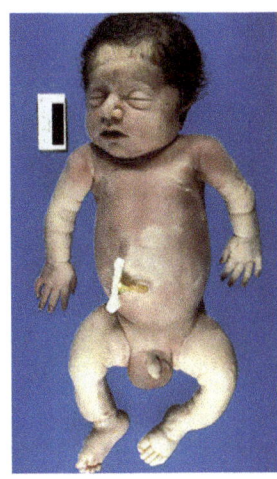

Fig. 127: *Congenital osteogenesis imperfecta (OI type II)*—Note multiple deformities secondary to intrauterine fractures, hypotelorism with beaking of the nose, extremely short, deformed and bent limbs, broad thighs, etc. X-ray studies reveal crumpled long bones and fractured and beaded ribs. The neonatal form is a lethal syndrome, incompatible with life. Around 50% are stillborn. The remaining 50% die soon after birth from respiratory insufficiency.

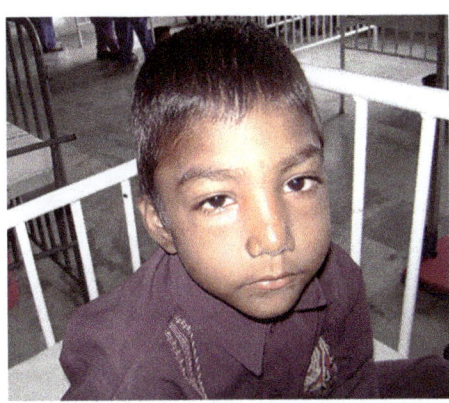

Fig. 128: *Acute glomerulonephritis*—The child presented with periorbital puffiness, fever, and hematuria with hypertension.

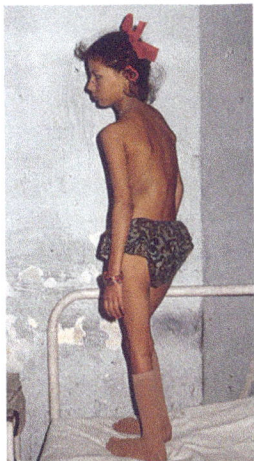

Fig. 129: *Pott's spine*—Note the kyphosis as a consequence of tuberculous spondylitis causing destruction of vertebral bodies.

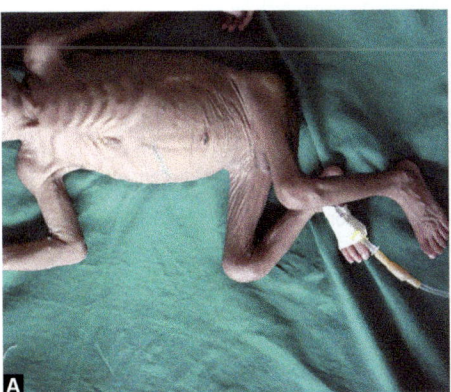
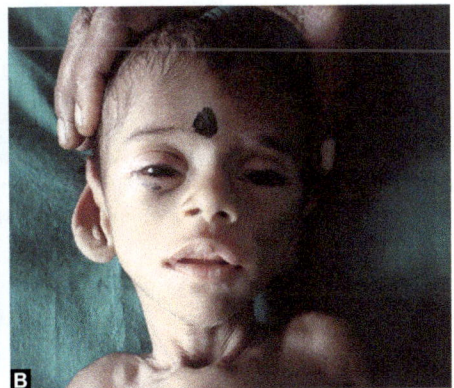

Figs. 130A and B: *Nutritional marasmus*—Note the remarkable wasting of both muscle and subcutaneous fat with absence of edema.

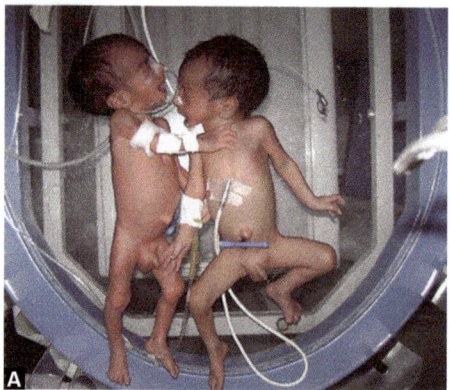
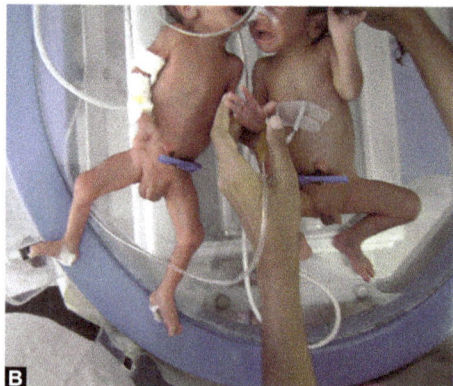

Figs. 131A and B: *Monozygotic twins with twin–twin transfusion (fetal transfusion syndrome)*—There was history of maternal hydramnios. Over and above treatment for asphyxia. Whereas the recipient twin needed an exchange blood transfusion, the donor twin was given an immediate blood transfusion for severe anemia.

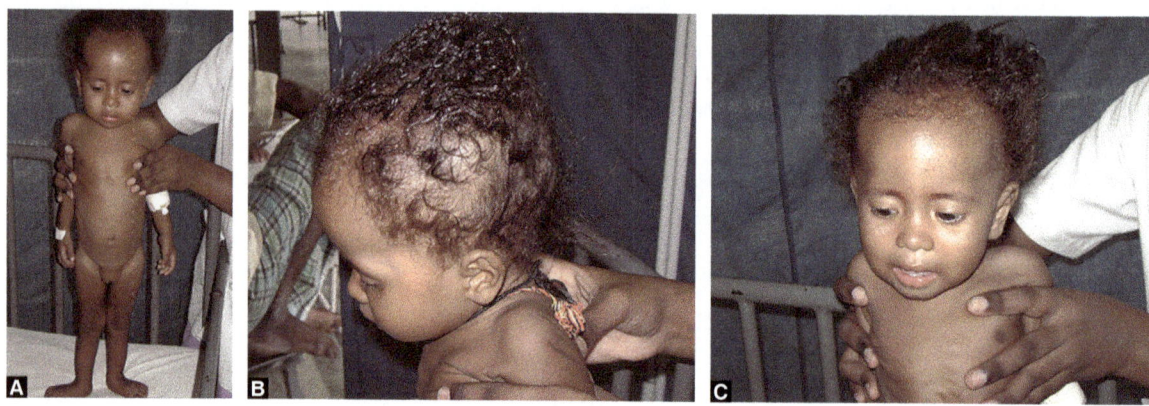

Figs. 132A to C: *Kwashiorkor*—Note the growth retardation, muscle wasting with retention of some subcutaneous adiposity, psychomotor change, and bilateral pedal edema. Hair changes, though not an essential feature of kwashiorkor, are clearly seen in this child.

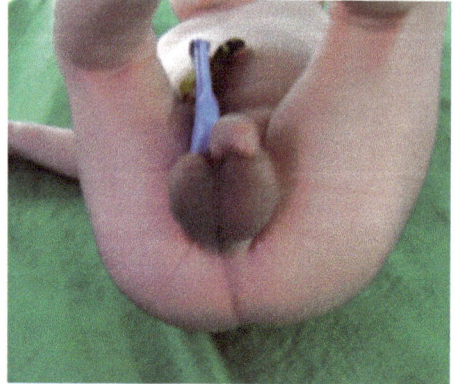

Fig. 133: *Imperforate anus*—An invertogram (with infant held upside down, suspended by legs) is needed for finding the level of the anorectal defect.

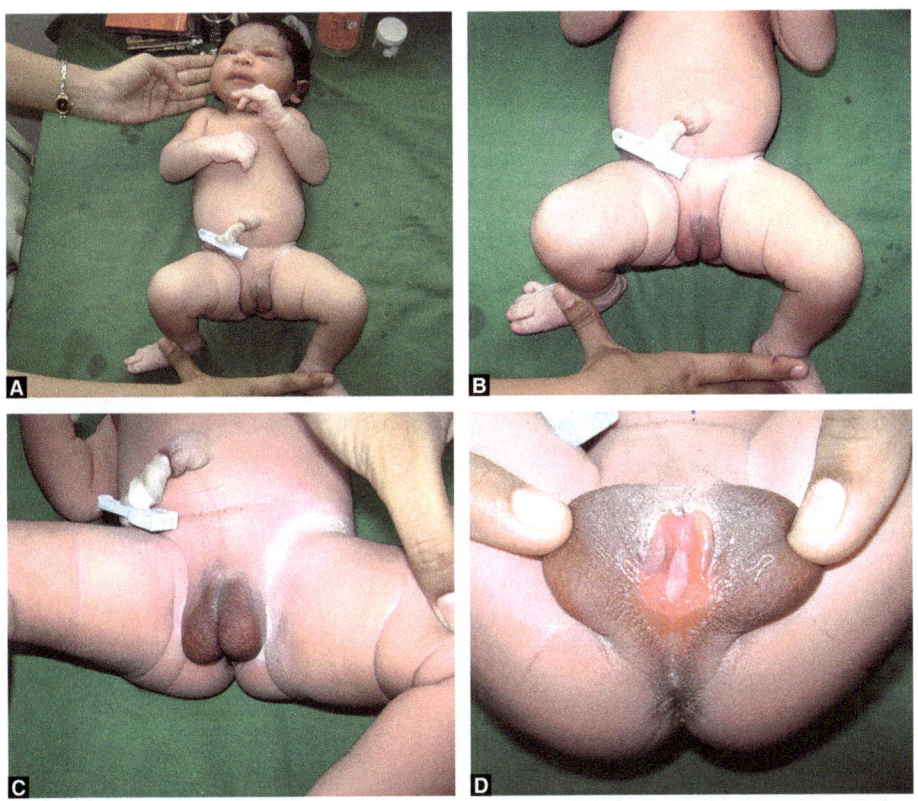

Figs. 134A to D: *Ambiguous genitalia*—Note the phenotype female. In case of suspicion of testicular feminization, it is important to screen the child with a buccal smear for barr bodies and appropriate genetic evaluation.

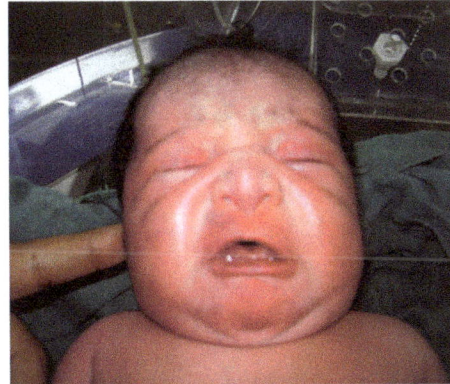

Fig. 135: *Natal teeth*—Note that the teeth are present right at birth unlike the neonatal teeth that erupt in the first month of life. These may exist as an isolated finding (often as a familial trait) or in association with cleft palate, Pierre-Robin syndrome, Ellisvan-Creveld syndrome, Hallermann–Stroff syndrome, congenital paronychia, and other congenital anomalies. These may be harmless but are prone to cause pain, refusal to feed, maternal discomfort, and, very infrequently, entry into the airways.

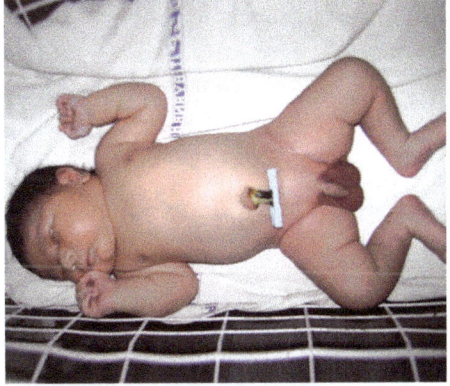

Fig. 136: *Infant of diabetic mother*—This baby was born to a mother with poorly controlled diabetes. Note the large-sized plum baby with puffy and plethoric facies despite birth at 38 weeks of gestation. Such an infant has enhanced chances of congenital anomalies [including congenital heart disease, e.g. ventricular septal defect (VSD), atrial septal defect (ASD), transposition of the great vessels (TGV), tricuspid atresia (TA), coarctation of the aorta (COA), etc.], respiratory distress syndrome, and hypoglycemia.

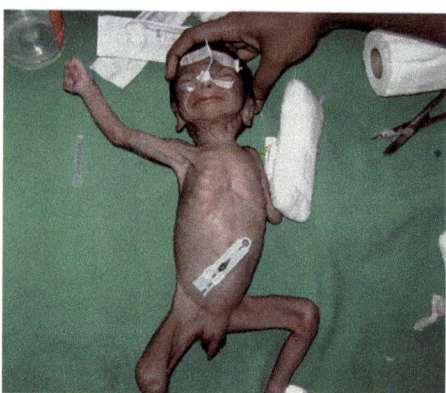

Fig. 137: *Intrauterine growth retardation (IUGR)*—Note the baby looks marasmic, long, and thin with skin losing its normal elasticity and hanging in folds (malnourished type). Differential diagnosis is from hypoplastic infant who is proportionally small in all parameters due to reduction in cell population.

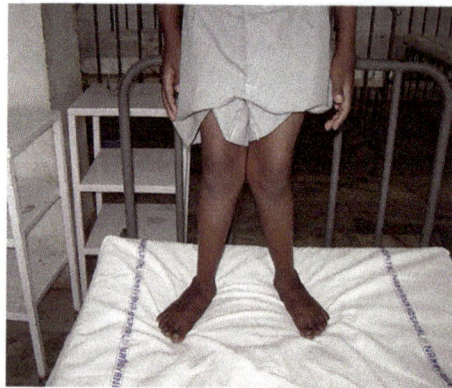

Fig. 140: *Advanced refractory rickets*—Note the gross knock-knee deformity (genu valgum) in a 7-year-old child with poorly controlled celiac disease despite massive doses of vitamin D with supplements of calcium and phosphorus.

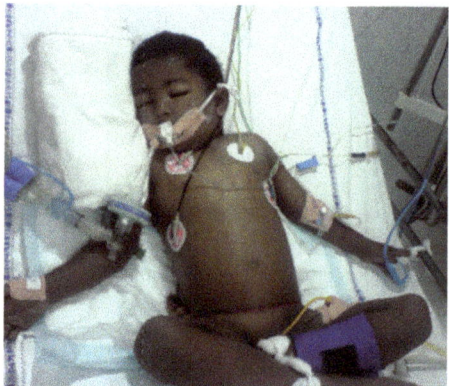

Fig. 138: *Transposition of great arteries (TGAs) with congestive cardiac failure and hospital-acquired bronchopneumonia*—Note that the infant is quite large in size, weighing 4.5 kg at birth. The mother was a known diabetic under treatment.

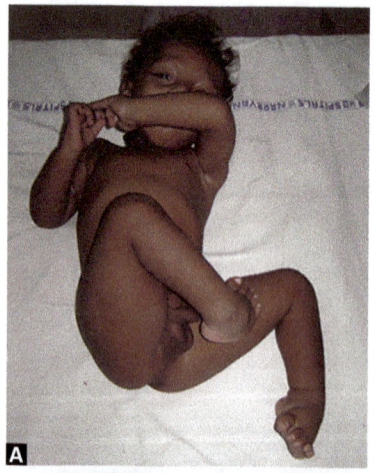

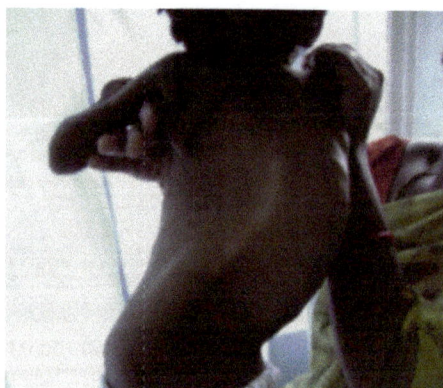

Fig. 139: *Scoliosis*—Note the severe lateral deformity of the spine (the angle of curvature, measured by Cobb's technique) being far beyond 10° in posteroanterior (PA) view of the X-ray of chest in a child who developed chest wall restriction, resulting in lung impairment in the form of decrease in vital capacity, forced expiratory volume in 1 (FEV1), work capacity, diffusion capacity, chest wall compliance, and partial pressure of arterial oxygen (PaO_2).

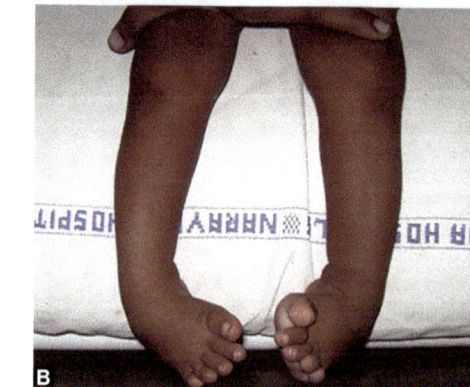

Figs. 141A and B: *Congenital talipes equinovarus (CTEV)*—Note the clubfoot deformity in the form of forefoot cavus and adductus and hindfoot varus and equinus. It is sound principle to examine the spine for occult dysraphism.

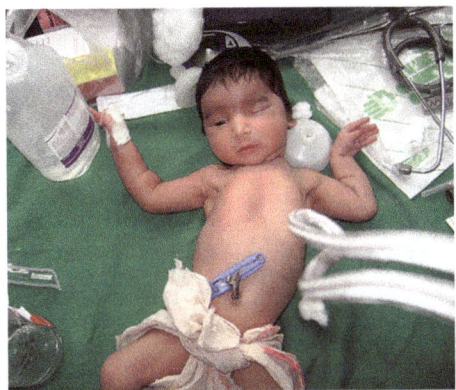

Fig. 142: *Facial palsy*—Note inability to close left eye following birth trauma. Facial palsy at birth is, as a rule, a compression neuropathy resulting from forceps application during delivery. In a large majority of the cases, it regresses in a matter of days or weeks.

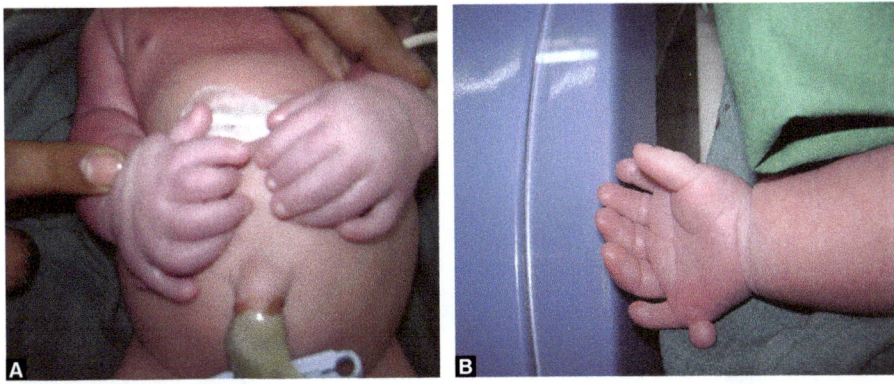

Figs. 143A and B: *Polydactyly*—Note the presence of supernumerary digits on the ulnar border of hands (preaxial). Association with many syndromes (e.g. Carpenter syndrome, Ellis–van Creveld syndrome, Meckel–Gruber syndrome, polysyndactyly, etc.) is known.

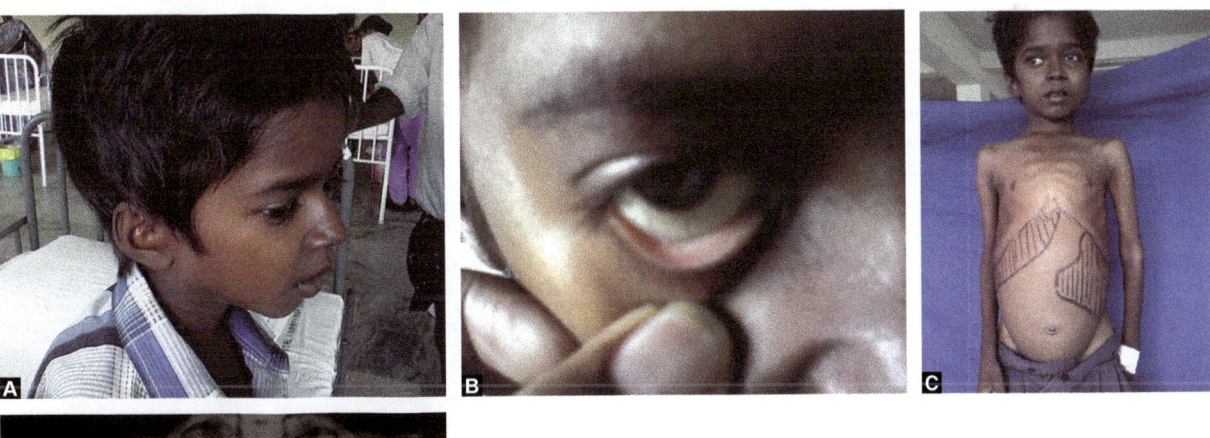

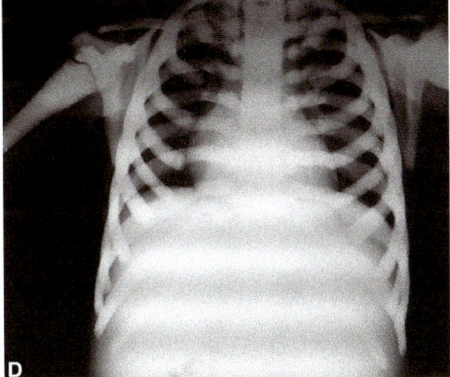

Figs. 144A to D: *Osteopetrosis (marble bone disease)*—This 10-year-old boy presented with (A to C) short stature and growth retardation (height 123 cm, weight 28 kg), anemia, hepatosplenomegaly, and lymphadenopathy. There was history of long bone fracture thrice in the past years following trivial trauma. (D) The diagnosis is established by radiology which shows remarkably high bone density with vertical striations of long bones and transverse bands in shaft and soft tissue opacities due to calcification. Differential diagnosis of radiological picture includes fluorosis, lead poisoning, and idiopathic hypercalcemia.

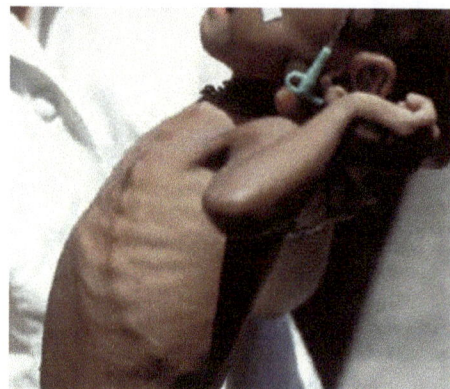

Fig. 145: *Scorbutic rosary*—Note that the costochondral beading in scurvy is sharp, angular, and tender against the smooth, rounded, and nontender costochondral beading seen in rickets.

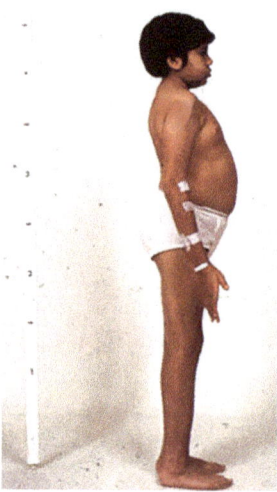

Fig. 146: *Pituitary dwarf*—The upper or lower segment ratio was 1:1 with an IQ of around 100. Response to therapy with growth hormone turned out to be remarkable.

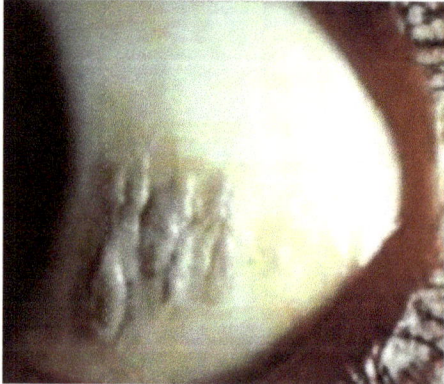

Fig. 147: *Bitot spot*—Note the more or less triangular spot with the base adjoining the corneal limbus. The finding corresponds to XIb stage of xerophthalmia as per World Health Organization (WHO).

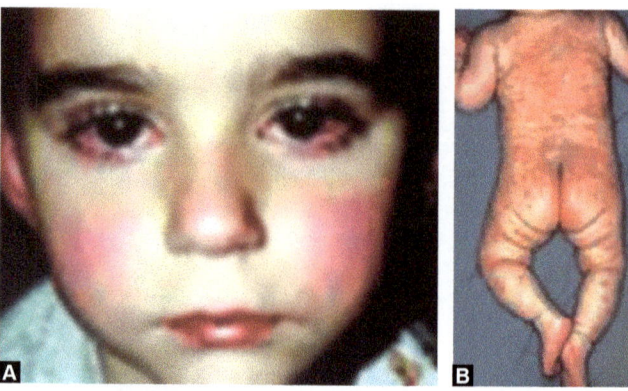

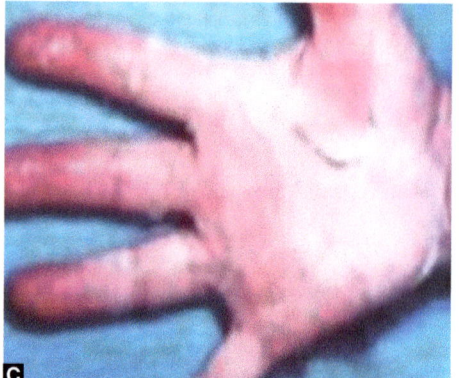

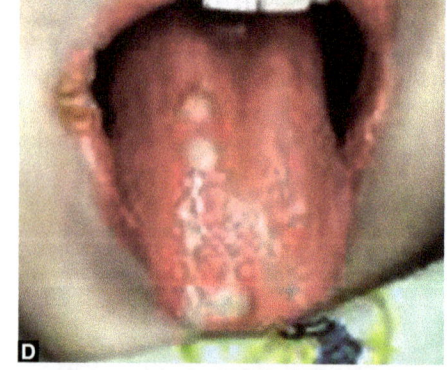

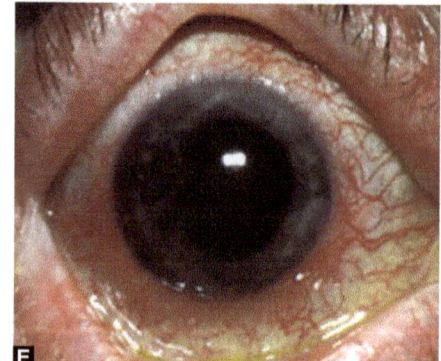

Figs. 148A to E

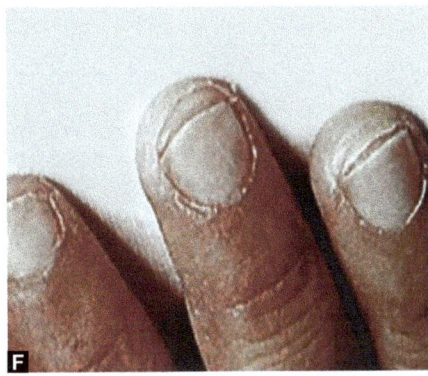

Figs. 148A to F: *Kawasaki disease*—Note the salient features such as typical rash involving (A) face, (B) body, (C) palms, (D) tongue, and (E) eyes. (F) Also note peeling of skin.

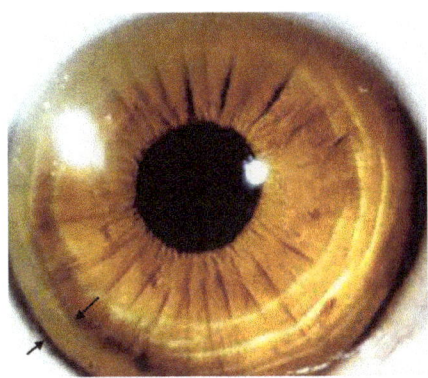

Fig. 149: *Kayser–Fleischer ring*—Note the brown ring around the limbus of cornea. The cause is copper deposition in the Descemet membrane in a 17-year-old teenager suffering from Wilson's disease who presented exclusively with neurological manifestations, including extrapyramidal signs like rigidity, dysarthria, dysphagia, drooling, and intellectual deterioration.

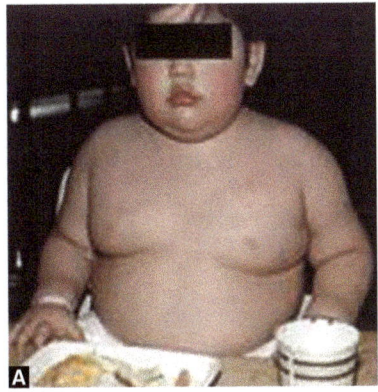 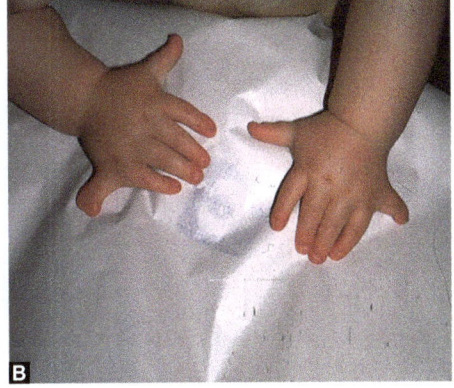

Figs. 150A and B: *Laurence–Moon–Biedl syndrome*—Note the obesity and polydactyly. The child also suffered from mental retardation, short stature, and hypogenitalism.

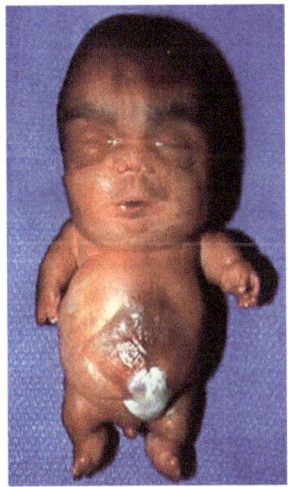

Fig. 151: *Rhizomelic chondrodysplasia*—Note the symmetrical rhizomelia, and craniofacial dysmorphism. The rare condition is an autosomal recessive disorder.

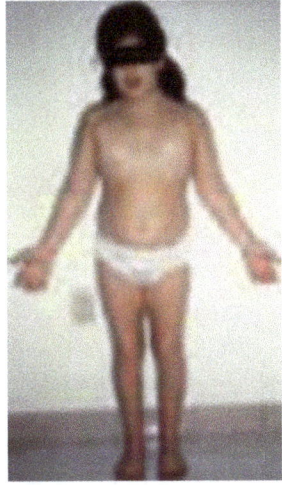

Fig. 152: *Turner syndrome*—Note the short stature, short webbed neck, shield chest with widely spaced nipples, and increased carrying angle (cubitus valgus) in this mentally challenged girl. She also suffered from coarctation of aorta, a well-known association with this syndrome. Cytogenetic studies confirmed 45XO chromosomal pattern.

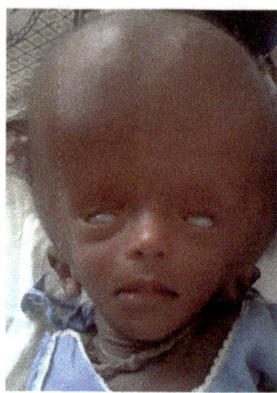

Fig. 153: *Congenital hydrocephalus*—Note the very large head size with sunset sign and scalp vein distention with taut skin over the scalp. The "sunset sign" is due to loss of upward conjugate gaze.

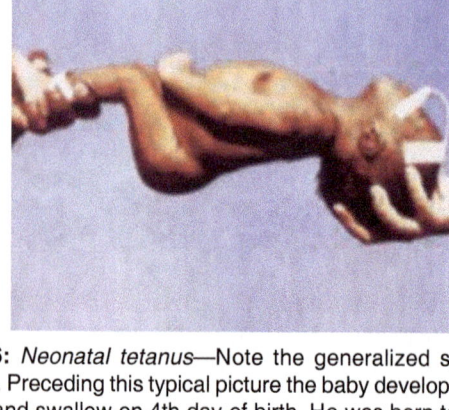

Fig. 156: *Neonatal tetanus*—Note the generalized spasm and stiffness. Preceding this typical picture the baby developed inability to suck and swallow on 4th day of birth. He was born to a mother who had not been immunized against tetanus. The delivery was conducted in unhygienic conditions. So was the management of umbilical cord. Terminally, the baby developed seizures and bronchopneumonia.

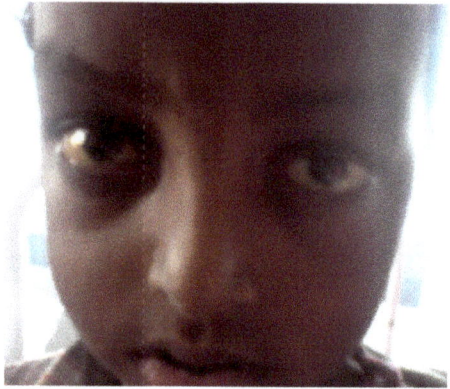

Fig. 154: *Viral hepatitis*—Note the jaundice in a child who presented with anorexia, nausea and vomiting, abdominal discomfort, and tender hepatomegaly.

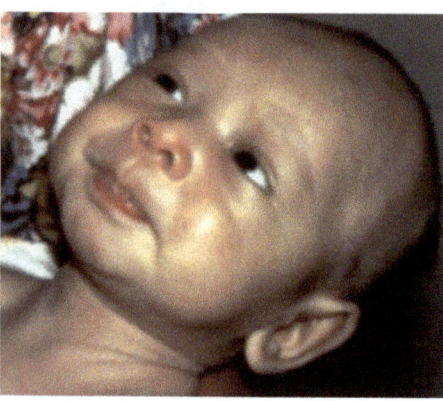

Fig. 157: *Neonatal tetanus*—Note the characteristic facial appearance during the course of a spasm.

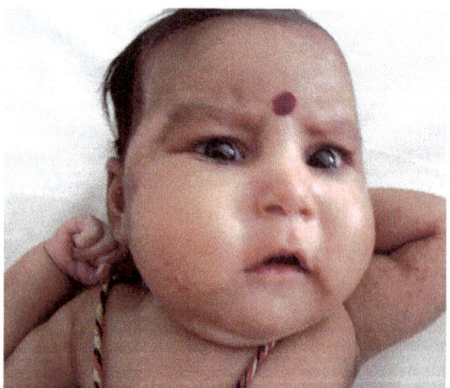

Fig. 155: *Von Gierke disease (Glycogen storage disease type I)*—Note the classical "doll face". The infant also had enlarged liver and kidneys, growth retardation. A tendency for hyperlipidemia, hypoglycemia, lactic acidosis, bleeding, and gout is common in these children.

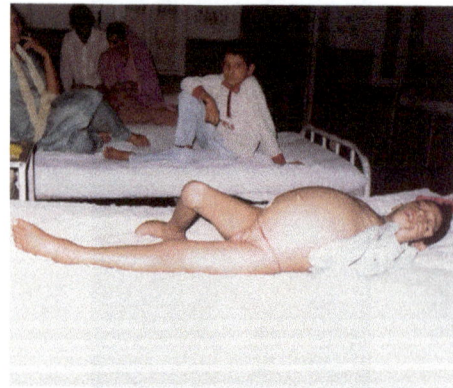

Fig. 158: *Japanese encephalitis (JE)*—An 8-year-old, known for exposure to night-biting mosquitoes in an endemic area during transmission season, convalescing from JE. After the acute onset of encephalitic manifestations, characterized by fast changing CNS signs, he passed through subacute stage. Diagnosis of JE was confirmed by demonstration of virus specific. Immunoglobulin M (IgM) antibodies in the serum on 3rd day of onset of manifestations.

Color Atlas 35

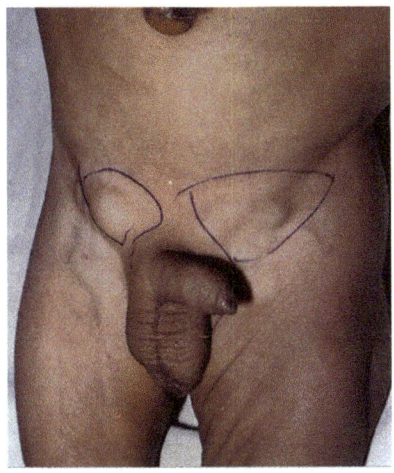

Fig. 159: *Bilateral inguinal lymphadenopathy (chronic)*—Note that though tuberculosis is the most common cause, differential diagnoses includes other infections, immunologic disorders, neoplastic disease, and drugs.

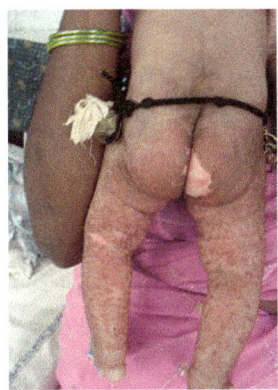

Fig. 160: *Flaky-paint dermatosis*—Note the characteristic skin lesions and pedal edema in an infant with kwashiorkor.

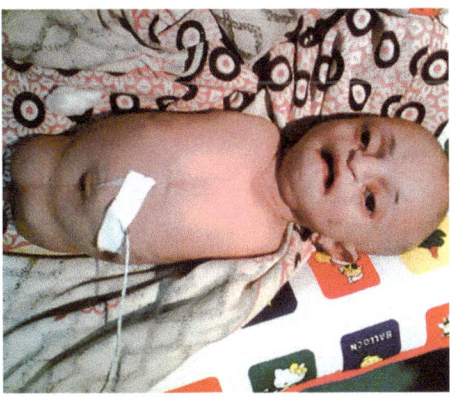

Fig. 161: *Amelia*—Note the complete absence of both upper and lower extremities in the neonate.

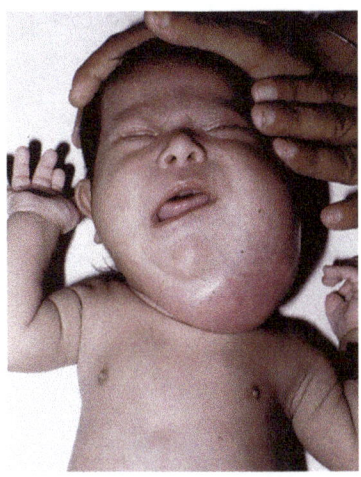

Fig. 162: *Large abscess*—Noteworthy differential diagnosis includes cervical lymphadenitis and cystic hygroma.

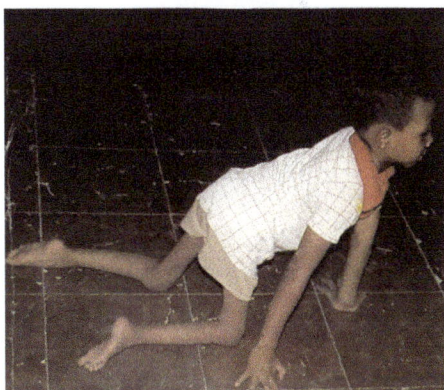

Fig. 163: *Postpolio residual paresis (PPRP)*—Currently this is the most common cause of childhood disability in India and other developing countries. With eradication of polio, the incidence of handicap from this disease will gradually wane.

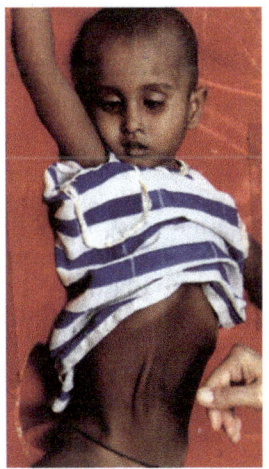

Fig. 164: *Severe dehydration*—Note loss of skin turgor (elasticity), listlessness, and sunken eyes in this child who was hospitalized with acute gastroenteritis, progressive drowsiness, and oliguria.

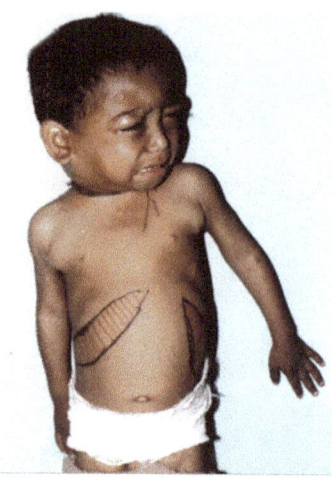

Fig. 165: *Disseminated tuberculosis*—Note the generalized lymphadenopathy, hepatosplenomegaly, and malnutrition. Mantoux was 30 mm × 30 mm. X-ray of chest showed miliary mottling.

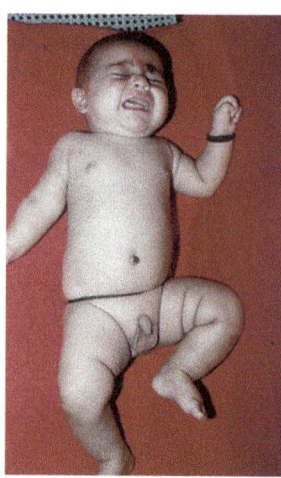

Fig. 168: *Turner syndrome*—Note the shield chest with widely apart nipples.

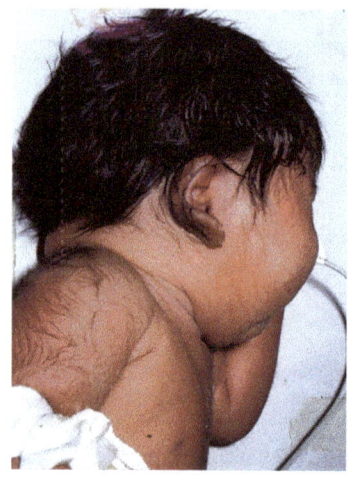

Fig. 166: *Infant of the diabetic mother*—Note the characteristic plethoric chubby appearance with hairy pinna.

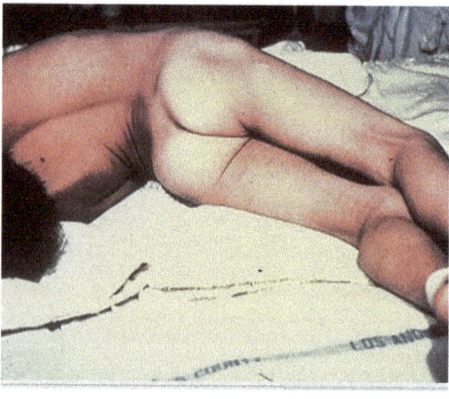

Fig. 169: *Opisthotonos*—Note the arching back of the body with the head thrown backward. Causes of opisthotonos include dystonia, tetanus, severe head injury, meningitis, brain tumor, Arnold–Chiari malformation, subarachnoid hemorrhage, seizures, and strychnine poisoning.

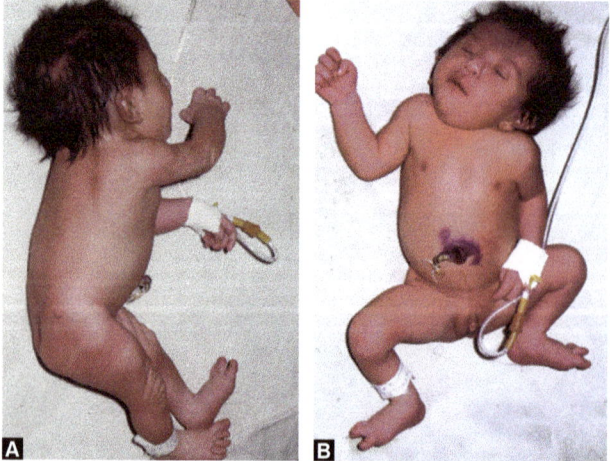

Figs. 167A and B: *Turner syndrome*—Note the short webbed neck, pedal edema, shield chest, and ambiguous genitalia. Karyotyping showed 45XO configuration.

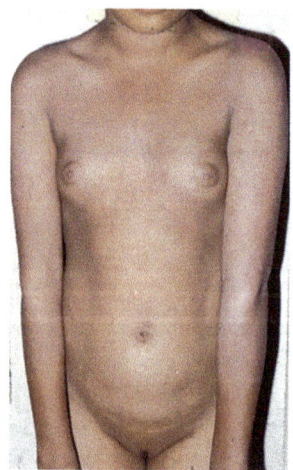

Fig. 170: *Precocious puberty*—Note the premature breast development (gynecomastia) in this 7-year-old girl.

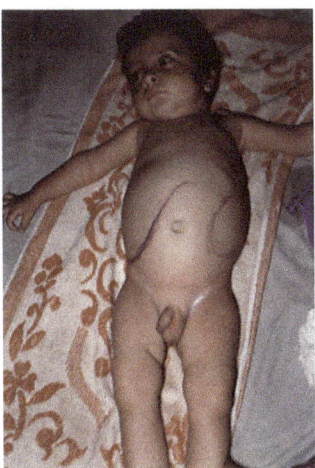

Fig. 171: *Glycogen-storage disease*—Note the massive hepatosplenomegaly.

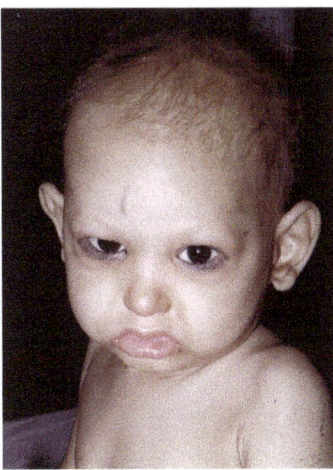

Fig. 172: *Anhidrotic ectodermal dysplasia*—Note the hypotrichosis with absence of eyebrows in this 15-month-old baby. There was yet no dental eruption. He was brought for unexplained pyrexia. Even in peak summer, he hardly exhibited any sweating.

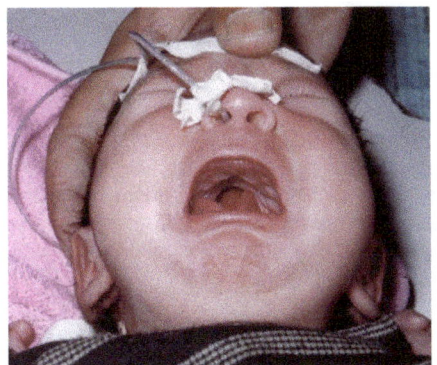

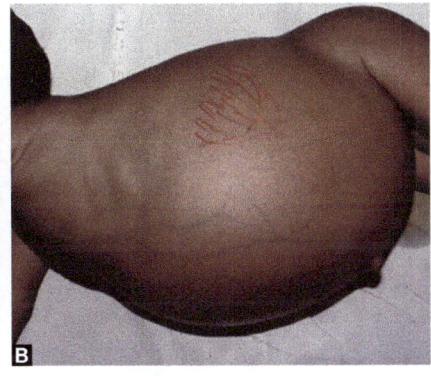

Fig. 173: *Pierre Robin syndrome*—Note the glossoptosis, micrognathia, and high-arched palate.

Figs. 174A and B: *Chronic liver disease with cirrhosis*—Note the massive ascites with hepatosplenomegaly. The history was strongly suggestive of neonatal cholestasis.

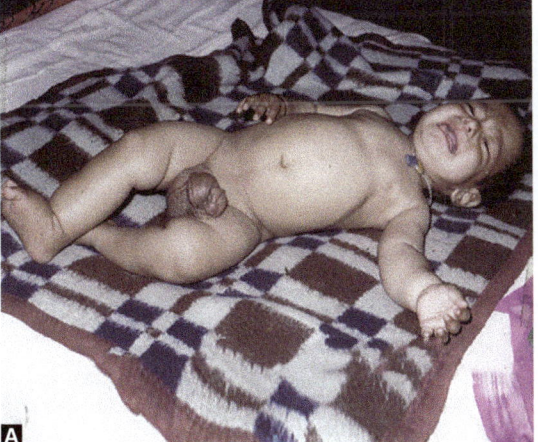
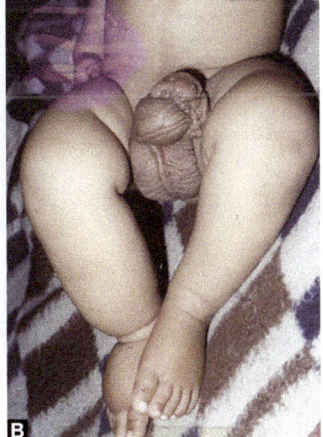

Figs. 175A and B: *Milroy disease*—Note the lymphedema which was present since birth and showed pitting only on firm pressure. Involvement of the external genitalia with disfigurement is also seen. This autosomal dominant disorder should be differentiated from lymphedema present in Turner syndrome and Noonan's syndrome (male Turner syndrome).

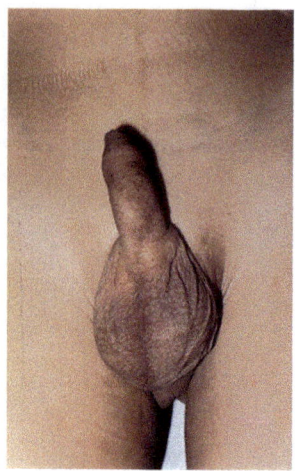

Fig. 176: *Priapism*—The modus operandi in this child with sickle-cell anemia was obstruction of venous outflow secondary to excessive pooling of blood in the corpora cavernosa. The differential diagnosis includes leukemias (especially chronic myeloid leukemia), sickle-cell disease, and perineal trauma. Impotence is among the important sequelae.

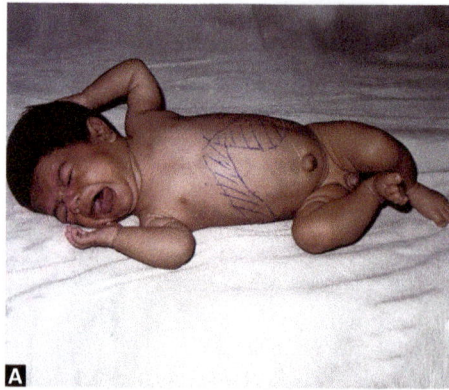
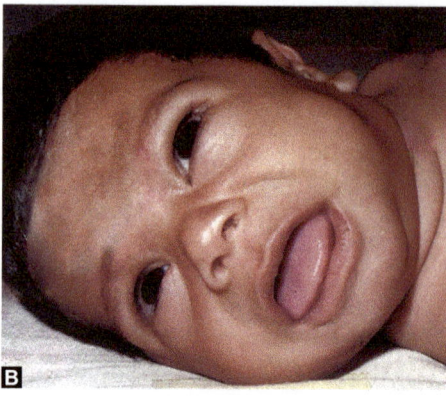

Figs. 178A and B: *Hurler syndrome (MPS-IH)*—Note the grotesque-like coarse facies, large protruding tongue, dwarfism, somewhat cloudy corneas, mental retardation, and hepatosplenomegaly. X-ray skull showed J-shaped sella turcica and X-ray spine demonstrated ovoid-shaped lower dorsal and upper lumbar vertebral bodies beak-like projections anteriorly.

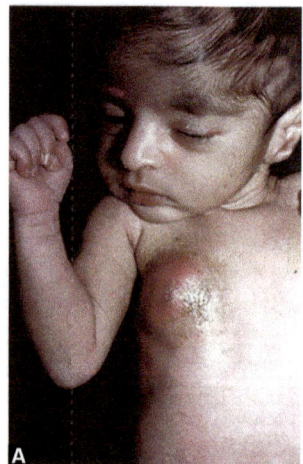
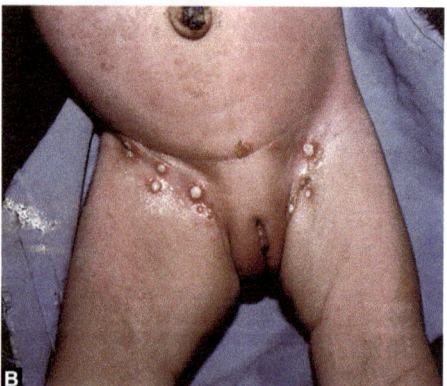

Figs. 177A and B: *Neonatal sepsis*—Note the large pyemic abscess and multiple pustules.

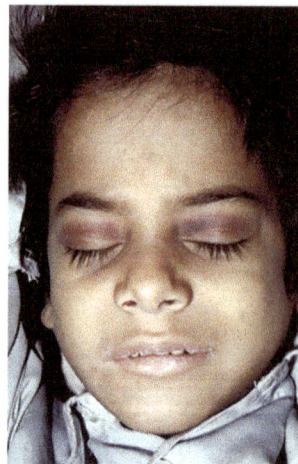

Fig. 179: *Acute lymphoblastic leukemia*—Note severe anemia with ecchymosis.

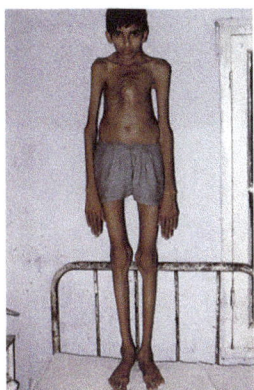

Fig. 180: *Marfan syndrome (arachnodactyly)*—Note the tall stature, slimness, pectus excavatum, pes planus, and arachnodactyly. Steinberg and wrist signs were positive.

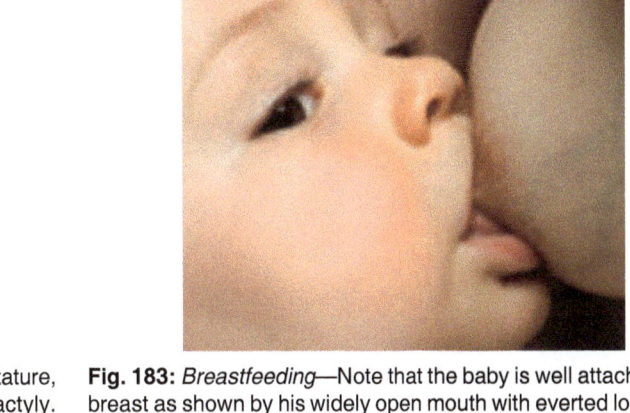

Fig. 183: *Breastfeeding*—Note that the baby is well attached to the breast as shown by his widely open mouth with everted lower lip so that he sucks not just the nipple but also the areola, nostrils are free enough to breathe properly and chin touches the breast. Semisitting position in mother's lap is the best for good breastfeeding.

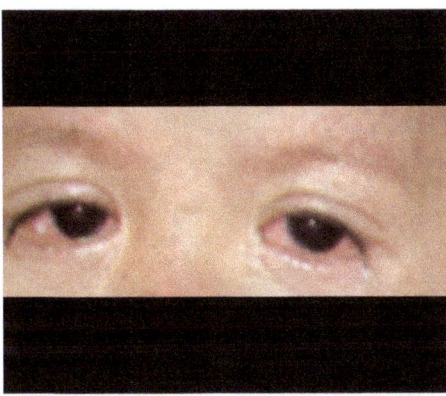

Fig. 181: *Antimongoloid slant*—Note the downward slant of the eyes (just opposite to that of Down syndrome). Differentials include Treacher Collins syndrome, Apert syndrome, Turner syndrome, Goldenhar syndrome, de Lange syndrome, and DiGeorge syndrome.

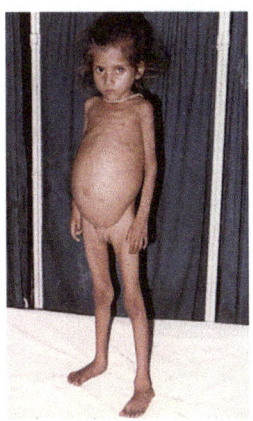

Fig. 184: *Celiac disease (gluten-induced enteropathy)*—Note the growth retardation with pot-belly and corneal opacity secondary to vitamin A deficiency (keratomalacia) that developed 6 months earlier. Besides investigations, elimination of gluten from diet and later challenge with it established the diagnosis.

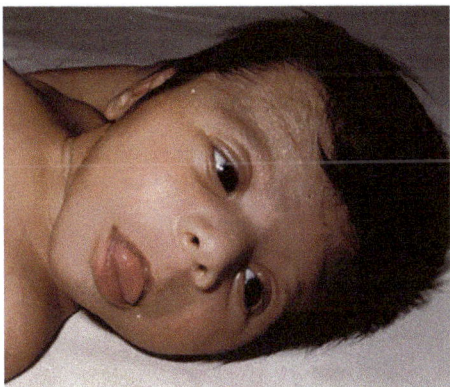

Fig. 182: *Treacher Collins syndrome*—Note the mandibulofacial dysostosis and antimongoloid slant of the eyes.

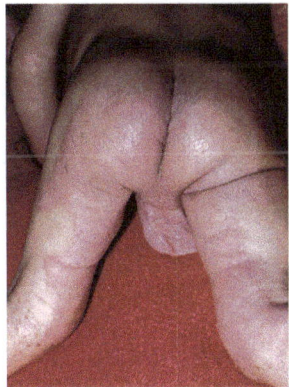

Fig. 185: *Acrodermatitis enteropathica*—Note the characteristic perineal lesions with symmetrical distribution. Other manifestations included perioral lesions, light-colored scalp hair, blepharitis, nail dystrophy, and chronic diarrhea. Response to oral zinc supplementation was dramatic.

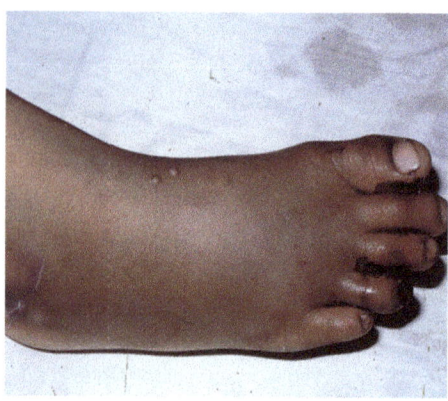

Fig. 186: *Snakebite*—Note the extensive inflammatory swelling of the foot and bleeding. The clotting time on admission was 25 min. The child showed full recovery following therapy, including 300 mL of antivenom serum (AVS).

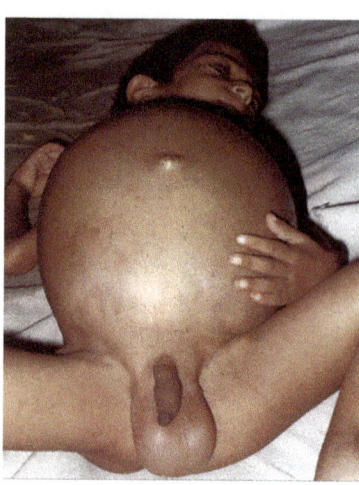

Fig. 187: *Massive abdominal distention*—The child had massive ascites with scrotal edema. Abdominal tap and other investigations clinched the diagnosis of tuberculosis.

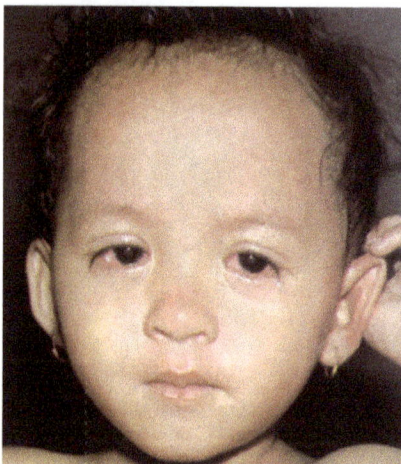

Fig. 188: *Measles*—Note the maculopapular rash (red blotchy pattern) over the face in the child who started with high fever, cough, coryza, and conjunctivitis. The rash then spreaded downward to the torso and extremities.

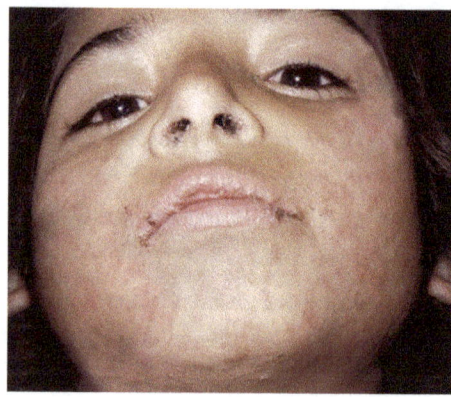

Fig. 189: *Measles*—Note the characteristic maculopapular rash in this unvaccinated girl.

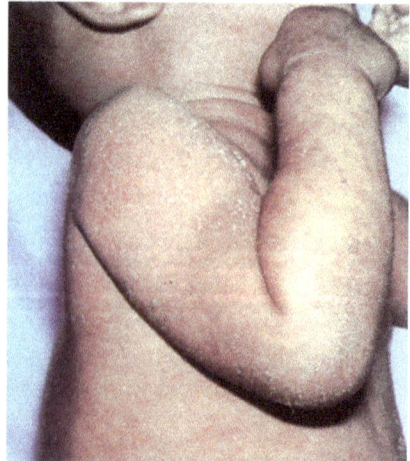

Fig. 190: *Measles*—Note the rash showing disappearance in the some progression as it evolved, leaving behind a fine desquamation (peeling) of skin.

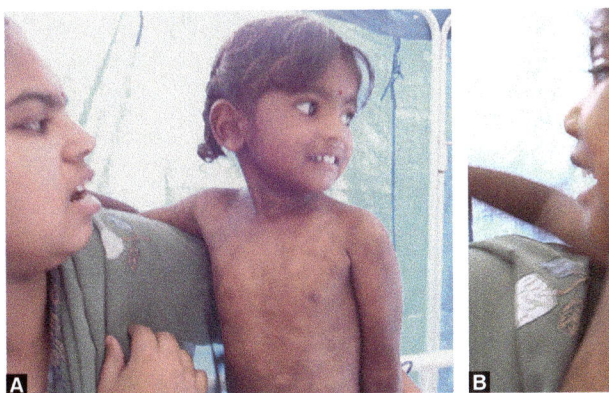
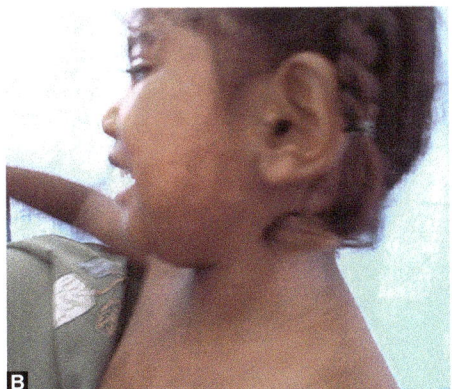

Figs. 191A and B: *Postmeasles pigmentation*—Note the darkened patches during convalescence.

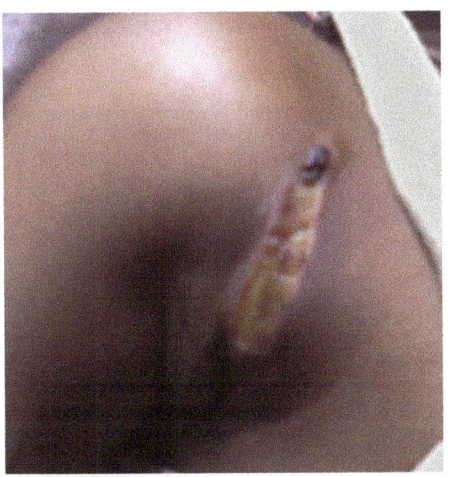

Fig. 192: *Child abuse*—Note the consequences of branding having roots in parents' firm faith in witchcraft.

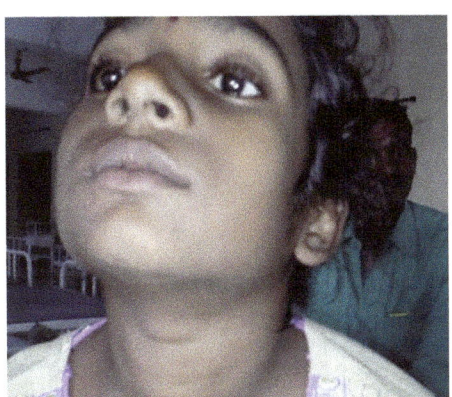

Fig. 193: *Goiter (stage 3)*—Note the clearly visible neck swelling.

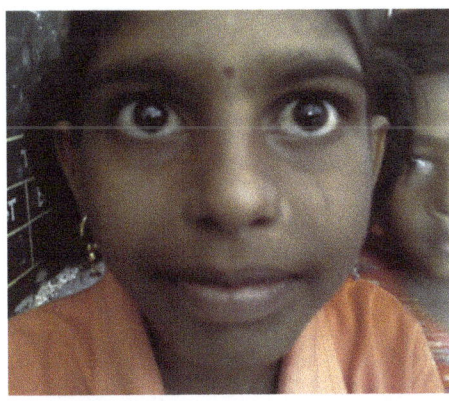

Fig. 194: *Hyperthyroidism*—Note the characteristic staring with wide palpebral fissures in a girl who presented for weight loss in spite of enormous dietary intake, excessive irritability, and poor school performance.

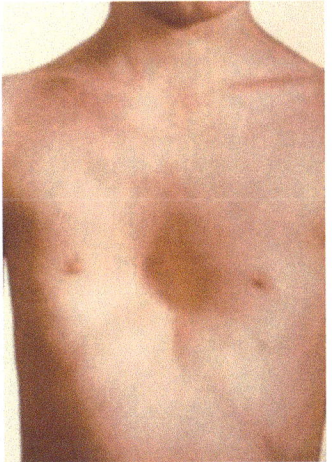

Fig. 195: *Pectus excavatum (funnel chest)*—Most frequently, it is a congenital defect. Infrequently, it may be secondary to rickets.

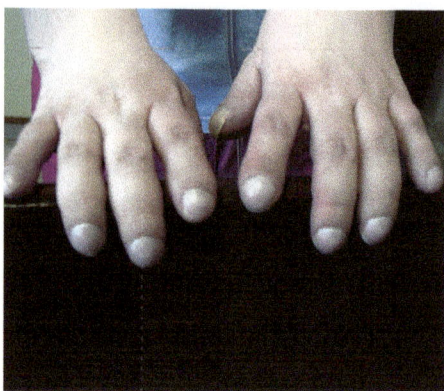

Fig. 196: *Clubbing and cyanosis in cystic fibrosis*—Recurrent respiratory infection, chronic diarrhea, and growth retardation dominated the clinical picture. Sweat chloride turned out to be 110 mEq/L against the normal of less than 60 mEq/L.

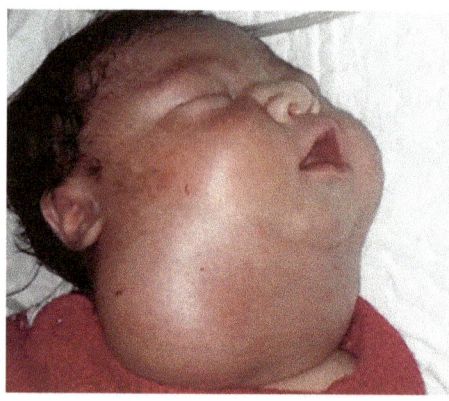

Fig. 199: *Cystic hygroma*—Note the large swelling involving almost the whole of right face and neck. Differentials include lymphadenitis, large abscess, and lymphoma.

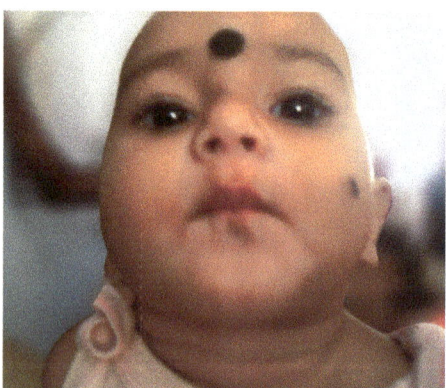

Fig. 197: *Microcephaly secondary to premature closure of all sutures*—Note the symmetrical reduction in head size and shape.

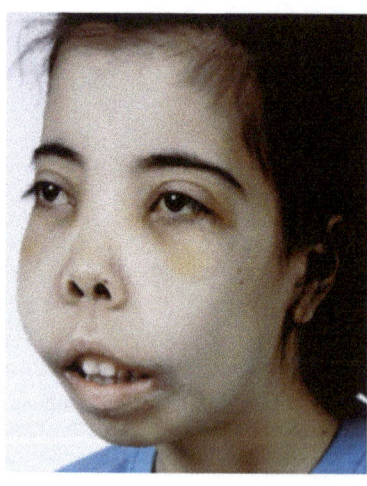

Fig. 200: *Hemolytic facies*—Note the depressed bridge of nose, widely apart eyes, open mouth with maloccluded teeth, etc.

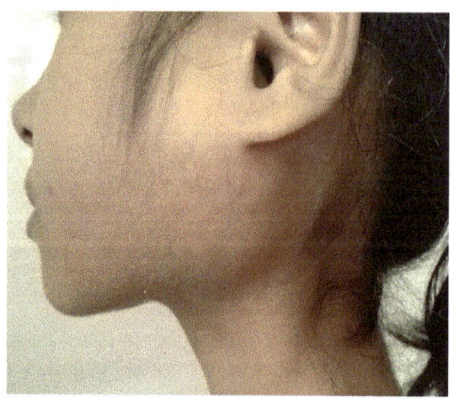

Fig. 198: *Mumps*—Note the left parotid swelling.

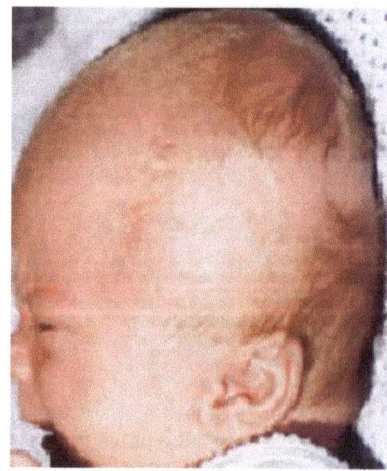

Fig. 201: *Craniosynostosis*—Note brachy turricephaly and low-set ears.

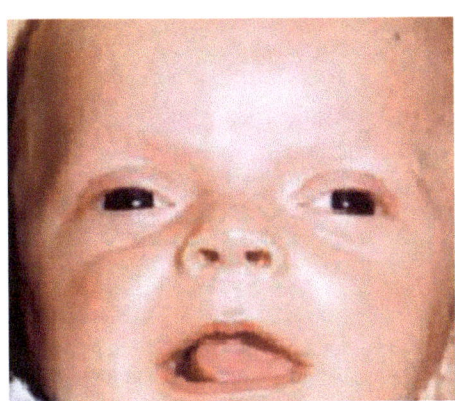

Fig. 202: *Smooth philtrum*—Note the flattening of the normal infranasal depression. Fetal alcohol and Prader–Willi syndromes figure among the conditions in which it is seen.

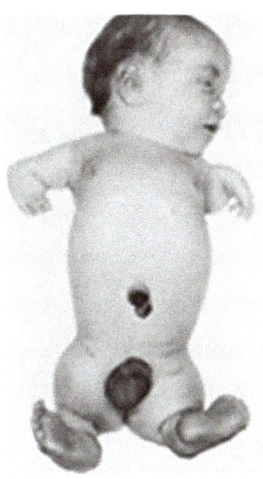

Fig. 203: *Phocomelia*—Note that the hands and feet are attached unusually close to the limbs. The condition is also termed "thalidomide baby".

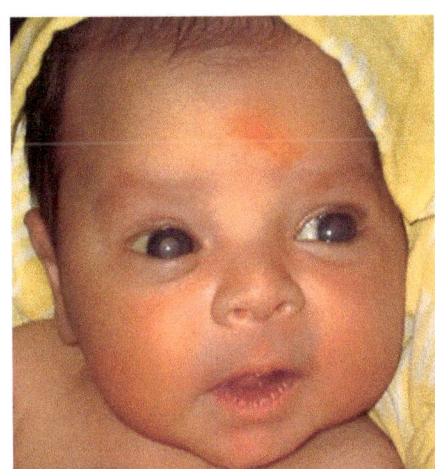

Fig. 204: *Primary congenital glaucoma*—Note corneal enlargement and opacification due to primary congenital glaucoma (both eyes).

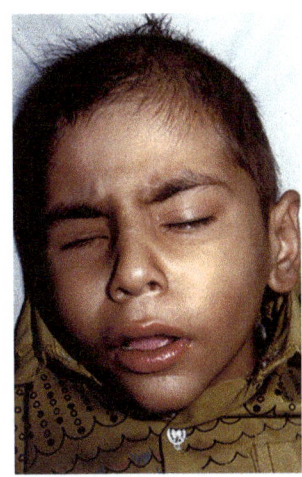

Fig. 205: *Toxic alopecia*—Note the acute loss of hair in a diffuse pattern during the initial treatment with cancer chemotherapy. Also termed as "anagen effluvium", it is a temporary condition. Hair regrowth occurs after the offending therapy is discontinued. The causes include, besides cancer chemotherapy (alkylating agents, antimetabolites, mitotic inhibitors), hypervitaminosis A, heparin, coumarins, boric acid, thallium, and thiouracil. Other causes of acquired diffuse alopecia include sudden severe weight loss, a febrile illness, psychiatric stress, surgery, acute blood loss/donation, and discontinuation of high dose steroid therapy.

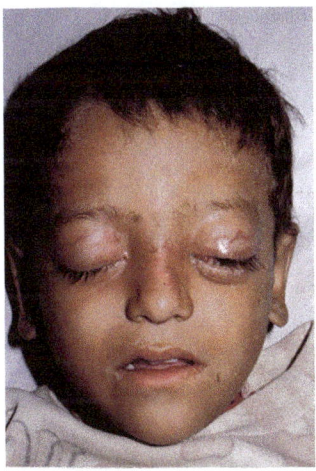

Fig. 206: *Cavernous sinus thrombosis*—Noteworthy conditions that need to be considered in differential diagnosis are periorbital cellulitis and subperiosteal abscess. In the former vision and eye movements are normal. In the latter, ophthalmoplegia is present and vision begins to diminish.

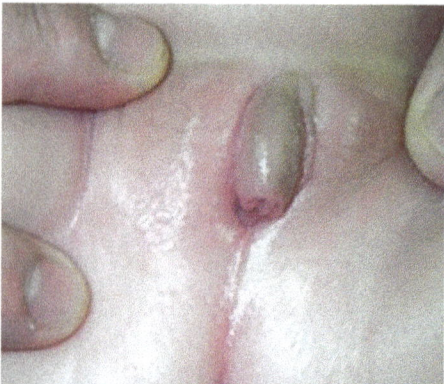

Fig. 207: *Ambiguous genitalia*—Note the hypertrophied clitoris in congenital adrenal hyperplasia (CAH).

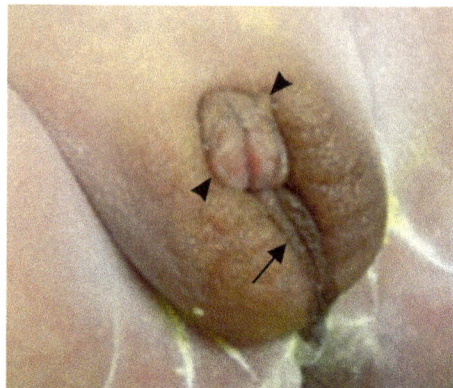

Fig. 208: *Ambiguous genitalia*—Note micropenis, hypospadias, and bifid scrotum.

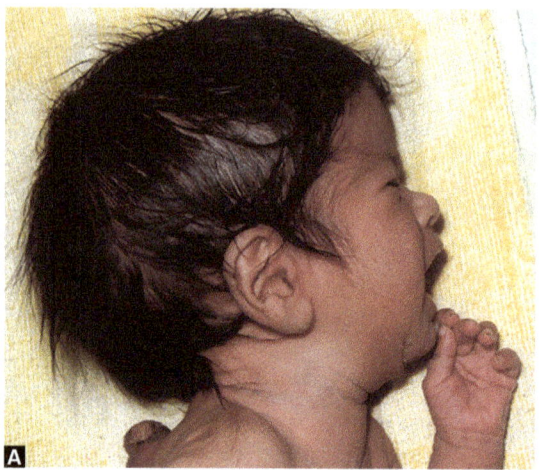
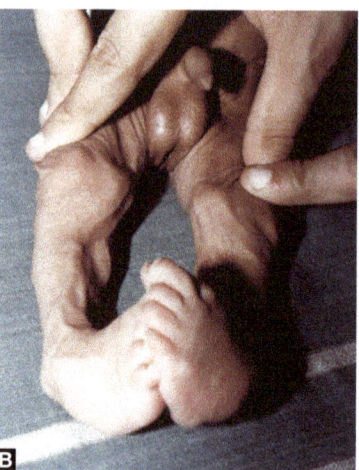

Figs. 209A and B: *Congenital hydrocephalus with meningomyelocele*—The infant also had congenital talipes equinovarus (CTEV) with additional features of arthrogryposis multiplex congenital.

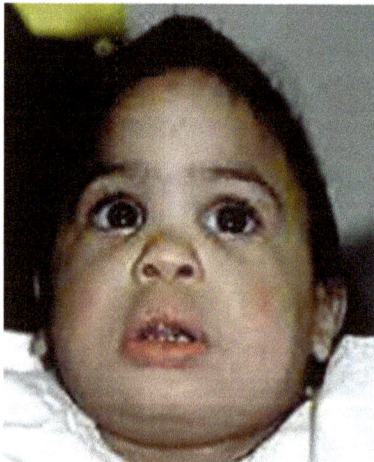

Fig. 210: *Trigonocephaly*—Note the conical front of head with hypotelorism as a result of craniosynostosis of metopic sutures.

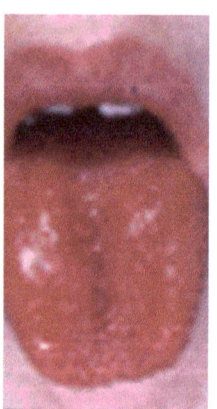
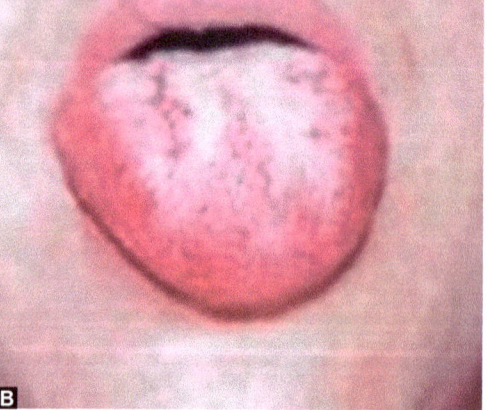

Figs. 211A and B: *Strawberry tongue*—Note the red and white strawberry tongue. It is a feature of Kawasaki disease, scarlet fever and toxic shock syndrome. In scarlet fever, it is white strawberry tongue which forms to red strawberry tongue in the next few days.

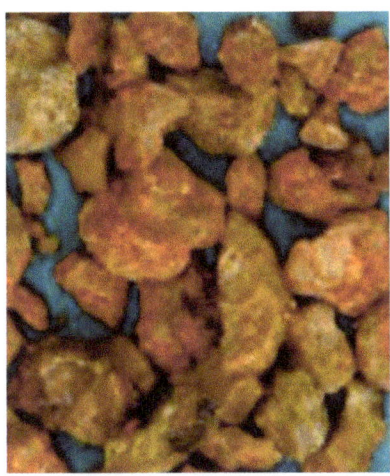

Fig. 212: *Fecolith*—The hard, dry, solid masses often cause abdominal distension and discomfort, anal fissure, and encopresis.

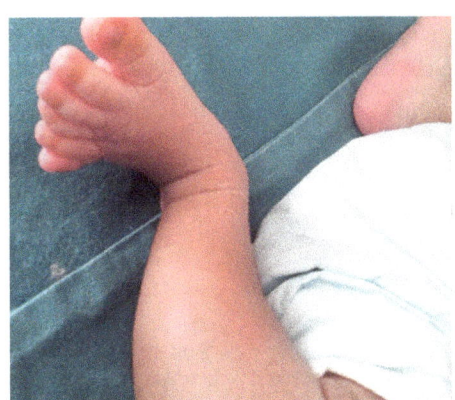

Fig. 215: *Polydactyly*—Note six toes.

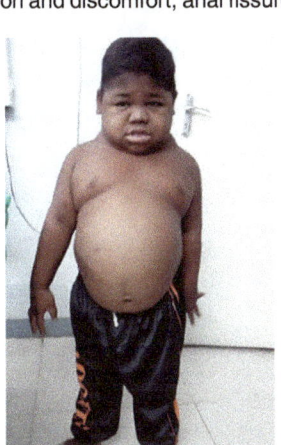

Fig. 213: *Hypothyroidism*—Note short stature, obesity, dull facies, and mental retardation.

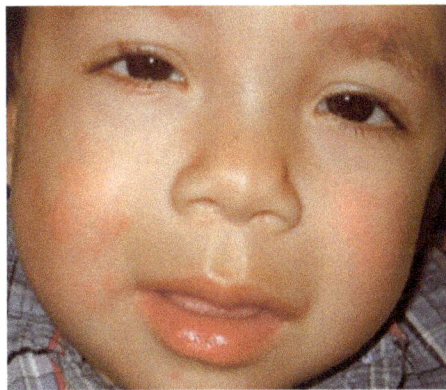

Fig. 216: *Redman syndrome*—Note the development of red facies following administration of vancomycin.

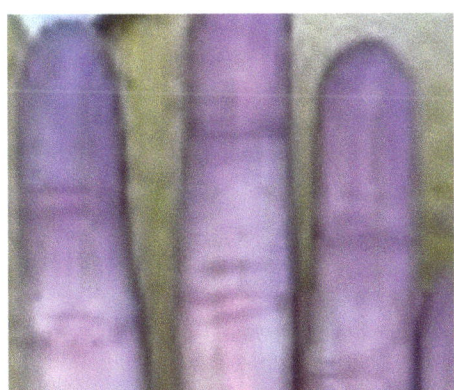

Fig. 214: *Cyanosis*—Note blue discoloration of fingers.

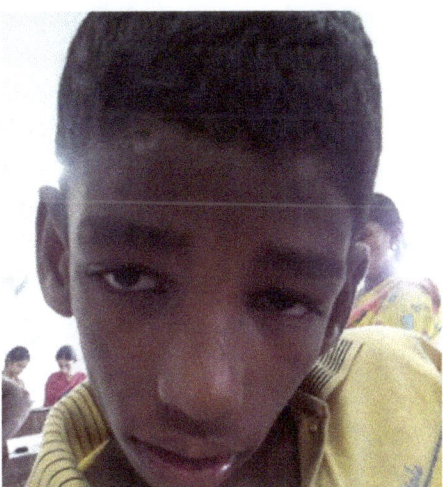

Fig. 217: *Triangular facies in Silverman–Russell syndrome*—Note the triangular-shaped face with a small jaw and a pointed chin. This child, born low birth weight (LBW) [small for gestational age (SFGA)], suffered from growth retardation with short stature and asymmetry of the body.

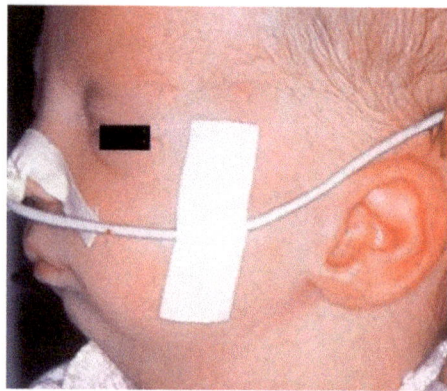

Fig. 218: *Pierre Robin syndrome*—Note the remarkably undersized jaw (micrognathia) in the infant who developed respiratory distress because of glossoptosis.

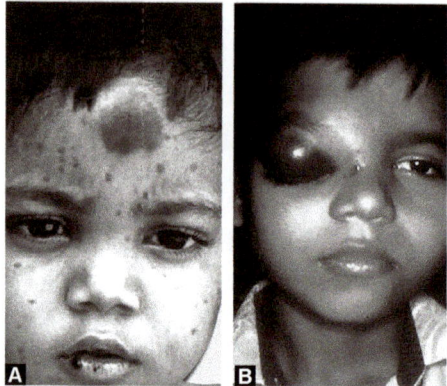

Figs. 219A and B: *Immune thrombocytopenic purpura (ITP)*—Note the skin bleeds in the form of petechiae, purpura, and ecchymosis.

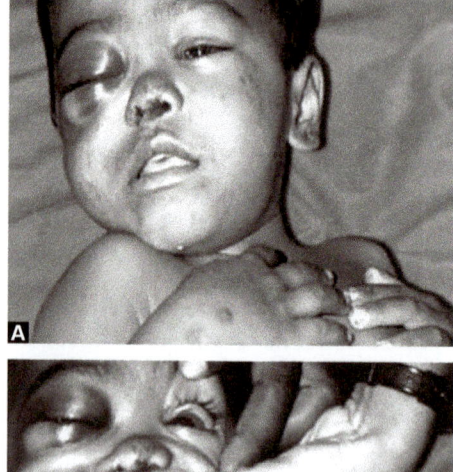

Figs. 221A and B: *Disseminated intravascular coagulation (DIC)*—Note the bleeding from nostrils and over skin.

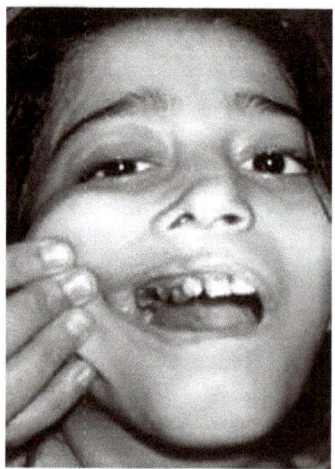

Fig. 220: *Immune thrombocytopenic purpura (ITP)*—Note the gum and oral mucosal bleed.

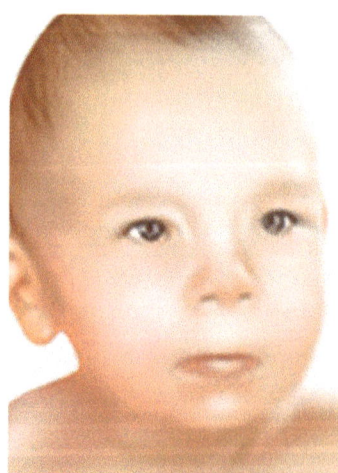

Fig. 222: *Fetal-alcohol syndrome*—Note the features such as smooth philtrum, thin upper lip, micrognathia, epicanthal fold, short palpebral fissure, and microcephaly in this physically and mentally retarded child whose mother consumed alcohol during pregnancy.

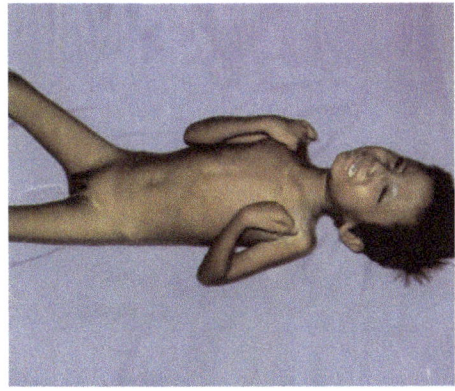

Fig. 223: *Tetanus*—Note the characteristic spasm following a provocative stimulus.

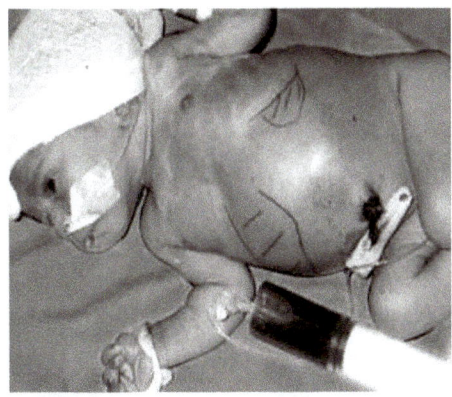

Fig. 224: *Disseminated intravascular coagulation (DIC)*—Note the purpura and hepatosplenomegaly in a neonate with sepsis.

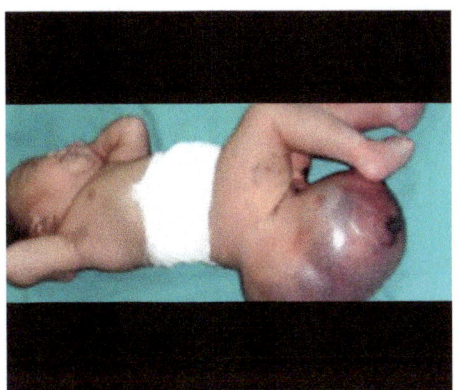

Fig. 225: Sacrococcygeal teratoma.

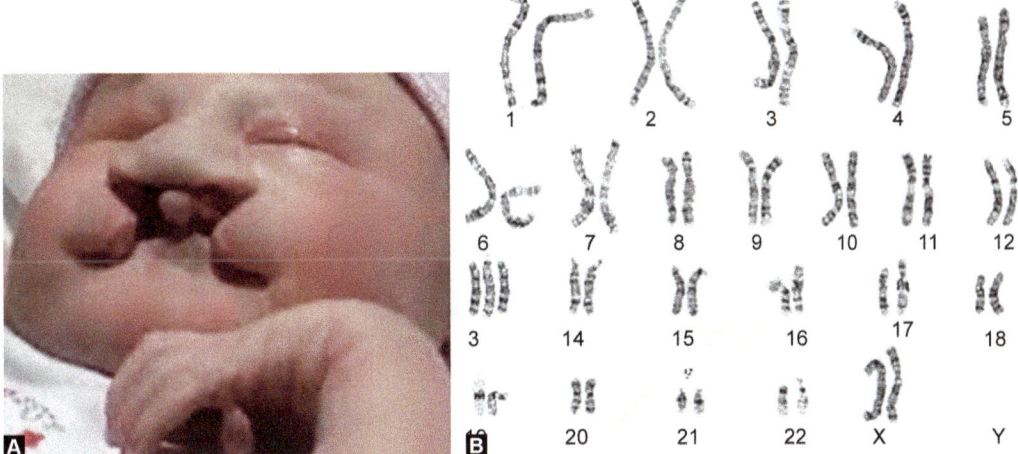

Figs. 226A and B: *Trisomy 13 (Patau syndrome)*—In addition to cleft lip and palate and rudimentary finger, the baby had multiple physical anomalies from eyes to foot.

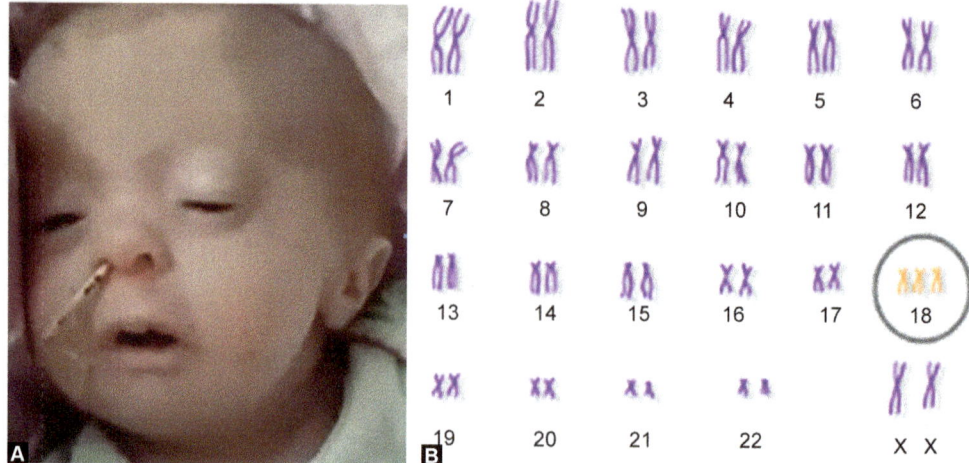

Figs. 227A and B: *Trisomy 18 (Edwards' syndrome)*—Note a microcephalic abnormally shaped head, a small mandible and mouth, low-set ears. The baby also had long overlapping fingers with underdeveloped thumbs and clenched fists, and smooth "rocker bottom" feet (with a rounded base). Often a cleft lip and palate are also present.

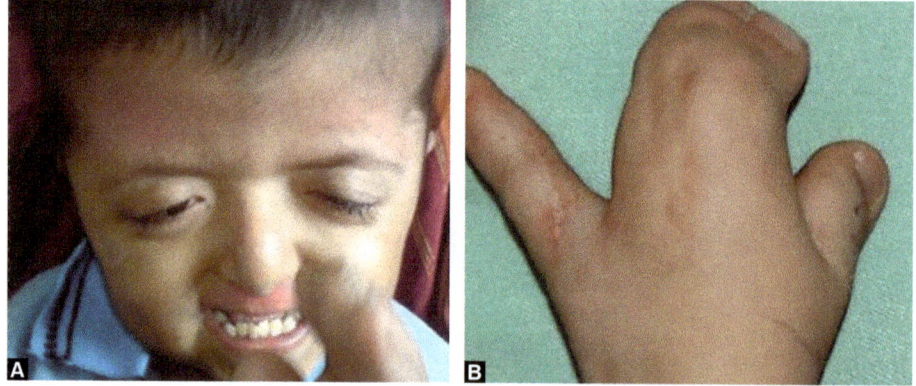

Figs. 228A and B: *Apert syndrome*—Note the microcephaly secondary to craniosynostosis, proptosis, antimongoloid slant of eyes and syndactyly in the intellectually deprived child. Mutation in fibroblast growth factor receptor 2 (FGFR2) on chromosome 10 appears to be the cause.

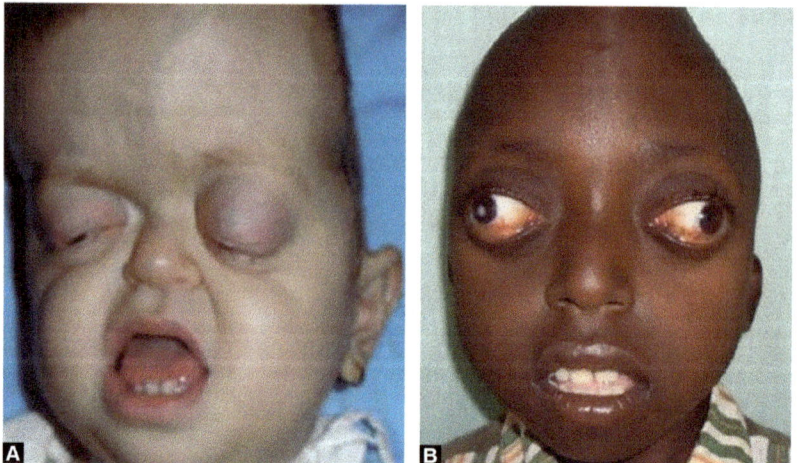

Figs. 229A and B: *Crouzon's syndrome*—Note the microcephaly secondary to craniosynostosis, proptosis with drooling of upper eyelids, antimongoloid slant of eyes, beaked nose, and hypoplastic maxilla. An autosomal dominant disorder, it results from mutation in fibroblast growth factor receptor 2 (FGFR2) on chromosome 10.

Color Atlas 49

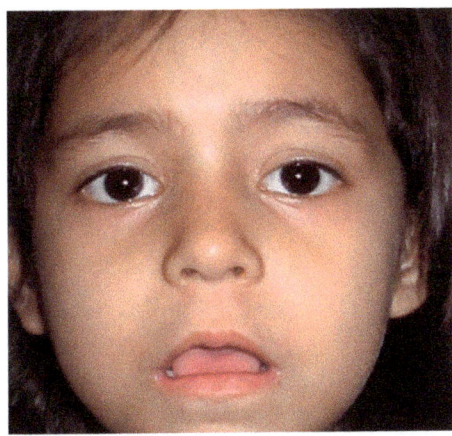

Fig. 230: *Adenoid facies*—Note the dull look and consistently open mouth to facilitate breathing. Hypertrophied lymphoid tissue at the nasopharynx keeps the nose blocked.

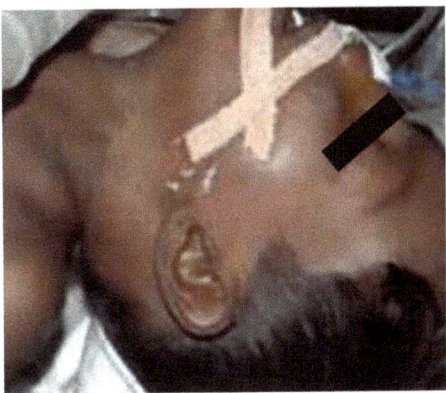

Fig. 234: *Snakebite*—Note the broken-neck sign following viper bite.

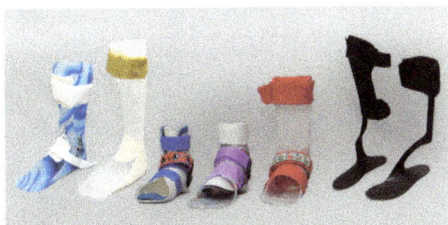

Fig. 231: *Orthoses in cerebral palsy*—Selection of the suitable orthosis is aided by computer gait analysis.

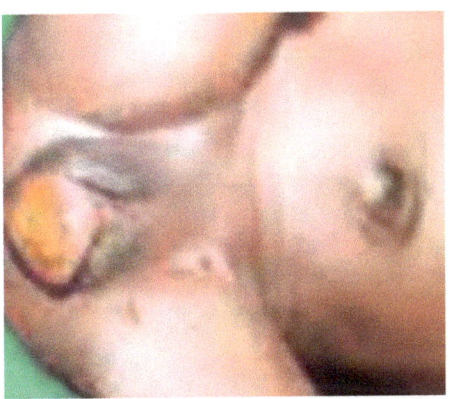

Fig. 235: *Rectal prolapse*—This followed severe dysentery in a malnourished child.

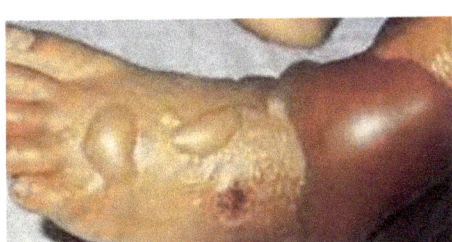

Fig. 232: *Snakebite*—Note the extensive bruising and blistering.

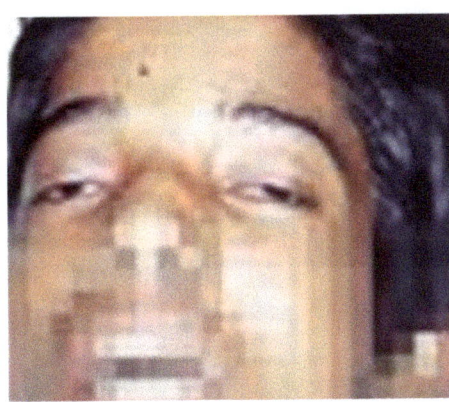

Fig. 233: *Snakebite*—Note the bilateral ptosis.

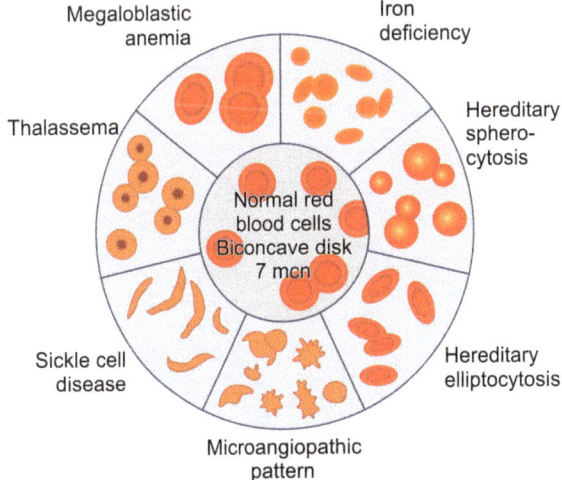

Fig. 236: Normal red blood cells and deviations in leading types of anemia.

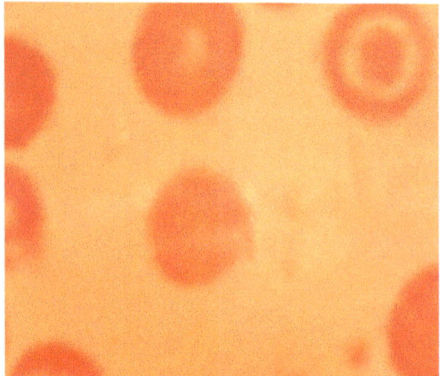

Fig. 237: Target cells.

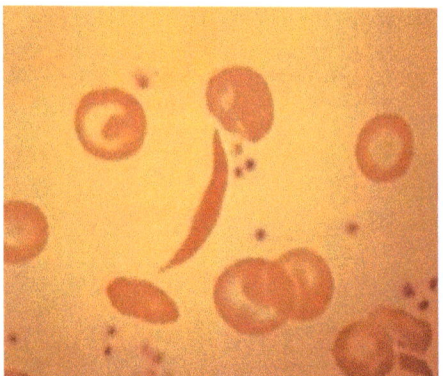

Fig. 238: Sickle cells.

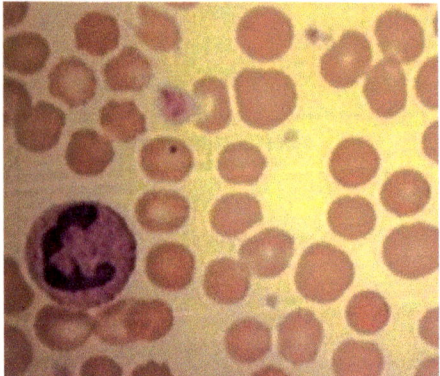

Fig. 239: Spherocyte.

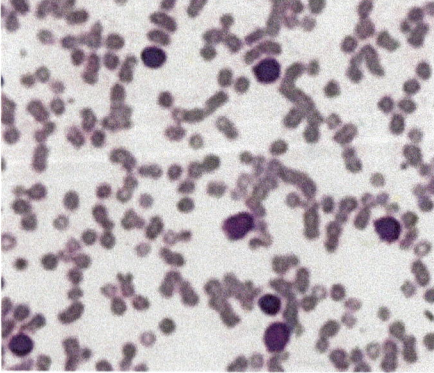

Fig. 240: Acute lymphocytic leukemia (ALL).

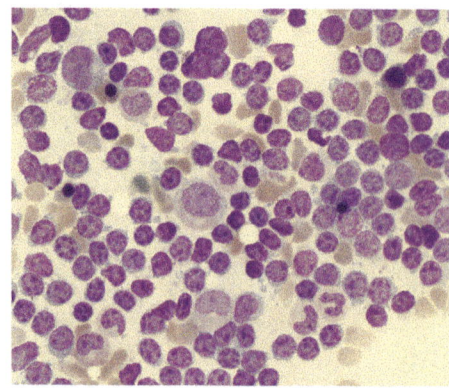

Fig. 241: Chronic lymphocytic leukemia (CLL).

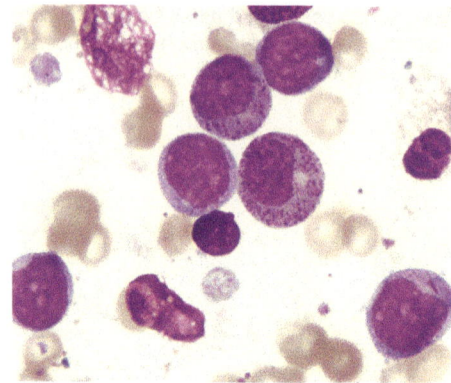

Fig. 242: Acute myeloid leukemia (AML).

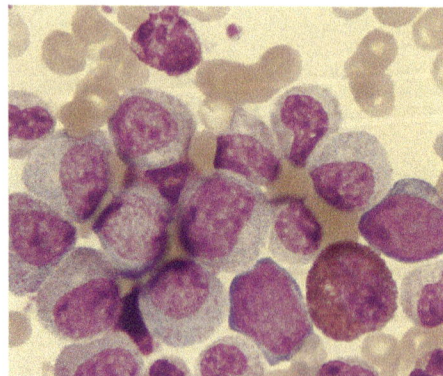

Fig. 243: Chronic myeloid leukemia (CML).

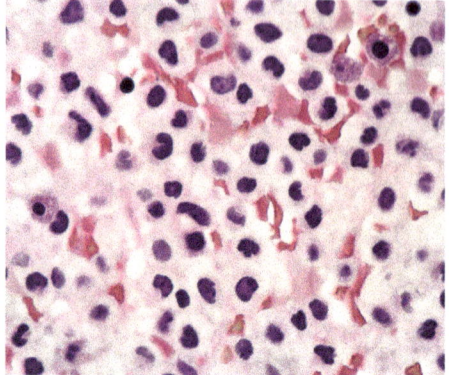

Fig. 244: Hairy cell leukemia.

Color Atlas 51

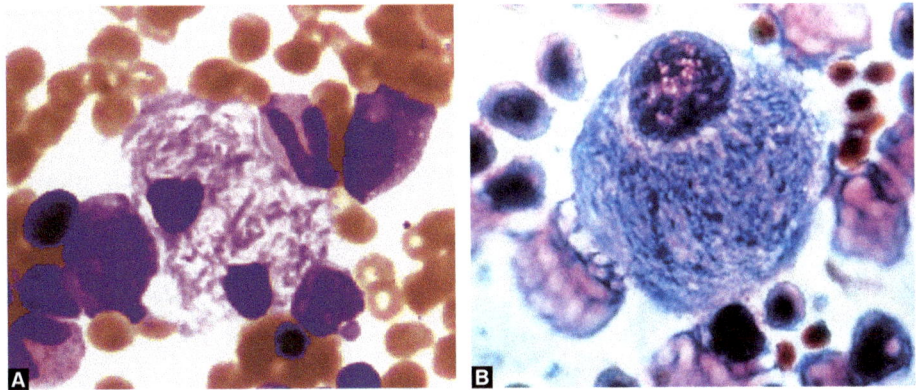

Figs. 245A and B: *Gaucher cells*—Note that the nucleus is pushed off to the side, the remainder of the cell getting filled with abnormal lipids.

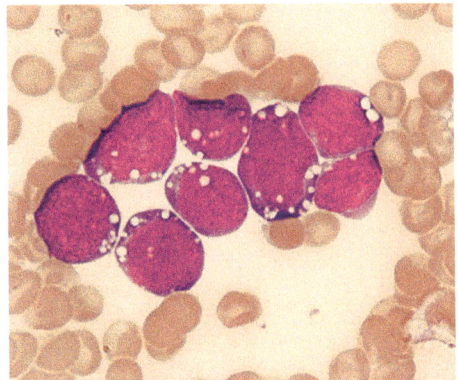

Fig. 246: Burkitt lymphoma.

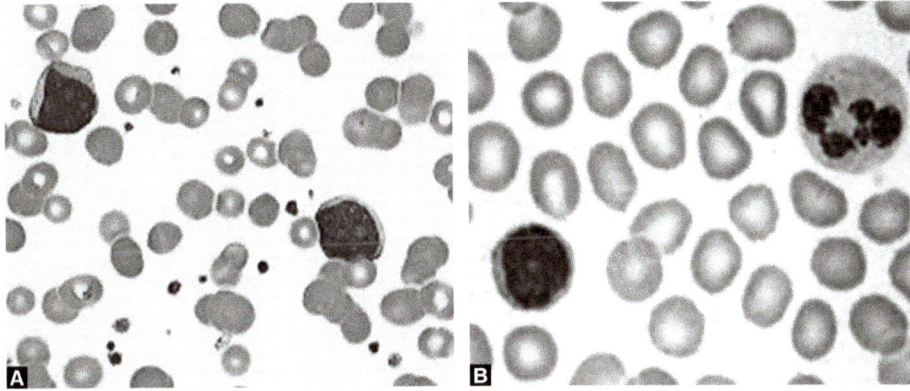

Figs. 247A and B: *Idiopathic thrombocytopenic purpura (ITP)*—Note the normal platelet count (A) and remarkable reduction in platelet count (B).

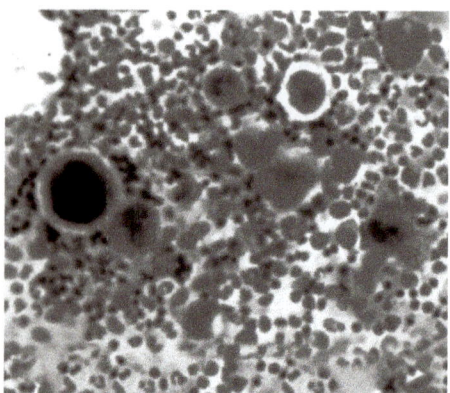

Fig. 248: *Idiopathic thrombocytopenic purpura (ITP)*—Note the increased megakaryocytes in bone marrow.

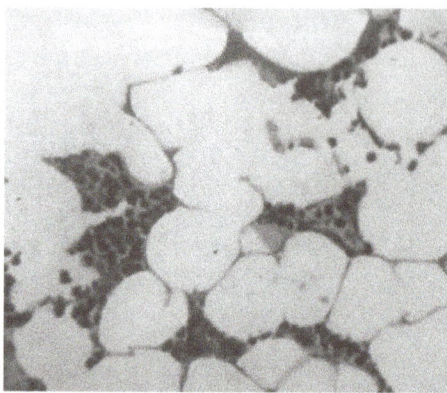

Fig. 250: *Aplastic anemia*—Note the morphologic changes and replacement of cellularity with fat.

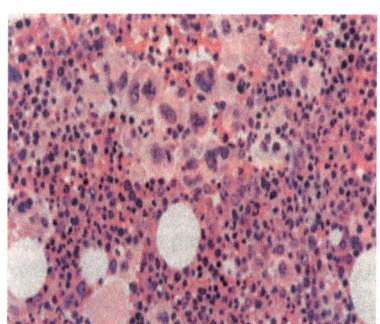

Fig. 249: *Thrombocytosis*—Note the increased platelet count as well as platelet clumping.

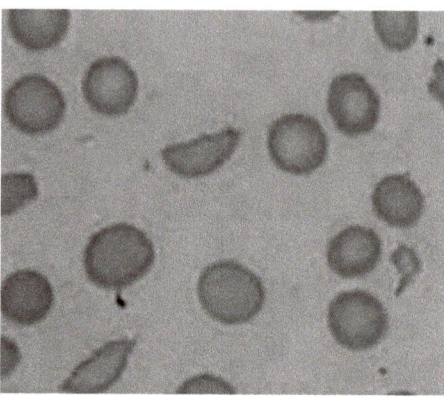

Fig. 251: Microangiopathic hemolytic anemia (Kin lymphoma).

SECTION 2

Differential Diagnosis of Common Pediatric Presentations

CHAPTER 1

Abdominal Distension

BACKGROUND

By definition, *abdominal distension* means enlargement or protuberance of abdomen out of proportion to the body size as a result of:
- Reduced tone of abdominal wall musculature
- Increased abdominal content, say fluid, gas or solid lump.

The term denotes a mere symptom that may not necessarily mean a disease. As for instance, many small infants swallow far-too-much of air when crying or during the course of a feed, particularly when sucking is quite prolonged for one or the other reason. A protuberant abdomen (potbelly) is a common finding in normal, healthy toddlers. It is related to relative hypotonia of abdominal rectus muscles and lumbar lordosis.

Ascites, i.e. fluid in the peritoneal cavity, tends to distend the abdomen both in flanks and anteriorly, provided that it is significantly large in quantity. In addition to fluid in the gut (usually from obstruction or imbalance between absorption and secretion), there is some accompanying gas as well (usually from swallowed air or action of endogenous bacteria or other flora). Audible gurgling noises may also be present.

Abdominal distension from gas in peritoneal cavity (pneumoperitoneum) which may be accompanied by a tympanic percussion note (yes, even on top of a solid organ like liver) points to a perforation of a viscera. Mobile, nontender fecal lumps, i.e. fecaliths, indicate severe constipation.

HISTORY

When confronting a child with abdominal distension, ask the respondent about the general health of the child. Has he been doing well, or not really been thriving satisfactorily? Is there a history of chronic/recurrent diarrhea and/or constipation? Any passage of worms in stools? Does he have feeding problem? Any history of colic? Any suggestion of swelling over face and legs? Is the mother aware of any lump within the abdomen? Any suggestion of emotional deprivation? Any drug intake? Any weight loss or failure to thrive?

In teenage girls, amenorrhea despite advanced puberty should point to imperforate hymen with hematocolpos.

A history of sexual activity should be obtained in view of the likelihood of pregnancy in female adolescents.

Points in history suggesting etiology of abdominal distension are presented in Table 1.1.

PHYSICAL EXAMINATION

Physical examination should aim at delineating if abdominal distension appears to be the result of poor tone of the

TABLE 1.1: Points in history suggesting etiology of abdominal distension.

Parameter	Likely cause
Healthy toddler without gastrointestinal complaints	Normal
Chronic diarrhea with fatty stools	Malabsorption syndrome
Chronic diarrhea with recurrent respiratory infections and failure to thrive despite good dietary intake	Cystic fibrosis
Clinical evidence of rickets	Rickets
Recurrent abdominal pain	Worm infestation
Acute diffuse, severe abdominal pain with progressively increasing distension	Intestinal obstruction
Acute diffuse, severe abdominal pain with fever	Peritonitis
Progressive asymptomatic distension with weight loss	Malignancy
Absolute constipation	Hirschsprung's disease
Amenorrhea in female adolescent	Imperforate hymen
Use of antimotility drug(s) such as diphenoxylate HCl or loperamide	Drug-induced

TABLE 1.2: Interpretation of physical findings.

Physical finding	Likely diagnosis
Healthy toddler with abdominal wall hypotonia	Physiologic
Rachitic rosary, widening of wrists, costochondral beading, genu valgus/varus	Vitamin D deficiency, rickets
Growth failure, delayed milestones, mental retardation, facial features, hypotonia, chronic constipation	Hypothyroidism
Tympanic abdomen	Intestinal obstruction, pneumoperitoneum, aerophagia, peritonitis
Silent abdomen (absent sounds), dehydration	Paralytic ileus
Fever, tenderness	Peritonitis
Ascites	Liver disease, renal disease, heart disease, malnutrition, tuberculosis
Lump other than liver and spleen	Wilms tumor, neuroblastoma
Massive spleen size	Tropical splenomegaly, chronic myeloid leukemia (CML), portal hypertension, thalassemia major, Cooley's anemia
Massive liver size	Hepatoblastoma

abdominal wall musculature, or it is secondary to gas, fluid or solid.

After overall inspection, palpation should take off from the lower quadrants, progressing upward. This assists in appreciating the lower edges of liver and spleen. Local or generalized tenderness, involuntary guarding (a sign of peritonitis), any lump (mass) and rebound tenderness need special attention. Presence of ascites must not be missed.

Interpretation of important clinical signs is presented in Table 1.2.

INVESTIGATIONS

Investigations, if at all required, depend on the merits of each case.

If abdominal distension does not appear to be benign and physiologic, it is appropriate to do:
- Routine hemogram, urine and stool examination
- Serum electrolytes
- Electrocardiogram (ECG) when hypokalemia is on the card.

When ascites is present and is not likely to be of nutritional, renal or cardiac etiology, it is usually advisable to carry out:
- Abdominal paracentesis
- Liver function tests
- Abdominal imaging: Ultrasonography, computed tomography (CT) scan
- Liver biopsy
- Tuberculosis profile.

In case of suspected portal hypertension, additional investigations include:
- Upper gastrointestinal endoscopy
- Portal angiography
- Splenic venoportogram.

IMPORTANT DIFFERENTIALS

Abdominal Distension in the Newborn

The causes at this age include intestinal obstruction, rupture of stomach or some other member of alimentary tract, biliary, or urinary tract, tracheoesophageal fistula, congenital megacolon, septicemia, peritonitis or necrotizing enterocolitis, congenital nephrotic syndrome, tumors and cysts, congenital heart disease, urethral obstruction, gray baby syndrome, etc.

Abdominal Distension in Infancy and Childhood

Aerophagy

Though decidedly common in infancy, aerophagy may sometimes occur in older children as well and cause abdominal distension.

Obesity

It is no longer uncommon in developing countries. Hence, unlike in the past, now it needs to be borne in mind in the differential diagnosis of abdominal distension.

Flabby Abdominal Muscles

Hypotonia of abdominal muscles are a common cause of abdominal distension, e.g. protein-energy malnutrition (both primary and secondary as in malabsorption syndrome), rickets (Fig. 1.1), hypothyroidism, Down's syndrome, floppy baby syndrome, cerebral palsy, etc.

Dehydration

Dehydration with or without electrolyte imbalance as in acute gastroenteritis is an important cause of abdominal distension.

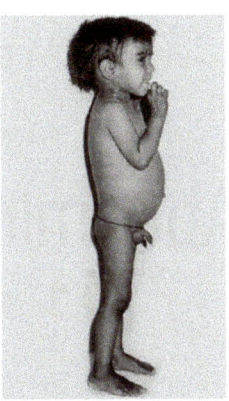

Fig. 1.1: Abdominal distension in a 4-year-old with growth retardation, chronic diarrhea and vitamin D deficiency rickets. The primary diagnosis in this child turned out to be celiac disease.

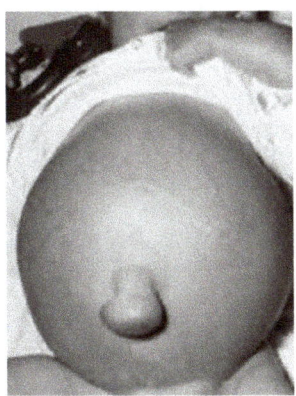

Fig. 1.2: Severe Abdominal distension secondary to biliary cirrhosis.

Ascites

Ascites is a cause of abdominal distension may occur in disorders involving the cardiovascular system (congestive cardiac failure), pericardium (constrictive pericarditis), kidneys (acute glomerulonephritis, nephrotic syndrome), liver [Indian childhood cirrhosis, portal hypertension (Fig. 1.2)], pancreas (chronic pancreatitis), inferior vena cava (thrombosis), lymphatics (tuberculosis, Hodgkin lymphoma) as also in hypoproteinemic states like nephrotic syndrome, protein-losing enteropathy, gross protein-energy malnutrition (Kwashiorkor type), cystic fibrosis and malabsorption states (celiac disease).

Remember, ascitic fluid is generally a transudate with a low protein concentration resulting from low plasma colloid pressure (in hypoalbuminemia), from high portal venous pressure or from both. Usually, development of ascites accompanies significant fall in serum albumin. Additional factors contributing to it include fluid leak from lymphatics and visceral peritoneal capillaries. Furthermore, as the ascitic fluid collects, sodium excretion in urine greatly falls. Thus, additional dietary sodium goes straight to the peritoneal cavity.

Infrequently, when ascitic fluid is an exudate, i.e. with high protein concentration, an inflammatory or malignant process must be suspected.

Drugs

Drugs such as diphenoxylate HCl, loperamide and indomethacin are known to cause abdominal distension in some subjects.

Remaining Causes

Remaining causes include paralytic ileus, intestinal obstruction, perforation, mesenteric cyst, peritonitis, liver cysts and tumors, hydronephrosis, polycystic kidney, renal vein thrombosis, nephroblastoma (Wilm's tumor), neuroblastoma, adrenal hemorrhage, anterior meningocele, pancreatic cyst, leukemia, tyrosinosis, Gaucher disease, porphyria, *Helicobacter pylori* infection, etc.

FURTHER READING

1. Belamarich PF. abdominal distension. In: Adam HM, Foy JM (Eds). *Signs and Symptoms in Pediatrics*, Illinois: American Academy of Pediatrics 2015:1-11.
2. Green M. *Pediatric Diagnosis*, 6th edn. Philadelphia: Saunders 1998.
3. Wyllie R. Major symptoms and signs of digestive tract disorders. In: Kliegman RM, St Geme III JW, Blum NJ. et al (Eds). *Nelson Textbook of Pediatrics*, 21st edn. Philadelphia: Elsevier 2020:1522-1528.

CHAPTER 2

Abdominal Pain

BACKGROUND

Abdominal pain may be acute or recurrent (now rechristened 'chronic'). The latter is encountered more frequently in pediatric practice. Mind you, acute abdominal pain does not imply that the pain has got to be continuous or persistent in all instances. As a matter of fact, it is characterized by pain-free gaps in most of the cases.

According to John Apley, the term *recurrent abdominal pain (RAP)* should be restricted to three or more attacks of abdominal pain severe enough to cause interference in the routine over a period of at least 3 months. According to him, a vast majority of cases (90%) have functional rather than organic abdominal pain. This may well be true for European children. In India and other resource-limited countries, quite a proportion of cases have abdominal pain, i.e. secondary to organic causes especially intestinal worm infestations such as *Giardia lamblia, Ascaris lumbricoides, Ancylostoma duodenale*, tapeworms, etc. Undoubtedly, 'functional' cases too are seen though in relatively less proportion compared to the West.

Currently Rome III criteria are recommended for functional bowel disorders associated with abdominal pain or discomfort in children. Following four classes are identified:
1. Functional dyspepsia
2. Irritable bowel syndrome
3. Childhood functional abdominal pain
4. Abdominal migraine.

In order to appreciate that abdominal pain may well be related to gastrointestinal motility which is under influence of autonomic nervous system, it is important to take a recourse to the gut-brain interaction (Fig. 2.1).

Box 2.1 presents list of common causes of acute abdominal pain.

Box 2.2 presents list of major causes of chronic abdominal pain.

Table 2.1 provides the general rules/guidelines for localization of abdominal pain.

Table 2.2 provides the list of clinical differences among three major types of recurrent abdominal pain, namely functional, organic and dysfunctional.

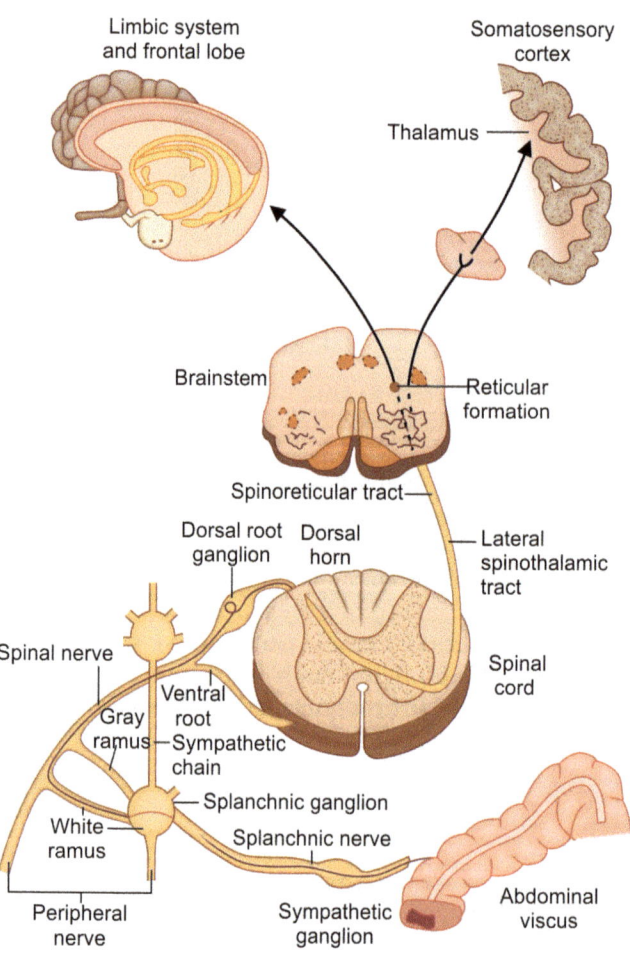

Fig. 2.1: Gut-brain intersection.
Source: Reproduced with permission from Tomar BS. Recurrent abdominal pain. In: Gupte S (Ed). *Recent Advances in Pediatrics: Gastroenterology, Hepatology and Nutrition*. New Delhi: Jaypee 2000:1-11.

BOX 2.1: Common causes of acute abdominal pain.

- Acute gastroenteritis/ acute gastritis
- Intestinal obstruction (massive ascariasis, intussusception)
- Urinary tract infection
- Mesenteric lymphadenitis
- Appendicitis
- Pancreatitis
- Viral hepatitis
- Liver abscess
- Sickle cell disease
- Cholecystitis/gallstone
- Irritable bowel syndrome

BOX 2.2: Major causes of chronic abdominal pain.

- *Gastrointestinal:* Worm infestation, gastroesophageal reflux (GER), lactose intolerance, cow's milk allergy, inflammatory bowel disease (IBD), celiac disease, chronic constipation, Helicobacter pylori gastritis, Meckel's diverticulum, malrotation with intermittent volvulus
- *Liver, gallbladder and pancreas:* Hepatitis, liver abscess, gallstones, recurrent pancreatitis
- *Genitourinary:* Calculus, urinary tract infection (UTI), dysmenorrhea, pelvic inflammation disease
- *Vascular:* Sickle cell crisis, Henoch-Schönlein purpura (HSP), angioneurotic edema
- *Malignant:* Hepatoblastoma, neuroblastoma, secondaries
- *Inborn error of metabolism (IEM):* Acute intermittent porphyria
- *Toxicity:* Lead poisoning

TABLE 2.1: General rules/guidelines for localization of abdominal pain.

Embryologic Origin	Adult structure	Spinal segments	Clinical pain location
Foregut	Distal esophagus, stomach, proximal duodenum, liver, biliary tree, pancreas	T5-T6 to T8-T9	Between xiphoid and umbilicus
Midgut	Small intestine, appendix, ascending colon, proximal two-third of transverse colon	T8-T11	Periumbilical
Hindgut	Distal one-third of transverse colon, descending colon, rectosigmoid	T11-L1	Between umbilicus and pubis

(*Source:* Adapted with permission from Gupta V. Recurrent abdominal pain. In: Gupte S (Ed). *Recent Advances in Pediatrics: (Special Vol 2: Tropical Pediatrics).* New Delhi: Jaypee 1998:193-217.)

TABLE 2.2: Clinical differences among functional, organic and dysfunctional recurrent abdominal pain.

Type	Examples	Diagnostic strategy	Therapeutic strategy
Functional	School phobia Complaint modeling Loss of significant person Secondary gain	Search for understanding of pain experience: Meaning of symptom to patient (significance) How symptom dealt with by patient, family, school Affective meaning of pain experience (pleasant or unpleasant)	Counseling (e.g. anticipatory guidance concerning developmental changes) Psychotherapy ± Environmental manipulation
Organic	Urinary tract infection Pyelonephritis Hydronephrosis Hiatal hernia Lead intoxication Inflammatory disease of intestine	Search for cause classic signs and symptoms of organ disease Organic-related questions Screening for occult organ disease Staged, selective investigation	Specific treatment indicated by diagnosis or Surveillance for organ disease Parental instruction reintercurrent organ disease
Dysfunctional	Chronic stool retention (common) Lactose intolerance Generalized autonomic imbalance (± anxiety) Intestinal gas syndromes Heightened awareness of normal motility Menses Mittelschmerz	Search for predispositions Constitutional factors (e.g. lactose deficiency) Environmental factors (e.g. high milk intake) Interaction between 1 and 2 Specific tests (e.g. abdominal radiograph, lactose tolerance test) Patients/parents going for investigations on their own Diary of associated events	Environmental manipulation (e.g. lactose, free diet, contact with school health personnel) Reassurance based on positive knowledge of known predispositions ± Counseling

(*Source:* Adapted with permission from Gupta V. Recurrent abdominal pain. In: Gupte S (Ed). *Recent Advances in Pediatrics: (Special Vol 2: Tropical Pediatrics).* New Delhi: Jaypee 1998:193-217.)

HISTORY

A meticulous history, though often it is second hand is mandatory. Since when the child has been suffering from pain? Is it continuous or shows periods of relief in between the episodes of pain? How about the previous attacks of abdominal pain over the months/years? Get details about the episodes/attacks.

What is the actual site of pain? Is it all over the abdomen or is restricted to paraumbilical area, epigastrium, etc.? Or does it show change in site from time to time? Lack of localization rather goes against the organic cause. Likewise, closer the pain occurs to umbilicus, less is the chance of organic disease.

What is the nature of pain? Is it stabbing, colicky or dull?

What is its behavior like? Is it getting worse or appears to be settling down?

It is important to know how pain started. Was there any preceding illness? Are there any associated symptoms like headache, vomiting, diarrhea, fever, passage of worms in stools, port-wine color of urine or dysuria?

Do not ever forget to ask especially in the case of an infant how he is being fed? Cow's milk allergy is well known to cause abdominal pain.

It is vital to obtain psychosocial history. How is the child doing in school and is he genuinely interested in going to school? Do rest of the family members have abdominal pain? Are the parents highly stung with tense personalities?

PHYSICAL EXAMINATION

While examining the child with abdominal pain, remember to check the whole child, not just the abdomen. Quite a few cases of abdominal pain have this problem secondary to an extra-abdominal ailment such as pneumonia or sickle cell anemia, etc. (Box 2.3). The physical workup should also include urethral and vaginal orifices and, if workable rectal examination.

Abdominal palpation is best begun from the lower quadrants and then moved upward so that the lower edges of liver and spleen are not missed. A careful observation for local or generalized tenderness and involuntary guarding (a sign of peritonitis), and rebound tenderness needs to be made.

In most children, physical examination reveals nothing abnormal. In these children, especially if no abnormal signals are present, chances of functional abdominal pain increase considerably.

INVESTIGATIONS

Investigations are indicated when history and physical examination suggest a nonfunctional etiology and their choice is usually guided by the differential diagnosis reached from clinical workup.

The screening laboratory tests include:
- Complete blood picture (CBP)
- Stool examination for ova and cysts.

Rather than a battery of tests in a go (often demanded by parents), special tests need to be opted after due consideration of the individual merits of the cases. As for example, ultrasound is warranted in the event of a suspected intussusception. If pancreatitis is on the card, it is advisable to go for serum amylase and lipase.

IMPORTANT DIFFERENTIALS

Acute Abdominal Pain

Acute Appendicitis

In acute appendicitis, the most common surgical cause of acute abdominal pain in infants and children, is that the pain is crampy and over the periumbilical area at the outset. Later, it comes to be located over the right iliac fossa in case the organ is in the typical position. It may be felt in the hypogastrium or within the pelvis, if the position is pelvic, and in the loin if it is retrocolic. What is noteworthy is that pain is only rarely severe. Along with complaint of pain, there is severe tenderness over the appendix, pyrexia and tachycardia. Vomiting follows shortly. The child becomes anorexic. The only indication of acute appendicitis in infancy may be general irritability and inclination to lie quietly with hips flexed.

An inflamed appendix may cause diarrhea by irritation of the adjacent colon, urinary frequency and urgency by irritation of the bladder, and lumbar lordosis with somewhat flexed hip by right psoas muscle spasm.

Remember, sudden relief in pain in a child with acute appendicitis may point to perforation.

Radiological visualization of fecalith in the appendix supports the diagnosis of appendicitis.

BOX 2.3: Nondigestive tract causes of abdominal pain.

- Pneumonia
- Endocarditis
- Child abuse and neglect (CAN)
- School phobia
- Abdominal migraine
- Sickle cell crisis
- Systemic lupus erythematosus (SLE)
- Porphyria
- Pelvic osteomyelitis
- Pelvic inflammatory disease (PID)
- Vertebral disk inflammation
- Angioedema
- Familial Mediterranean fever
- *Drugs:* Nonsteroidal anti-inflammatory drugs (NSAIDs) like aspirin, ibuprofen, mefenamic acid, indomethacin, diclofenac, celecoxib

Acute Peritonitis

Acute primary peritonitis, a bacterial infection of the peritoneal cavity without demonstrable intra-abdominal cause is characterized by fever, abdominal pain, vomiting and prostration. Abdomen is distended and shows diffuse tenderness with doughy resistance. Rebound tenderness and rigidity together with sluggish or absent bowel sounds establish the diagnosis clinically. Leukocytosis with 90% polymorphonuclear response is noteworthy.

Acute secondary peritonitis is usually due to entry of enteric bacteria into the peritoneal cavity from an inflamed appendix, intussusception, volvulus, rupture of Meckel's diverticulum, incarcerated hernia, peptic ulcer, ulcerative colitis, pseudomembranous enterocolitis, meconium ileus, necrotizing enterocolitis, etc. Diffuse abdominal pain, fever, nausea, and vomiting are the usual presenting complaints. The physical findings include rebound tenderness, abdominal wall rigidity, sluggish or absent bowel sounds, and shock. Eventually, the child may develop progressive toxemia. Leukocytosis with predominance of polymorphonuclear cells is characteristic.

Mesenteric Lymphadenitis

This condition, in which there is swelling and inflammation of the mesenteric lymph glands in the ileocecal region in particular may be clinically indistinguishable from acute appendicitis. Among the causative agents rank viruses, *Yersinia enterocolitica, Escherichia coli, Salmonella* and *Shigella.*

The patient is usually a child above 3 years of age. Following an upper respiratory catarrh, he develops abdominal pain (periumbilical or in the right iliac fossa), nausea, vomiting, diarrhea or constipation (usually former) and fever. The pain is intermittent. The remissions last a few hours. During remission, the child is comfortable.
The following points may help in differential diagnosis from appendicitis:
- Shifting of the point of maximum tenderness on turning the child on his side favors mesenteric adenitis.
- Temperature tends to be higher in mesenteric adenitis than in appendicitis.
- Tenderness is felt nearer the umbilicus and is less well localized in mesenteric adenitis than in appendicitis.
- Muscle guarding/rigidity over the right iliac fossa in mesenteric adenitis is not true but only voluntary.
- In a proportion of cases of mesenteric adenitis, it may be possible to palpate the enlarged glands.
- Leukocytosis is infrequent in mesenteric adenitis.

In doubtful instances, one may have to resort to laparotomy for establishing the diagnosis.

Finally remember that appendicitis and mesenteric lymphadenitis may well coexist.

Acute Pancreatitis

Accompanying mild to severe abdominal pain are fever, vomiting, and abdominal tenderness. In advanced cases, paralytic ileus, shock, jaundice, blue discoloration of umbilicus and flanks, disseminated intravascular coagulopathy (DIC), renal failure and disturbances of potassium and calcium metabolism may complicate the picture.

In suspected cases, diagnosis needs to be established by demonstrating raised serum amylase. Plain X-ray abdomen shows ileus. Barium meal reveals duodenal displacement.

Remember that though acute pancreatitis may result from several causes, including viral infection, trauma, drugs (corticosteroids, azathioprine, thiazides), and malnutrition, its most common cause in pediatric practice remains mumps. Manifestations of acute pancreatitis follow 3 days or 4 days after the swelling of parotid gland(s).

Intussusception

This condition characterized by telescoping of one of the portions of intestine into a more distal portion resulting in necrosis of the involved segment is the most frequent cause of acute abdominal pain and intestinal obstruction during the first 2 years of life.

Clinical features include episodic pain, vomiting and rectal passage of bloody mucus (currant jelly stools). Fever and prostration are usually present sooner or later. Abdomen is tender and distended. A sausage-shaped mass may be palpable in the upper abdomen in early stages. Rectal examination may show a cervix-like mass and blood on the examining finger.

Plain X-ray abdomen may reveal absence of bowel gas in the right lower quadrant and dilated loops of small bowel.

Barium enema may reveal the intussusception as an inverted cap and an obstruction to the progression of barium. In the area of intussusception, there may be a ceiling-spring appearance to the column of barium.

Conservative hydrostatic reduction gives good results in an overwhelming majority of the patients. It should be avoided in the presence of strangulation, perforation, or severe toxicity.

Surgical reduction may become necessary in some cases.

Acute Gastritis

In acute gastritis, regardless of origin, epigastric pain, tenderness and sensation of pressure and fullness especially intensifying after food consumption occur. Nausea, vomiting, belching and lack of appetite are other symptoms.

Viral Hepatitis

Nonspecific pain, localized in the right upper quadrant may occur in some children at the onset of viral hepatitis. Accompanying features include anorexia, jaundice, tender hepatomegaly, and fatty food intolerance. If jaundice is yet to make its appearance but diagnosis of hepatitis is suspected, you must test urine for bile salts and pigments followed by other liver function test, if necessary.

Liver Abscess

Besides pain in the right hypochondrium (often referred to the right shoulder), the patient is febrile. The liver is enlarged and tender.

Screening shows raised and immobile diaphragm. Demonstration of *Entamoeba histolytica* in stool and aspiration of characteristic anchovy* sauce (chocolate colored) pus from liver swelling establishes the diagnosis of amebic liver abscess.

Subphrenic Abscess

Subphrenic abscess of whatsoever origin (usually it is bursting of a liver abscess, appendicitis, colitis) causes pain and tenderness in the right or left hypochondrium with radiation to the corresponding shoulder. The subject is toxic. Screening reveals a raised and immobile diaphragm with gas under it. Aspiration of pus confirms the diagnosis.

Cholecystitis

Abdominal pain may rarely be a manifestation of cholecystitis in children. Tenderness and pain may be in the right upper abdomen, right lower abdomen, periumbilical area, or entire abdomen. Abdominal distention, vomiting, fever, anorexia, and slight icterus may also be present.

Pyelonephritis

Besides nonspecific pain in the loins (flanks) or suprapubic region, urinary tract infection (UTI) may cause high fever (often accompanied by chills), urinary frequency, dysuria, vomiting, anorexia and irritability. Demonstration of pyuria on microscopic examination establishes the diagnosis.

Acute Glomerulonephritis

The onset of acute glomerulonephritis may be heralded by flank or midline abdominal pain. Associated manifestations include periorbital edema, dark-colored urine, oliguria, low-grade fever and hypertension. There is a preceding history of pharyngitis or impetigo. Urine microscopy shows hematuria and red cell and granular casts.

Anaphylactoid Purpura

Also called Henoch-Schönlein purpura, the disorder occurs most frequently about 5–6 years of age. Abdominal pain occurs in the Henoch type. Associated features include urticaria, petechiae over extensor surface of the limbs and around buttocks, bleeding from gut and nephritis. Hess capillary test, bleeding time, clotting time and platelet count are all normal.

Porphyria

In this disorder, colicky abdominal pain is precipitated on administering a barbiturate or sulfa drug. Most frequent site of abdominal pain is epigastrium or iliac fossa. Diffuse tenderness of abdomen is present. Vomiting, fever and constipation usually accompany the abdominal pain. Leukocytosis is often present. Hoesch's test for porphobilinogen (PBG) is positive.

Extra-abdominal Causes

Lower lobe pneumonia and pleurisy may cause referred upper abdominal pain synchronous with respiration.

Pleurodynia (Bornholm's disease, epidemic myalgia, devil's grip), a group B Coxsackie virus infection may cause severe colicky abdominal pain. History of illness in other family members especially during summer or fall helps in arriving at this diagnosis.

Acute tonsillitis or other respiratory infections may cause abdominal pain.

Hiatal hernia may lead to reflux esophagitis and pain in the area of xiphoid process.

Severe coughing, vomiting and diarrhea may strain the abdominal muscles and cause pain.

Drugs and Heavy Metals

These include tetracyclines, erythromycin, lincomycin, cephalosporins, ethionamide, para-aminosalicylic acid (PAS), rifampicin, trimethoprim, vincristine, azathioprine, corticosteroids, niclosamide, dichlorophen, amitriptaline, carbamazepine, chlordiazepoxide, ergotamine, gentian violet, iodides, iron, nystatin, diphenylhydantoin, piperazine, primidone, troxidone and lead.

Chronic Abdominal Pain

Colic

This is perhaps the most common cause of RAP in infancy. The attacks come in paroxysms and are accompanied by severe crying.

---

*Small fish for the herring family having a strong flavor, it used for sauce, paste, etc.

Aerophagy or *excessive* wind in the gastrointestinal tract is due to prolonged sucking, more so on an empty breast, far-too-narrow a hole in the feeding bottle teat, or inadequate burping constitutes an important cause of abdominal pain.

Three-month colic, also called *evening colic*, is characterized by paroxysms of abdominal pain (mild to severe) lasting a few minutes at a time and occurring usually in the evening or late in the afternoon. During the paroxysm, the face is often flushed, or there is circumoral pallor. The legs are drawn up over abdomen and the feet are cold and the hands clenched. The abdomen is tense and distended. The infant cries incessantly. The attack dies down only when the infant is exhausted or passes flatus or stools. This is followed by a quiet period in which he may have a nap only to be awakened by another paroxysm.

The observation that the paroxysms have characteristic rhythmic timing and one can hear loud borborygmi during their course strongly suggests that the condition has intestinal origin. Since the colic occurs late in the afternoon or in the evening, it has been suggested that events in the household routine, leading to excitement, anxiety, fear or anger, may have something to do with the occurrence of 3-month colic.

Cow's milk allergy may be responsible for colic in a small proportion of infants. Vomiting, diarrhea (usually watery), skin rash (infantile eczema or urticaria), rhinitis, otitis media, chronic cough with wheeze (just as in bronchial asthma), anemia and failure to thrive are the other accompanying manifestations. Smear from rectal mucus shows eosinophils. Withdrawal of cow's milk is followed by disappearance of the manifestations. Its reintroduction leads to reappearance of them within 48 hours.

Intestinal Worm Infestation

Intestinal infestation with *G. lamblia, E. histolytica*, roundworm, hookworm, *Strongyloides stercoralis, Trichuris trichiura*, or tapeworms constitutes by far the most frequent cause of RAP in later infancy and childhood in resource-limited populations. Accompanying manifestations include change in bowel habit, change in appetite, failure to gain weight and even loss of weight. Each and every child with RAP must have at least 3 (preferably 5) meticulous stool check-ups on successive days to exclude worm infestation.

Helicobacter pylori Infection

That *H. pylori* may be responsible for RAP in a proportion of children has been highlighted only recently. It appears that the spiral-shaped Gram-negative bacteria with unipolar flagella causes RAP through its remarkable ability to cause chronic gastric inflammation, i.e. chronic gastritis, and duodenal ulcer disease.

Diagnosis of RAP secondary to *H. pylori* infection can be confirmed by noninvasive investigations like urea breath test and serology. Nonetheless, the most reliable test is flexible gastrointestinal endoscopy to obtain biopsy of the gastric mucosa for histopathology, culture or rapid urease test.

It should particularly be suspected in cases of RAP from underprivileged communities with clustering in families and institutions for mentally retarded and orphanages.

There is as a rule no evidence of infection. In a small proportion, there may be evidence of epilepsy.

Abdominal Epilepsy

Abdominal epilepsy is characterized by recurrent but sudden attacks of abdominal pain lasting a few minutes and followed by sleep. The diagnosis may be collaborated by an electroencephalogram (EEG) and/or gratifying response to diphenylhydantoin sodium (phenytoin) in full therapeutic doses.

Constipation

Excessive drying of feces leading to impaction and partial intestinal obstruction may be responsible for RAP. The constipated child may experiences some difficulty and pain in passing a hard, dry stool.

Food Allergy and Lactose Intolerance

Cow's milk allergy has been blamed for infantile colic in some cases. It has been postulated that such an allergy may be responsible for RAP in childhood as well. Similarly, it has been argued that allergy to some other foods may also cause abdominal pain.

Recently, considerable evidence has supported the hypothesis that many cases of RAP may be related to lactose intolerance. Even sucrose intolerance has been blamed for such a pain.

Crohn's Disease

In this chronic inflammatory disorder of unclear etiology, full thickness of segments of bowel wall usually terminal ileum is involved. The disease occurs only infrequently in childhood.

When it manifests with abdominal pain, the latter is crampy and exacerbated by eating but somewhat reduced after defection. Among associated features rank chronic diarrhea (at times with bloody mucopurulent stools), malnutrition, palpable abdominal masses, perianal lesions, aphthous stomatitis, polyarthritis, clubbing and erythema nodosum.

Diagnosis is confirmed by sigmoidoscopy, rectal biopsy, endoscopy, and radiologically by upper and lower gastrointestinal barium studies.

Ulcerative Colitis

This is a chronic diffuse inflammatory and ulcerative disease involving mainly the mucosa and submucosa of colon and rectum. As with Crohn's disease, etiology is not yet known. The incidence is very low in childhood particularly in the first year of life.

Abdominal pain in this disorder is in the form of intermittent mild crampy bouts related to the bowel movements. Other manifestations include bloody diarrhea, anorexia, anemia, weight loss, arthralgia, clubbing and growth retardation.

Diagnosis is confirmed by rectal examination, sigmoidoscopy, endoscopy and barium enema.

Sickle Cell Anemia

In this inherited abnormality of hemoglobin 'S' limited to dark population, the patient may suffer from repeated crises, lasting up to a week. During the crisis, the child may have severe abdominal pain, backache or joint pain with vomiting, anorexia and fever. Accompanying features of the disease include pallor, intermittent jaundice and hepatosplenomegaly (in older children, spleen is shrunk due to repeated infarctions, the so-called 'autosplenectomy').

Diagnosis is corroborated by demonstration of sickle-shaped red cells in the blood film, reticulocytosis, increased resistance of red cells to osmotic lysis and an abnormal electrophoretic pattern showing dominantly hemoglobin 'S'.

Urinary Tract Infection

Despite claims that UTI may cause RAP, it appears that such a situation occurs only when UTI accompanies obstructive uropathy (usually pelviureteric).

Psychogenic Pain Abdomen

In a considerable proportion of children with RAP, no organic cause may be detected despite painstaking investigations.

It has been argued that in some of these cases, abdominal pain may be simply a sort of *attention-seeking device*. The child senses parents' much-too-much anxiety over his tummy pain. He knows that his raising an alarm would bring the whole family around him, everybody wanting to do one or the other thing for him. This gives him immense joy and he wants to have more of it, again and again. This is the background of recurrence of pain.

Children whose parents frequently complain of one or the other bodily pain may demonstrate their anxiety as well as sympathy by imitating and feeling the same pain as that of the parent. This so-called *imitation pain* occurs far more than what is indeed appreciated.

Recurrent abdominal pain may well be related to worries and tension. In the so-called *Monday morning pain*, the child who has had a nice holiday a day before simply does not want to make it to school as the Monday morning comes and complains of pain in the tummy. The reasons for wanting to avoid going to school may include unpleasant experience such as bullying, teasing and beating by a teacher and/or schoolmates.

Periodic syndrome refers to periodic occurrence of certain symptoms such as colicky abdominal pain, nausea and vomiting, headache (often of migrainous type), diarrhea or constipation, marked pallor or flushing, fever and prostration present in any combination. Premonitory visual, auditory, sensory or mental symptoms may be present. What is remarkable is that in between the attacks the child is perfectly all right. Most of the subjects are emotional, highly strung, obsessional and perfectionists. Their parents' expectations are far too lofty. A quarrel in the family or school examination often precipitates the attack.

Remaining Causes of Recurrent Abdominal Pain

The causes of recurrent abdominal pain are peptic ulcer, hydronephrosis, lead poisoning, periodic peritonitis, hereditary angioneurotic edema, chronic relapsing pancreatitis, porphyria, etc.

FURTHER READING

1. Croffie JM, Fitzgerald JE, Chong SK. Recurrent abdominal pain in children—a retrospective study of outcome in a group referred to a pediatric gastroenterology practice. *Clin Pediatr (Phila)* 2000;39:267-274.
2. Gupta V. Recurrent abdominal pain. In: Gupte S (Ed). *Recent Advances in Pediatrics: Tropical Pediatrics.* New Delhi: Jaypee 1998:193-217.
3. Loizides AM, Orellana KA, Thomson JF. Abdominal pain. In: Adam HM, Foy JM (Eds). *Signs and Symptoms in Pediatrics.* Illinois: American Academy of Pediatrics 2015:12-26.
4. Wyllie R. Major symptoms and signs of digestive tract disorders. In: Kliegman RM, St Geme III JW, Blum NJ, et al (Eds). *Nelson Textbook of Pediatrics,* 21st edn. Philadelphia: Elsevier 2020:1522-1528.

CHAPTER 3

Ambiguous Genitalia (Intersex)

BACKGROUND

The term, a*mbiguous genitalia,* denotes discrepancy between the actual sex and the bizarre external genitalia (Box 3.1). The external genitalia are characteristic of neither a male nor a female. The entity is also called *hermaphroditism* (*herm* referring to "good" and *aphroditism* to "goddess").

Ambiguity results from excessive virilization of a female (female hermaphroditism) or defect in masculinization of a male (male hermaphroditism).

Hermaphroditism must be suspected in any male child with a small penis, hypospadias and undescended testes. Any girl with a doubtful mass in the labia majora or groin needs to be examined to be certain if the mass could be testes.

BOX 3.1: Broad classification of ambiguous genitalia (intersex).

46, XX intersex (46, XX—virilized)
Androgen exposure:
Fetal source—21-hydroxylase deficiency, 11-beta-hydroxylase deficiency
Maternal source—virilizing ovarian or adrenal tumor, androgenic drugs
Ambiguous source—in association with genitourinary or gastrointestinal malformations

46, XY intersex (46, XY—undervirilized)
Testicular differentiation defects:
- WAGR syndrome
- Denys-Drash syndrome

Testicular hormone deficiency:
- Persistent Müllerian duct syndrome
- Receptor defects for anti-Müllerian hormone
- Leydig cell aplasia

Androgen action defect:
- Androgen receptor defects
- Androgen insensitivity syndrome, both partial and complete
- Smith-Lemli-Opitz syndrome
- 5-alpha reductase II mutations

True gonadal intersex:
XX, XY, XX/XY, chimeras

HISTORY

The history should trace the presence of intersex siblings or such other close relatives and the mode of inheritance. A history of consanguinity is of vital importance. Was the mother on hormonal therapy during the pregnancy? What was the time sequence of appearance of secondary sex characters in the child with ambiguous sex problem?

PHYSICAL EXAMINATION

The physical examination should confirm the presence or absence of testes (in the scrotum or inguinal canal), the degree of labioscrotal fusion, size of penis or clitoris, hypospadias, and uterus through rectal examination. Search should also be made for renal, anal and other congenital anomalies.

Presence of two labioscrotal masses confirms the existence of two testes. Possibility of female pseudohermaphroditism is thereby immediately rule out.

INVESTIGATIONS

Investigations include the following:
- Buccal smear to know the real gonadal sex (negative in male hermaphroditism and positive in true hermaphroditism and female pseudohermaphroditism)
- 17-ketosteroids and pregnantriol in urine
- Serum electrolytes
- Chromosomal studies
- Radiologic studies
- Gonadal biopsy is a must when gonads are in the abdomen and in certain other vague cases.

In many instances, laparotomy may be warranted to be certain of the diagnosis.

Flow chart 3.1 presents a diagnostic approach to ambiguous genitalia.

Flow chart 3.1: Algorithmic approach to diagnosis of ambiguous genitalia.

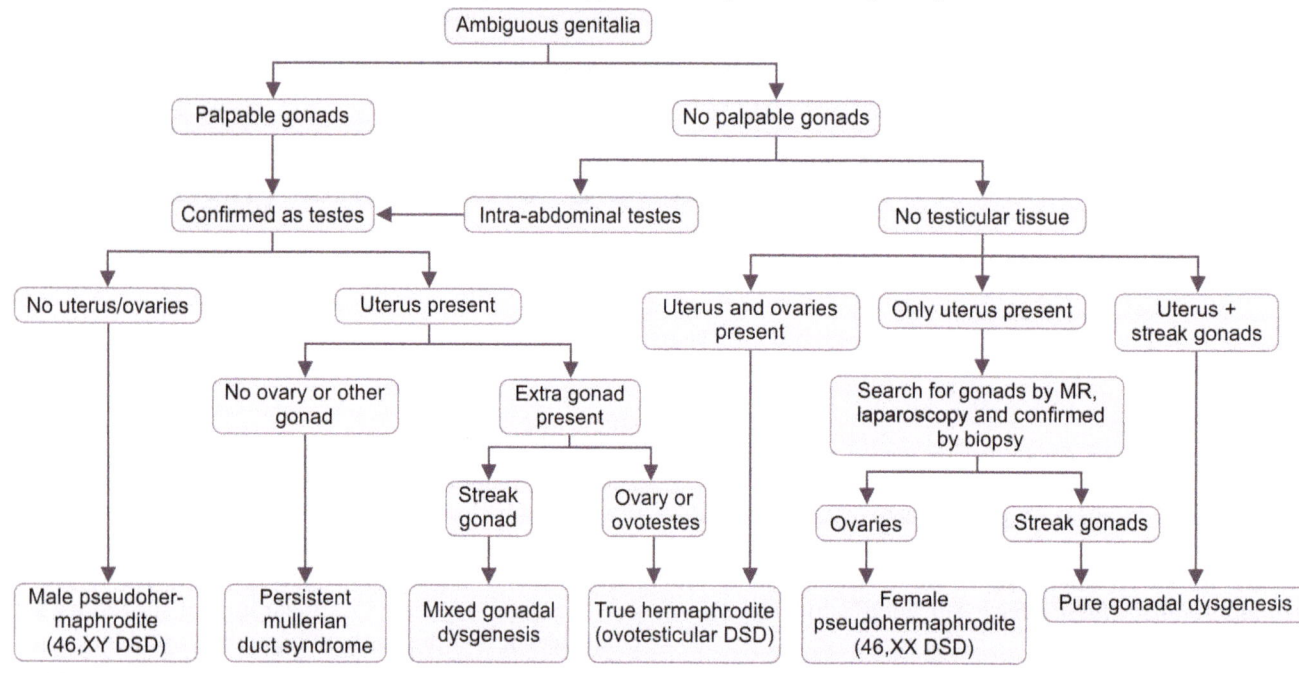

(*Source:* Adapted with permission from Chavhan GB, Parra DA, Oudjhane K, et al. Imaging of ambiguous genitalia: classification and diagnostic approach. *Radiographic* 2008;28:1891-1904)

IMPORTANT DIFFERENTIALS

True Hermaphroditism

This condition is quite rare. A sheer over 500 cases are on record. In this state, both ovarian and testicular tissues are present either in the same or in the opposite gonads. The external genitalia are usually ambiguous. The phenotype may, however, be male or female. Ovotestis is the most frequently seen gonad in true hermaphroditism. The testicular tissue in such an ovotestis is, however, defective. As a result, secretion of androgens and anti-Müllerian hormone is grossly inadequate. A true hermaphrodite is best brought up as a female with selective removal of testicular tissue.

Male Pseudohermaphroditism

This condition is generally characterized by male phenotype. The penis is small with hypospadias (Fig. 3.1). Testes are undescended. Labioscrotal folds are fused. A casual look gives an impression of female genitalia. The genotype is XY. Incomplete virilization of the external genitalia is the main problem. Its causes include defects in testicular differentiation Its causes include defects in testicularharacterized by differentiation (Campomelic syndrome characterized by sex reversal i.e. chromosomally

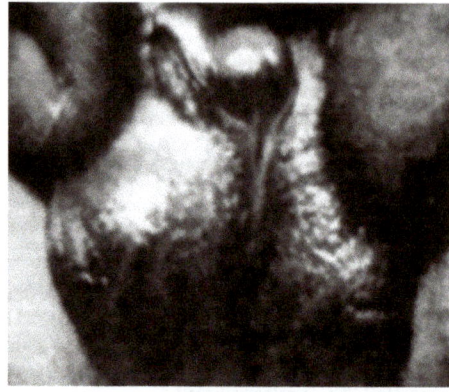

Fig. 3.1: Male pseudohermaphroditism. Note that the external genitalia are confusing. Whether the child has a small penis with hypospadias or it is indeed a virilized clitoris is apparently not clear. What indeed clinched the diagnosis in this child was palpability of two testes in the so-called "labioscrotal" sac. Gonadal biopsy showed purely testicular tissue that was dysgenetic.

male but have female genitalia and reproductive system in association with skeletal dysplasia), pure gonadal dysgenesis (Swyer syndrome characterized by one X chromosome and one Y chromosome, normally present in males, have a female appearance), gonadal agenesis (embryonic testicular regression syndrome), and defects in testicular hormones (uterine hernia syndrome), and defects in androgen action (5-alpha reductase deficiency, testicular feminization syndrome, Reifenstein syndrome). In one-third male hermaphrodites, no cause is determined.

Female Pseudohermaphroditism

This is the most common type of hermaphroditism. It is characterized by masculinization of the genetically female child. Ovaries are present. Clitoris is large enough and looks like penis. Labia majora is large and may be fused, giving the appearance of a scrotal sac. Its causes include excessive intake of androgens by the mother, congenital adrenal hyperplasia and maternal virilizing tumors.

Congenital adrenal hyperplasia is by and large the most common cause of female hermaphroditism. Masculinization may be to the extent of development of a false penile urethra. The child looks a male with cryptorchidism. Degree of virilization is greater in salt-losers than nonsalt-losers. It is highest with 21-hydroxylase and 11-beta-hydroxylase defects.

FURTHER READING

1. Chavhan GB, Parra DA, Oudjhane K, et al. Imaging of ambiguous genitalia: classification and diagnostic approach. *Radiographics* 2008;28:1891-1904.
2. Rapaport R. Intersex. In: Kliegman RM, St Geme III, Blum NJ, et al (Eds). *Nelson Textbook of Pediatrics*, 21st edn. Philadelphia: Elsevier 2020:2394-2403.
3. White PC, Speiser PW. Congenital adrenal hyperplasia due to 21-hydroxylase deficiency. *Endocr Rev* 2000;21:245-291.

CHAPTER 4

Anemia

INTRODUCTON

Anemia (Greek: an—not, haima—blood) is defined as a quantitative or qualitative deficiency of red cells or hemoglobin concentration in circulation. The term is, by no means, always synonymous with pallor. Many infants and children look pale though there is no anemia at all. The vice versa too is true. Often in mild anemia, it is virtually impossible to be sure about the diagnosis unless and until hemoglobin level is ascertained.

HISTORY

History should contribute to reaching the probable cause of anemia. Specific questioning should be done about loss of blood, dietary consumption, drug intake and infection. What is the roundabout length of time the child has been suffering from anemia? Is he tolerating it well? Or, does he get fatigued easily? Of late, is there history of dyspnea and development of edema over feet and legs? Any suggestion of intestinal worm infestation? A family history of hemoglobinopathies suggests a hereditary anemia such as thalassemia, sickle cell anemia, spherocytosis, etc.

PHYSICAL EXAMINATION

In the physical examination, pallor is the classic finding suggestive of anemia. One should look for it in nail beds, palpebral conjunctiva, buccal mucosa, skin and palmar creases. Additionally, one should specifically look for jaundice, petechiae, purpura, ecchymosis, hepatosplenomegaly, injuries, etc. Association of anemia with splenomegaly and icterus are suggestive of a hemolytic etiology. Anemia plus hepatosplenomegaly, bruising and fever strongly point to acute leukemia.

Table 4.1 presents clinical grading of anemia.

Table 4.2 presents the World Health Organization (WHO) grading of anemia.

TABLE 4.1: Clinical grading of anemia.

Grade	Clinical parameters
Mild	Pallor of conjunctiva and/or mucous membrane
Moderate	Above plus pallor of skin
Severe	Above plus pallor of palmar creases

TABLE 4.2: WHO grading of anemia.

Hemoglobin range	Grade
10 g/dL—cut-off point for ages*	Mild
7–10 g/dL	Moderate
Below 7 g/dL	Severe

*Below 2 weeks 13 g/dL, up to 6 months 9.5 g/dL, 6 months to 12 years 11 g/dL, above 12 years 12 g/dL.

INVESTIGATIONS

It is important to have complete blood picture (CBP) with special reference to hemoglobin level, red blood cell (RBC) count, peripheral blood film, reticulocyte count, etc.

Additional investigations are guided by the individual merit of the case and suspected diagnosis. For instance, in thalassemia, it is a must to do electrophoresis and determination of actual fetal hemoglobin (HbF) level. Supportive investigations include osmotic fragility and skull X-ray for hair-on-end appearance. In megaloblastic anemia, Schilling test may be needed. In leukemias, bone marrow becomes mandatory. In some cases of nutritional anemia, serum ferritin may be needed.

Box 4.1 presents an excellent clinical approach to differential diagnosis of anemia in a child.

> **BOX 4.1:** Clinical approach to differential diagnosis of anemia in a child.
>
> *Is anemia associated with other hematologic abnormalities? If yes, consider*
> - Aplastic anemia
> - Leukemia
> - Other bone marrow replacement disorders
>
> *Is anemia associated with reticulocytosis? If yes, consider*
> - Bleeding disorder
> - Ongoing hemolysis
>
> *Is there associated hyperbilirubinemia or increased serum lactate dehydrogenase? If yes, consider*
> - Hemolytic anemia
> - In this situation, review the peripheral blood film (PBF) for:
>   - *Spherocytes:* Hereditary spherocytosis, autoimmune hemolytic anemia, Wilson's disease
>   - *Sickle cells:* Sickle cell anemia/disease, sickle beta-thalassemia
>   - *Target cells:* Hemoglobin SC disease
>   - *Hypochromic RBC, nucleated RBC:* Homozygous beta-thalassemia, hemoglobin E beta-thalassemia
>   - *Microangiopathy:* Hemolytic uremic syndrome, thrombotic thrombocytopenia
>   - *Bite/blister cells:* Glucose-6-phosphate dehydrogenase (G-6-PD) deficiency
>
> *Is anemia associated with a lower than appropriate reticulocyte response? if yes, assess RBC size*
> - *Microcytic RBC:* Iron deficiency, thalassemia trait, hemoglobin E disorder, lead poisoning
> - *Macrocytic RBC:* Folic acid/vitamin B_{12} deficiency, inborn error of metabolism (if neutrophil hypersegmentation, i.e. megaloblastic change), Diamond-Blackfan anemia, congenital dyserythropoietic anemia, Pearson syndrome (if no such change)
> - *Normocytic RBC:* Anemia of chronic conditions, anemia of renal disease (renal failure), transient erythroblastopenia of childhood, anemia associated with hypothyroidism

> **BOX 4.2:** Causes of iron deficiency anemia.
>
> *Inadequate iron stores at birth*
> - Grossly undernourished mother
> - Low birth weight (LBW)/prematurity/twinning
> - Perinatal bleeding
> - Far-too-early ligation of umbilical cord
>
> *Inadequate iron supply*
> - Delayed introduction or semisolids and solids
> - Massive intestinal parasitosis (e.g. giardiasis, ancylostomiasis)
>
> *Inadequate iron absorption*
> - Persistent/recurrent/chronic diarrhea
> - Malabsorption state preponderance of dietary components that inhibit iron absorption (tea, coffee, legumes, spinach, cereals, egg yolk, phytates, etc.)
> - Poor intake of vitamin C
>
> *Heightened requirements*
> LBW exhibiting catch-up growth
>
> *Heightened tosses*
> - Blood loss (both occult and overt)
> - Massive ancylostomiasis or trichuriasis
> - Cow milk protein (CMP) allergy
> - Cow milk (unheated) consumption of first year, especially in first 6 months of life
> - Recurrent diarrhea

IMPORTANT DIFFERENTIALS

Nutritional Anemia

Iron deficiency is the most common etiologic factor in nutritional anemias. Firstly, it is especially common in infancy because both breast and cow's milk are incapable of meeting infant's requirements of iron. Secondly, poor iron stores in premature babies predispose to further deficiency so that, at about third month (the time of maximal physiologic reduction of hemoglobin), there may result marked iron deficiency in case they are not given iron supplements. Twins commonly become iron deficient.

In older children, causes include inadequate intake malabsorption, infection, and chronic blood loss as in hookworm infection and cow's milk protein allergy. Nutritional anemia, dominantly iron deficiency, nearly always accompanies vitamin D deficiency rickets and scurvy (Box 4.2).

Low mental development index (MDI) and low infant behavior record (IBR) as manifested by unhappiness, lack of cooperation and short attention span are noteworthy features of iron deficiency anemia.

Clinical features include progressive pallor, irritability, anorexia, tiredness, failure to thrive, pica and koilonychia. Diarrhea is often present. Occasionally, especially in severe anemia, hepatosplenomegaly may be detected. A hemic murmur (soft systolic, having maximal intensity over the base and changing with patient's position) is commonly heard.

Most infants and children learn to adapt to nutritional anemia of prolonged duration. Some, however, end up with congestive cardiac failure, more so in the presence of an added stress.

Anemia from Blood Loss

In the newborn, causes of anemia include placental/umbilical cord bleeding, fetofetal transfusion (bleeding of one twin into the other), hemorrhagic disease of the newborn, cephalhematoma, and subaponeurotic hemorrhage.

Trauma, epistaxis, esophageal varices, hiatal hernia, hemangiomas, ulcerative colitis, polyps, Meckel's diverticulum, cow's milk allergy, hematuria, Henoch-Schönlein purpura, hemophilia and malignancy are other causes of anemia due to blood loss.

Hookworm infestation is an important cause of chronic anemia in tropical settings such as ours. Each adult worm is claimed to suck the host of little over 0.1–0.5 mL of blood daily. The dominant clinical features are progressive anemia, anorexia, pain abdomen and malnutrition. Pica is often present. Advanced cases may have gross anemia with hypoproteinemia leading to edema and even anasarca. Diarrhea, alternating with constipation, may also be present. Some degrees of malabsorption, as a result of histological as well as functional damage to the small intestinal epithelium, occurs in many cases.

Many drugs are known to be potent cause of gastrointestinal bleeding. These include aspirin, chlortetracycline, acetazolamide, thiazides, indomethacin, methotrexate and antimetabolites. In recent years, aspirin, when given frequently, has emerged as an important cause of gastrointestinal bleeding and anemia. Besides causing gastrointestinal bleeding, it may lead to hypoprothrombinemia or thrombocytopenia.

Hemolytic Anemia

Hemolytic anemia is characterized by sustained reticulocytosis above 2% (indicative of increased bone marrow activity in response to shortened peripheral survival of red cell) together with continued problem in the hemoglobin level. Associated findings may include light rise in serum bilirubin (indirect) but frank jaundice usually does not occur unless, of course, hepatic function too is significantly impaired, abnormal peripheral smear and splenomegaly with some hepatomegaly. In chronic hemolytic process only, striking X-ray changes may be observed in skull, long bones, metacarpals and phalanges.

Hemolytic disease of the newborn must be seriously considered if the newborn manifests anemia and jaundice on the very first day of life. Hepatosplenomegaly is present. In Rh hemolytic disease, the foremost investigation is to demonstrate that the mother is Rh negative whereas the baby is Rh positive. Direct Coombs' test on infant's red cells is positive and anti-Rh titer of mother is high. Other investigations show high serum bilirubin (indirect), reticulocytosis, and anti-Rh agglutinins and hypoglycemia.

ABO hemolytic disease is generally mild, manifesting as anemia, jaundice and hepatosplenomegaly. Jaundice is frequently delayed until 48–72 hours after birth, in the case of ABO incompatibility, mother's blood group is O and infant's A or B. Mother, depending on infant's group, develops anti-A or anti-B antibodies in her blood.

Hereditary spherocytosis (congenital acholuric jaundice, congenital hemolytic anemia) is characterized by family history of acholuric jaundice or unexplained anemia, onset of anemia and jaundice in neonatal period or infancy, splenomegaly usually becoming evident after infancy, and characteristic spherocytic cell (which is smaller than the normal red cell and lacks the central pallor of the biconcave disk) and reticulocytosis. Osmotic fragility and autohemolysis tests are of immense value in establishing the diagnosis.

Remember that acquired spherocytosis may be encountered in autoimmune hemolytic anemia, hemolytic disease of the newborn from Rh or ABO incompatibility, and thermal injury to red cells as in extensive burns.

Thalassemia major (Cooley anemia) is characterized by progressive severe anemia with grow splenomegaly noticed during the second 6 months of first year and typical hemolytic facies due to thickening of the bones of face and skull (Fig. 4.1). Blood picture shows a microcytic hypochromic anemia (usually the hemoglobin level between 4 g/dL and 9 g/dL range), anisocytosis, poikilocytosis, moderate basophilic stippling, nucleated and fragmented red cells (target cells), large number of normoblasts and striking reticulocytosis. Osmotic fragility test shows reduced fragility. HbF usually exceeds 40%.

Radiologic findings include thinning of the cortex, widening of the medulla (due to marrow hyperplasia) and coarsening of trabeculations in the long bones, metacarpals and metatarsals. Skull X-ray shows the "hair-on-end" appearance due to vertical striations from widening of the diploic space and atrophy of the outer table (Fig. 4.2).

Sickle cell anemia is characterized by severe chronic hemolytic anemia, irreversible sickled cells in peripheral blood smear and a clinical course marked by episodes of pain (crises) on account of occlusion of small blood vessels by spontaneously sickled red cells. Spleen is significantly

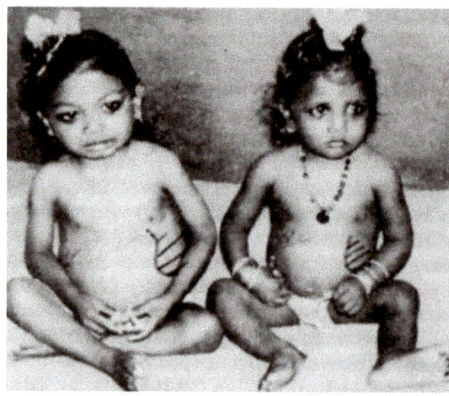

Fig. 4.1: Thalassemia major. Note the facial appearance and splenohepatomegaly in the two siblings suffering from chronic hemolytic anemia. Fetal hemoglobin in the child on the right was 60% and in that on the left 52%.

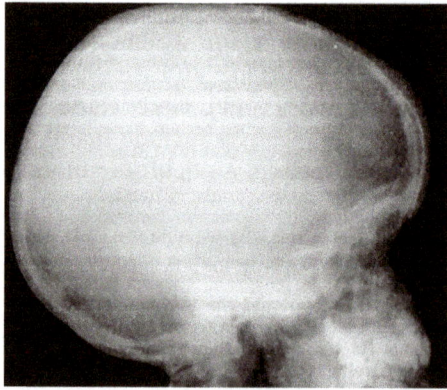

Fig. 4.2: Thalassemia major. X-ray of skull showing hair-on-end appearance (caused by vertical trabeculae) in thalassemia major. Also note that the diploic spaces are significantly widened. Such a roentgenographic picture may occasionally be seen in chronic iron deficiency anemia (IDA).

enlarged but usually shrinks in later childhood. Jaundice results from progressive impairment of liver function. Cerebral strokes, impaired renal function and gallstones together with greatly enhanced incidence of superadded infections, as severe as pneumococcal meningitis and septicemia, are the well-known features of patients with sickle cell anemia.

Glucose-6-phosphate dehydrogenase (G6PD) deficiency may lead to hemolytic anemia when certain drugs are administered (primaquine, nitrofurantoin, furazolidone, phenacetin, diphenhydramine, sulfas, salicylates, vitamin K), when certain foods (broad beans) are eaten, and when infection (viral hepatitis, infectious mononucleosis) occurs.

Drugs such as antimalarials, chloramphenicol, sulfas, cyclophosphamide, nitrofurantoin, penicillins, rifampicin, phenacetin, mefenamic acid, cephaloridine and vitamin K may cause hemolysis even when there is no G6PD deficiency.

Hemolytic uremic syndrome is characterized by hemolytic anemia, bloody diarrhea, renal failure and thrombocytopenia. The blood smear shows characteristic burr cells with bizarre shape.

Autoimmune hemolytic anemia results from production by the patient of abnormal antibodies directed against his own red cells. Direct Coombs' test is usually positive. The cause may be an underlying disease such as systemic lupus erythematosus (SLE), lymphoma or immunodeficiency, or drugs such as penicillin, cephalosporins, phenacetin, quinidine and methyldopa. In around 20% instances, it is idiopathic.

In the acute transient variety, a respiratory infection precedes prostration, anemia, jaundice, fever, hemoglobinuria and splenomegaly. This variety occurs mostly in infants and young children and shows excellent response to corticosteroid therapy.

In the chronic variety, hemolysis goes on over prolonged period—months or a year. Response to corticosteroid therapy is variable.

Anemia from Inadequate Red Cell Production

This implies that bone marrow is unable to produce sufficient number of new red cells to replace those removed from circulation. Low reticulocyte count is the hallmark of this variety of anemia.

Congenital hypoplastic anemia may be of two types. The Fanconi's syndrome is characterized by presence of associated multiple congenital anomalies such as microcephaly, mental retardation, microphthalmia, squint, nystagmus, short stature, hypogonadism, defects of radius and thumb, brown pigmentation of skin, congenital heart disease, webbed neck and renal abnormalities. In congenital pure red cell anemia, called Diamond-Blackfan syndrome, profound anemia manifests by 2-6 months of age. Associated congenital anomalies such as triphalangeal thumbs have been described in some cases. Without blood transfusions and/or corticosteroid therapy, congestive cardiac failure and death are more or less a rule.

Acquired hypoplastic or aplastic anemia may result from viral, bacterial or parasitic infections, infiltration of marrow by malignant tissue as in leukemia, Niemann-Pick disease, Gaucher disease, osteoporosis (marble bone disease), irradiation, or chemicals and drugs (chloramphenicol, antimetabolites, phenylbutazone, lead).

FURTHER READING

1. Glader B. The anemias. In: Kliegman RM, St Geme III, Blum NJ, et al (Eds). *Nelson Textbook of Pediatrics*, 21st edn. Philadelphia: Elsevier 2020:1604-1606.
2. Nathan DG, Orkin SH. Nathan and Oski's Hematology of Infancy and Childhood, 5th edn. Philadelphia: Saunders 2002.
3. Sobti P, Chandra J, Gupte S. Pediatric hematology. In: Gupte S (Ed): *The Short Textbook of Pediatrics*, 13th edn. New Delhi: Jaypee 2020.

CHAPTER 5

Ataxia

INTRODUCTION

Ataxia (Greek: lack of order) means, lack of cooperation or coordination of separate muscles or groups or muscles in order to accomplish a definite act. The poorly coordinated drunken gait is, perhaps, the most common way in which ataxia manifests.

HISTORY

Enquiry should ascertain how ataxia started. Was it preceded by a rash, ingestion of drugs, infectious illness or a neurologic disease involving sensorium and causing, among others, seizures?

PHYSICAL EXAMINATION

Physical examination should make it clear whether ataxia is cerebellar or sensory. In cerebellar ataxia, Romberg sign (failure to maintain standing attitude while standing on tip-toes and knees bent when eyes are closed) is usually negative whereas cerebellar signs like nystagmus, dysarthria, hypotonia and pendular jerks may be positive. The child's movements become slow, awkward and incomplete (adiadochokinesia).

In sensory ataxia due to posterior column lesion, Romberg sign is positive and there may be other evidence of sensory loss.

INVESTIGATIONS

Special investigations that may be needed as per the requirement of the clinical impression include lumbar puncture, computed tomography (CT) scan and magnetic resonance imaging (MRI).

IMPORTANT DIFFERENTIALS

Acute Cerebellar Ataxia

The condition usually occurs in 1–5 years age group, following a viral infection such as chickenpox, poliovirus type 1, influenza A and B, echovirus and coxsackie type B, or results from an autoimmune response to a variety of agents.

Onset of ataxia is always acute. In half of the cases, a nonspecific infection precedes it by about 3 weeks or so. The most dominant feature of the clinical picture is the severe ataxia, resulting in rapid deterioration of gait.

The disease is self-limiting, ataxia clearing in just a week or so in mild cases and in about 2 months in a large majority of the full-blown cases.

Drug Toxicity

Ataxia as a drug reaction may occur in case of piperazine, phenytoin, antihistaminics, chlordiazepoxide, diazepam, colistin, streptomycin, indomethacin, ethanol, vincristine and meprobamate. Solvent sniffing is now emerging as an important cause of ataxia amongst school children and adolescents even in Indian subcontinent.

Hypoglycemia

Ataxia resulting from hypoglycemia is accompanied by one or more of such symptoms as pallor, vertigo, diaphoresis, tachycardia, tachypnea, seizures and coma.

Acute Labyrinthitis

Acute labyrinthitis after mumps is an important though rare cause of acute ataxia. In such cases, vertigo always coexists.

Encephalitis

Ataxia may occasionally be a manifestation of encephalitis. The accompanying manifestations include change in sensorium (varying from lethargy to coma), fever, vomiting, seizures, bizarre behavior, altered speech, headache, irritability and feeding difficulty. An inflammatory reaction of meninges may produce some meningeal signs. Clinical picture shows rapid variation from hour-to-hour. Cerebrospinal fluid (CSF) is essentially normal, except that it flows under high pressure.

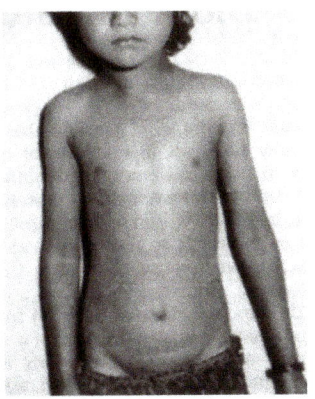

Fig. 5.1: Refsum's syndrome. Note ichthyosis in this girl with progressive ataxia (cerebellar). She also suffered from progressive deafness and polyneuritis. Funduscopy showed bilateral retinitis pigmentosa.

Brain Tumors

Ataxia as a manifestation of brain tumors develops rather gradually. Accompanying manifestations may include vomiting headache, diplopia, personality changes, speech disturbances, irritability and decline in intellect. Papilledema and hydrocephalus are common findings.

Astrocytoma occurs in 3–8 years age group. It is characterized by unilateral cerebellar signs. Besides ataxia, the child may have nystagmus, hypotonia, areflexia and tilting of the head to the side of lesion.

Medulloblastoma occurs in 3–5 years age group, mostly in males. Ataxia, usually, is severe.

Pontine glioma of brainstem occurs in 6–8 years age group. Besides ataxia, the child may demonstrate bilateral multiple cranial nerve involvement (usually 6th and 7th), pyramidal signs and absent or only minimal signs of raised intracranial pressure.

Friedreich Ataxia

This spinocerebellar degenerative disorder, usually manifesting in late childhood or adolescence, begins with a progressive gait defect. All too soon, incoordination of upper limbs follows. The classical triad of ataxia, positive Babinski's sign and absent ankle jerks is more or less pathognomonic.

The skeletal deformities encountered in these conditions include high arched foot (pes cavus), hammer toes, and scoliosis. Cardiovascular system (CVS) defects are cardiomegaly, arrhythmias and congestive cardiac failure.

Ataxia-Telangiectasia

This, another spinocerebellar degenerative disorder, manifesting in infancy, begins with delayed walking and ataxia. Later, other manifestations like progressive dysarthria, intention tremors, nystagmus and choreoathetosis appear. Involuntary eye movements are normal but control over voluntary movements is lost. Tendon reflexes are sluggish and may even be absent.

Telangiectasia makes appearance over bulbar conjunctiva and skin (ears, nasolabial folds, flexor creases of limbs) by 5 years of age. Variable immunologic deficiencies usually occur. By adolescence, the patient may develop dementia and malignancy.

Refsum's Syndrome

This inborn error of metabolism, manifesting usually in later childhood or adolescence, is characterized by progressive cerebellar ataxia, ichthyosis, retinitis pigmentosa, polyneuritis and deafness (Fig. 5.1).

Abetalipoproteinemia (acanthocytosis, Bassen-Kornzweig syndrome) is characterized by malabsorption (manifesting in infancy), slowly progressive ataxia (manifesting later in childhood), retinal degeneration (manifesting in adolescence) and red cells with multiple spiny projections.

Remaining Causes of Ataxia

Remaining causes of ataxia are hypothyroidism, Hartnup disease, maple syrup urine disease, disseminated sclerosis, mumps, migraine, cerebral abscess, Guillain-Barré syndrome, cerebral palsy, hysteria, head injury, etc.

FURTHER READING

1. Belamarich PF. Abdominal distention. In: Adam HM, Foy JM (Eds). *Signs and Symptoms in Pediatrics*. Illinois: American Academy of Pediatrics 2015:1-11.
2. Harris MC, Bernbaum JC, Polin JR, et al. Developmental and follow-up of breastfed term and near-term infants with marked hyperbilirubinemia. *Pediatrics* 2001;107:1075-1080.
3. Johnston MV. Movement disorders. In: Kliegman RM, St Geme III, Blum NJ, et al (Eds). *Nelson Textbook of Pediatrics*, 21st edn. Philadelphia: Elsevier 2020:2488-2493.
4. Paulson H, Ammache Z. Ataxia and hereditary disorders. *Neurol Clin* 2001;19:759-782, viii.

CHAPTER 6

Blood in Stools

BACKGROUND

Blood in stools is a cause of considerable alarm to the parents. It may be fresh (hematochezia) or chemically altered black in color (melena*). In doubtful cases, it is important to confirm if the red color in the stools is indeed due to blood. Ingestion of iron or bismuth-containing preparations or eating earth or charcoal (pica) may simulate melena. It is a good practice to confirm the presence of blood chemically.

HISTORY

What is the amount of blood detected in stools? Is it mixed with mucus? Or, is it in the form of a simple coating or streaks over a well-formed stool, any accompanying diarrhea, constipation, painful defecation, abdominal pain, vomiting, fever, epistaxis, or bleeding from other sites? Any history of worm infestation, pica, drugs or surgery on tonsils?

PHYSICAL EXAMINATION

Physical examination should determine, if the child is in shock due to excessive blood loss. Always look for evidence of portal hypertension, hemangioma, purpura, telangiectasia, intestinal obstruction, and blood dyscrasias. Nasal passages should be carefully inspected for signs of epistaxis and anus and rectum for fissure, polyp, and hemorrhoids. In case of acute abdomen, you must search for signs of abdominal trauma.

You must inspect not only the stools but also urine. Hematuria may well be the cause of blood staining of the napkin.

In case of evidence, favoring rectal polyp or colitis, it is advisable to do sigmoidoscopy.

---
*Greek: melena means black.

INVESTIGATIONS

Newborn
- Apt test for swallowed blood in case of a newborn
- Abdominal imaging for necrotizing enterocolitis (NEC), intussusception, etc.

Latter age group
- Stool microscopy, especially for *Entamoeba histolytica*
- Antibody blood test for *E. histolytica*
- Stool culture, especially for *Shigella* (in selected cases)
- Sigmoidoscopy or colonoscopy
- Liver function test (LFT) in suspected portal hypertension
- Splenoportogram for localizing the level of obstruction in portal hypertension.

IMPORTANT DIFFERENTIALS

Swallowed Maternal Blood

This is the most common cause of blood in stools in a newborn, particularly during the first 3-4 days of life. The blood is swallowed during delivery, or later while the baby sucks the nipple. It is usually red, intermingled in the meconium. The general condition of the baby appears fine.

To be sure if it indeed is maternal blood, you may filter the material and add one part of 0.25 N (1%) NaOH to five parts of supernatant fluid. In case of maternal blood, the color changes to yellow. If the color remains as such, it is fetal blood, pointing to the hemorrhagic disease of the newborn.

Hemorrhagic Disease of the Newborn

Blood in stools is accompanied by other manifestations like epistaxis, hematemesis, and bleeding from umbilical cord and skin as well in the viscera. Prothrombin time is prolonged. Clotting time may also be prolonged in majority of the cases. The disease manifests on 2nd or 3rd day of life. Vitamin K deficiency appears to be the probable etiologic factor.

Necrotizing Enterocolitis

In this disorder, the baby (usually low birth weight, born before term) develops, besides bloody diarrhea, lethargy, vomiting, abdominal distention, hypothermia, and apnea. The infant is extremely ill and may terminally go into cardiovascular collapse.

Predisposing factors include maternal fever, amnionitis, sepsis, respiratory distress syndrome (usually of mild type), umbilical artery catheterization in exchange transfusion, and oral feeding with high osmolar (hypertonic) stuff.

Diagnostic radiologic findings include air-fluid levels, dilated loops of gut, separation of loops of gut, and linear streaks of intraluminal air, *pneumatosis intestinalis*.

Dysentery

In older infants and children, dysentery remains by far the most common cause of blood in stools.

The usual form results from *Shigella* infection. The accompanying tenesmus, toxemia, fever, abdominal pain, and distention are characteristic features. Other bacilli causing similar but mild clinical picture include *Salmonella* and *Escherichia coli*.

Intestinal infestation with *E. histolytica, Giardia lamblia, Hymenolepis nana, Strongyloides stercoralis*, and *Trichuris trichiura* may manifest with dysentery. Bilharzia is a pre-eminent cause of bloody diarrhea in certain areas. Hookworm is an important cause of blood loss in stools (usually in melena) but not that of dysentery.

Gastritis

Gastritis (inflammation of gastric mucosa) may be responsible for blood in stools—fresh in young children and melena in older ones. Ryle's tube trauma and stress ulcer are well-known cause of gastrointestinal bleeding.

Polyp

Internal polyp, especially rectal polyp, usually causes moderate but painless bleeding. The diagnosis is by suspicion and should be led to rectal examination, rectosigmoidoscopy and barium enema. The most common site is about 10 cm above the anus.

Intussusception

Rectal passage of bloody mucus is accompanied by episodic abdominal pain, vomiting, fever, and prostration. Abdomen is tender and distended. A sausage-shaped lump may be palpable in the upper abdomen in early stages. Rectal examination may show a cervix-like mass and blood on the examining finger.

Plain X-ray of abdomen may show absence of bowel gas in the right lower quadrant and dilated loops of small bowel.

Barium enema may demonstrate the intussusception as an inverted cap and an obstruction to the progression of barium. In the area of intussusception, there may be a ceiling-spring appearance to the column of barium.

Conservative hydrostatic reduction gives good results in a large majority of the cases, provided that there is no evidence of strangulation, perforation or severe toxicity.

Meckel Diverticulum

In this condition, there is acute loss of large amount of blood (usually dark red) in stools. Abdominal pain, if present, is slight. The patient, usually under 2 years of age, looks quite pale and may be in shock due to loss of lot of blood. Meckel diverticulum is frequently found in children with Turner syndrome. Diagnosis, highlighted by high sense of suspicion, can only be established by laparotomy.

Anal Fissure

If a child passes small amount of bright red blood that appears to form a sort of coating over the hard stools and the parents say that the child experiences painful defecation, you must seriously entertain the diagnosis of anal fissure. The condition may result either from hard stools or use of rectal thermometer. Diagnosis may be established on examination of the anus.

Blood Dyscrasias

Profuse blood loss in stools may occur in idiopathic thrombocytopenic purpura (ITP), anaphylactoid purpura (Henoch–Schönlein purpura), leukemias, hemolytic uremic syndrome, and disseminated intravascular coagulopathy (DIC).

Antibiotic-associated Pseudomembranous Colitis

Invariably caused by the toxins produced by *Clostridium difficile*, the clinical spectrum of pseudomembranous colitis (PMC) may range from a mild, nonspecific diarrhea to severe colitis. Relatively, a lower incidence is seen in children. Ampicillin, amoxicillin, cephalosporin (second- and third-generation), and clindamycin are the most likely antibiotics associated with it.

Remaining Causes of Blood in Stools

Cow's milk allergy, ulcerative colitis, Crohn's disease, intestinal hemangiomas, hiatal hernia, esophageal reflux, esophageal varices, peptic ulcer, hypertrophic pyloric stenosis, intestinal duplication, hemorrhoids, and foreign bodies.

FURTHER READING

1. Patwari A, Gupte S, Anderson RA. Pediatric gastroenterology. In: Gupte S (Ed). *The Short Textbook of Pediatrics*, 13th edn. New Delhi: Jaypee 2020.
2. Green M. Pediatric *Diagnosis and Interpretation of Symptoms and Signs in Children and Adolescents*. Philadelphia: Saunders 1998.
3. Horvath K, King J. Major manifestations of gastrointestinal disease. In: Gupte S, Horwoth K (Eds). *Pediatric Gastroenterology, Hepatology and Nutrition*. New Delhi: Jaypee 2009:6-14.
4. Wyllie R. Major symptoms and signs of digestive tract disorders. In: Kliegman RM, St Geme III JW, Blum NJ, et al (Eds). *Nelson Textbook of Pediatrics*, 21st edn. Philadelphia: Elsevier 2020:1522-1528.

CHAPTER 7

Chest Pain

BACKGROUND

Most children complain of some kind of chest pain at one or the other time. Fortunately, in a vast majority of the cases, it is benign, usually either psychogenic or what is known as "stitch". However, in the wake of parents' anxiety, concern, and pressure, often the pediatrician's efforts get focused on excluding cardiac disease via certain investigations that may not be really necessary.

HISTORY

Symptomatic enquiry must include information on the exact site of pain. It is not infrequent for the child or the parents to point to the epigastrium and yet call it chest. Is the onset sudden or insidious? What does the pain seem like? Is it made worse by movements? Does it follow exertion after a meal? When does it occur; while working or during sleep? Any history of chest injury? Is there past history of surgery on the chest or disease such as bronchial asthma? Any family history of chest pain or heart disease? Box 7.1 presents the "red flags" in history.

PHYSICAL EXAMINATION

An examination of chest wall may show skin lesion or musculoskeletal cause. One should always exclude a cardiac, pulmonary, and abdominal pathology as a cause of chest pain. These need to be considered "red flags" in physical examination (Box 7.2).

BOX 7.1: "Red flags" in history.

- Foreign body aspiration
- Syncope
- Fever
- Chills
- Tightness in chest
- Underlying sickle-cell disease, Kawasaki disease, cystic fibrosis, hypertrophic obstructive cardiomyopathy, Turner's syndrome, Marfan's syndrome
- Palpitations
- Trauma.

BOX 7.2: "Red flags" in physical examination.

- Dyspnea
- Cyanosis
- Pathologic heart murmur(s)
- Tachycardia
- Pleural rub
- Pericardial rub.

INVESTIGATIONS

A careful history and physical examination often rules out the need for any investigation or guide the appropriate test(s) that may be needed.
- Chest X-ray for pneumonia, pleural effusion/empyema, pneumothorax, etc.
- Electrocardiogram (ECG) for pericarditis, angina, etc.
- Spirometry for bronchospasm as in asthma.

DIFFERENTIALS

Benign Chest Pain

Stitch

The condition refers to cramp-like pain on one side of the lower chest or upper abdomen. It occurs usually on exertion after meals. The cause is strain on peritoneal ligaments attached to the diaphragm.

Psychogenic

Older children with autonomic dysfunction may imitate anginal pain in a senior family member. The manifestations do not fit into any known pattern. Chest pain may be paroxysmal or recurrent. Just a distraction may cause relief. Other symptoms include palpitations, giddiness, and such breathing troubles as air hunger and yawning. Psychogenic hyperventilation may often accompany in which case the condition is called *Da Costa or effort syndrome.*

In psychogenic chest pain, the problem seldom occurs during sleep or play period. Further, blood pressure may show a tendency to hypertension on a psychogenic basis. ECG is normal.

Organic Chest Pain

Skin

Herpes zoster is characterized by crops of vesicles (as a rule confined to a dermatone) and neurologic pain in the area of involved dermatone. Fever and local tenderness with regional lymphadenitis are usually present.

Muscles

Quite a common cause of chest pain in childhood is muscular pain, which may result from contusion secondary *to injury or viral myalgia*. The pain is sudden. It is usually "point pain" and tenderness may be present. There is no associated illness.

The well-known entity, *pleurodynia*, also called *epidemic myalgia, devil's grip or Bornholm disease* is caused by Coxsackie virus (group B). It is characterized by severe paroxysmal and stabbing or shooting pain that is aggravated with the respiratory movements. Muscles are frequently tender and swollen. Fever and headache may coexist. Rest of the family members may be affected.

Dermatomyositis, trichinosis or cysticercosis are responsible for a small proportion of cases of chest pain.

Skeleton

Crack or fracture of a rib, osteitis (usually costochondritis), *periostitis, osteomyelitis, hematoma or tumor* may cause localized pain and tenderness, swelling, redness, and raised temperature, usually at the costochondral junction.

Tietze syndrome (costochondral osteopathic costalis tuberosa) is characterized by painful, tender swelling of the costochondral junction, more so of the second, third, and fourth ribs of the right side. There may be spontaneous pain during respiratory movements. It sometimes radiates to shoulder and arm. Paresthesia may accompany it. A probable physical strain may well be the cause.

Diseases of vertebral column such as tuberculosis, rheumatoid arthritis, or osteomyelitis may cause neuralgia, leading to chest pain.

Pleura and Lungs

Pleurisy and pneumonia complicated by direct or indirect involvement of pleura cause severe knife-like stabbing pain that is worse on respiratory exertion and that may radiate to shoulder.

Pulmonary embolism/infarction, though rare in childhood, may cause substernal or pleuritic pain that radiates to the shoulder. Associated manifestations include tachycardia, tachypnea, dyspnea, bloody sputum, and shock. If embolism is large enough, crepitations and pleural friction rub may be heard.

Cardiovascular System

Pericarditis, as in rheumatic fever, tuberculosis, or pyogenic infection, is the most common cause of precordial pain in children. The pain is usually dull and poorly localized and may be referred to shoulder or neck. It worsens on swallowing and on exaggerated respiratory movements. A friction rub may accompany the pain. The nib is synchronous with the heartbeat. Neck veins are congested. Heart sounds are distant.

Myocarditis or pancarditis may also cause precordial pain through acute dilatation of the heart.

Angina, though rare in childhood, may cause dull persistent precordial pain which may occasionally be interrupted by stabbing sensation. It may be referred to the shoulder or arm.

Esophagus

Retrosternal or substernal pain may result from esophagitis secondary to ingestion of irritants, hiatal hernia, foreign body, peptic ulcer, esophageal ulcer or achalasia cardia. It is aggravated by swallowing, recumbent position or stooping forward. Associated symptoms include dysphagia, regurgitation hematemesis, melena, and excessive salivation.

Remaining Causes of Chest Pain

Viral hepatitis, peritonitis, hemoperitoneum, diaphragmatic pain, gallbladder disease, sickle-cell anemia, cystic fibrosis, splenic or liver capsule rupture, stretching of renal capsule, pneumothorax, lung abscess, aortic valve disease (rheumatic), aortic stenosis, etc.

FURTHER READING

1. Coleman WL. Recurrent chest pain in children. *Pediatric Clin North Am* 1984;31:1007-1026.
2. Green M. *Pediatric Diagnosis*, 6th edn. Philadelphia: Saunders 1998.
3. Loughlin GM. Chest pain. In: Loughlin GM, Figen H (Eds). *Respiratory Disease in Children: Diagnosis and Management.* Baltimore: William and Wilkins 1994:207-214.
4. Schroeder SA. Chest pain. In: Adam HM, Foy JM (Eds). *Signs and Symptoms in Pediatrics*. Illinois: American Academy of Pediatrics 2015:111-118.

CHAPTER 8

Child Abuse and Neglect

BACKGROUND

Child abuse and neglect (CAN) is defined as maltreatment of children by the parents, guardians or other caretakers. Almost 75% of abuse recognized in the hospitals is physical. Rest of the 25% cases are of psychologic/emotional abuse, sexual abuse or nutritional deprivation leading to failure to thrive.

HISTORY

As and when you encounter a child in whom it is clear that the history of injuries, etc. narrated by the attendants is at variance with the actual observations made by you, you must suspect child abuse.

In particular, consider this diagnosis when the child presents with multiple hematomas, multiple fractures and scars, multiple cuts, bruises and abrasions, burns, strap marks, cord marks, trauma to genitals, and malnutrition (in a child who appears to be unwanted).

A large majority of parents who abuse their children are the ones who had experienced physical or other abuse as children. They are neither criminals nor psychopaths, but just unhappy adults (because of some family crisis) living under tremendous stress and strain. The susceptible child is one who has negativism, a difficult temperament and offensive behavior such as enuresis, soiling, habitual crying, and spilling. Usually, there is a considerable delay in seeking medical advice.

PHYSICAL EXAMINATION

Physical examination should proceed methodically and carefully with inspection and palpation of all body surfaces.

All bruises (Fig. 8.1) and burns should, in particular, be noted and described in terms of location, size, shape, and color.

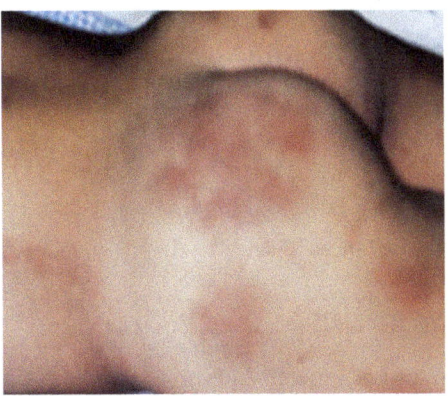

Fig. 8.1: Child abuse and neglect (CAN)—Bruising of varying time frame.

Areas of tenderness may point to occult trauma. Radiological evaluation is, therefore, necessary.

Moreover, careful measurements need to be taken and photographed. It should be noted if bruises resemble a particular instrument pattern (say, belt buckle, cord, cigarette but, fingers).

Careful attention should be paid to the oral cavity, groin, and scalp for signs of occult trauma.

Funduscopic examination is an often overlooked part of the evaluation when physical abuse is suspected. Retinal hemorrhages are highly suspicious for abuse resulting from "shaken-baby syndrome". Infants who are forcibly shaken may present with unexplained injuries, seizures or a decreased level of consciousness.

Such nonspecific symptoms such as vomiting, irritability or abnormal respiration may be manifestations of abusive head injury—the diagnosis which is easily overlooked. Remember, head injury needs to be kept in mind if facial or scalp bruises are present.

Presence of xanthochromic cerebrospinal fluid via nose may suggest an old intracranial bleed.

Box 8.1 lists some of the physical indicators of CAN.

BOX 8.1: Physical indicators of child abuse.

- Bruises on uncommonly injured body surfaces
- Blunt instrument marks or burns
- Human hand marks or bite marks
- Multiple injuries at different stages of healing
- Evidence of poor care or failure to thrive
- Circumferential immersion burns (Fig. 8.2)
- Unexplained fundal (retinal) hemorrhages.

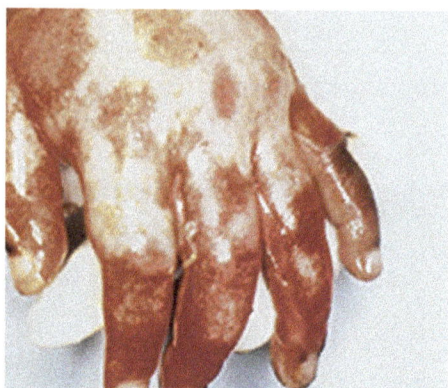

Fig. 8.2: Child abuse and neglect (CAN)—Immersion burns.

INVESTIGATIONS

Skeletal fractures must be interpreted in the context of the child's developmental ability and the history of injury.

A transverse long-bone fracture in a 2-month-old infant is highly suspicious for physical abuse but may be unremarkable in an 8-year-old child.

Certain fractures are relatively more specific for nonaccidental trauma. Fractures involving parts of the skeletal system or caused by mechanisms of injury, which are unlikely to be from accidental trauma, need to cause suspicion.

IMPORTANT DIFFERENTIALS

Physical Abuse

The most important clue to physical abuse is that the injury is unexplained—often far-too-much for the history of a minor accident. Injuries usually seen include bruises, welts, lacerations, and scars. The arms may reveal finger and thumb impressions of the abuser. Thrashing with a belt, sticks or ruler may leave lash marks on the body. Bite marks are seen as crescent-shaped bruises. Slap marks are visible as two to three parallel bruises, usually over the cheeks. The neck may reveal choke marks. Strings or ropes tied round ankle or wrists leave circumscribed marks. Occasionally, the shape of a bruise may point to the instrument used to cause it.

An important point to remember in physical injury as a result of abuse is that bruises are found at various stages of healing.

Inflicted burns are usually caused by holding the child forcibly in hot water as a punishment for bedwetting or failure in bowel control. A circular type of burn involving only the buttocks or thighs and waist is the most frequently seen in hot water injury. Cigarette burns, usually found over hands and feet are seen as punched out circular lesions of nearly the same size. Hot solid burns produced by placing the child against a hot plate or heating develop characteristic shape.

Child abuse may result in as dangerous an injury as subdural hematoma, manifesting with convulsions and coma owing to the increased intracranial pressure. In half of the cases, skull fracture(s) may also be detected. Fundoscopy almost always shows presence of retinal hemorrhages. Since cases of subdural hematoma in battering are usually the result of violent shaking injuries, you may be able to locate grab mark bruises of upper limbs, shoulders, and chest.

Another type of dangerous injury in battering is the blow injury over the abdomen, causing rupturing of liver or spleen. Infrequently, tear injury of duodenum or jejunum may occur. The child with intra-abdominal injury presents with recurrent vomiting, abdominal distention, tenderness, sluggish or even absent bowel sounds and shock.

Remember, it is advisable to have a good radiologic bone survey including skull, long bones, and thorax, and if indicated, pelvis and spine. Such findings as chip fractures or multiple bone injuries at various stages of healing due to repeated assaults are very helpful in reaching the diagnosis.

Sexual Abuse

Sexual abuse occurs from three sources. First, sexual maltreatment by a family member, usually the father or an uncle, on a child who may well be an adopted or a step one. Second, sexual abuse by friends and acquaintances of the child or family. Third, sexual abuse by strangers. Molestation, intercourse, and rape are the three types of sexual abuse encountered in practice. Since in a large majority of the cases of sexual abuse, there are no definitive physical findings, a sensitive and tactful handling of history taking is needed. The physician ought to learn child's vocabulary and use dolls and pictures to clarify body parts and to build-up the story rug-by-rug. Skin, mouth, rectum, and external genitals should be especially examined for signs of trauma. A hymenal opening of 5 mm or more is to be considered abnormal in a prepubertal girls.

Nonorganic Failure to Thrive

An unwanted and unplanned child's feeding may be terribly neglected. Emotional and nutritional deprivation eventually leads to malnutrition. The examination of such a child shows, besides signs of nutritional deficiencies, stark hygienic neglect as evidenced by a nappy rash, impetigo or scabies, unwashed skin, uncut finger and toe nails, and dirty clothing.

When such a child is admitted to the hospital and fed generously on a diet appropriate for age in the new setting and is also given enough of love for at least a week, his weight gain becomes remarkably impressive.

Some Other Differentials

Scurvy, no doubt, produces subperiosteal hemorrhage in the lower third of the femur, leading to pain and pseudoparalysis and thus confusion with battering. The presence of spongy, swollen, bluish purple gums, scorbulic rosary, follicular hyperkeratosis with minute hemorrhages at the root of hair follicles together with radiologic bony changes* at and around knee joint are classical of scurvy. Moreover, signs in scurvy are usually bilateral.

Syphilis may manifest in the form of tender swelling in connection with bones and Parrot's pseudoparalysis as a result of osteochondritis. Radiologic findings include destruction, thickening, and irregular borders of metaphysis, destructive changes at diaphysis, transverse bands at metaphysis, and subperiosteal thickening with hyperostosis. Serological tests for syphilis are positive.

Caffey disease, also called *infantile cortical hyperostosis*, manifests with fever followed by marked swelling of soft tissues of face and jaws and progressive thickening of flat and long bones such as scapula, clavicle, and tibia. The course is characterized by waxing and waning. After several years, spontaneous cure occurs.

Chronic hypervitaminosis A may present as tender swellings of bones. The accompanying symptoms include failure to thrive, anorexia, irritability, alopecia, seborrhea, angular stomatitis, craniotabes, desquamation of palms and soles, hepatomegaly, and pseudotumor cerebri. History of excessive intake of vitamin A and hyperostosis of long bones, best seen about the middle of the shaft in X-ray, confirm the diagnosis.

Osteogenesis imperfecta tarda often presents with fractures resulting from minimal trauma. Presence of findings such as blue sclerae, skeletal deformities, short stature, and deafness helps in reaching this diagnosis.

FURTHER READING

1. Alexander R, Levitt C, Smith W. Abusive health trauma. In: Reece R, Ludwig S (Eds). *Child Abuse: Medical Diagnosis and Management*, 2nd edn. Philadelphia: Lipincott, William and Wilkins 2001.
2. Kundra S, Singh T, Gupte S. Child abuse and neglect. In: Gupte S (Ed). *The Short Textbook of Pediatrics*, 13th edn. New Delhi: Jaypee 2020.
3. Mehta MN. Physical abuse of abandoned children in India. *Child Abuse Negl* 1982;6:171-175.
4. Mishra D, Aggarwal K. Child abuse and neglect. In: Gupte S (Ed). *Recent Advances in Pediatrics-16*. New Delhi: Jaypee 2006:370-400.
5. Srivastava RN. *Child Abuse and Neglect*. New Delhi: Jaypee 2013.

---

*Radiologic bony changes simulating scurvy are seen in Menkes Kinky hair disease as well.

CHAPTER 9

Clubbing

BACKGROUND

The term, *clubbing*, refers to loss of natural angle between nail plate and nail bed with boggy fluctuation of the nail bed. The depth of the finger at the base of nail bed becomes equal or more than that at the distal interphalangeal joint. In advanced cases, there is an increase in the curvature of the nail from top downward and swelling or enlargement of the distal end of the finger, giving it an appearance of a drumstick. The cause is altered prostaglandin metabolism, leading to an increase in the connective tissue. Hippocratic nail is its other name.

HISTORY

Attempt should be to get information about history of other member(s) in the family having clubbing, symptoms suggestive of congenital heart disease, chronic lung disease (cystic fibrosis, tuberculosis, etc.), suppurative disease (lung abscess), steatorrhea (cystic fibrosis, celiac disease, tropical sprue, etc.), etc.

PHYSICAL EXAMINATION

In doubtful cases, the following clinical maneuvers are helpful in demonstrating clubbing:
- Normally, depth at the base of the nail is smaller than depth at the distal interphalangeal joint. If it becomes equal or more, digital clubbing is present. This is supposed to be the best method of identifying clubbing (Fig. 9.1).
- *Schamroth (diamond) sign*: Normally, if we approximate the nails of two fingers, a diamond, i.e. rhomboid-shaped window is left out. Disappearance of window indicates existence of clubbing. This sign is quite sensitive even for slight clubbing. The reason for disappearance of the window is hike in amount of soft tissue under the base of the nails (Fig. 9.2).
- *Lovibond profile sign*: The increase of the angle between curved nail plate and proximal nail fold (viewed from

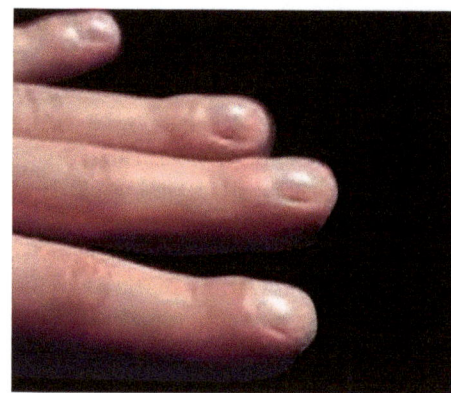

Fig. 9.1: *Digital clubbing*: Note that the depth of the base of the nail is much more than the depth at the interphalangeal joint.

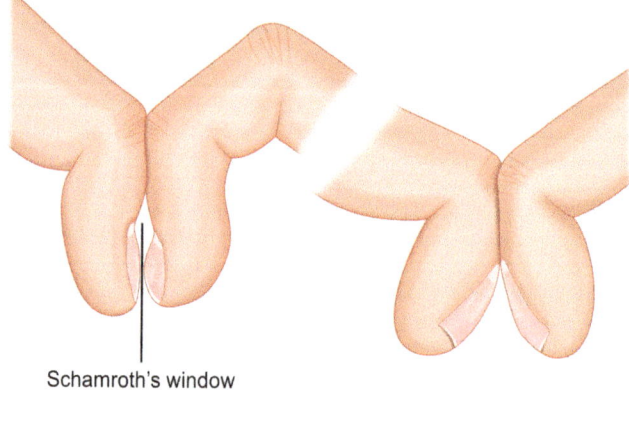

Fig. 9.2: *Schamroth (diamond) sign*: Note the diamond-shaped.

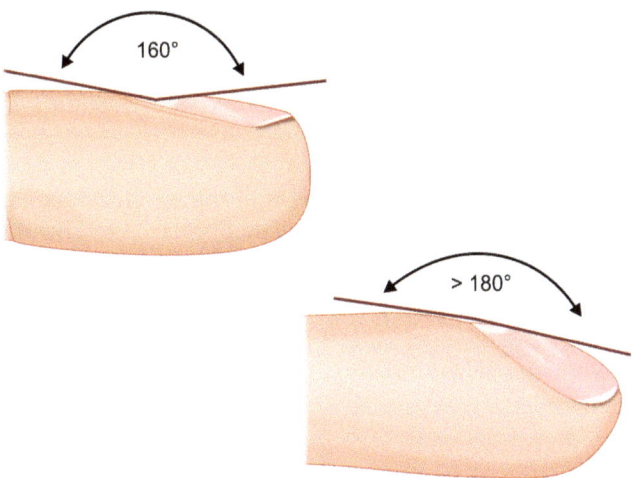

Fig. 9.3: *Lovibond profile sign:* Note the increase of the angle between curved nail plate and proximal nail fold to more than 180° (right) from the normal or the decrease to less than 160° from the normal (left).

lateral side) to more than 180° from the normal or decrease to less than 160° from the normal (Fig. 9.3).
- *Curth's modified profile sign:* The decrease of the angle between middle phalanx and terminal phalanx at interphalangeal joint to less than 160° from the normal, which is equal to 180°.
- *Fluctuation sign:* Clubbing may also be elicited by rocking the nail on its bed with examiner's index finger and thumb. It seems to float.

IMPORTANT DIFFERENTIALS

Pulmonary Disorders

Chronic Suppuration

Bronchiectasis: Clubbing is an important feature of bronchiectasis, which is usually associated with tuberculosis, congenital anomalies of bronchi or bronchioles, aspiration of a foreign body that remained unattended or chronic/recurrent chest infection in the presence of a disease, such as cystic fibrosis, ciliary dyskinesia or an immune system defect. The symptoms include chronic cough with purulent sputum, foul-smelling breath, i.e. halitosis, recurrent chest infection, and failure to thrive. Auscultatory findings include wheeze and crepitations, which may be localized due to a foreign body or may be generalized (cystic fibrosis).

Empyema: Clubbing develops in case of long-standing empyema when anemia and other manifestations of malnutrition also coexist. Manifestations are usually those of pneumonia, but they may be absent. Chest signs include diminished movements of the affected side, widening and dullness at times, (even edema) of the intercostal spaces, dull percussion note, diminished air entry, and shift of the mediastinum to the opposite side. In addition to an X-ray chest, a diagnostic pleural tap must be done.

Lung abscess: Clubbing may develop in a case of chronic lung abscess when the subject remains without appropriate treatment for a long time. Onset is usually insidious with fever, persistent cough, and foul-smelling sputum. Occasionally, dyspnea and chest pain may occur. Chest signs are usually those of consolidation with bronchial breathing. X-ray of the chest shows characteristic opacities; the cavities reveal fluid levels.

Pulmonary Tuberculosis

Significant clubbing occurs in a proportion of children with progressive pulmonary tuberculosis, especially of fibrocaseous type.

Cystic Fibrosis

Presence of clubbing in association with gross malnutrition despite good appetite and good dietary intake, recurrent diarrhea, and recurrent chest infections ever since early infancy, must arouse suspicion of cystic fibrosis. Steatorrhea is notably pancreatogenous. Demonstration of high sweat chloride (over 60 mEq/L) clinches the diagnosis.

Other Pulmonary Causes

Pulmonary alveolar proteinosis, alveolar-capillary block syndrome, Hamman–Rich syndrome, chronic fibrosing alveolitis, emphysema, chronic pneumonia, mesothelioma, and malignancy, especially of bronchus.

Cardiovascular Disorders

Infective Endocarditis

Clubbing is an important feature of infective endocarditis in which it is often accompanied by tender transient swellings which are pea-sized, in the pulp of fingers and toes (Osler nodes) and also splinter hemorrhages, beneath the nails. Anemia, splenomegaly, low-grade fever, and microscopic hematuria are also present. Diagnosis is established by positive blood cultures which are taken every 6 hours for 36 hours, and by demonstration of the vegetations by echocardiography in advanced cases. Underlying lesion is always rheumatic or congenital heart disease.

Cyanotic Congenital Heart Disease

In transposition of great arteries (TGA), the child usually develops some clubbing by 6 months. In tetralogy of Fallot (TOF), it takes almost 2 years for clubbing to be noticeable.

Gastrointestinal Disorders

Steatorrhea

Clubbing may be encountered in some children suffering from significant steatorrhea such as celiac disease, tropical sprue, gross protein-energy malnutrition, iron-deficiency anemia, and ancylostomiasis.

Ulcerative Colitis

Clubbing is an important component of the extraintestinal manifestations of ulcerative colitis which include arthralgia, erythema nodosum, pyoderma gangrenosa, iritis, hepatitis, peripheral hypoproteinemic edema, phlebitis, hemolytic anemia, etc.

Crohn's Disease (Regional Ileitis)

Clubbing, as in the case of ulcerative colitis, may figure among the extraintestinal manifestations of this inflammatory bowel disease, which is usually characterized by segmental transmural involvement of distal ileum and colon.

Multiple Polyposis

In this disease with involvement of the colon, clubbing may coexist with painless bright red rectal bleeding, usually after the age of 3–5 years. Even after surgical excision through a sigmoidoscopy, 25% subjects show recurrence. Some patients may develop malignancy.

Hepatic Disorders

Clubbing may be seen in cases of biliary cirrhosis, i.e. extrahepatic biliary atresia, cystic fibrosis, and chronic active hepatitis.

Other Causes of Clubbing

Congenital (idiopathic), thyrotoxicosis, Hodgkin's lymphoma, etc.

FURTHER READING

1. Darmstadt GL, Sidbury R. Disorders of the nails. In: Kliegman RM, St Geme III JW, Blum NJ, et al (Eds). *Nelson Textbook of Pediatrics*, 21st edn. Philadelphia: Elsevier 2020:2731-2733.
2. Gupte S, Smith R. Pediatric history-taking and physical (clinical) examination. In: Gupte S (Ed). *The Short Textbook of Pediatrics*, 13th edn. New Delhi: Jaypee 2020.
3. Silverman BA. Nail defects. In: Eichenfield LF, Frieden LJ, Esterly NB (Eds). *Textbook of Neonatal Dermatology*. Philadelphia: Saunders 2001:504-510.

CHAPTER 10

Coma

BACKGROUND

Coma (Greek: *koma*—a deep sleep) is a state of profound and prolonged unconsciousness from which the individual cannot be aroused except for short periods.

Four stages of depressed consciousness are recognized:
- *Stage 1 (stupor)*: The patient can be aroused for brief periods, during which he may be able to make simple verbal and voluntary motor responses. Stupor (unconsciousness) may alternate with delirium (mental confusion, disorientation, irrational conversation, and motor excitement).
- *Stage 2 (light coma)*: The patient cannot be aroused, except with painful stimuli. However, moaning and semi-purposeful avoidance movements may be noticed.
- *Stage 3 (deep coma)*: Painful stimuli now fail to produce a response, or they lead to extension and pronation of arms (decerebrate posturing).
- *Stage 4 (brain death)*: The patient is flaccid and apneic. All brainstem functions are lost though some spinal reflexes may still be intact.

The modified Glasgow coma scale (Table 10.1) is of considerable help in evaluating progress of the child with altered consciousness.

TABLE 10.1: Modified Glasgow coma scale.

Score	Over 1 year	Under 1 year
		Eyes opening
4	Spontaneous	Spontaneous
3	To verbal command	To shout
2	To pain	To pain
1	No response	No response
		Best motor response
6	Obeys	Spontaneous
3	Localizes pain	Localizes pain
4	Flexion-withdrawal	Flexion-withdrawal
3	Flexion-abnormal (decorticate rigidity)	Flexion-abnormal (decorticate rigidity)
2	Extension (decerebrate rigidity)	Extension (decerebrate rigidity)
1	No response	No response

Score	Over 5 years	2–5 years	0–23 months
		Best verbal response	
5	Oriented and converses	Appropriate words and phrases	Smiles, coos appropriately
4	Disoriented and converses	Inappropriate words	Cries, consolable
3	Inappropriate words	Persistent cries or screams	Persistent inappropriate crying or screaming
2	Incomprehensible sounds	Grunts	Grunts, agitated or restless
1	No response	No response	No response

HISTORY

History has got to be second hand. Yet, pertinent information obtained rapidly helps in arriving at provisional diagnosis. Interrogate about any recent trauma or accident (head injury), poisoning, drug overdose, and prior disease such as diabetes mellitus, epilepsy, central nervous system (CNS) disease, liver disease, kidney disease, etc. A history of acute febrile illness, especially if accompanied by convulsions, points to meningitis, encephalitis, cerebral malaria, or typhoid encephalopathy. Coma in association with hyperpyrexia in hot weather may mean heatstroke.

PHYSICAL EXAMINATION

Physical examination should be rapid, focusing on the following:
- *Respiration Cheyne-Stokes:* Involvement of thalamus (deep cerebral or diencephalon lesion)
- *Irregular hyperventilation:* Damage to brainstem (midbrain or pons)
- *Slow and deep:* Raised intracranial pressure, CNS infection, or after a convulsive episode
- *Ataxic:* Damage to medulla. Respiratory arrest usually follows
- *Slow, shallow, and periodic:* Narcotics
- *Acetone smell:* Diabetic ketoacidosis
- *Foul breath:* Uremia
- *Blowing out of one check only:* Ipsilateral facial paralysis
- *Deep, rapid, gasping:* Acidosis.

Pattern of pupillary reaction:
- *Widely dilated but fixed:* Third nerve paralysis, resulting from tentorial herniation
- *Widely dilated but reactive:* Postictal state or deep plane of anesthesia
- *Pinpoint:* Drug intoxication (opiates, barbiturates, etc.) or brainstem involvement
- *Unilateral dilated, fixed:* An expanding lesion on the same side (it may well be a false localizing sign)
- *Mid-position fixed:* Midbrain lesion
- *Roving non-conjugate deviation:* Light plane of anesthesia
- *Conjugate deviation:* Cerebral lesion of same side or an irritative process on the opposite side
- *Nystagmoid movement:* Posterior fossa lesion of same side.

Eye movements are tested by what is known as *doll's head maneuver* or *doll's eye phenomenon.* Turn the head briskly from side to side while patient's eyes are open. You would notice that the eyes move conjugately to the opposite side. Absence of the response, (*oculocephalic response*), or its depression implies that the lesion is at the level of brainstem or midbrain. If this results in deviation of the eye down and laterally, third nerve dysfunction due to tentorial herniation must be considered. Oculocephalic response needs third, sixth, and vestibular component of eighth nerve intact.

Head and Body

Quickly examine for injury marks and evidence of ingestion of poisonous agents.

Limbs

Failure to move one side or asymmetrical movements suggest paralysis/paresis. Remember that, in hemiplegia, the paretic leg lies in external rotation and moves less than the other leg, spontaneously as also in response to painful stimuli. When lifted and allowed to fall back, it drops limply.

Decorticate posturing, characterized by arms which are flexed over the chest, hands which are fisted, and legs which are extended, points to severe, diffuse cerebral cortex lesion.

Decerebrate posturing, characterized by rigid extension and pronation of arms and extension of legs, as such or in response to pain, suggests midbrain lesion. Unilateral decerebrate posturing, often accompanied by contralateral third nerve paralysis, is usually a sign of tentorial herniation.

Fever

Hypothermia indicates possibility of barbiturate or alcohol intoxication, or shock. High fever suggests acute infection, toxic encephalopathy, heat stroke, intracranial hemorrhage or postictal state.

Neck Rigidity

It suggests meningitis. Subarachnoid hemorrhage or herniation of cerebral tonsils may also manifest as nuchal rigidity. However, remember that it may be absent in a comatosed child though he is decidedly suffering from one of the earlier causes.

Reflexes

Absence of corneal reflex or tonic neck reflex suggests severe brain damage. A consistently positive Babinski sign may be of value.

Fundoscopy

Fundoscopic examination is a must for evidence of papilledema. Since papilledema takes almost 24–48 hours to manifest, its absence on examination cannot be taken to exclude raised intracranial pressure. Early signs of high intracranial pressure are absence of venous pulsations and distention of retinal veins.

Detection of preretinal hemorrhages points to the probability of subarachnoid or subdural bleeding.

Diagnostic possibilities, depending upon presence or absence of focal signs and raised or normal intracranial pressure, may be categorized as follows:
- Focal signs present
  - Raised intracranial pressure
    - *Trauma:* Subdural, epidural or intracerebral hemorrhage, subdural contusion, etc.

- Intracranial tumor
        - *Central nervous system infection:* Brain abscess, subdural empyema, encephalitis, etc.
        - *Vascular lesion:* Arteriovenous malformation
    – Normal intracranial pressure
        - *Vascular lesion:* Cerebral arterial occlusion
        - *Central nervous system infection:* Encephalitis
        - *Trauma:* Cerebral contusion
        - *Epilepsy:* Postictal state with Todd paralysis
- Focal signs absent
    – Raised intracranial pressure
        - *Metabolic encephalopathy:* Lead poisoning, water intoxication, Reye syndrome, severe anoxia, etc.
        - *Central nervous system infection:* Meningitis, encephalitis, etc.
        - *Trauma:* Subdural hemorrhage in infants, subarachnoid hemorrhage, etc.
        - Intracranial tumor
        - Hydrocephalus
    – Normal intracranial pressure
        - *Metabolic encephalopathies:* Most of them
        - *Drug intoxication*
        - *Central nervous system infection:* Meningitis encephalitis
        - *Trauma:* Concussion
        - *Epilepsy:* Postictal state.

IMPORTANT DIFFERENTIALS

Diabetic Ketoacidosis

There may or may not be positive history of diabetes mellitus. Other manifestations may include nausea, vomiting, dehydration with dry skin, weakness, polyuria, confusion, tachypnea, soft eyeballs, and convulsions. Tendon reflexes are absent or poorly elicited. The diagnosis is established, if there is smell of acetone in breath, slightly flushed cheeks, glycosuria, acetonuria, and high blood sugar (Fig. 10.1).

Nonketotic Hyperosmolar Coma

This rare but important entity is characterized by minimal or absent ketoacidosis, very high blood sugar, severe dehydration (hypernatremic), and rising blood urea nitrogen (BUN) (azotemia). High cerebrospinal fluid (CSF) sodium content causes cerebral edema which is responsible for coma and convulsions.

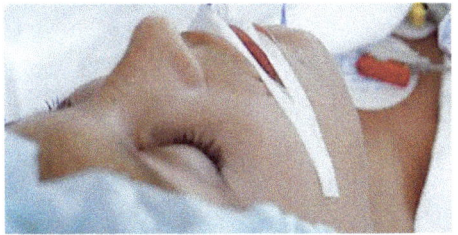

Fig. 10.1: Diabetic ketoacidosis.

Hypoglycemic Shock

Hypoglycemia, usually from overdose of insulin, reduced glucose intake or excessive exercise in a known diabetic patient, may cause coma which requires to be differentiated from that resulting from ketoacidosis. An enquiry reveals that coma was preceded by change in personality with temper tantrums, crying or outbursts of laughing, dizziness, headache, sudden hunger, flushing, convulsions or transient squint. In contrast to the picture in diabetic ketoacidosis, eyeballs are rather tense and tendon reflexes active to exaggerated.

Head Injury

Here, history of injury is available. Progressive focal neurologic signs suggest intracranial bleeding, say subdural hematoma. Periods of unconsciousness or amnesia following injury suggest concussion.

Seizure Disorder

Coma in seizure disorder may occur in the following situations: (i) postictal state in which coma may occur in association with Todd paralysis, (ii) status epilepticus, and (iii) overdose of antiepileptic drug(s).

Drugs and Poisons

Drugs and poisons which may cause coma only when consumed in large amount include barbiturates, opiates (morphine), alcohol, carbon monoxide (exposure to coal smoke in a closed, stuffy room during winter), kerosene oil, lead, tricyclic antidepressants (haloperidol), diphenoxylate, salicylates, amphetamines, antihistaminics, phenothiazines, organophosphates, piperazine, diphenylhydantoin sodium, and solvent sniffers.

It is advisable to make a note of the signs which indicate poisoning. For instance, small constricted pupils point to opiate, barbiturate or phenothiazine poisoning. Dilated pupils may mean belladonna, amphetamine or antihistamine poisoning. Odor of alcohol is obvious in breath, whereas perspiration may suggest salicylate, organophosphate or lysergic acid diethylamide (LSD*). A hot dry skin may be a sign of belladonna poisoning.

---

*Also known as "acid", it is a highly potent psychedelic drug. It is manufactured illegally from lysergic acid, which is found in the ergot fungus that grows on rye and some other grains.

Hyperventilation with respiratory alkalosis may point to salicylate poisoning. Needle marks, especially in adolescents, suggest narcotic poisoning as a part of drug abuse. Nystagmus may point to barbiturate or diphenylhydantoin poisoning.

Central Nervous System Infections

Cerebral malaria, typhoid encephalopathy, meningitis, and encephalitis are important causes of coma. Pointers in clinical profile together with investigative findings contribute in arriving at specific diagnosis.

Dehydration and Electrolyte Imbalance

Dehydration and electrolyte imbalance, especially in tropical climate, may *per se* cause loss of consciousness in early childhood. The most common cause is undoubtedly gastroenteritis. But a cause likely to be forgotten is diabetes insipidus in which inadequate fluid intake may result in coma due to hyperosmolarity.

Liver Disease

Viral hepatitis and Indian childhood cirrhosis may end up in a coma. There usually is history suggestive of liver disease preceding coma. The presence of smell of raw liver, called "fetor hepaticus", hepatosplenomegaly, ascites, and hemorrhagic tendency assist in arriving at the diagnosis.

Reye's syndrome is characterized by sudden onset of vomiting, irritability, and coma preceded by a mild respiratory infection. Liver is palpable. In spite of marked liver dysfunction, jaundice is, as rule, minimal or absent. Hypoglycemia is always present. Preceding history of administration of aspirin to the child with an exathemanta (usually, chickenpox) is usual.

Uremic Coma

There usually is a fairly long preceding history of renal disease. Before coma manifests, signs such as pallor, puffiness of face, pretibial edema, and fetid odor of breath become apparent. Often, it is the routine detection of hypertension that points to the renal origin of coma before suggestive urine findings, high blood urea nitrogen (BUN) or creatine results are available.

Hysteria

Absence of organic disease on clinical work-up and investigations, especially in prepubertal girls demonstrating alteration in consciousness, may suggest the probability of dissociative type of hysterical neurosis. One must demonstrate positive evidence of hysteria—at least that the subject has psychopathic personality—before finally reaching this diagnosis.

Syncopal Attacks

During such an attack, the subject loses consciousness only for a brief period. The history of labile vasomotor system, as indicated by earlier attacks induced by cough, strain or emotions, helps in establishing this diagnosis. One must rule out a cardiac disorder, including paroxysmal tachycardia.

Remaining Causes of Coma

Gram-negative septicemia, anaphylaxis, hypovolemia, etc.

FURTHER READING

1. Gulat S, Singh LR, Gupte S, Chowdhary B. Pediatric neurology. In: Gupte S (Ed). *The Short Textbook of Pediatrics*, 13th edn. New Delhi: Jaypee 2020.
2. Kapoor A. Coma. In: Gupte S (Ed). *Textbook of Pediatric Emergencies*, 2nd edn. New Delhi: Peepee 2008:184-189.
3. Nair RR. Coma. In: Gupte S (Ed). *Recent Advances in Pediatrics*. New Delhi: Jaypee 2004:1-14.
4. Singhi PD, Singhi SC. The comatose child. In: Singhi M (Ed). *Medical Emergencies in Children*. New Delhi: Sagar Publications 2000:208-218.
5. Wong CP, Forsyth RJ, Kelly TP, et al. Incidence, etiology and outcome of nontraumatic coma: a population-based study. *Arch Dis Child* 2001;84:193-199.

CHAPTER 11

Constipation

BACKGROUND

Constipation (Latin: constipare—to press together) refers to a difficult or painful passage of small hard, dry stools that contain mainly solids and minimal water. Infrequency of defecation is usually associated. But that is not always so. The commonly held belief that constipation means infrequency of defecation is, therefore, not correct.

It is of value to understand that all pelvic and abdominal muscles play an important role in defecation. Nevertheless, three muscular sphincters surrounding the anus and the rectum (internal and external sphincters and puborectalis) are the most important (Fig. 11.1). When the conditions are conducive for defecation, the striated muscles of the pelvic flow and external sphincter are relaxed voluntarily, the anorectal angle is diminished and the abdominal muscles contract to facilitate the downward passage of stools. The main propulsive activity comes through the nonperistaltic mass contraction of the colon.

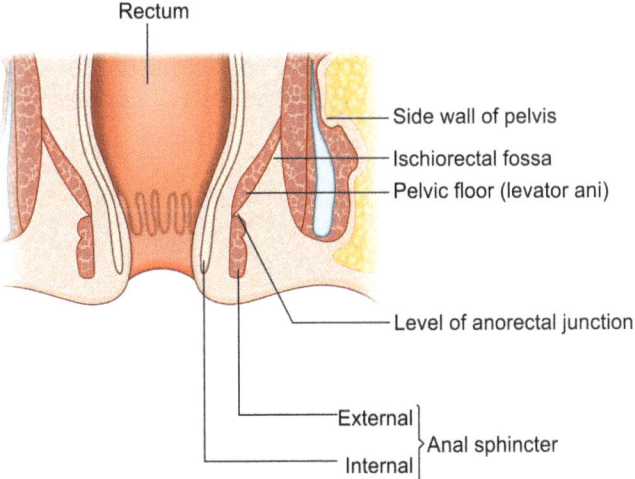

Fig. 11.1: Muscle involved in defecation.
Source: Sarin YK, Kaur G, Singh T. Constipation. In: Gupte S (Ed). *Recent Advances in Pediatrics (Special Vol 6: Gastroenterology, Hepatology and Nutrition)*. New Delhi: Jaypee 2000:213-226.

Two fundamental factors contributing to constipation are: (i) defects in emptying the rectum and (ii) defects in filling the rectum.

Defects in emptying the rectum, leading to stool retention, may result from interference with defecation reflex initiated by pressure receptor in the rectal muscles. Lesions of the rectal muscles, sacral spinal cord afferent fibers, and the pelvic floor and abdominal muscles, and lesions that prevent adequate relaxation of anal sphincter fall in the group.

Defective rectal filling may be encountered whenever there is poor gut peristalsis (hypothyroidism, diphenoxylate, loperamide opiate use, etc.), or there is mechanical structural lesion (Hirschsprung's disease).

Both in defective emptying and filling, excessive drying of the stools follows. Hard, dry stools are rather painful to evacuate, leading to further retention. Thus, a vicious cycle is set up. Constipation, therefore, tends to be self-perpetuating.

It is the anxiety on the part of the parents that may render constipation to have adverse effects (primarily on child's emotional health) and not the constipation per se.

HISTORY

The following clarifications in the history are helpful in reaching the diagnosis: How long has the problem of constipation been? Is it ever since birth or occurred later? What is the child's usual bowel habit and in which way has it changed? Is the passage of stool painful? What is the frequency and consistency of motions? What are the feeding habits? Can the constipation be explained by the kind of diet? Any relationship with drugs, particularly laxatives or purgatives? Is there any associated pain with defecation or in the abdomen? What is the color of stools? Is there any vomiting? Any history of passage of worms in stools? Any fecal incontinence?

In the newborn history, it should be enquired if the baby passed the meconium within first 24 hours or not.

In toddlers and preschool children, history of any problem in toilet training needs to be obtained.

In infants on much-too-much of cow's milk, constipation is common.

PHYSICAL EXAMINATION

In general physical examination, assess about the overall growth and development and nutritional status.

It is important to examine the abdomen for undue distention and palpable hard masses (fecoliths). Anus and rectum in particular need to be inspected for any fecal impaction, placement of anal orifice, skin tags, soiling, fissures, etc.

Examination of spine for a dimple, hair tuft, a palpable vertebral deformity, etc. is important.

INVESTIGATIONS

- Functional constipation does not need any tests.
- Thyroid profile is required for suspected hypothyroidism as the cause of constipation in a particular child.
- A plain X-ray abdomen may be done to confirm the presence of fecolith that is felt on palpations a mass.
- Rectal biopsy is needed for confirming the diagnosis of Hirschsprung's disease.

DIFFERENTIALS

Neonatal and Early Infancy

Benign

Breastfeeding: In the later neonatal period and early infancy, breastfed babies may pass stools only once in a few days. But, mind you, these stools are rather loose (like those the breastfed infant passes in early neonatal period) and seldom dry and solid. In true sense, this is not constipation.

If a breastfed infant's mother is consuming much-too-much of fats and proteins, his stools may be firmer and pultaceous.

Artificial feeding: It contributes to development of constipation through the following factors:
- Inadequate fluid intake, especially in hot weather
- Excessive sweating due to overclothing
- Inadequate sugar in the milk feed.

Delayed weaning: Inadequate or delayed introduction of semisolid foods.

Medication: Abuse of laxatives or purgatives over a prolonged period by the parents obsessed by the desirability to have daily bowel movement, causing diarrhea alternating with constipation.

Drugs like isoniazid, chlordiazepoxide, imipramine, amitriptyline, and vincristine may cause constipation.

Organic

Obstructive/mechanical lesions: Imperforate anus is characterized by a cutaneous collection of meconium in the perineal region, presence of an anal fissure in place of opening and usually a fistulous opening in the perineum, into vulva or urethra.

Anorectal stenosis occurs usually in association with other congenital anomalies and in preterm infants. There may be history of passage of stools resembling expelled toothpaste. A rectal examination needs to be done to confirm the diagnosis.

Ectopic anus placed anteriorly may well be a common cause of constipation.

Meconium plug syndrome is characterized by passage of a sticky white plug of mucus followed by flatus and liquid meconium or delay in passage of meconium beyond 36 hours. Insertion of the little finger into the rectum releases the *meconium plug*.

Meconium ileus, a common presentation in cystic fibrosis of pancreas, is characterized by feeding difficulty, abdominal distention, bilious vomiting between 34 hours and 48 hours of birth and fecal pellets (Fig. 11.2). Abdominal examination may reveal a palpable lump. X-ray abdomen (plain film) may show uneven dilated loops of bowel, air-fluid levels, and a bubbly granular density. Barium enema may show microcolon from disuse.

Small left colon syndrome, resembling *meconium plug* syndrome, may occur mostly in infants of diabetic mothers and is due to disturbance of peristalsis.

Functional ileus of the newborn is characterized by manifestations of intestinal obstruction in the absence of any anatomical obstruction. It is secondary to septicemia, pneumonia, electrolyte imbalance, and certain metabolic abnormalities. The condition is purely functional and occurs more often in the preterm infants.

Hirschsprung's disease usually manifests in the first week of life with failure to pass meconium, abdominal distention,

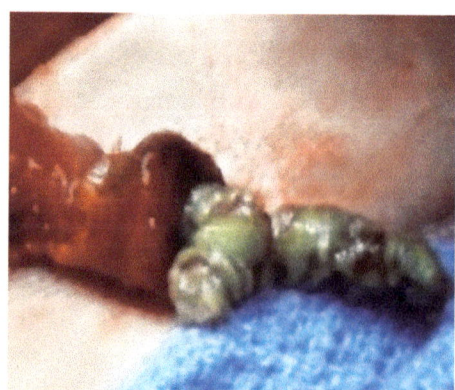

Fig. 11.2: Fecal pellets in meconium ileus.

bilious vomiting, and feeding difficulty. Later, the pictures may be complicated by diarrhea secondary to enterocolitis. The infant fails to thrive satisfactorily. Rectal examination shows no fecal matter and the canal may feel narrow and tight. X-ray abdomen (plain film) shows gaseous distention whereas barium enema reveals a narrow distal segment and a dilated proximal segment of the colon and residual barium that may be detected 12–48 hours after the initial examination. The characteristic radiologic changes may manifest after 6 weeks of life. The diagnosis needs to be confirmed by rectal biopsy which demonstrates agangliosis, i.e. absence of ganglion cells of the submucous (Meissner's) and intramural (Auerbach's) plexuses.

Pseudo-Hirschsprung's disease is a very rare cause of constipation in infancy. It usually manifests some years after birth. It results from poor tone of the colon, leading to dilatation but, unlike true Hirschsprung's disease, here the rectum is full, bowel does not have a narrow segment and agangliosis is not seen. Encopresis (fecal soiling) is an important manifestation.

Severe vomiting, as encountered in congenital pyloric stenosis or possetting, may also cause constipation.

Polyuria as in diabetes insipidus (nephrogenic), renal acidosis or hypercalcemia usually due to hypervitaminosis D, renal tubular defects or hyperparathyroidism.

Hypokalemia may be responsible for constipation in infants who suffer from dyselectrolytemia following an attack of diarrhea.

Hypothyroidism should be suspected in an infant who is constipated and also has feeding difficulty, prolonged physiological jaundice, hypothermia, hypotonia, poor mother activity, and umbilical hernia with or without facial features of the disease. Radiologically, retarded bone age help to reach the diagnosis.

Severe hypotonia as in prune-belly syndrome characterized by congenital absence of the abdominal muscles.

Lead poisoning should be suspected in infants exposed to lead (say, lead paint flakes, artist's paints, kajal or surma, fumes from batteries, etc.) and suffering from constipation in association with transient pain abdomen, resistant anemia, weight loss, irritability, vomiting, headache, personality changes, and ataxia. A lead line over the gums is typical. Urine lead level of more than 85 µg/24 hours is diagnostic.

Later Infancy and Childhood

Benign

Poor dietary intake: Inadequate dietary roughage and large amounts of milk are by far the most common cause of constipation in later infancy and childhood. A therapeutic trial can demonstrate it.

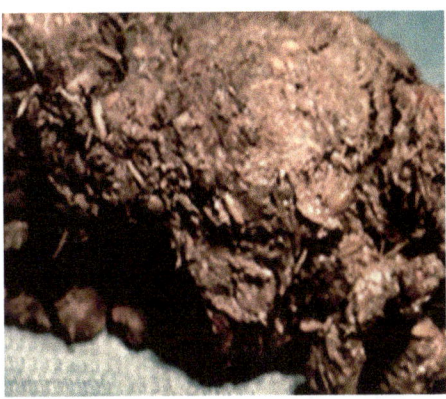

Fig. 11.3: *Fecolith*: Note the extreme form of fecal impaction, a hardening of feces into lump(s). It may occur anywhere in the intestinal tract but is typically found in the colon.

Abuse of laxatives and purgatives: Parents, who are eager that the child must have a bowel movement daily, indulge in frequent administration of laxatives or purgatives to the child. As a result, he begins to be dependent on such a medication and unless it is given as a daily "ritual" he may pass constipated stools, the so-called "Fecolth" (Fig. 11.3).

Poor toilet training: Parents, overanxious about the daily bowel movement, may force the child to sit on the "pottie" far too long against child's wish. Others may examine each and every stool that the child passes quite critically, inducing the child to refuse to empty his bowels. Reactive constipation secondary to poor toilet training is most often seen in children whose mothers are overprotective, tense, anxious, and indulgent and having tendency to use coercive methods. The fathers, on the other hand, are fond of exerting excessive discipline.

Organic

Intestinal parasitosis: Though most parasitic infestations are known to cause diarrhea, at least *Giardia lamblia* and hookworm may well cause constipation alternating with diarrhea. Since both the infestations are quite common in tropical settings, intestinal parasitosis should always be excluded in cases of constipation unless, of course, the cause is very obvious.

Anal fissure: An anal fissure causes pain during defecation and thus, may lead to withholding of the stools. Later, even if the child tries he finds it difficult to empty such a heavily loaded rectum. There may follow dilatation of the colon proximal to it. Anal fissure may result from hard scybala per se.

Hirschsprung's disease: Already described in this chapter.

Pseudo-Hirschsprung's disease: Already described in this chapter.

Hypothyroidism: Already described in this chapter.

FURTHER READING

1. Bellamarich PF. Constipation. In: Adam HM, Foy JM (Eds). *Signs and Symptoms in Pediatrics.* Illinois: American Academy of Pediatrics 2015:119-133.
2. Dave S, Gupta DK. Hirschsprung's disease and associated neuronal intestinal malformations. In: Gupte S (Ed). *Recent Advances in Pediatrics-12 Hot Topics.* New Delhi: Jaypee 2002:47-65.
3. Horvath K, King J. Major manifestations of gastrointestinal disease. In: Gupte S, Horvalh K (Eds). *Pediatric Gastroenterology, Hepatology and Nutrition.* New Delhi: Jaypee 2009.
4. Thapa BR. Constipation and encopresis. In: Gupte S (Ed). *Recent Advances in Pediatrics.* New Delhi: Jaypee 2004: 413-423.
5. Wyllie R. Major symptoms and signs of digestive tract disorders. In: Kliegman RM, St Geme JW III, Blum NJ, et al; (Eds). *Nelson Textbook of Pediatrics,* 21st edn. Philadelphia: Elsevier 2020:1522-1528.

CHAPTER 12

Seizures

BACKGROUND

The term, *seizure*, denotes a temporary disturbance of brain function manifested by involuntary motor, sensory, autonomic or psychic phenomenon, alone or in any combination. Some change in sensorium is usually present. Though a wide variety of central nervous system (CNS) disorders can cause seizures, the fundamental defect remains irritation of the CNS in each one of them.

Seizures are relatively more common in infancy and childhood than at any other period of life, the peak incidence occurring during the first 2 years. The overall incidence in childhood is stated to be 8%, among mentally retarded children (except those with Down syndrome) 20%, and among those suffering from one or the other type of cerebral palsy 35%.

HISTORY

Clinical workup must, in the first place, clarify if what has been described as seizure is indeed seizure or not. Disorders simulating recurrent seizures include breath-holding spells, narcolepsy, abdominal epilepsy, hysterical fits, syncope, apneic spells and migraine.

In the newborn, it is infrequent to see seizures in the form of typical tonic-clonic movements. On the other hand, such apparently minor manifestations as twitching, conjugate deviation of eyes, hypertonus in a twitching limb, irregular jerky movements and nystagmus, startling, pallor and hypotonia, slow and irregular respiration with periods of apnea and feeble cry, and cyanotic attacks may well mean seizures.

Symptomatic inquiry should include all the details about the attack: Was the onset sudden or gradual? Were the seizures local or generalized? Where did they begin? In which fashion did they progress to rest of the bodily parts? Did the child micturate or defecate during the attack? How long did the attack last? Was there fever preceding or following the attack? Did he sleep after the attack? Or, did the attack lead to headache, automatism or paralysis? Any associated manifestations like neck stiffness, vomiting, behavioral problems, or discharging ear?

In case of recurrent seizures, ask the attendants to give a clinical account of the first attack and the age at which it occurred. What is the minimal and maximal gap between the attacks? Is there any aura preceding the attack? Does the attack ever occur during sleep? Does the child bite his tongue, injure himself, micturate or defecate during convulsions? Does he lose consciousness? Are there any such manifestations as persistent headache, automatism or pseudoparalysis (Todd's paralysis) after the episode?

PHYSICAL EXAMINATION

In recurrent seizures, secondary to organic brain damage, you must look for evidence of such conditions as tuberous sclerosis, hydrocephalus, Sturge-Weber syndrome, cysticercosis, toxoplasmosis, syphilis, mental retardation, cerebral palsy, etc.

INVESTIGATIONS

- Funduscopy
- Blood sugar, calcium, and phosphorous
- Lumbar puncture
- *Cranial imaging:* Skull X-ray, computed tomography (CT) scan, magnetic resonance imaging (MRI), pneumoencephalography, arteriography radioisotope brain scan in persistent localized seizures.
- Electroencephalogram.

IMPORTANT DIFFERENTIALS

Seizures in the Newborn

Following conditions need to be considered when encountering seizures in the newborn:

First and second day: Perinatal problems such as birth injury, asphyxia, hypoxia, intracranial (especially intraventricular) hemorrhage; drug withdrawal syndrome; pyridoxine dependency; accidental injection of anesthesia into baby's scalp during labor; inborn errors of metabolism such as phenylketonuria.

Third day: Hypoglycemia.

Fourth day and onward: Fulminant infections such as septicemia, meningitis; hypocalcemic tetany, hypo- or hypernatremia, hypomagnesemia; kernicterus; tetanus; congenital malformations like arteriovenous fistulae, pomocephaly; intrauterine infections like toxoplasmosis, rubella, cytomegalic inclusion disease, herpes simplex (TORCH/STORCH).

Perinatal Problems

Birth trauma, following difficult delivery, may result in anoxia together with cerebral edema and microhemorrhages in low birth weight newborns and massive hemorrhages in mature babies. In the former situation, convulsions may present as tonic spasms preceded by some clonic jerks on first day only. In the later situation, convulsive manifestations usually appear between 2 days and 7 days of birth. These are unilateral and are accompanied by retinal hemorrhages, dyspnea, bulging anterior fontanel, skull fracture and cephalhematoma, and blood-stained or frankly bloody cerebrospinal fluid (CSF).

Hypocalcemia

Hypocalcemic tetany, the most common biochemical cause of neonatal seizures, occurs usually in babies on cow's milk formula rich in phosphates. Manifestations occur either on first day or about the seventh day of birth. These include, besides convulsions, jitteriness, laryngeal spasm, tremors, muscular twitching and carpopedal spasm. The infant remains all right in between the attacks.

Serum calcium is invariably under 8 mg% and phosphorus high.

Intravenous administration of calcium gluconate (5–10 mL of 10% solution) leads to dramatic response.

Hypoglycemia

Convulsions due to hypoglycemia are likely to occur in infants who suffer from intrauterine growth retardation, in infants of toxemic mothers, in infants of diabetic or prediabetic mothers, in smaller of the twins, and in infants with idiopathic respiratory distress syndrome, kernicterus, Beckwith-Wiedemann syndrome, infections, adrenocortical hyperplasia and glycogenosis.

Manifestations include, besides seizures, tremors, twitching, cyanosis and apneic spells.

Blood glucose level is under 30 mg% in term infants and 20 mg% in preterm ones.

Infections

Pyogenic meningitis as such or as a complication of septicemia is an important cause of neonatal convulsions. The most common complaint is that the infant is just not well with refusal to feed, lethargy, irritability and restlessness. Umbilicus is often septic. Neck stiffness is usually absent and anterior fontanel may or may not be bulging. Lumbar puncture is essential to establish the diagnosis.

Tetanus is likely to occur in newborns in whom umbilical cord is cut under septic conditions and mud, dung or such other harmful substances are applied to the navel at birth or soon after it. It usually manifests at 5 days or 6 days after birth with difficulty in sucking, stiffness of jaws, and generalized spasticity, spontaneously or in response to external stimuli. Risus sardonicus is a classical manifestation.

Malaria in neonatal period, though rare, may manifest with convulsions either on account of cerebral involvement or hyperpyrexia.

Pyridoxine Dependency

The newborn of a mother who has had prolonged administration of pyridoxine during pregnancy may develop convulsions which are resistant to various treatments. Such a pyridoxine dependency may also occur in newborns suffering from a hereditary metabolic defect leading to unusually large needs of pyridoxine.

The infant is restless between convulsive attacks, reacting to external stimuli (acoustic and mechanical) with twitching. He blinks the eyes, moving in an uncoordinated fashion.

A dramatic response to a 25 mg dose of pyridoxine is a rule.

Drug Withdrawal Syndrome

The newborn of a mother addicted to narcotics (morphine, heroin) or alcohol is prone to develop withdrawal symptoms which include seizures, irritability and excessive drooling.

Accidental Injection of Anesthesia

During labor, as the mother is being given paracervical block, baby's scalp may be accidentally injected. Such a newborn develops intractable seizures.

Electrolyte Imbalance

Both hypo- and hypernatremia, following dehydration or its incorrect treatment with parenteral fluids and electrolytes, may cause severe convulsions with permanent neurologic damage.

Hypomagnesemia

A newborn with convulsions associated with established hypocalcemia not showing response to calcium therapy must arouse suspicion of hypomagnesemia.

Metabolic Disorders

You must consider possibility of an inborn error of metabolism if convulsions are resistant and there is a history of such a disorder in the family.

Galactosemia is characterized by occurrence of convulsions following ingestion of milk. Presence of jaundice and hepatosplenomegaly supports the diagnosis.

Fructose intolerance is characterized by occurrence of hypoglycemic seizures or coma immediately after ingestion of such foods as contain fructose, say carrot, fruits juices, milk formulas containing sucrose, or cane sugar.

Maple syrup urine disease (MSUD) is characterized by hypoglycemic seizures in association with feeding difficulty, marked metabolic acidosis, progressive neurologic and mental deterioration and odor of maple syrup in urine.

Congenital Malformations of Central Nervous System

A newborn presenting with seizures and facial asymmetry, microcephaly or any other obvious malformation should be suspected of an underlying developmental defect of CNS, say arteriovenous fistula, congenital hydrocephalus, porencephaly, microgyria, corpus callosum agenesis or hydrancephaly*.

Aicardi syndrome is characterized by trio of infantile spasms resistant to therapy, chorioretinopathy and agenesis of corpus callosum. Additional features include mental retardation and vertebral and costal abnormalities. Its cause appears to be a newly-mutated X-chromosomal-dominant gene lethal to males in utero. Naturally, all patients are females. Prognosis is poor, most subjects dying in early life.

Drugs

If mother has had large doses of phenothiazine(s) as a part of management of toxemias of pregnancy, the newborn may suffer from phenothiazine poisoning. Though jitteriness is the most common manifestation, he may have seizures, thamide administered for neonatal asphyxia if given even in a marginally higher than the recommended doses, may be responsible for convulsions.

Seizures in Later Infancy and Childhood

Acute (Nonrecurrent) Seizure Disorders

Febrile seizures: The term refers to seizures occurring at the onset of acute extracranial infection or in association with high environmental temperature.

This is the most common cause of seizures between 3 months and 5 years with peak between 6 months and 3 years of age. Outside this age range, it is infrequent to have febrile seizures. Boys are affected nearly twice as frequently as girls. Family history of convulsions and higher incidence in twins and children born of consanguineous unions are noteworthy.

The remaining salient features of the condition are:
- It is usually associated with rapid rise in body temperature. There is, therefore, preceding history of the child having been unwell a few hours prior to the onset of seizures.
- Generalized rather than focal seizures are nearly a rule.
- The attack lasts less than 10–15 minutes and in no case more than 20 minutes.
- There is no recurrence before 12–18 hours of the attack accompanying rapid rise of body temperature.
- There is no residual paralysis of a limb following the attack.
- Cerebrospinal fluid after the attack is normal.
- Electroencephalogram (EEG) after the attack is normal.

Seizures associated with fever (not of CNS infection) but not satisfying the above criteria are often labeled "atypical" rather than "typical" febrile convulsions. This condition is now considered a precursor of idiopathic epilepsy.

Central Nervous System Infections

Pyogenic meningitis may manifest suddenly with seizures in association with high fever, restlessness, irritability, vomiting, headache and neck stiffness. Cranial nerve palsies and papilledema are present in some cases. The presence of a generalized purpuric rash points to meningococcal meningitis.

Encephalitis manifests with change in sensorium (varying from lethargy to coma), fever and vomiting in addition to seizures. Whereas an infant may show gross irritability, headache is a common symptom in older children. Remaining manifestations may include peculiar behavior, hyperactivity, altered speech and ataxia. There is rapid variation in the clinical picture from hour-to-hour.

Cerebral abscess (Figs. 12.1A to D) is characterized by headache, vomiting and visual disturbances from high intracranial pressure, focal neurologic manifestations such as seizures, cranial nerve palsies, ataxia, visual field defects and hemiparesis from local pressure, high or low irregular fever, chills, rigors and leukocytosis from toxemia, and irritability, behavioral problems, drowsiness, and weight loss from intracranial suppuration. The presence of a septic focus such as otitis media, lung abscess, empyema, bronchiectasis, infective endocarditis, or cyanotic congenital heart disease lends support to the diagnosis.

Cerebral malaria, a life-threatening complication of *Plasmodium falciparum* infection, is characterized by

---

*Destruction of the cerebral hemispheres which are transformed into a sort of membranous sac filled with cerebrospinal fluid (CSF) and the renerants of cortex and white matter.

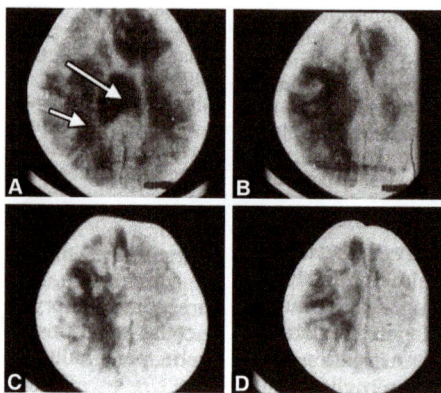

Figs. 12.1A to D: Computed tomography (CT) scan showing multiple cerebral abscesses in an infant suffering from suppurative otitis media (SOM).

meningeal signs, seizures and coma. CSF is more or less within normal limits.

Toxic Factors

Tetanus has a sudden onset with muscle spasm and cramps, particularly about the location of inoculation, back and abdomen. In the next 48 hours, clinical picture worsens. Neck rigidity, positive Kernig sign and trismus become prominent. The face assumes atypical expression, "risus sardonicus", which consists of clenching of jaws, laterally drawn lips and raised eyebrows. There is increasing stiffness of upper limbs and legs. The former are kept flexed and the latter hyperextended.

A typical tetanic spasm lasts 5–10 seconds and consists of agonizing pain, stiffness of the body which gets almost arched backward with retraction of head (opisthotonos) and clenching of jaw. As the disease progresses, a very simple stimulus also precipitates an attack. In advanced cases, spasms may become almost a continuous and constant phenomenon.

High fever is uncommon but a low-grade fever is usually present.

Lead encephalopathy, occurring late in the course of plumbism is characterized by seizures, high intracranial pressure and coma. A preceding history of transient abdominal pain, resistant anemia, weight loss, irritability, vomiting, constipation, headache, personality changes and ataxia is usually elicitable.

A lead line over the gums is characteristic of plumbism.

Urine lead level of over 80 μg/dL/24 hours is diagnostic.

Shigellosis, which usually manifests in the form of bacillary dysentery, may also cause in 1 in 10 subjects seizures together with such CNS symptoms as headache, delirium, neck stiffness and fainting.

Nontyphoidal salmonellosis, though commonly a cause of gastroenteritis (particularly the outbreaks occurring in late summer and early fall), may also be responsible for very high fever, headache, confusion, change in sensorium, meningismus and seizures.

Anoxic state, as a result of such factors as inhalation anesthesia or sudden severe asphyxia, may cause convulsions.

Biochemical Defects

Hypocalcemic tetany in the postneonatal period occurs in subjects suffering from such predisposing conditions as vitamin D deficiency rickets, malabsorption syndrome, alkalosis or hypoparathyroidism which may be idiopathic or secondary to operative damage in thyroidectomy done for thyrotoxicosis.

The diagnosis of tetany associated with rickets is not difficult. The patient shows usual evidence of rickets such as delayed closure of anterior fontanel, rachitic rosary and widening of wrists. X-ray of wrist shows cupping, fraying and fragmentations of the epiphyseal ends of radius and ulnar and increased distance between the epiphysis and carpal bones. Serum alkaline phosphatise and phosphorus are elevated. Serum calcium is low.

In idiopathic hypoparathyroidism, tetanic seizures occur in infants suffering from defective dental enamel, brittle nails, cataract, recurrent diarrhea susceptibility to fungal infection, hypocalcemia and hyperphosphatemia. This combination is named DiGeorge syndrome. Remarkable lymphocytopenia and immunologic deficiencies constitute its hallmark.

In another form of idiopathic hypoparathyroidism, hypocalcemic convulsions are superimposed on such associations as short stature, mental retardation and shortening of the ulnar metacarpal bones so that the index finger becomes the longest finger. This form is tended pseudohypoparathyroidism.

Hypomagnesemia tetany must be suspected if in spite of adequate therapy with calcium, the patient's hypocalcemic state fails to respond clinically, biochemically or both.

Hypoglycemia in the postneonatal period may be due to insulin overdose, hyperplasia of islets of Langerhans, hypopituitarism, adrenocortical insufficiency, liver disease, glycogenoses or fructose intolerance.

Manifestations include early morning seizures preceded by pallor, sweating and weakness.

Electrolyte Imbalance

Hypo- or hypernatremia, usually in association with dehydration or its careless correction, may cause seizures even in later infancy and childhood as in neonatal period.

Cerebral Edema

Convulsions may complicate the clinical profile in a child with acute nephritis, burns or allergic edema of the brain. The development may well be related to cerebral edema.

Drugs

A large number of drugs are suspected of causing convulsions. The list includes phenothiazines, aminophylline, antihistamines, acetazolamide, diphenoxylate, strychnine, propoxyphenes, hexachlorophene, steroids, amitriptyline, amphetamine, imipramine, pyrimethamine, chloroquine, carbamazepine, nalidixic acid, metoclopramide, and isoniazid.

Chronic or Recurrent Seizure Disorders

Epilepsy: The term refers to "various symptom complexes characterized by recurrent, paroxysmally attack of unconsciousness or impaired consciousness, usually with a succession of tonic or clonic muscular spasms or other abnormal behavior". It may be organic (secondary or symptomatic) or idiopathic.

Organic epilepsy: It is frequently accompanied by cerebral palsy, mental retardation and electrocardiogram (ECG) abnormalities. Various conditions that may cause it are:

- *Post-traumatic*: Direct damage to brain tissue.
- *Posthemorrhagic*: Injury to brain at birth or afterward, bleeding diathesis, rupture of miliary aneurysm, pachymeningitis.
- *Postanoxic*: An after-effect of severe neonatal asphyxia.
- *Postinfectious*: Meningitis, encephalitis, cerebral abscess, sinus thrombophlebitis.
- *Post-toxic*: Kernicterus, chronic poisoning with lead, arsenic, etc.
- *Postmetabolic*: Hypoglycemic brain damage.
- *Degenerative*: Intracranial neurofibromatosis, cerebromacular degeneration, subacute sclerosing panencephalitis (SSPE).
- *Congenital*: Arteriovenous aneurysm, Sturge-Weber type of vascular anomaly, cerebral aplasia, porencephaly, hydrocephalus, tuberous sclerosis.
- *Parasitosis*: Cysticercosis (Figs. 12.2A and B), hydatid disease, ascariasis, toxoplasmosis, syphilis.

Idiopathic epilepsy: Also called cryptogenic, primary, essential or genuine epilepsy, it may be of genetic or acquired type.

Classification of epilepsy as per the International League Against Epilepsy is presented in Box 12.1. Conventional semantics, wherever applicable, are mentioned in brackets.

Grand mal epilepsy is characterized by generalized tonic-clonic seizures which are predominantly tonic during

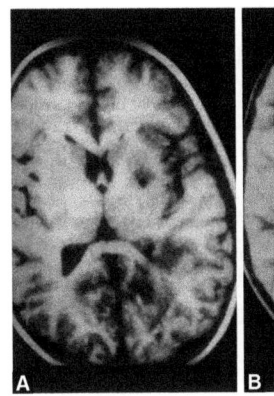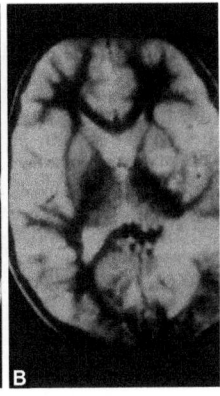

Figs. 12.2A and B: Neurocysticercosis. Magnetic resonance imaging (MRI), T1- and T2-weighted axial images showing degenerating parenchymal cysts.

BOX 12.1: International league against epilepsy classification of epilepsy.

Generalized
- Tonic-clonic (grand mal)
- Tonic
- Clonic
- Absence (petit mal)
- Atonic/akinetic (minor motor)
- Bilateral epileptic myoclonus syndromes

Idiopathic
- Benign neonatal
- Childhood absence
- Juvenile absence
- Juvenile myoclonic
- Grand mal on awakening
- Generalized idiopathic

Cryptogenic
- West syndrome (infantile spasms)
- Lennox-Gastaut syndrome (childhood epileptic encephalopathy)
- Myoclonic-astatic seizures
- Myoclonic absences

Localized (Partial) Seizures
- Simple partial (without impaired consciousness):
  – Motor symptoms
  – Sensory symptoms
  – Autonomic symptoms
  – Mixed symptoms
- Complex partial (with impaired consciousness):
  – Simple partial, but loss of consciousness
  – With automation

Syndromes
- Symptomatic:
  – Chronic progressive epilepsy
  – Epilepsia partialis continua
- Idiopathic:
  – Benign childhood focal epilepsy with centrotemporal spikes (rolandic epilepsy)
  – Epilepsy with occipital paroxysms

Undetermined Syndromes
- Neonatal seizures
- Severe myoclonic epilepsy of infancy
- Epilepsy with continuous spike waves during slow-wave sleep
- Acquired epileptic aphasia

infancy. The attack in one-third cases preceded by an "aura", manifests suddenly. During the tonic phase, lasting less than 20-40 seconds, the child usually loses consciousness. His face becomes pale and gets distorted with rolling of the eyeballs upward or to one side. The pupils dilate and corneas become insensitive to touch. The head is thrown backward or to a side. Rapid contraction of jaw muscles may cause biting of the tongue. Rapid contraction of the diaphragm and intercostal muscles may force the air out of the lungs through the closed glottis, causing a characteristic "starving cry". Rapid contraction of abdominal muscles may cause micturition, and less often, even defecation. As the tonic phase progresses, inadequate respiration results in cyanosis.

The clonic phase, which may not be quite perceptible in infancy, follows tonic phase, lasting over a variable period.

After the attack, the patient usually sleeps. The postconvulsive sleep is followed by the so-called "postictal reactions" in the form of confusion, headache and stupor. Occasionally, Todd's paresis/paralysis (usually for 12-24 hours but infrequently for a week or so), and prolonged automatism may follow.

Petit mal epilepsy (absences, dizzy spells, lapses, fainting turns) is characterized by brief transient loss of consciousness, lasting up to 30 seconds, without any preceding aura, any convulsive movements or any postictal sleep. Classically, a child, busy in writing or reading, suddenly stops the activity, resuming it after the attack is over in some seconds, usually less than 20-30 seconds. During the attack, he is likely to drop the pen or notebook held in hand. Falling on ground, as in the case or grand mal seizures, is rare. The child is usually unaware of the attack. Factors that precipitate an attack include exposure to blinking light and hyperventilation. The frequency may be one or two episodes a month, or hundreds of them a day.

Typically, petit mal seldom occurs before the age of 3 years and often settles without any treatment by puberty. The peak incidence in childhood occurs between 4 years and 8 years. The incidence in girls is higher than in boys.

Electroencephalogram shows a characteristic 3 per second spike and wave pattern.

Focal epilepsy, though usually of postorganic origin, may occasionally be idiopathic. It may be sensory or motor, the latter being the dominant variety seen in childhood.

In the motor variety, called Jacksonian epilepsy, seizures are typically clonic, involving muscles that are usually brought into action or voluntary movements. Thus, hands, face and tongue are more frequently affected than feet and trunk. By the term "Jacksonian march" is meant that focal convulsions in a particular part progress too others in a fixed pattern. For instance, convulsions beginning in thumb would spread to fingers, wrist, arm, face and leg on the same side in this fixed order. A point meriting mention is that, in focal epilepsy, consciousness is usually not affected unless, of course, when its spread is rapid and extensive.

Psychomotor epilepsy (temporal lobe epilepsy) is characterized by visceral symptoms like nausea, vomiting or epigastric sensations, followed by short period of increased muscular tonicity and, later, semipurposive movements during a period of impaired consciousness or amnesia. Vasomotor manifestations such as circumoral pallor are frequently present. Some children may have slight aura in the form of a "shrill cry" or an indication for "help".

The episode usually remains for 1-5 minutes. The postictal period is often marked by a brief spell of sleep or drowsiness. Thereafter, the child resumes normal activity.

The EEG is often normal, except during the episode of seizure.

Infantile myoclonic epilepsy (infantile spasm, salaam seizures, lightning major, jackknife epilepsy, West syndrome) is characterized by massive attacks of sudden dropping (flexion) of the head and flexion of the arms, once or as many as several hundred times a day. The affected child is under 2 years of age, usually under 6 months. Significant developmental as well as mental retardation is more or less a rule in both primary (seizures occurring before 4 months or developmental level low right from beginning as in congenital cerebral defect) and secondary (following unrecognized encephalitis or an underlying defect in cerebral metabolism) types.

The EEG changes are in the form of random high-voltage slow waves and spikes, suggesting a disorganized state. *Hypsarrhythmia* is the name given to this EEG pattern.

Epilepsy-simulating States and Epileptic Equivalents

Narcolepsy: This disorder, simulating epilepsy, occurs only rarely in childhood. Boys suffer more often than girls. The attack is characterized by diurnal episodes of irresistible sleep, usually precipitated by sudden emotional upheaval. The patient, while working, talking, swimming, driving or walking, suddenly stops activity and falls asleep. The sleep is shallow and he can easily be aroused. After waking up, he is quite alert.

Narcolepsy usually becomes chronic though spontaneous cure, or, at least, improvement occurs more often in it than in the case of true epilepsy.

Hysteria

Also called hysterical fits or psychogenic epilepsy, the condition occurs in children usually above 6 years, with a typical neurotic background. During the attack, such characteristic features of true epilepsy as dilation of pupils, pallor of skin and mucous membrane, true loss of consciousness, loss of sphincter control and bodily injury are absent. Further, the attack lasts fairly long (half-an-hour or so) and during its course the patient exhibits bizarre crying, moaning and irrelevant talk.

Breath-holding Spells

This common condition of early childhood with onset between 6 months and 18 months of age is sometimes accompanied by tonic and clonic convulsions in which case differentiation from true epilepsy becomes essential. First, in breath-holding spells, an obvious precipitating factor such as a disciplinary conflict between the child and the parents (which may manifest in one or the other form) can invariably be elicited. Secondly, cyanosis in spells precedes convulsions whereas in epilepsy it appears after the convulsions have progressed. Thirdly, EEG in spells is invariably normal.

Syncope

Simple fainting spell, often complicated by tonic and clonic convulsive reactions involving face and arms, may follow a pinprick, a sudden fright or some such situation, provided that the child is in sitting or standing position. Such a subject has a defect in reflex regulation of the vascular system. As a result, with precipitation from one of the factors, sudden relaxation of the visceral venous system occurs, leading to bradycardia and hypotension. Note that if you make the child lie flat on table, or if you make him cry vigorously before and during a minor surgical procedure such as drawing a blood sample, chances are that he would not have fainting spell.

Remaining causes of fainting, chiefly due to transient cerebral anemia, include hyperventilation in upright position, Stokes-Adams syndrome, paroxysmal tachycardia, hyperactive carotid sinus reflex (as in sick sinus syndrome resulting from myocarditis or cardiac surgery), posterior fossa tumor, cough syncope (as in asthma) and extension of neck in a child with fused cervical vertebrae.

Migraine

Some authorities regard migraine as a variant of epilepsy on account of its episodic nature often preceded by an aura, its chronicity, its genetic features, its occurrence in association with epilepsy in the same family, and occasional replacement of migraine by typical epilepsy in due course.

FURTHER READING

1. Bains HS, Mittal S. Febrile seizures. In: Gupte S (Ed). *Recent Advances in Pediatrics (Special Vol 18: Pediatric Neurology)*. New Delhi: Jaypee 2007:334-340.
2. Greydanus DE, Van Dyke DH. Epilepsy in adolescents. In: Gupte S (Ed). *Recent Advances in Pediatrics (Special Vol 19: Developmental and Behavioral Pediatrics)*. New Delhi: Jaypee 2007:300-339.
3. Gulati S, Singh LR, Gupte S, et al. Pediatric neurology. In: Gupte S (Ed). *The Short Textbook of Pediatrics*, 13th edn. New Delhi: Jaypee 2020.

CHAPTER 13

Cough

INTRODUCTION

The term, *cough*, refers to the violent and noisy expulsion of air from the lungs. Ordinarily, it is a normal reflex and aims at clearing the tracheobronchial tree. In the presence of a pathological condition, it may assume a magnitude that is quite disturbing, both to the sufferer and the people around.

The stimulus for producing cough is of two types. First, exogenous as in smoke, dust, or foreign body. Second, endogenous as in bronchitis, bronchiolitis, pneumonia, respiratory airway edema, excessive production of mucus, and stimulation of vagus nerve by mediastinal tumors, aneurysms or aortic arch anomalies.

Cough may be acute or chronic in nature.

HISTORY

The diagnostic possibilities are narrowed down considerably from clarification on the following points in the history: Is the cough acute or chronic? Acute episodes of cough may accompany acute bronchitis, bronchiolitis or pneumonia. If hoarseness and cough coexist, viral laryngotracheobronchitis is a sound possibility. Is the cough productive or nonproductive? What is description of sputum? When did cough start? Is it barking or brassy? Is it accompanied by wheezing? Any associated fever or other constitutional manifestations? Any relationship to food? Any upper respiratory congestion? Is there any history of allergy, heart disease, asthma or tuberculosis?

PHYSICAL EXAMINATION

Physical examination should, among other things, pointedly find out if the chest, nose and throat are normal or abnormal. Inspiratory stridor indicates laryngeal disease. Widespread rhonchi indicate major airway obstruction (bronchospasm). Fine crepitations favor pneumonia or pulmonary edema in which fluid fills the alveoli. Is there any localized or generalized lymphadenopathy? Any evidence of congenital or acquired heart problem? Whether liver and spleen are palpable? Whether there is rhinorrhea, blocked nose or tonsillitis?

INVESTIGATIONS

Acute short-lived cough usually does not need investigations. In chronic cough, investigative evaluation becomes mandatory.
- Complete blood picture
- Chest X-ray
- Sputum examination
- Mantoux test
- Sweat chloride
- Alpha-1 antitrypsin level
- Immunologic studies.

IMPORTANT DIFFERENTIALS

Upper Respiratory Tract Infections

Acute infection of the upper airway (frequently viral: adenovirus, enterovirus, myxovirus) is often accompanied by dry cough. Other symptoms include blocked or running nose, earache or sore throat. Chest examination usually reveals no abnormal finding, except for conducted sounds from the upper respiratory tract. Usually, the disease is self-limited.

Lower Respiratory Tract Infections

Pneumonias, both bacterial and viral, are invariably accompanied by cough. Fever, varying degrees of respiratory distress, prostration and, on auscultation, crepitations may be present. Decreased breath sounds with localized crepitations and dullness of percussion note favor consolidation. Remember, manifestations in viral pneumonia are not as severe as in bacterial pneumonia.

Acute bronchitis is characterized by dry cough that is worst at night, mild constitutional symptoms and wheezing. Cough may become productive in a span of about 5 days. Some tachypnea and widespread rhonchi are present.

Acute bronchiolitis usually follows an upper respiratory tract infection and is characterized by onset of rapid shallow breathing and prostration. Cough is usually mild; so is the fever. Marked dyspnea may lead to cyanosis, dehydration and respiratory acidosis. Chest signs include intercostal and suprasternal retraction, hyper-resonant percussion note, diminished breath sounds, characteristic wheezing and crepitations at the end of inspiration and early expiration.

Bronchial Asthma

Attack is characterized by marked dyspnea, bouts of cough and expiratory wheezing. Cyanosis, pallor, sweating, exhaustion and restlessness are often present and the pulse is rapid. The disease should be seriously considered if the cough occurs in the early morning hours because of exposure to house dust, before the child falls asleep or is induced by, physical exertion, particularly if cough has a paroxysmal pertussis-like character.

Pleuritis

It may present as dry cough. But, then, there usually is a unilateral pain or friction rub.

Mouth-Breathing

In case of adenoids or thumb sucking, it may be accompanied by dry cough. At night, cough becomes worse since the air breathed through the mouth is neither filtered nor moistened and irritates the tracheal mucosa, causing cough and susceptibility to superimposed recurrent infection.

Congestive Cardiac Failure

It may lead to congestion of the pulmonary circulation. This causes dry cough to begin with but, as pulmonary edema increases, cough too becomes productive.

Neuropathic State

It may lead to compulsive dry cough as an attention-seeking device. It is a sort of "tic".

I see about a dozen of such cases a year. Of course, I make sure organic etiology (especially, bronchial asthma) is carefully excluded.

Bronchiectasis

It is characterized by an insidious onset with persistent or recurrent cough productive of copious, mucopurulent sputum which is foul-smelling and has postural relationship. In advanced cases, dyspnea, cyanosis, clubbing and hemoptysis may also be present. Classical auscultatory finding is the "localized crepitations" repeatedly found over the affected area. Other signs suggestive of collapse-consolidation may also be present.

Lung Abscess

Acute abscesses may develop during the course of staphylococcal pneumonia.

Chronic abscesses have insidious onset with fever, persistent cough and foul-smelling sputum. At times, dyspnea and chest pain may occur. Clubbing develops in a patient who has remained without adequate treatment over a prolonged period. Chest signs are usually those of consolidation with bronchial breathing.

Foreign Body

Aspiration of peanut, almond, popcorn, groundnut seed, grains or pulses may cause a sudden paroxysm of cough in a subject who was earlier otherwise well. There is congestion of the face and a state of almost suffocation. Partial obstruction of the main bronchus results in massive emphysema; the complete obstruction causes massive collapse. A few days later, the child may be brought to the hospital with signs and symptoms of pneumonia. Further delay may lead to development of lung abscess or bronchiectasis. Diagnosis is from history of a sudden paroxysm of violent cough, clinical findings of pneumonia, collapse, emphysema, etc. bronchoscopy and radiology.

Pertussis (Whooping Cough)

Three stages, each stage lasting around 2 weeks, are known. The first, i.e. catarrhal stage, consists of catarrhal manifestations in the form of rhinitis, sneezing, lacrimation, fever and irritating cough that is nocturnal to begin with but later becomes diurnal. The second, i.e. paroxysmal (spasmodic) stage is characterized by severe paroxysmal coughing which consists of repeated series of coughing (expiratory), followed by sudden deep, violent inspiration with characteristic crowing sound called "whoop" due to laryngospasm. There is associated suffocation, congested face with or without cyanosis, anxious look and bulging of eyes. Sweating, congestion of neck veins and confusion may follow the spells. Periorbital edema, subconjunctival hemorrhages, ulcer of frenulum of tongue, exhaustion, dehydration and convulsion may complicate the clinical picture. The third, i.e. convalescent stage is characterized by slow resolution of the paroxysms. The so-called "habit pattern of coughing" may, however, linger on and on over subsequent weeks and months. Remember, in previously immunized infants and in children below 6 months of age, the characteristic symptom-complex may not be encountered.

Remaining Causes of Cough

The remaining causes of cough are smoking, cystic fibrosis, tracheoesophageal fistula, hiatal hernia, stenosis of esophagus, megaesophagus due to achalasia, congenital heart disease, alpha-1 antitrypsin deficiency, repeated aspiration as in cerebral palsy, compression of trachea by enlarged mediastinal glands or vascular anomalies.

FURTHER READING

1. Dani VS, Mogre SS, Saoji R. Evaluation of chronic cough in children: clinical and diagnostic spectrum and outcome of specific therapy. *Indian Pediatr* 2002;39:63-69.
2. Deep A, Ganu S. Persistent cough. In: Gupte S (Ed): *Recent Advances in Pediatrics*. New Delhi: Jaypee 2006:205-217.
3. Gupte S, Forfar R, William ME. Cough in infants, children and adolescents. In: Gupte S, Gupte SB, Gupte M (Eds). *Recent Advances in Pediatrics: Infectious Diseases-II*. New Delhi: Jaypee 2015:304-322.
4. Marcus MG. Cough. In: Adam HM, Foy JM (Eds). *Signs and Symptoms in Pediatrics*. Illinois: American Academy of Pediatrics 2015:135-143.
5. Parks DP, Ahrens RC, Humphries CT, et al. Chronic cough in childhood: approach to diagnosis and treatment. *J Pediatr* 1989;115:856-862.

CHAPTER 14

Cyanosis

BACKGROUND

Cyanosis means bluish-purple discoloration of the skin and mucous membrane due to an increase in the level of reduced hemoglobin of arterial blood (congenital heart disease), or accumulation of abnormal hemoglobin (methemoglobinemia).

Central cyanosis is the result of inadequate oxygenation of blood (congestive cardiac failure, certain lung conditions), or mixture of arterial and venous blood (right to left shunt, venous-arterial shunt). Such a cyanosis is generalized though the involvement of tongue is characteristic.

Peripheral cyanosis is due to high reduction of oxyhemoglobin occurring in capillaries as and when blood flow is slow (cold injury, heart failure, venous obstruction). In this situation, tongue remains unaffected and limb is cold. Remember that cyanosis associated with heart failure may well be of mixed type.

Since cyanosis is recognized when at least 5 g/dL of reduced (unsaturated) hemoglobin is present in the systemic arterial blood, one may fail to detect it in individuals with severe anemia. On the other hand, subjects with polycythemia may manifest it more easily. Skin color and thickness, and also blood flow influence the determination of cyanosis.

HISTORY

Age of the patent is important. Persistent cyanosis in a newborn often points to the diagnosis of cyanotic congenital heart disease [transposition of great arteries (TGAs), respiratory distress syndrome, amniotic fluid inhalation or congenital anomalies of upper airway].

When was cyanosis first noticed: right at birth or subsequently? Cyanosis appearing some weeks after birth may well be suggestive of tetralogy of Fallot (TOF).

Is it present all the time or only at times?

If persistent, does it become worse sometimes? Hypercyanotic spells of TOF are a glaring example of such a situation.

Any suggestions of respiratory illness (cystic fibrosis, severe asthma) or heart disease (right to left shunt in congenital heart disease)?

Any suggestion of poisoning from nitrite, aniline dyes or drugs like phenacetin, sulfonamides, dapsone, etc. causing methemoglobinemia. In this condition, cyanosis does not have the usual bright blue color.

PHYSICAL EXAMINATION

While examining a patient for cyanosis, it is a must to do so in good light (preferably daylight) and also to have a normal control for comparison (Fig. 14.1). Once it is clear that the subject has central cyanosis, it needs to be clear if it is secondary to a cardiac or a respiratory disease (Fig. 14.2).

INVESTIGATIONS

- Arterial blood gas analysis and blood oxygen saturation by pulse oximetry.
- A complete blood picture (CBP) helps detect features like anemia, polycythemia, etc. High total leukocyte count (TLC) is indicative of infections.
- Chest X-ray to detect lung pathologies like pneumonia, severe bronchiolitis, pleural effusion, etc.
- Electrocardiogram (ECG) to detect abnormalities of the heart rhythm and rate.
- Echocardiography.

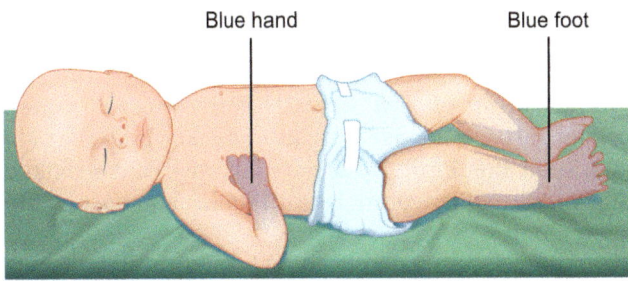

Fig. 14.1: Acrocyanosis in a newborn. It is common even in healthy newborns.

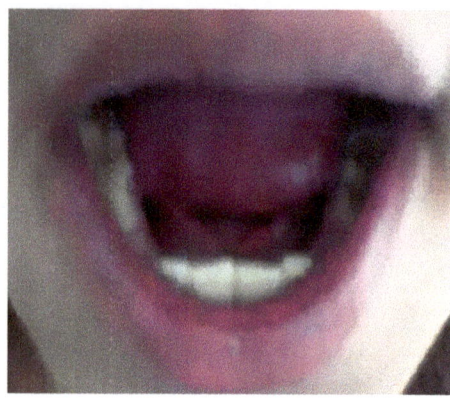

Fig. 14.2: Central cyanosis. It is always indicative of a pathologic condition.

- Transesophageal echocardiogram (TEE).
- Cardiac Doppler with echo or ultrasound.
- Cardiac or chest computed tomography (CT) scan and magnetic resonance imaging (MRI) scan.
- Cardiac catheterization.

IMPORTANT DIFFERENTIALS

Cyanosis of Respiratory Origin

Upper Airway Obstruction

Deficient oxygenation of arterial blood may occur in congenital anomalies of larynx, trachea and vascular ring, or from aspiration/inhalation of amniotic fluid, mucus or foreign body. Inspiratory stridor and suprasternal and intercostal retraction are characteristic.

Defect in Diffusion

Acute respiratory distress syndrome, including hyaline membrane disease, is the most important cause of cyanosis in the newborn.

Pneumonia may cause cyanosis from diffusion defect at any age.

Wilson-Mikity syndrome causes cyanosis and respiratory distress a week or 2 after birth.

Cyanosis of Cardiac Disease Origin

Congenital Heart Disease

Transposition of great arteries is the most common congenital heart disease that causes marked cyanosis right at or soon after birth. Dyspnea, congestive cardiac failure and failure to thrive occur later. Clubbing also develops in a few months.

It occurs predominantly in male infants (male-female ratio 4:1). These infants are of relatively large birth weight though they gain poorly subsequently. Incidence of diabetes mellitus in the grandparents is high.

Examination reveals a remarkably enlarged heart. Auscultation shows no classical pattern of murmurs which are usually related to the type of coexisting communication without which transposition of great vessels (TGV) is incompatible with life.

Radiology shows enlarged heart (not on the first day but by the end of first week) which may appear "egg-shaped", and plethoric lung fields.

The ECG reveals right ventricular hypertrophy (RVH), right axis deviation and often P-pulmonale. Signs of left ventricular hypertrophy (LVH) may be seen in case of accompanying pulmonary hypertension or ventricular septal defect (VSD).

Cardiac catheterization and selective angiography are necessary to confirm the diagnosis of exact type of transposition.

Tetralogy of Fallot (pulmonary stenosis, VSD, RVH, dextroposition and overriding of aorta) is the most common cause of persistent cyanosis that usually begins after the third month of life. Along with cyanosis, the infant also has dyspnea. As he grows, he feels comfortable in squatting or lying down position only. Anoxic, hypoxic or cyanotic spells may occur due to cerebral anoxia. Such spells consist of dyspnea and cyanosis with or without unconsciousness. By the age of 2 years, some clubbing becomes obvious.

Auscultation reveals a loud short systolic murmur that is best heard at left sternal border in the third space. The louder or harsher the murmur, the less is the degree of severity of the disease. The murmur is usually not accompanied by a thrill. P2 is usually single.

Blood studies show polycythemia.

Chest X-ray reveals oligemic (poorly vascularized due to diminished pulmonary blood flow) lung fields, a small boot-shaped heart with the tip of the boot turned up above the diaphragm (because of RVH), and concavity of the pulmonary artery segment (small pulmonary conus). Aortic arch is on right side in 20–25% of the cases.

The ECG shows RVH and beaked P waves. Two-dimensional echocardiography reveal anterior-superior displacement of the outflow ventricular septum, causing stenosis of the subpulmonic right ventricular outflow.

Cardiac catheterization and selective angiocardiography are of vital importance to elucidate anatomic anomalies in doubtful cases.

Tricuspid atresia is characterized by appearance of severe cyanosis together with dyspnea and hypoxic spells shortly after birth.

Auscultation reveals a systolic or continuous murmur at the base or the apex due to atrial or VSD.

The ECG shows P waves, LVH with left axis deviation and A-V block.

X-ray chest shows oligemic lung fields. There is marked predominance of the left heart. The base of the heart is narrow and right border is straight because of absent or hypoplastic right ventricle, provided that right atrium is not markedly dilated.

Truncus is characterized by presence of marked cyanosis at birth. Auscultation reveals a loud systolic murmur.

X-ray shows cardiomegaly and oligemic lung fields, provided that associated pulmonary atresia is not present.

Total anomalous pulmonary venous return (TAPVR) is characterized by marked cyanosis as a result of right-to-left shunt. ECG reveals RVH. Incomplete bundle branch block may or may not be present.

Eisenmenger complex is characterized by reversal of the shunt from left-to-right to right-to-left in cases of such defects as ventricular septal or patent ductus arteriosus, thereby causing marked cyanosis. The condition carries poor prognosis.

Congestive Heart Failure

Here, cyanosis is predominantly peripheral as a result of delayed venous return. Remaining manifestations of heart failure are: right-sided raised jugular venous pressure (JVP), hepatomegaly, splenomegaly in infants, edema, basal crepitations; left-sided tachypnea, orthopnea, chest retraction, cough, sweating over head in infants.

Cyanosis Related to Abnormal Hemoglobin

Methemoglobinemia may produce a blue tint that is less bright and more leaden than cyanosis encountered in respiratory or cardiac disease.

Its causes in infants include poisoning from nitrite, aniline dyes or drugs like phenacetin, sulfonamides and dapsone.

In older children, nitrobenzene-containing drugs may be responsible for methemoglobinemia.

There is a condition, familial congenital methemoglobinemia, that results from abnormal hemoglobin M. Inheritance shows autosomal dominant pattern.

Deficiency of nicotinamide adenine dinucleotide (NADH)-methemoglobin reductase (diaphorase) is an autosomal recessive disorder with cyanosis.

FURTHER READING

1. Green M. *Pediatric Diagnosis*, 6th edn. Philadelphia: Saunders 1998.
2. Singh MK, Kumar V. The newborn with cyanosis and tachypnea. In: Gupte S, Saxena A (Eds). *Recent Advances in Pediatrics (Special Vol 16: Pediatric Cardiology)*. New Delhi: Jaypee 2006: 105-126.
3. Ushay HM. Cyanosis. In: Adam HM, Foy JM (Eds). *Signs and Symptoms in Pediatrics*. Illinois: American Academy of Pediatrics 2015:145-159.

CHAPTER 15

Deafness

BACKGROUND

The term *'deafness'* denotes inability to hear with or without amplification. The term *'hearing loss'* means impairment of hearing ability. The deafness is rarely complete. The disability may have significant effect on normal speech and social development of the child. The overall incidence of hearing impairment is around 1–2/1,000 children. In our busy pediatric outpatient department (OPD) at Jammu, I was, on an average, seeing a dozen cases or so a week. Admittedly, a much larger number apparently goes to the ear, nose and throat (ENT) OPD or remains undetected. According to a conservative estimate, in India alone, there are around 35 million children with hearing impairment of varying grades.

Deafness may well be congenital or acquired, temporary or permanent, organic or nonorganic, peripheral or central, conductive, and mild, moderate or profound.

It is customary to think of deafness as central or peripheral. Central deafness results from auditory deficit originating along central nervous system (CNS) from the proximal eighth nerve to the cortex from such insults as seizures, tumors, demyelinating disease, Landau-Kleffner syndrome, etc.

Peripheral deafness refers to dysfunction in sound transmission through the external or middle ear as also its conversion into neural cavity at the inner ear and eighth nerve. It may be of three types:
1. Conductive in which the disease affects the sound-conducting mechanism of the ear, say middle or the external ear as in impacted wax, foreign body, perforation of tympanic membrane, otitis media with effusion, cholesteatoma, and osteosclerosis, etc.
2. Sensorineural in which the disease involves the perceiving apparatus, say cochlea, eighth nerve or any other area up to the brainstem as in lesion of acoustic division of eighth nerve or destruction of hair cells in inner ear.
3. Mixed in which conductive and sensorineural deafness coexist.

Remember, only around 6% hearing-impaired children have profound hearing loss. Others manage to retain some hearing. Nevertheless, even mild or unilateral deafness has a detrimental effect on development and performance of the child. In particular, deafness occurring early in life is likely to affect the development of speech, behavior, attention, academic attainment, social development and emotional development.

All infants and children suspected of deafness may not really be deaf. For instance, a child may apparently appear to be deaf just because he is unmindful of commands from his intense involvement in play or certain such activities. Such a response may also be encountered in a child with bad manners and indiscipline. A mentally subnormal child may well be slow in his hearing response though he may not actually be deaf. Inadequate social responsiveness, as in autism, often makes the child appear deaf.

Early identification of deafness is through high index of suspicion (high-risk register criteria) and screening methods. For this, it is important to have a sound knowledge of the timetable of development of normal hearing and speech (Box 15.1).

BOX 15.1: Timetable of development of various phases of hearing and speech.

0–3 months	Startles to loud noise, awakens to sounds, blink reflex or eye widening to noise
3–4 months	Quietens to mother's voice, stops playing and starts listening to new sounds, looks for source of new sounds that are not in sight
6–9 months	Enjoys musical toys, coos and gurgles with inflection, says "mama", "papa"
12–15 months	Responds to his name, responds to "no", follows simple requests, develops an expressive vocabulary of 3–5 words, imitates certain sounds
18–24 months	Knows body parts, develops expressive vocabulary at least 20–50 words, uses 2-word sentences, half of speech intelligible for strangers
36 months	Develops expressive vocabulary of 500 words, uses 4–5 word sentences, speech 80% intelligible for strangers, understands some words

HISTORY

History should include information on maternal infections (STORCH), consumption of drugs by the mother during pregnancy, birth asphyxia, severe hyperbilirubinemia, septicemia, meningitis, administration of ototoxic drugs during neonatal period, etc. Developmental delay, particularly in speech, should be a wakeup call for evaluation for hearing loss.

PHYSICAL EXAMINATION

In a young child, it is important to exclude wax in the external ear employing an auroscope.

As a rule, all infants, especially the high-risk ones (various in utero infections like rubella, use of ototoxic drugs during pregnancy, perinatal hypoxia, congenital deafness in the family, CNS infections), should be screened in early weeks of life and, in any case, by 3–4 months of age. The usual neonate responses include a loud noise by a startle reaction, a facial grimace, blinking, gross motor movements, quieting of crying or crying when quiet, opening the eyes when closed, inhibiting suckling responses, a catch in respiration, and a change in the heart rate. A 3- to 4-month infant responds by turning his head toward the sound. A good screening test consists in a rattle held 25 cm away from the neonate's ear, on a level with the ear, the movements of the eyes or head in response to sound are noted.

SPECIAL TESTS

Following screening procedures, a resort to sophisticated audiographic evaluation in a diagnostic setting is warranted. It comprises auditory brainstem response (ABR) test/brainstem electric response audiometry (BERA) in which electrical signals are picked up by surface electrodes originating from acoustic signs passing to the brainstem from the cochlear nerve.

IMPORTANT DIFFERENTIALS

Congenital Deafness

Genetic

Familial (early onset):
Syndromal: Waardenburg syndrome, characterized by white forelock, lateral displacement of inner canthi, broad nasal bridge, heterochromia of iris and deafness (Fig. 15.1), is an important cause of congenital deafness. Other syndromes accompanied by deafness include Pendred, Usher, Treacher

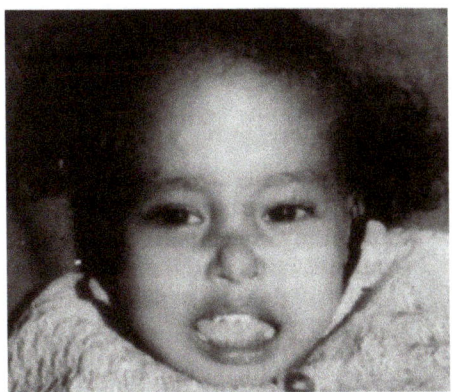

Fig. 15.1: Waardenburg syndrome (type 1). Note the white forelock, lateral displacement of inner canthi, broad nasal bridge and heterochromia. The child had sensorineural deafness as well.

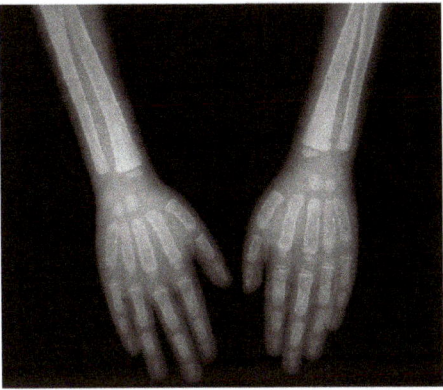

Fig. 15.2: Hypothyroidism. Note that only two carpal bones are visualized in this 2.5 years old child (who presented with delayed milestones, coarse facial features and hearing loss). Bone age is, therefore, just 1 year, i.e. retarded. Diagnosis of hypothyroidism was supported by T_4, and thyroid-stimulating hormone (TSH) levels.

Collins, Pierre Robin, Crouzon, Klippel-Feil, trisomy 13 (Patau), 16 (Edwards), and 21 (Down).

Congenital defects: Association with cleft palate.

Nongenetic

Drug teratogenicity: Quinine, thalidomide, aminoglycosides, vancomycin, neomycin, irradiation.

Intrauterine infections: Rubella, cytomegalovirus (CMV), syphilis, human immunodeficiency virus (HIV). About one-third infants of mothers who had rubella in the first 3 months of pregnancy are likely to suffer from hearing impairment which may well be unilateral or partial. Just because no history of rubella during pregnancy is forthcoming is not a good reason to exclude this infection.

Metabolic/endocrinal: A proportion of infants with hypothyroidism (Fig. 15.2) may suffer from hearing impairment.

Postnatal

Genetic

Familial (late onset):

Syndromal: Hunter-Hurler, von Recklinghausen, Alport, and Alström.

Nongenetic

Mechanical: Wax and foreign body are important causes of partial deafness. These block the conduction of hearing by mechanical obstruction.

Infections: Meningitis, encephalitis, measles, mumps, syphilis, and recurrent otitis media are important causes of acquired deafness.

Drugs: Aminoglycosides, ibuprofen, quinine, chloroquine, salicylates, vancomycin, vincristine, furosemide, macrolides and platinum.

Toxic: Severe neonatal hyperbilirubinemia, regardless of the etiologic factor, is a potential precursor of deafness. Though it is usually accompanied by other signs of kernicterus such as athetosis, at times, deafness may be the only finding.

Brain damage: Cerebral palsy, mental retardation, very-low-birth-weight (VLBW), severe asphyxia, and prolonged mechanical ventilation are frequently accompanied by deafness. According to one estimate, one-fifth to one-fourth children with cerebral palsy suffer from hearing loss, the incidence being higher in athetotic than in spastic cerebral palsy.

FURTHER READING

1. Katbamna B, Crumpton T. The child with hearing loss. In: Gupte S (Ed). *Recent Advances in Pediatrics*. New Delhi: Jaypee 2002:395-420.
2. Smith RJ. Deafness: from bedside to bench and back. *Lancet* 2002;360:656-657.
3. Tharpe AM, Sladen DP, Rothplete A. Hearng loss. In: Adam HM, Foy JM (Eds). *Signs and Symptoms in Pediatrics*. Illinois: American Academy of Pediatrics 2015:451-458.

CHAPTER 16

Delayed Puberty

BACKGROUND

The term, *delayed puberty*, denotes absence of onset of puberty (signs of sexual development in the form of increase in volume of testes in boys and breast budding in girls) by 14 years in boys and 13 years in girls.

We must remember that environmental and genetic factors have significant influence on onset of puberty. In America, for instance, white girls have relatively delayed puberty as compared to their white counterparts. The group of girls in whom strenuous physical exercise and slimness are the hallmark (e.g. athletes, sports girls, gymnasts, ballet dancers, etc.) are known to have quite a delayed puberty.

HISTORY

History and physical examination should obtain information on significant nutritional deficiencies (both primary and secondary), chronic illnesses such as chronic diarrhea/malabsorption, tuberculosis, asthma, anosmia, etc. and chronic consumption of drugs such as steroids, family history of delayed puberty [constitutional delay of growth and puberty (CDGP)].

PHYSICAL EXAMINATION

Besides, a good general and systemic examination, attention needs to be given to testicular size, phallic size, pubic hair, breast development, growth velocity, etc. Whereas growth velocity is all right for child's chronologic age, it is subnormal in hypogonadotrophic hypogonadism. In the latter, pubertal progression too is slow compared to the normal in CDGP.

It is of value to record Tanner's pubertal staging, height measurement, body proportions, weight, etc. as also to identify accompanying obesity, if any.

INVESTIGATIONS

Special investigations include:
- Determination of bone age
- Endocrinal studies with special reference to basal levels of sex hormones, gonadotropins, adrenal androgens, prolactin gonadotropin-releasing hormone (GnRH) stimulation and human chorionic gonadotropin (hCG) stimulation tests
- Karyotyping
- Testicular biopsy
- Pelvic ultrasonography (girls)
- Vaginal smears in girls (girls).

DIFFERENTIALS

Constitutional Delay of Growth and Puberty

Genetic factors may cause delayed development and delayed puberty because of slow onset in gonadotropin release. There is frequently a positive history of "late maturers" in the pedigree chart of the index case. In due course, maturation begins to proceed normally. There is, therefore, as a rule, no role of any therapy, except for the psychotherapy for the associated psychological problems usually secondary to the associated short stature.

Delayed Puberty Associated with Chronic Systemic Illnesses

Chronic systemic disorders such as chronic malnutrition, chronic diarrhea/malabsorption syndrome (celiac disease, tropical sprue, cystic fibrosis, etc.), chronic anemia, and anorexia nervosa.

Hypogonadotropic Hypogonadism (Failure of GnRH and/or Low FSH and LH)

Two varieties are recognized. In the congenital or genetic variety, lack of gonadotropin causes delayed testicular maturational. The subjects with this condition are tall but have small histologically immature testes. It is encountered in Kallmann syndrome (eunuchoid stature, infantile genitalia, color blindness, anosmia, and Leydig cell hypofunction), Pasqualini syndrome or fertile eunuch (eunuchoid stature, normal genitalia or a normal penis with small testes and reduced number of Leydig cells), Laurence-

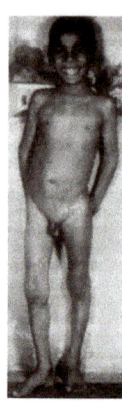

Fig. 16.1: Delayed puberty of acquired variety in a 17-year-old boy with hypothyroidism.

Moon–Biedl syndrome, congenital anomalies, and primary gonadotropin deficiency (hypopituitarism).

In the acquired variety, the operative factors include intracranial tumors, inflammatory and traumatic lesions, irradiation of hypothalamic-pituitary region, hypothyroidism (Fig. 16.1), and hyperprolactinemia.

Hypergonadotropic Hypogonadism/Primary Gonadal Failure (High FSH and LH)

In the congenital or genetic variety, etiologic conditions include Turner syndrome (45 XO), Klinefelter syndrome (47XXY), and Noonan syndrome.

In the acquired variety, causative factors include mumps-related orchitis, anticancer therapy for gonads, vanishing testes syndrome, testosterone biosynthetic defects, infiltrative or autoimmune diseases of gonads.

FURTHER READING

1. Gupte S, Koff AW. Pediatric endocrinology. In: Gupte S (Ed). *The Short Textbook of Pediatrics*, 13th edn. New Delhi: Jaypee 2020.
2. Kelnor CJ, Butler GE. Abnormal puberty. In: Mcintosh N, Helms PJ, Smyth RL (Eds). *Forfar and Arneil's Textbook of Pediatrics*, 6th edn. New York: Churchill Livingstone 2003: 489-496.

CHAPTER 17

Diarrhea

BACKGROUND

Diarrhea ranks among the "three chief killers" of our infants and children. Almost 10% of preschool mortality and 25% of infant mortality is ascribed to diarrhea (Fig. 17.1). The magnitude of the morbidity too is considerable.

In terms of stool volume, diarrhea is defined as loose stools of more than 10 mL/kg/day in infants and more than 200 g/24 hour in subsequent ages. In view of the logistic difficulty to accurately measure the volume of the stool in clinical environment, diarrhea may be defined as the passage of more than or equal to three watery stools per day.

Acute diarrhea is defined as an increase in frequency, fluidity, and volume of stools of short duration. It is responsible for around 20% of pediatric admissions in India and other developing countries. In the peak diarrheal season (summer and rainy seasons), 75% of pediatric beds may be occupied by children suffering from it (Box 17.1).

Persistent diarrhea means an acute episode of diarrhea (invariably infective) that persists for 2 weeks or beyond. Major malabsorptive disorders such as celiac disease, cystic fibrosis or endemic tropical sprue do not fall under this domain.

The risk factors for an acute attack of diarrhea or gastroenteritis persisting beyond 2 weeks period include:
- Six months to 1-year-age group of patients; after 2 years of age, persistent diarrhea is infrequent.
- Low birth weight (LBW), prematurity, and malnutrition, especially when accompanied by vitamin A deficiency
- Artificially fed infants
- Diarrheal episode accompanied by blood and mucus in stools, e.g. disease caused by enteropathogenic or aggressive adherent *Escherichia coli*, *Shigella*, *Campylobacter jejuni*, and rotavirus, especially in infants under 3 months.
- Indiscriminate use of oral rehydration salts (ORS), especially with high content of sugar and intake of fruit juices and carbonated drinks.
- Lactose intolerance
- Cow milk protein (CMP) allergy
- Sepsis and other systemic infections
- A preceding diarrheal episode in the recent past. Deterioration in nutritional status, insult to small bowel mucosa, contamination of artificial formula feed, and osmotic diarrhea are some of the factors that may

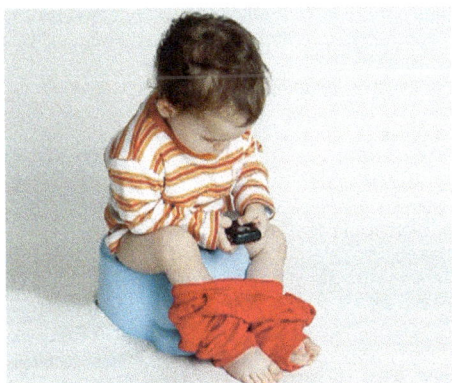

Fig. 17.1: Diarrheal disease is a leading cause of morbidity and mortality in infancy and childhood.

BOX 17.1: Causes of acute diarrhea.

Etiology of acute diarrhea

- *Enteric infections*
  - *Bacteria:* Escherichia coli, Shigella, Salmonella, Staphylococcus, Cholera vibrio, Yersinia enterocolitica, Campylobacter jejuni, Clostridium difficile, Aeromonas hydrophila, Vibrio parahaemolyticus, Plesiomonas shigelloides
  - *Viruses:* Rotavirus, Norwalk and allied viruses, enterovirus, influenza virus, measles virus, etc.
  - *Parasites:* Entameba histolytica, Giardia lamblia, Cryptosporidium, Cyclospora cayetanensis, Isospora, Hymenolepis nana, Trichuris trichiura, malarial parasite
  - *Fungi:* Candida albicans
  - *Parenteral:* Upper respiratory tract infection (URI), otitis media, tonsillitis, pneumonia, urinary tract infection, etc.
- **Drugs:** Antibiotics
- *Dietetic/nutritional:* Overfeeding, starvation, food allergy, food poisoning, etc.
- Nonspecific

singularly or in combination contribute to causation of persistent diarrhea
- *Intestinal parasitosis*: Heavy giardiasis is an important factor in tropical settings.

Three clinical patterns of persistent diarrhea have been recognized. These are:
1. Several motions per day without any adverse effect on nutritional status growth and development.
2. Several motions without dehydration, but with malnutrition, growth retardation, etc.
3. Several motions with dehydration that is difficult to control with ORS.

Such associated manifestations as progressive weight loss, malnutrition, anorexia malabsorption, and secondary infections are usual.

Chronic diarrhea has been differently defined by various authorities. There is, however, some consensus that this designation should be restricted to "diarrhea of at least 2-week duration, or three attacks of diarrhea during the last 3 months". Significant malabsorption as in celiac disease, cystic fibrosis or tropical sprue is usual and is a glaring feature of this condition. Box 17.2 list the overall etiology of chronic diarrhea. Box 17.3 lists common causes of chronic diarrhea in India. This should be appreciated that, though a large number of conditions can cause chronic diarrhea, in practice only some select conditions monopolize the situation in India.

HISTORY

Acute Diarrhea

History must, in the first place, verify the main complaint of diarrhea for its accuracy. Are stools indeed several in number with increased fluidity and volume? Subjects with loose watery stools exceeding 10/24 hours in number are in danger of developing dehydration, particularly if intake is restricted.

Remember that often diarrhea is overdiagnosed in newborns and infants who are entirely on breastfeeding. Babies on only breast milk not only pass frequent motions–frequently after each feed; at times even 24/24 hours–but the stools are also loose (unless he is suffering from Hirschsprung's disease). The color of stools may be bright green. There may also be curd in stools in early weeks.

Many babies are brought to the doctor with complaint that they pass frequent green small motions. The cause is almost always underfeeding. Hence, the name "starvation stools". They need to be adequately fed rather than managed with antidiarrheal drug(s).

How long has the child had diarrhea? Any vomiting? Any blood in stools? Is there any abdominal pain? Any relationship with feeding? Did it start following any special food item, say ice cream? Any history of fever? Does he pass worms in stools or vomitus?

BOX 17.2: Etiology of chronic diarrhea.

Intestinal mucosal causes
- Altered integrity
  - Infections/infestations: Viral, bacterial, fungal, parasitic, etc.
  - Cow's milk protein allergy/intolerance
  - Soy protein allergy/intolerance
  - Inflammatory bowel disease
- Altered immune function
  - Human immunodeficiency virus (HIV) or acquired immunodeficiency syndrome (AIDS)
  - Autoimmune enteropathy
- Altered function
  - Abetalipoproteinemia
  - Acrodermatitis enteropathica
  - Tropical sprue
  - Selective folate deficiency
  - Defects in Cl^-, HCO_3^-, Na^+/H^+
- Altered digestive function
  - Cystic fibrosis
- Altered surface area
  - Celiac disease
  - Malnutrition
  - Iron deficiency anemia
  - Endemic tropical sprue
  - Hookworm infestation
- Altered secretory function
  - Enterotoxin—producing bacteria
  - Vasoactive peptides—secreting tumors
- Altered anatomical structures
  - Congenital megacolon
  - Partial small bowel obstruction
- Altered motility
  - Malnutrition
  - Diabetes mellitus
  - Intestinal pseudo-obstruction
  - Scleroderma

Intestinal intraluminal causes
- Excessive intake of carbonated drinks
- Excessive intake of sorbitol, lactulose, magnesium salts
- Carbohydrate malabsorption
- Congenital monosaccharide malabsorption

Pancreatic causes
- Cystic fibrosis
- Chronic pancreatitis

BOX 17.3: Causes of chronic diarrhea in Indian children.

- Protein-energy malnutrition (PEM)
- Iron deficiency anemia
- Excessive consumption of fluids (carbonated drinks, fruit juices, etc.)
- Intestinal parasites (*Giardia lamblia, hookworm, roundworm, Entamoeba histolytica, Strongyloides stercoralis, Trichuris trichiura, tapeworms*, etc.)
- Intestinal infection (enteropathogens, *Mycobacterium tuberculosis*, etc.)
- Celiac disease
- Cystic fibrosis (CF)
- Endemic tropical sprue
- Carbohydrate intolerance
- Irritable colon syndrome
- Ulcerative colitis
- Miscellaneous (regional ileitis, anatomic defects, protein-losing enteropathy, etc.)

Is there any weight loss, drowsiness, abdominal distention, oliguria or anuria? Information on these points is important to evaluate severity of dehydration, if any.

Always enquire if there is previous history of recurrent diarrhea? The apparently acute diarrhea may well be related to the chronic problem such as malabsorption syndrome, intestinal infestations or irritable bowel syndrome.

Persistent Diarrhea

It is important to obtain the following information:
- How was the acute diarrheal episode handled?
- Any history of intake of much-too-much of ORS, carbonated drinks or fruit juices?
- Any suggestion of a systemic infection, including sepsis.
- Any history of cow's milk or other food intolerance.

Chronic Diarrhea

The importance of a carefully taken history cannot be overemphasized. Most valuable pointers and clues are likely to be obtained from answers to the following question:
- Did the symptoms appear early in infancy (cystic fibrosis), or after the first 6 months of life (celiac disease)?
- Was there any relationship between onset of symptoms and introduction of supplementary feeds (lactose intolerance), or cereals (celiac disease)?
- Is there a family history of chronic diarrhea (cystic fibrosis, celiac disease, hereditary lactose intolerance, etc.)?
- Is there any history of intolerance to an item of food, i.e. wheat, barley, rye (celiac disease), or milk (lactose intolerance)?
- Was the child failing to thrive from early infancy, or did he start growth failure after introduction of a semisolid food? The latter situation is very much suggestive of celiac disease?
- How is the appetite? It is generally increased in cystic fibrosis and in some children suffering from giardiasis. In celiac disease, it is invariably lost. Mothers of celiacs often express surprise "as to how children who eat so little can pass such voluminous stools".
- Does the mother feel that the child eats like a glutton? When, in spite of this observation, the child is suffering from failure to thrive, one must entertain the possibility of cystic fibrosis. We have encountered this situation in some children suffering from symptomatic giardiasis as well.
- What do the stools look like? Large, pale, frothy, and very foul-smelling stools are highly suggestive of steatorrhea. Characteristically, white, fatty stools with plenty of undigested material are most often a feature of giardiasis.
- Was the persistent diarrhea preceded by an attack of acute gastroenteritis? This situation is highly indicative of secondary lactose intolerance. The condition is fairly common and the stools in it are watery, profuse, accompanied by excess of flatus, and have very foul odor. The perianal area appears raw and red in a great majority of these children.
- Is there history of excessive consumption of fluids (carbonated soft drinks, fruit juices, etc.)?

PHYSICAL EXAMINATION

Acute Diarrhea

The major thrust is on evaluation of hydration status as per the World Health Organization (WHO) guidelines and nutritional status.

Persistent Diarrhea

The major thrust is on assessment of nutritional status (which is invariably affected) and presence of superimposed dehydration (which is less frequent).

Chronic Diarrhea

Thrust is on assessment of growth and development in view of chronic impact on nutrition which is likely to be hampered.

RELEVANT INVESTIGATIONS

Acute Diarrhea

- Serum electrolytes
- Stool microscopy for ova and cysts
- Stool culture.

Persistent Diarrhea

- Meticulous stool microscopy for ova and cysts on at least 6 successive days.
- Stool culture
- Stool for reducing substances.

Chronic Diarrhea

- Every child with chronic diarrhea must have meticulous microscopic examinations of stools at least on 3 (preferably 6) consecutive days before one rules out presence of intestinal infestations.
- The presence of numerous large fat globules, after staining with Sudan-III or eosin, is indicative of steatorrhea.
- Chemical examination of stools for 24-hour stool fat is, however, a more reliable index of steatorrhea.
- Remaining tests include:
  – D-xylose test
  – Endoscopic jejunal biopsy
  – Intestinal radiology
  – Schilling test
  – Sweat chloride test
  – Tryptic activity
  – Lactose tolerance test, etc.

The choice of test(s) is dictated by the clinical situation.

IMPORTANT DIFFERENTIALS

Acute Diarrhea

Infective Diarrhea

Enteric infections are undoubtedly responsible for a large majority of pediatric diarrhea cases. *Enterobacteriaceae* responsible for diarrhea include *E. coli* (strains such as enteropathogenic, diarrheagenic, enterotoxigenic, and enteroinvasive), *Shigella, Salmonella, Staphylococcus, Vibrio cholerae, Yersinia enterocolitica, Campylobacter, Clostridium difficile, Klebsiella,* and *Pseudomonas aeruginosa.*

Antibiotics such as lincomycin, clindamycin, and ampicillin may precipitate pseudomembranous enterocolitis, often from growth of *C. difficile*. Manifestations are sudden onset of diarrhea (as such or bloody), abdominal distention, and fever. Gross fluid loss kills 50% of the patients in spite of treatment.

Virus such as rotavirus, Norwalk-like agent, Hawaii virus, adenovirus, asteroid virus, calicivirus, coronavirus, enterovirus, and minirotavirus have been found to be responsible for majority of the cases of acute infective diarrhea.

Rotavirus is the most frequently encountered virus in diarrheal stools in nearly all areas in which it has been pointedly looked for. The peak incidence occurs in the age group 9–12 months. Excepting newborns, it has been observed to have a predilection for winter months in India as well as abroad. Transmission is by feco-oral route. The incubation period is usually less than 48 hours (range 1–7 days). The average duration of illness is 5–7 days. Its important clinical feature is that vomiting usually precedes the onset of diarrhea. About 30–50% cases show slight fever, 25% mucus in stools, and just an occasional case shows blood in stools.

Norwalk and Norwalk-like agents are associated with outbreaks of generally mild gastroenteritis occurring in school, community or family settings. The incubation period is around 48 hours. The attack is usually mild and self-limited, lasting 12–24 hours in majority of the cases. Vomiting, abdominal pain, anorexia, headache, myalgia, and malaise are important features of diarrhea associated with these viruses.

Parasites responsible for acute diarrhea include *Giardia lamblia* and *Entamoeba histolytica*.

The usual presentation in symptomatic giardiasis is with vague abdominal pain, acute on chronic diarrhea, poor appetite, failure to thrive, and nutritional deficiencies. Occasionally, acute dysentery-like manifestations may occur. Even transient ulcerative colitis has been described.

In amebiasis, the symptoms range from mild gastrointestinal upset to acute diarrhea/dysentery or chronic colitis. Unlike adults, who may have only loose motions, children usually pass mucus (free of pus) together with blood. The latter is generally not mixed with fecal matter or mucus. Abdominal pain and tenesmus may also accompany.

Cryptosporidiosis in immunocompromised hosts may cause severe diarrhea.

Strongyloidiasis, though uncommon in our country, may manifest with severe diarrhea, pain in abdomen, mild itching, and urticaria at the site of penetration into the skin and chest manifestations simulating Loeffler syndrome.

Trichuriasis is characterized by prolonged diarrhea with blood-streaked stools, right lower abdominal pain, tenesmus, malnutrition with anemia, rectal prolapse, and allergic manifestations like eosinophilia, and Charcot-Leyden crystals in stools. In case of heavy infestation, numerous worms may be seen on the surface of the prolapsed rectal mucosa.

Dwarf tapeworm (*Hymenolepis nana*) infestation may manifest with sudden onset of mucus or bloody diarrhea with abdominal pain.

Severe ascariasis may cause allergic necrotizing hemorrhagic enteritis. Manifestations include diarrhea, abdominal pain, vomiting, and gross flatulence.

Fungi such as *Candida albicans* may cause acute diarrhea in children suffering from a serious illness, particularly when on prolonged antibiotic therapy.

Parenteral diarrhea may occur secondary to infections such as upper respiratory tract infection (URI), otitis media, tonsillitis, pneumonia, urinary tract infection, malaria, septicemia, or peritonitis especially accompanying appendicitis.

Antibiotic-associated diarrhea (pseudomembranous colitis) may result from growth of *C. difficile, Staphylococcus aureus* or *C. perfringens*, following therapy with clindamycin, ampicillin, penicillin or cephalosporins. All antibiotics with exception of vancomycin stand implicated in its etiology.

Noninfective Diarrhea

Dietary factors include overfeeding, starvation, food allergy, and food poisoning.

Osmotic diarrhea may occur in infants consuming a very large amount of sugar in the feed. The overwhelming osmotic load in the intestine pulls lot of water into the lumen, causing diarrhea. Such a diarrhea, unless it is allowed to become protracted, causes no such problem as dehydration or undernutrition.

Drugs causing diarrhea include ampicillin, iron, para-aminosalicylate (PAS), phenothiazines, nalidixic acid, thiabendazole, carbamazepine, niclosamide, dichlorophen, and overdose of thyroxine. Antibiotic induced pseudomembranous enterocolitis, in which *C. difficile* is usually cultured, is described under "infective diarrhea" in this very chapter.

Persistent Diarrhea

Causes of acute diarrhea are yet not clear. All that we know is that certain risk factors makes the child, usually an infant, vulnerable to it. The illness is preventable through attention to risk factors and manageable, through predominantly dietary manipulation.

Chronic Diarrhea

Protein-energy Malnutrition

This is by far the most common cause of chronic diarrhea in developing countries. The causes of diarrhea in protein-energy malnutrition (PEM) include:
- Recurrent superimposed gastrointestinal tract (GIT) infections, including infestations;
- Effect of PEM *per se* on intestinal mucosa, causing reversible villus atrophy and malabsorption, inhibition of enzyme disaccharidase mainly lactase which results in disaccharide intolerance (mainly lactose), and damage to pancreas; and
- Iron deficiency anemia (a common accompaniment of PEM) which can, on its own, lead to enteropathy by damaging the intestinal epithelium.

Iron-deficiency: Anemia

As it is mentioned earlier, chronic iron-deficiency anemia (no matter whether it occurs as such or in association with PEM) is capable of causing villus atrophy, resulting in absorptive defect and chronic diarrhea.

Intestinal Parasitic Infestations

Giardia lamblia, Entamoeba histolytica, H. nana, and *Ancylostoma duodenale* are now known to be responsible for a significant proportion of cases of chronic diarrhea. In addition, *Trichuris trichiura, Strongyloides stercoralis, Taenia solium, T. saginata,* and infrequently *Ascaris lumbricoides* may account for a small proportion to cases.

The widespread occurrence of PEM, iron-deficiency anemia, and intestinal infestations in our settings demands that, in our approach to chronic diarrhea in pediatric practice, these three causative entities are carefully excluded. Then, and only then, the child should be subjected to a battery of investigations, most of which are cumbersome.

Endemic Tropical Sprue

Classically, the patient is a grown-up child with chronic diarrhea, malabsorption, considerable malnutrition, and anemia.

Steatorrhea is usually moderate to gross. D-xylose test shows poor intestinal absorption. Partial or subtotal villus atrophy is present. Schilling test is almost always abnormal, indicating that intestinal mucosal atrophy and absorptive dysfunction are not limited to the upper gut but are present in the ileum as well.

Response to folic acid, tetracyclines, or both are gratifying.

Celiac Disease

Though one of the most common causes of chronic diarrhea in the West, celiac disease is relatively less frequent in pediatric population in our settings.

Also termed as gluten-sensitivity and gluten-induced enteropathy, the disorder usually manifests a few months after introduction of gluten-containing foods often a wheat preparation in the feeding program. Chronic diarrhea with large, pale, highly foul-smelling stools, which stick to the "pottie". Growth failure, anemia and other vitamin and nutritional deficiencies, potbelly, irritability, and anorexia are the classical presenting features.

To establish functional and histological defect of small intestinal mucosa, you must demonstrate abnormally high 24-hour stool fat, poor absorption in D-xylose test, and villus atrophy in peroral jejunal biopsy. Serologic markers are now being increasingly employed in screening and diagnosis of chronic diarrhea.

Responses to elimination of gluten from diet and, later, to gluten challenges are essential to establish the diagnosis.

Cystic Fibrosis

This condition is a common cause of chronic diarrhea, beginning fairly early in infancy, in the European countries. Its recognition in Indian children is a recent happening.

In this genetic disorder, involving the exocrine pancreas and other exocrine glands, the child manifests with chronic/recurrent diarrhea and respiratory infections (especially from early infancy), failure to thrive despite exceptionally good appetite, and multiple nutritional deficiencies. Stools are characteristically steatorrheic but may be loose. An obstinate catarrhal cough or "frog in the throat" may be present ever since first week of life. Abdominal distention, palpable liver, clubbing and higher incidence of rectal prolapse, and nasal polyps are the other findings.

An important observation by the mother is "a line of salt on the forehead after sweating" or "the baby tastes salty when kissed".

Clinical suspicion must lead to fat balance studies and D-xylose test to establish that steatorrhea is not enterogenous in origin. Poor tryptic activity lends support to clinical diagnosis. But, a high sweat chloride (>60 mEq/L) is a "must" to confirm the diagnosis.

Carbohydrate Malabsorption

Disaccharide malabsorption, secondary to conditions such as acute gastroenteritis, PEM, cow's milk allergy, cystic fibrosis, celiac disease or drugs like neomycin, has emerged as a common cause of protracted diarrhea. Besides watery diarrhea (stools contain very little solid matter and are acidic), the patient has excoriation of perianal area and buttocks, abdominal distention and abdominal pain. Response to withdrawal of the offending sugar from the diet, points favorably to this diagnosis.

Confirmation of diagnosis is from:
- Low pH of stools (<6) while the patient is on modest dietary intake of the offending sugar(s)
- Presence of reducing substances in stools
- Disaccharide (usually lactose) tolerance test
- Breath test involving measurement of H^+
- *Barium meal*: The suspected sugar is added to a barium meal. Defect in its absorption causes fluid retention in intestinal lumen, intestinal hurry, and coarsening of the mucosal folds
- Peroral jejunal biopsy for assay of the enzyme(s).

Monosaccharide malabsorption, secondary to several conditions, has also been emerging as an important factor in causation of protracted diarrhea. Exclusion of glucose and galactose from diet with intravenous feeding for some days in serious cases gives gratifying response.

Cow's Milk Allergy

About 1–2% infants may have hypersensitivity to cow's milk (beta lactoglobulin in most; casein, lactalbumin, bovine serum globulin, and albumin in some).

Manifestations include protracted diarrhea (usually watery), vomiting, colic, skin rash (eczema or urticaria), rhinitis, otitis media, chronic cough with wheeze, anemia, and poor weight gain.

Eosinophilia, glucosuria, sucrosuria, lactosuria, aminoaciduria, renal tubular damage, and acidosis may occur in some cases. Smear from rectal mucus shows eosinophilia.

Response to omission of cow's milk from feeding regime is excellent.

Irritable Bowel Syndrome (Toddler's Diarrhea)

The term refers to a group of children, aged 1–3 years, who suffer from recurrent diarrhea and abdominal pain. Yet, they thrive well.

Since recurrences occur at the time of psychological stress and strain (say, departure of mother on a journey), and in view of a strong familial tendency, the condition is believed to be of psychogenic origin.

Crohn's Disease

This occurs rarely in children. Manifestations, besides chronic diarrhea, include crampy abdominal pain (worse on eating and reduced after defecation), malnutrition, palpable abdominal masses, perianal lesions, aphthous stomatitis, polyarthritis, clubbing, and erythema nodosum.

Sigmoidoscopy, rectal biopsy, endoscopy, and upper and lower GI barium series are needed to establish the diagnosis.

Ulcerative Colitis

In this rare disorder of childhood, manifestations include recurrent bloody diarrhea, intermittent bouts of crampy abdominal pain, anorexia, weight loss, arthralgia, and growth retardation.

Rectal examination, sigmoidoscopy, endoscopy, and barium enema are required to confirm the diagnosis.

Acrodermatitis Enteropathica

Also called Brandt's syndrome, this familial condition, manifesting at the time of weaning, is characterized by chronic diarrhea, symmetrical bullous lesions, paronychia, and loss of hair. Skin lesions are most marked over the buttocks as also around anus and mouth, blepharitis, and conjunctivitis are frequent accompaniments.

Acquired Immunodeficiency Syndrome

Diarrhea in association with anorexia and malnutrition is often a serious problem in children with AIDS and other immunodeficiency disorders. Microorganisms (pathogenic opportunistic as well as otherwise nonpathogenic under ordinary circumstances) play an important role in the causation of chronic diarrhea and malabsorption. Cryptosporidium, an intestinal protozoan, has now emerged as an important cause of chronic diarrhea in AIDS. To begin with, diarrhea is produced watery; it tends to become chronic with unrelenting severity. Cryptosporidiosis is confirmed by identifying oocytes in feces following acid-fast staining, or in stained jejunal biopsy as round eosinophilic bodies. No drug shows encouraging anti-cryptosporidium effect.

FURTHER READING

1. Gupte S, Singh UK, Gupta RK. Antibiotic-related diarrhea. In: Gupte S (Ed). *Recent Advances in Pediatrics-12*. New Delhi: Jaypee 2002:41-48.
2. Horvath K. Chronic diarrhea and malabsorption. In: Gupte S (Ed). *Recent Advances in Pediatrics-13*. New Delhi: Jaypee 2003:1-22.
3. Patwari A, Gupte S, Anderson RA. Pediatric gastroenterology. In: Gupte S (Ed). *The Short Textbook of Pediatrics*, 13th edn. New Delhi: Jaypee 2020:549-587.
4. Ulshen MH. Diarrhea and steatorrhea. In: Adam HM, Foy JM (Eds). *Signs and Symptoms in Pediatrics*. Illinois: American Academy of Pediatrics 2015.
5. Vohra P. Inflammatory bowel disease. In: Gupte S (Ed). *Recent Advances in Pediatrics-12*. New Delhi: Jaypee 2002:23-39.

CHAPTER 18

Dyspnea

BACKGROUND

The term, *dyspnea*, refers to an uncomfortable awareness of difficulty in breathing. Quite often, it is noticed by the parents. Respiratory distress is a better term in case of dyspnea in infants and young children.

According to the New York Heart Association, dyspnea is graded as follows:
- *Grade 1*: Dyspnea on unaccustomed exertion
- *Grade 2*: Dyspnea on ordinary exertion
- *Grade 3*: Dyspnea on less than ordinary exertion
- *Grade 4*: Dyspnea at rest.

According to the American Thoracic Society, dyspnea grading is as follows:
- *Grade 0*: No breathlessness except with strenuous exercise.
- *Grade 1*: Breathlessness when hurrying on the level or walking up a slight hill.
- *Grade 2*: Walks slower than people of the same age on the level because of breathlessness or has to stop for breath when walking at own pace on level.
- *Grade 3*: Stops for breath after walking about 100 yards (96 m) or a few minutes on the level.
- *Grade 4*: Too breathless to leave the house or breathless when dressing or underdressing.

The term, *orthopnea*, denotes dyspnea in recumbent position but relieved as soon as the subject sits upright. The modes operandi revolves around increased venous return causing fall in vital capacity and increased diaphragm causing fall in end-expiratory volume during recumbent posture.

The term, *platypnea*, denotes dyspnea in sitting position.

The term, *trepopnea*, means dyspnea in decubitus position. The change to the opposite side, however, causes relief. It points to a unilateral lung disease say pleural effusion, increased empyema or a foreign body.

HISTORY

History should ascertain whether it is present at rest or occurs only on exertion. In the latter situation, what is the degree of exertion that is necessary to produce it? Does it compel the patient to sit up? Is there any cough? Is there any chest pain or fever? Any edema feet?

It is pertinent to ask for aspiration of a foreign body. Any recent trauma? Any ingestion of large amounts of agents such as salicylates?

Has there been any prior history of similar dyspnea, asthma, allergy, heart disease, trauma and drugs?

In case of the newborn, find out the precise postnatal "time" of occurrence of dyspnea. Is it accompanied by frothy blood oozing from mouth and nose? Was it a difficult delivery? Is the baby preterm or full-term? Any history of maternal diabetes, drug intake, or febrile illness? Any history of premature prolonged rupture of membranes? Is there a suggestion of aspiration of amniotic fluid, blood or meconium?

PHYSICAL EXAMINATION

Physical examination should, in particular, evaluate the respiratory, cardiovascular, and central nervous systems.

World Health Organization has in recent years been laying considerably stress on the usefulness of respiratory rate threshold for identifying pneumonia. Respiratory threshold are set at 60 for infants under 2 months, 50 for 2–12 months, and 40 for 1–5 years.

Respiratory rate is a useful predictor of lower respiratory infection in young infants. However, for hypoxia, subcostal retraction is a better predictor.

INVESTIGATIONS

In addition to the routine tests, especially complete blood picture (CBP), two basic investigations are:

1. *Radiology:* Chest X-ray
2. *Evaluation of status of ventilation:* Arterial blood gas measurement
   - Pleural tap in selected cases
   - Pulmonary function tests are helpful in critically ill patients.

Box 18.1 gives various steps of approach in differential diagnosis of respiratory distress in children.

DYSPNEA IN THE NEWBORN

Idiopathic Respiratory Distress Syndrome

Also called as *hyaline membrane disease (HMD)*, this condition, supposed to result from absence or reduction of surfactant, occurs in preterm babies, in babies born by cesarean section, and in babies of diabetic mothers.

It usually manifests within the first hour of birth with progressively increasing respiratory distress. Grunting respiration, flaring of alae nasi, retraction of ribs and sternum, and cyanosis are usually prominent. Low blood pressure, hypothermia, and hemorrhagic manifestations may complicate the clinical picture.

Auscultatory findings include poor air entry and widespread crepitations over both lungs.

Chest X-ray shows a characteristic picture ground-glass appearance and prominence of bronchial air shadows, the so-called "air bronchogram" pattern (Fig. 18.1). Generalized but patchy atelectasis occurs little later. In advanced stage, X-ray may reveal a completely opaque picture, the so-called "whiteout lung".

Table 18.1 gives the grading of findings of chest X-ray in HMD. Table 18.2 gives differential diagnosis of HMD. Gastric shake test is negative.

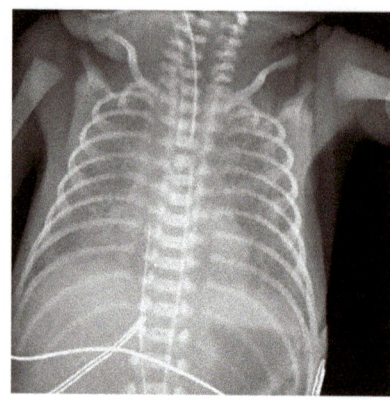

Fig. 18.1: *Respiratory distress syndrome.* Note the classical picture—bell-shaped chest, reticulogranular mottling, and air bronchogram.

TABLE 18.1: Grading of chest X-ray findings in respiratory distress syndrome (RDS).

Grade	Observation
1	Fine reticulogranular mottling with good lung expansion
2	Mottling with air bronchogram
3	Diffuse mottling, heart borders just discernible, prominent discernible air bronchogram
4	Whiteout lung in which there is a bilateral confluent opacification of lung

Massive Aspiration

Prenatal or natal aspiration of massive amount of amniotic fluid, blood or meconium occurs in situations such as postmature infants, small-for-date (SFD) infants, infants delivered by forceps or breech (fetal hypoxia, or asphyxia), prolonged labor, antepartum hemorrhage (APH), placental insufficiency, cord prolapse, and passage of meconium in utero.

At birth, the baby is asphyxiated and shocked. Within 3–4 hours, she becomes dyspneic with inspiratory intercostal retractions and expiratory grunt. High-pitched cry and absent or brisk, Moro's response may be noticed, pointing to brain damage.

Complications include atelectasis and/or emphysema, leading to pneumothorax, often with pneumonia.

Postnatal aspiration may occur in situations where the baby can suck well but his swallowing is inadequate (glossoptosis as in Pierre Robin syndrome, macroglossia, cleft palate, esophageal tumor, pharyngeal membrane, retropharyngeal tumor, etc.).

During a feed, the baby gets choked or regurgitates. This is followed by sudden dyspnea and cyanosis. Chest examination shows localized crepitations and evidence of collapse.

BOX 18.1: Various steps of approach in differential diagnosis of respiratory distress in children.

Step 1: ABC (assessment of the airway, breathing, and circulation, i.e. is the patient stable?)
Step 2: Think broadly about the differential diagnosis. Is the cause psychiatric, respiratory, or cardiovascular? Does the patient have a fever that indicates a possible infectious etiology?
Step 3: Now, gather basic information from the history:
- How old is the patient (newborn vs toddler vs adolescent)?
- How long has the shortness of breath been present?
- Sudden or insidious onset?
- Preceding events?
- Is this the first time?
- Associated symptoms?
- Underlying cardiovascular, respiratory or psychiatric problems?
- Ask whatever else seems relevant given the context, and you should have a good feeling about which of the three broad categories to pursue. Now remind yourself of the differential for that category and use it to narrow down the diagnostic possibilities. Remember, though, to keep an open mind.

Step 4: Physical examination
Step 5: Laboratory investigations/imaging
Step 6: Differential diagnosis.

TABLE 18.2: Differential diagnosis of respiratory distress syndrome (RDS).

Condition	Gestational age	History	Examination	Time of presentation	Chest X-ray
Hyaline membrane disease (HMD)	Preterms	Onset within 4 hours of birth	Tachypnea, chest indrawing, grunting, cyanosis	<6 hours	Hypoinflation, air bronchogram, reticulogranular mottling
Transient tachypnea	Term > preterms	Often operative delivery	Tachypnea, indrawing	<6 hours	Hyperinflation, prominent chest perivascular markings, interlobular septal edema
Meconium aspiration syndrome (MAS)	Term, post-term aspiration	Meconium-stained liquor at resuscitation	Meconium-stained baby with respiratory distress	<6 hours	Reticulonodular opacities in lower zone
Pneumothorax	Term > preterms	Resuscitation at birth	Transillumination test +ve, mediastinal shift	>6 hours, rarely <6 hours	Hyperlucent with collapsed lung
Pulmonary hemorrhage	Any—mostly preterms	Asphyxia, heart failure, bleeding tendency	Crepitations with marked pallor	>6 hours, rarely <6 hours	Unhelpful, whiteout
Infection	Any	Temperature instability	Not helpful	Any	Patchy changes
Congenital malformation	Term > preterms	Usually normal delivery	Depending on the malformation	<6 hours, rarely >6 hours	Diagnostic
Congenital heart disease	Term > preterms	Usually normal delivery	Cyanosis, murmurs, shock ±	>6 hours	Useful in some cases

(*Source:* Vishnu Bhat B, Serane VT. Hyaline membrane disease (HMD). In: Gupte S (Ed). *Recent Advances in Pediatrics (Special Vol 8: Emergency Pediatrics).* New Delhi: Jaypee 2001:348-365).

Meconium Aspiration Syndrome

The condition refers to the symptom-complex as a result of aspiration of meconium into the lungs in utero, during delivery or soon after birth.

In addition to respiratory distress persisting for days to weeks, the baby (usually postmature, SFD) has staining of nails, skin, and umbilical cord with meconium.

Complications include air leak syndromes (pneumothorax, emphysema, pneumomediastinum, pneumopericardium, pneumoperitoneum, etc.), hypoxic ischemic encephalopathy (HIE), persistent pulmonary hypertension (PPH), pulmonary or cerebral hemorrhage, superadded sepsis and subglottic stenosis. X-ray of chest shows overinflation (air trapping, focal emphysema, etc.), diffuse opacities (nodular), bilateral pneumonia, flat diaphragm, and retrosternal lucency. There may be evidence of air leak syndromes (Fig. 18.2).

Acute Respiratory Distress Syndrome

This condition, assort of noncardiac pulmonary edema, is caused by a diffuse lung injury [triggering factors include shock, near-drowning, septicemia, drug overdose,

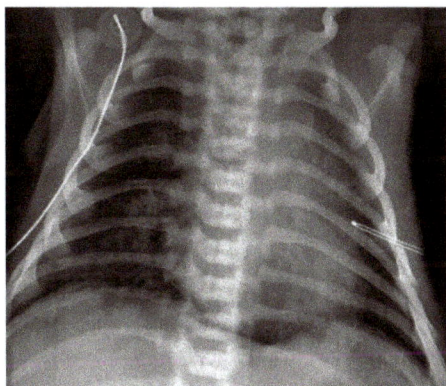

Fig. 18.2: *Meconium aspiration syndrome (MAS)*: Note the diffuse, coarse, nodular opacities, air trapping, and areas of focal emphysema.

aspiration, inhalation injury, disseminated intravascular coagulation (DIC), etc.] and may be encountered in as young an infant as 1–2-week-old neonate.

Manifestations include initial mild respiratory distress and hyperventilation giving way in 4–24 hours to hypoxemia, enhanced respiratory distress, cyanosis, and inspiratory crepitations. At this point, a large intrapulmonary shunt may be demonstrated. Without assistance from supplementary oxygen and/or mechanical ventilation, fatality may follow because of increasing hypoxemia and hypercapnia.

Pneumonia

Intrauterine pneumonia may occur in babies with history of prolonged premature rupture of membranes, febrile maternal illness, difficult delivery, and birth asphyxia.

The baby is ill, depressed, and lethargic at birth, and shows very little inclination to suck, she may vomit. Temperature is raised or subnormal. About 12–48 hours after birth, she becomes dyspneic without any cough. Respiration is often grunting.

Gastric aspirate cytology shows more than five polys per high power field or polys count more than three times the epithelial cell count.

Postnatal pneumonia, usually the result of aspiration from defective nasopharyngeal mechanism, or as a part of septicemia, occurs 48 hours after birth. Dyspnea, grunting respiration, and intercostal recession should warrant an immediate chest X-ray.

Group B Streptococcal Infection

When such an infection occurs early in neonatal period, the respiratory distress may result. The predisposing factors include prematurity, prolonged premature rupture of membranes, and maternal febrile illness.

The baby manifests the disease by the time she is 3 hours old with dyspnea, apnea, and shock.

Chest X-ray shows findings similar to those seen in idiopathic respiratory distress syndrome (IRDS) with or without coarse lower lobe opacities and exaggerated interstitial markings.

Gastric aspirate cytology shows polys and cocci.

Transient Tachypnea of Newborn

Also termed as *type II RDS* and *wet lung disease,* it occurs in approximately 1% of neonates, both term and preterm.

This is more or less a benign condition and is characterized by occurrence of slight respiratory distress in a full-term baby a few hours after birth. The general condition of the baby remains good and he becomes all right within 2–3 days. Infrequently, the condition may be accompanied by myocardial failure, pulmonary hypertension or right-to-left shunt.

Typical findings in the chest film are hyperinflated lung fields, perihilar opacities, exaggerated vascular markings, fluid in transverse fissure, and a minimal pleural fissure and an effusion (Fig. 18.3).

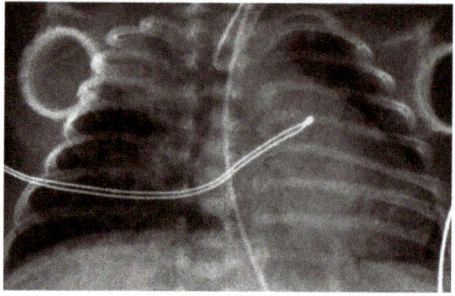

Fig. 18.3: *Transient tachypnea of the newborn*: Note the hyperaeration [against the hypoaeration of hyaline membrane disease (HMD)] and reticulogranular densities that disappear following ventilation (against HMD where disappearance takes a few days).

Massive Pulmonary Hemorrhage

This more or less fatal condition occurs in situations like intrauterine growth retardation, Rh incompatibility, IRDS, maternal diabetes, DIC, and acute left heart failure leading to hemorrhagic pulmonary edema and injection soda bicarbonate (hyperosmolar) leading to capillary insult.

The manifestations include abrupt onset of dyspnea (sometimes just apneic attacks) with frothy blood oozing from mouth and nose.

Wilson–Mikity Syndrome

This self-limited condition of uncertain etiology is characterized by occurrence of nonprogressive dyspnea, cyanosis, cough, and wheeze in a low birth weight infant (under 1,500 g) a week or two after birth. The condition subsides without any treatment in the next few weeks or months.

Pneumothorax

Pneumothorax occurs in the newborn more often than at any other age. The predisposing factors include fetal distress or difficult delivery leading to aspiration of meconium, and/or over-enthusiastic resuscitation, IRDS, and pneumonia.

Manifestations include occurrence of dyspnea and cyanosis soon after breathing gets established. At times, the baby seems to be in pain.

Clinical signs include mediastinal shift away from the affected side, hyperresonance, poor air entry, widened intercostal spaces, and depressed diaphragm.

Chest X-ray [posteroanterior (PA) and lateral films with the baby supine] shows a large pneumothorax as translucent air shadow without any lung marking, collapse and air in anterior mediastinum (Figs. 18.4 and 18.5). A small pneumothorax is often missed.

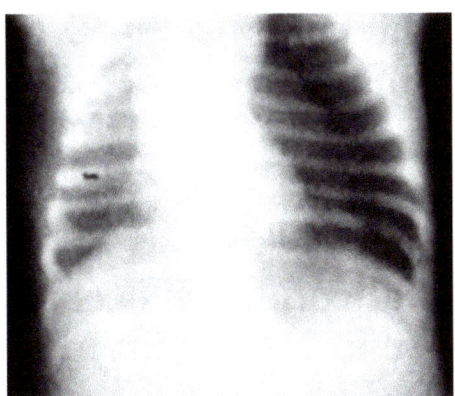

Fig. 18.4: *Neonatal pneumothorax:* Note pneumothorax with collapse and shifting of the mediastinum.

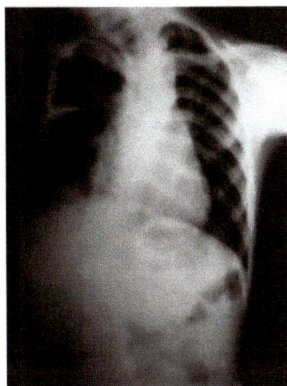

Fig. 18.5: Pneumothorax.

Pleural Effusion

The most common cause in a newborn is chylothorax though it may also accompany pneumonia, hydrops fetalis or Turner's syndrome. The infant presents with dyspnea shortly after birth.

Heart Failure

Heart failure (secondary to fibroelastosis, congenital heart disease (CHD), myocarditis, heart block, paroxysmal tachycardia, septicemia, glycogen storage disease, etc.) may well present with dyspnea. Remaining manifestations include feeding difficulty, cyanosis in excess of dyspnea and showing worsening on crying, edema as evidenced by puffiness or sudden weight gain, cardiomegaly, significant heart murmur(s), and enlarging liver.

Paralysis of Diaphragm

It may develop as such but is associated with Erb's paralysis in a vast majority of the cases. Mostly, right side is involved.

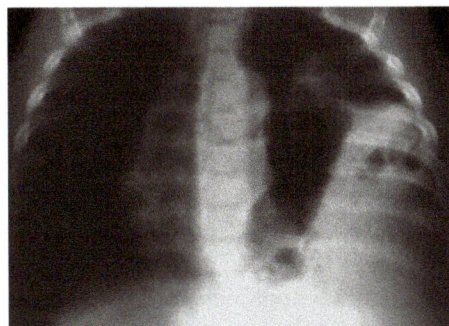

Fig. 18.6: A large diaphragmatic hernia.

The usual story is that following a difficult breech delivery, the newborn develops respiratory distress. On the affected side, respiratory movements are diminished. Mediastinum tends to be displaced to the opposite side.

Screening of chest shows paradoxical movements of the paralyzed leaf of the diaphragm with each respiration.

X-ray of chest may show slight elevation of the involved dome of diaphragm with heart displaced to the opposite side.

Choanal Atresia

In this condition, posterior nasal airway is blocked by a bony or membranous septum. It is the bilateral complete atresia that presents as a respiratory emergency in the newborn. There is absence of nose breathing despite considerable respiratory efforts, leading to cyanosis. Momentarily, the baby then takes a few galloping inspirations through mouth, thereby lessening the cyanosis temporarily. Asphyxia often causes death.

Diagnosis is supported by the presence of thick jelly-like nasal contents and absence of breath sounds while listening over the nostrils with a stethoscope. It is confirmed by inability to pass a fine catheter through each side of nose.

Diaphragmatic Hernia

A large diaphragmatic hernia, usually left-sided and through posterolateral segment, is an acute emergency, causing severe respiratory distress (Fig. 18.6). There is difficulty in establishing spontaneous breathing at birth. Right at birth or later, the baby develops labored gasping breathing and cyanosis.

The chest appears overfilled whereas abdomen may be flat or scaphoid. The air entry is diminished and one may be able to hear tinkling peristaltic sounds on the left side of chest. The heart is shifted to the right.

X-rays of chest (PA and lateral) show fluid and air-filled bowel loops in the thorax. The mediastinum is shifted to the opposite side.

Tracheoesophageal Fistula

It nearly always occurs in association with esophageal atresia. Incidence of accompanying CHD and other gastrointestinal tract (GIT) anomalies is high. There is often maternal hydramnios and single umbilical artery.

The newborn develops excessive drooling (salivation), the so-called "blowing bubbles", coughing, gagging, and even choking and cyanosis on the very first feed. The milk and saliva may regurgitate and enter into the lungs, causing aspiration pneumonia.

Once this diagnosis is suspected, a stiff radio-opaque rubber catheter should be passed into the stomach. It gets arrested at a distance of 8–10 cm from mouth. This may be demonstrated radiologically as well. Gas in the form of an air bubble is seen in the stomach in C type of fistula in which there is a communication between trachea and lower part of esophagus.

Pulmonary Agenesis

Unilateral agenesis, particularly involving right side, may cause cyanosis, dyspnea, and feeding difficulty in the newborn. The chest appears asymmetrical.

X-ray of chest reveals an abnormal opacity occupying the lung site with the mediastinum and the other lung shifted to the empty hemithorax. The diagnosis is confirmed on bronchoscopy, bronchography, and angiography.

Bilateral pulmonary hypoplasia usually occurs with renal agenesis, the so-called Potter's syndrome. The additional features of the syndrome are antimongoloid slant, low-set ears, depressed bridge of nose, and retrognathia (Potter's facies).

Unilateral pulmonary hypoplasia is usually associated with congenital diaphragmatic hernia.

Congenital Pulmonary Lymphangiectasia

In this disease, lymphatic ducts in the whole of the lung are greatly dilated as a primary defect (type I), secondary to pulmonary venous obstruction (type II) or as a part of generalized disease (type III).

It is usually symptomatic with respiratory distress and cyanosis in the neonatal period.

Chest X-ray shows punctate and reticular densities. Short of lung biopsy, diagnosis remains equivocal.

Congenital Lobar Emphysema

In this disease, a part or all of a lobe (usually left upper) gets involved from a check-valve type of obstruction of congenital origin. It may cause gross dyspnea and cyanosis in the newborn. X-ray of chest reveals a radiolucent lobe and mediastinal shift to the opposite side.

Persistent Pulmonary Hypertension of the Newborn

Persistent pulmonary hypertension of the newborn (PPHN), previously termed as *persistent fetal circulation (PFC)*, may be associated with primary factors such as anatomic malformations (alveolar capillary dysplasia, pulmonary hyperplasia, etc.), genetic differences in pulmonary smooth muscle development, chronic intrauterine stress, intrauterine closure of ductus or abnormal levels of vasoactive agents. It may be secondary to CHD, infections, polycythemia or upper airway obstruction.

Manifestations in a term neonate become apparent in first 12 hours. These include respiratory distress with retractions, grunting and nasal flaring, cyanosis, tachypnea, and hypoxia. Hypoxia may be refractory to oxygen therapy. Hypocalcemia and hypoglycemia may complicate the picture.

Chest X-ray reveals only minimal changes, which are no match to the severe respiratory distress. Cardiomegaly (due to right ventricular afterload caused by pulmonary hypertension) or characteristic findings of meconium aspiration syndrome (MAS) may be seen.

Prognosis is bad. Survivors, following treatment with such modalities as high oxygen therapy, assisted ventilation, high frequency ventilation, extracorporeal membrane oxygenation (ECMO), vasodilator drugs (tolazine), inhaled nitric oxide, and phosphodiesterase inhibitors are usually left with neurologic deficit. This may be in the form of impaired neurologic development, cerebral infarction, intraventricular hemorrhage (IVH), neurosensory loss, and convulsions.

Lung Cysts

Newborns with congenital lung cysts, believed to result as a developmental defect of the bronchial buds, may present with respiratory distress and tachypnea at birth or later, or with recurrent or persistent pneumonia.

More often, lung cysts are acquired, rather than congenital, following an infection (usually staph) or overinflation causing rupture of alveoli. Symptomatology and behavior remain similar in both types of cysts.

DYSPNEA IN POSTNEONATAL PERIOD

Pulmonary Causes

Bronchial Asthma

In this disorder, temporary narrowing of the bronchi by bronchospasm, mucosal edema, and thick secretions leads to characteristic bouts of dyspnea.

The onset of a paroxysm is usually sudden, often occurring at night. Occasionally, it is preceded by the so-called asthmatic aura in the form of tightness in chest, restlessness, polyuria or itching.

A typical attack consists of marked dyspnea, bouts of cough, and expiratory wheezing. Cyanosis, pallor, sweating, exhaustion, and restlessness are often present. Pulse is invariably rapid. The attack may subside in an hour or so, sometimes with vomiting or "coughing up" of viscid secretions. Some expiratory wheezing may persist for several days though the child is otherwise comfortable.

Acute Bronchiolitis

This serious inflammatory disease of bronchioles, in all probability of viral origin, occurs in infants with the peak incidence at around 6 months of age (Fig. 18.7).

Following upper respiratory catarrh, the child develops dyspnea and prostration. The breathing is rapid and shallow. Cyanosis and mild-to-moderate fever are usually present. Dehydration and respiratory acidosis frequently supervene. Cough, if present, is minimal.

Chest signs include intercostal and suprasternal retraction, hyperresonant percussion note, diminished breath sounds and crepitations, rhonchi and wheeze. Upper border of liver is often pushed down as a result of emphysema.

With prompt care, prognosis is very good.

Pneumonia

Dyspnea of sudden onset, if accompanied by high fever, chills, and cough, may mean pneumonia. In this situation, child may show active movements of alae nasi, grouting expiration, and lower costal recession with some cyanosis.

Chest signs include dullness, diminished breath sounds, bronchial breathing, and crepitations. In case of lobar pneumonia, the signs are restricted about the consolidation.

Chest X-ray assists in delineating the exact type (Figs. 18.8 to 18.12) and extent of pneumonia.

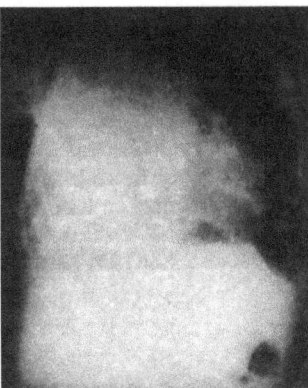

Fig. 18.8: *Massive consolidation*: Note that there is no shift of the mediastinum.

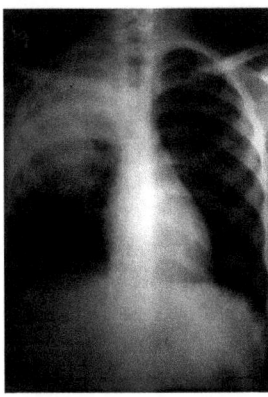

Fig. 18.9: Pneumonic consolidation of right upper lobe.

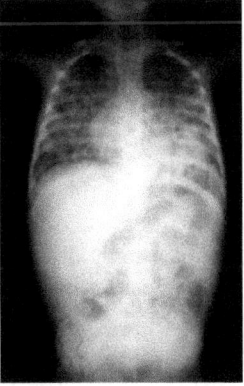

Fig. 18.10: Bronchopneumonia.

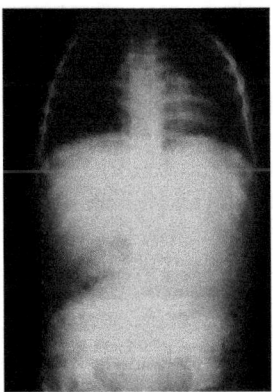

Fig. 18.7: *Acute bronchiolitis*: Note the massive air trapping and hyperinflation of the lungs. The lateral view in this condition is likely to show increased anteroposterior diameter of the chest. In a proportion (1/3rd) of the cases, presence of scattered areas of consolidation may render differentiation from early bronchopneumonia difficult.

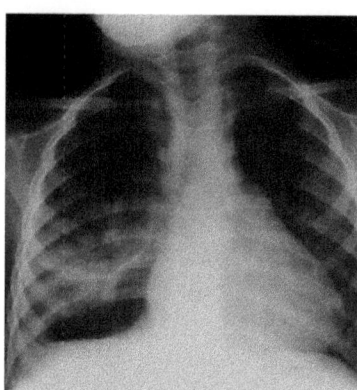

Fig. 18.11: Pneumatocele in staphylococcal pneumonia.

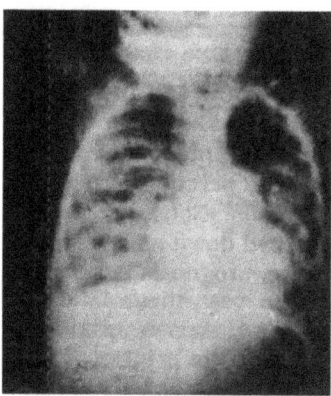

Fig. 18.12: Staphylococcal pneumonia with multiple pneumatoceles.

Asthmatic Bronchitis

Dyspnea may be a feature of asthmatic bronchitis, a nomenclature still recognized by some authorities as somewhat distinct from asthma. The disorder usually occurs in first 2 years of life. With an upper respiratory catarrh, child develops significant bronchospasm (manifested as "wheeze") and exudation similar to those encountered in older children with bronchial asthma.

Tropical Eosinophilia

This disease, probably an allergic response to filarial infection, may manifest in children beyond 1 year of age with some exertional dyspnea, persistent cough, wheeze, low fever, anorexia, growth failure, and malaise. At times, vague abdominal manifestations may be present together with enlargement of liver and lymph nodes. These manifestations tend to persist for months at a stretch without any significant systemic disturbances.

Total eosinophil count varies between 4,000/cmm and 50,000/cmm.

Chest X-ray usually shows increased reticular markings, coarse mottling (especially at the bases), and hilar prominence with clear peripheral lung fields.

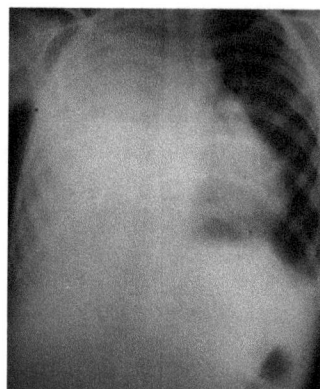

Fig. 18.13: Massive pleural effusion (right).

Pleural Effusion

Almost always occurring in children beyond 5 years of age, it is supposed to result from discharge of caseous material of a peripheral (subpleural) primary focus or enlarged regional lymph node.

Symptoms other than dyspnea include fever, weight loss, and chest pain.

Decreased chest movements, mediastinal shift toward the opposite side, dullness of percussion note, pleural rub, decreased breath sounds and vocal fremitus, and resonance are reliable signs of pleural effusion.

X-ray of chest reveals a uniform opacity with a curved fluid line (Fig. 18.13) which may become horizontal when air is also coexisting.

Aspiration of fluid confirms the presence of effusion. Straw-colored fluid with mostly lymphocytic response strongly favors tuberculosis pathology.

Empyema

Collection of thick pus in the pleural cavity (usually of staphylococcal etiology) may present with dyspnea, fever, cough, chest pain (which may be referred to the abdomen), and toxemia. In case of marked dyspnea, cyanosis may develop. Longstanding cases may have associated clubbing, anemia, and other manifestations of malnutrition.

Chest signs include diminished movements on the affected side, widening and fullness (at times edema) of the intercostal spaces, stony dull percussion note, diminished air entry, and mediastinal shift to the opposite side.

Chest X-ray shows diffuse density. In most cases, opacities are basal and costophrenic angle is obliterated. Loculated empyema may occur in fissures or at apex.

Diagnostic tap is needed in order to obtain pus for biochemical and bacteriological examination.

Löffler's Syndrome

Also called as eosinophilic pneumonia, it manifests with paroxysmal attacks of coughing, dyspnea, and, often, little fever and hepatomegaly. It is most often a manifestation of allergy produced by helminths, say *Ascaris lumbricoides*.

Blood eosinophilic count may be as high as 70%.

Chest X-ray shows widespread infiltration which may mimic miliary tuberculosis.

Atelectasis

A large atelectasis, particularly when it develops suddenly, may manifest with dyspnea, tachycardia, and cyanosis.

Chest appears flat over the affected area or side. Also, respiratory movements are decreased and the area is dull on percussion unless compensatory expansion of adjacent lung tissue has occurred.

Auscultation reveals decreased or absent breath sounds.

X-ray of chest establishes the diagnosis.

Emphysema

Congenital lobar emphysema, as it is said earlier, usually causes dyspnea in newborn. Infrequently, however, it may manifest in later months and even after several years. The child may present with dyspnea and cyanosis following compression of the normal lung by the emphysematous lung. The mediastinum may be displaced to the opposite side.

Chest X-ray shows a radiolucent lobe and a mediastinal shift.

Generalized obstructive emphysema, occurring mostly in infants suffering from respiratory infections, cystic fibrosis of pancreas, aspiration of zinc stearate powder, CHD with congestive cardiac failure (CCF), and miliary tuberculosis, manifests with expiratory dyspnea. Besides cyanosis, there is overaction of the accessory muscles of respiration, leading to suprasternal, supraclavicular, intercostal, and subcostal retraction.

Chest examination shows a hyperresonant percussion note, a relatively prolonged and roughened expiratory phase and fine or medium crepitations.

Chest X-ray shows low and flattened diaphragm, widening of intercostal spaces and poor density of lung fields.

Screening shows restriction in movements of diaphragm.

Pneumothorax

Except in the neonatal period, pneumothorax is uncommon in childhood. When it occurs, the predisposing factor is thoracentesis, pneumonia, empyema, lung abscess, emphysema lung gangrene or cyst, foreign body bronchial asthma, cystic fibrosis of pancreas, Ehlers–Danlos disease or Marfan syndrome. Spontaneous pneumothorax is infrequent. It is nearly always unilateral. Associated serous effusion will make it hydropneumothorax (Figs. 18.14 and 18.15) and a purulent effusion pyopneumothorax.

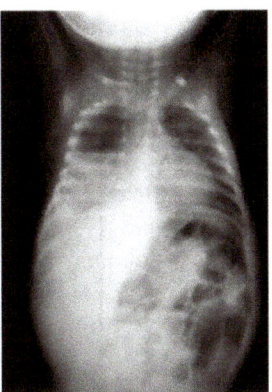

Fig. 18.14: Hydropneumothorax.

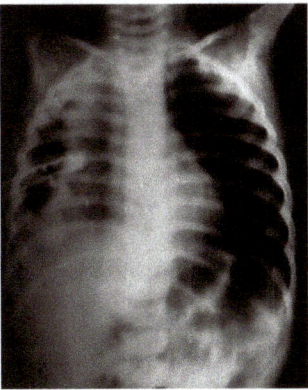

Fig. 18.15: Hydropneumothorax with pulmonary collapse.

Manifestations of an extensive pneumothorax include dyspnea, chest pain, and cyanosis.

Besides chest retractions, breath sounds are diminished over the affected lung and percussion note is tympanic. Mediastinum is shifted to the opposite side.

X-ray of chest shows air in the affected pleural cavity with partial collapse of the related lung and shift of the mediastinum to the unaffected side.

Aspiration of Foreign Body

Sudden coughing, choking or dyspnea in a healthy child should always raise the probability of aspiration of a foreign body such as peanut.

Examination reveals signs of collapse.

Chest of X-ray may reveal an area of collapse or a radiopaque foreign body.

Diaphragmatic Hernia

Congenital diaphragmatic hernia usually manifests soon after birth as a medical–surgical emergency. Infrequently, it may become symptomatic in infancy and childhood with vomiting, colicky abdominal pain, discomfort after eating, and constipation, as also dyspnea. Even intestinal obstruction may occur.

Obesity

In extreme exogenous obesity, fat accumulation on chest wall causes elevation of the diaphragm and restriction in expansion of the thoracic wall. As a result, alveolar hypoventilation with fall in pulmonary, tidal, and expiratory reserve volumes leads to severe cardiorespiratory distress. Pickwickian syndrome (after the obese boy in Charles Dicken's "Pickwick papers") is the name given to this disease.

Manifestation includes shortness of breath, cyanosis, periodic somnolence, and apneic spells. Cardiomegaly with or without CCF and polycythemia are common.

Hyperventilation

Hyperventilation syndrome is characterized by dyspnea, tightness or stabbing pain in chest, headache, abdominal pain, muscle pains, paresthesia, palpitations, dryness of mouth, vertigo, choking, weakness, blurred vision, confusion, and syncope. The manifestations appear in episodes.

Hyperventilation may also be a feature of uremia, hypernatremic dehydration, diabetic ketoacidosis, Reye's syndrome, and salicylate poisoning.

Chest Deformity

Severe chest deformity, irrespective of the cause, may be responsible for dyspnea.

Alpha-1-antitrypsin Deficiency

This rare but important cause of pulmonary disease (panacinar emphysema) may manifest in childhood with dyspnea, wheeze, and cough on top of growth failure and clubbing.

Anteroposterior diameter of chest is increased. Percussion note is hyperresonant; presence of infection may cause crepitations. Liver and spleen are palpable.

X-ray of chest shows overinflation and depressed diaphragm.

Serum trypsin inhibitory capacity is low.

Low alpha-antitrypsin level is confirmed by immunoassay.

Hamman–Rich Syndrome

Also called as idiopathic diffuse interstitial fibrosis of the lung, this rare disease has an insidious onset with dyspnea and cough (dry or productive of blood) followed by anorexia, weight loss easy fatigability, cyanosis, clubbing, and CCF (cor pulmonale). Death occurs from a fulminant intercurrent infection.

Chest X-ray shows progressive widespread granular or reticular mottling, or small nodular opacities.

Pulmonary Hemosiderosis

In this group of disorders (idiopathic or secondary), abnormally large amounts of hemosiderin are accumulated in the lungs.

Manifestations of idiopathic pulmonary hemosiderosis include chronic iron deficiency anemia refractory to iron therapy, cough, dyspnea and wheeze, hematemesis, melena or hemoptysis, clubbing, intermittent jaundice, and hepatosplenomegaly. Cardiac involvement (left bundle branch block) may occur in some patients.

Laboratory investigations show hypochromic anemia, eosinophilia, reticulocytosis, positive fecal occult blood and excessive number of iron-bearing macrophages (siderocytes or siderophages) in sputum, gastric washings or lung biopsy.

Chest X-ray shows infiltration simulating miliary tuberculosis.

Pulmonary Alveolar Proteinosis

In this very rare condition, occurring in association with immunologic deficiencies, tuberculosis and mycosis, eosinophilic protein and phospholipid-containing material occupy the alveoli, causing extensive consolidation.

Several months period of nonspecific symptoms like weight loss and anorexia is followed by cough, dyspnea, and cyanosis.

Chest X-ray shows a feathery density of butterfly distribution.

Lung biopsy confirms the definitive diagnosis.

Pulmonary Alveolar Microlithiasis

This rare familial disorder is characterized by deposition of minute chalky calculi in the alveoli.

Symptoms of progressive respiratory failure and cor pulmonale only infrequently appear in later childhood.

Chest X-ray shows bilateral, fine granular infiltrates.

Pulmonary Veno-occlusive Disease

This rare disease is characterized by pulmonary venous thrombosis and recanalization with intimal fibrosis.

Manifestations include exertional dyspnea and orthopnea, weight loss, fainting and ankle edema.

Physical findings include signs of pulmonary hypertension, CCF, and tricuspid incompetence.

Electrocardiography (ECG) shows right atrial and ventricular hypertrophy. Chest X-ray shows cardiomegaly, pulmonary arterial dilatation, and pulmonary edema. Cardiac catheterization reflects pulmonary arterial hypertension.

High Altitude Hypoxia

High altitude above 3,000 m (over 9,000 ft) may cause pulmonary edema in some subjects within hours of exposure.

Manifestations include cough, shortness of breath, chest pain, and vomiting. Within 48 hours, recovery occurs.

Chest X-ray shows bilateral patchy infiltration.

Pulmonary Embolism and Infarction

Pulmonary embolism in children may occasionally occur in association with surgical procedures, intravenous (IV) infusion, prolonged immobilization (inactivity), sickle-cell anemia, cyanotic CHD, severe dehydration, infective endocarditis, therapeutic bypass, shunts for hydrocephalus, accidental bone trauma, and longstanding nutritional deficiency states.

Clinical manifestations include sudden chest pain, dyspnea, tachycardia, hemoptysis, and collapse.

A sufficiently large infarct may cause impaired resonance and a pleural friction rub, distant or absent breath sounds, and moist crepitations.

Mortality rate is high.

Cardiac Causes

Paroxysmal Atrial Tachycardia

If a paroxysm of atrial tachycardia (usually in the range of 300/minute) ends up in CCF, lasting 6–24 hours or more, the infant becomes acutely ill. Dyspnea, cyanosis, restlessness, and irritability dominate the picture. In addition, there may be hepatomegaly, fever, and leukocytosis.

Congestive Cardiac Failure

Congestive cardiac failure, a common pediatric emergency, may result from several diseases. Besides dyspnea at rest (orthopnea) or on exertion, child has tachycardia, raised jugular venous pressure (JVP), tender hepatomegaly, bilateral basal crepitations, edema, peripheral cyanosis, and gallop rhythm.

Myocarditis

Clinical manifestations are similar in myocarditis of bacterial, viral, fungal, protozoal, parasitic, toxic or allergic origin. These include dyspnea, fever, malaise, arrhythmias (heart block-partial or complete), and CCF.

X-ray of chest shows cardiomegaly.

Congenital Heart Disease

Large ventricular septal defect (VSD) causes exertional dyspnea besides recurrent chest infections, CCF and failure to thrive. Heart is moderately or grossly enlarged (usually biventricular). The characteristic murmur is loud pansystolic, best heard over the left sternal border (third, fourth, and fifth spaces). A thrill usually accompanies it. Pulmonary second sound (P_2) may be split and accentuated due to pulmonary hypertension. A pulmonary diastolic murmur (Graham Steell murmur) may also be heard. X-ray of chest shows a large left-to-right shunt with enlarged heart (both ventricles and left atrium), enlarged pulmonary artery, and plethoric lung fields (over-vascularity) with or without hilar dance (Fig. 18.16).

Atrial septal defect (ASD) in older children may manifest with dyspnea, chest infection, bulging of the chest (due to enlargement of right ventricle), and growth failure. The typical murmur is ejection systolic, soft, and best heard over upper left sternal border (usually second space). It is preceded by a loud first sound and may be radiated to the apex and back. P_2 is widely split and fixed.

Chest X-ray shows atrial and ventricular enlargement, increased pulmonary vascularity, enlarged pulmonary artery, and rather small left ventricle and aorta.

Electrocardiography shows right ventricular hypertrophy (RVH) and right axis deviation.

Patent ductus arteriosus (PDA) may manifest with exertional dyspnea, left ventricular failure, CCF, and growth retardation. Occasionally, precordial pain and hoarseness (due to involvement of recurrent laryngeal nerve) may be present.

Pulse pressure is wide. As a result, water hammer pulse and prominent arterial corrigan's pulsations in the neck may be present. Differential cyanosis, in which left arm and both feet are involved, may be observed. A classical machinery murmur localized to second left intercostal space or transmitted to left clavicle or lower down, i.e. left sternal border is usually accompanied by a thrill. There may be paradoxical splitting of P_2.

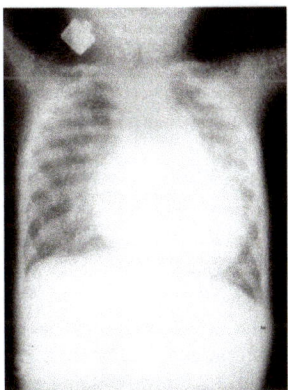

Fig. 18.16: *Ventricular septal defect (VSD)*: Note the cardiomegaly with pulmonary plethora.

Chest X-ray shows biventricular enlargement, prominent aortic knob and pulmonary artery and plethoric lung with hilar dance.

Electrocardiography is usually normal but may show ventricular hypertrophy. Deep Q-waves may be seen in left ventricular leads.

Tetralogy of Fallot presents with dyspnea and cyanosis that usually become evident after the closure of the ductus arteriosus, i.e. after third month of life. As the child grows, he feels comfortable while lying down or in squatting position only.

Anoxic, hypoxic or blue (cyanotic) spells consisting of dyspnea and cyanosis with or without unconscious may occur due to cerebral anoxia. By the age of 2 years, the child has usually developed some clubbing. CCF is unusual (Fig. 18.17). The typical murmur is loud short systolic, at left sternal border in third space. It is generally not accompanied by a thrill. P_2 is usually single.

Chest X-ray shows oligemic lung fields (poorly vascularized), a small boot-shaped heart with the tip of the boot turned up above the diaphragm (because of RVH) and concavity of the pulmonary artery segment (small pulmonary conus). One in every four to five cases has right aortic arch. ECG shows RVH with beaked P waves.

Transposition of great vessels (TGV) presents with severe cyanosis (differential with legs being less cyanotic than the arms) appearing at or shortly after birth followed by dyspnea and CCF. It constitutes hallmark of TGV. Clubbing takes a few months to develop. Clinically, heart is always enlarged. Murmurs are dependent on the coexisting communication. X-ray of chest shows cardiomegaly and grossly plethoric lung fields. ECG shows RVH, right axis deviation, and often P-pulmonale.

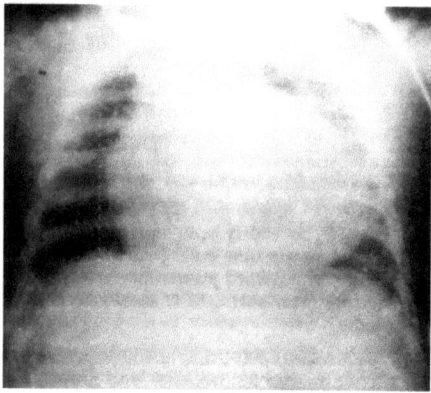

Fig. 18.17: Congestive cardiac failure (CCF) in a child with tetralogy of Fallot (TOF). Differential diagnosis of this unusual association includes presence of iron-deficiency anemia, restrictive ventricular septal defect (VSD) with TOF, hypertension, valvular regurgitation, infective endocarditis, myocarditis, additional shunt, valvular regurgitation, and absent pulmonary valve.

Coarctation of aorta syndrome of "preductal" type may manifest with dyspnea, feeding difficulty, failure to thrive, pitting edema, gallop rhythm, and rarely differential cyanosis due to PDA. Heart murmurs, depending on the associated cardiac conditions such as VSD may be heard. A systolic murmur is usually heard over the interscapular area. In "postductal" type, manifestations developing in later childhood may include fatigue, cramps, intermittent claudication, headache, weakness, and exertional dyspnea. In some cases, overgrowth of upper limbs and chest may occur. The most dependable physical finding is the weak, delayed, and even absent femoral arteries compared to the strong brachial arteries. The blood pressure in the arms is much higher than in the legs, provided the child is beyond 1 year of age. Occasionally, due to involvement of the left subclavian artery, left brachial pulse may be weaker, and the blood pressure in the left arm is lower than that on the right side. Dilated and tortuous collaterals may be seen over the interscapular area in older children. This is called as Suzman's sign. An ejection systolic murmur (grade 2/6) is heard at the aortic area and the lower left sternal border. A systolic murmur in the interscapular area is considered pathognomonic.

X-ray findings include some left ventricular enlargement, notching of the ribs caused by intercostal collaterals and "E" sign on barium swallow.

Electrocardiography may suggest RVH, particularly in infants.

Aortic stenosis of significant severity may be responsible for exertional dyspnea. Remaining manifestations include easy fatigability, precordial pain induced on exercise, and spells of unconsciousness. CCF may occur early in infancy. Systolic blood pressure and pulse pressure are low. A systolic thrill is present. Auscultation reveals a loud, harsh murmur in the second or third right intercostal space with transmission to neck.

X-ray shows slight left ventricular enlargement.

Electrocardiography may reflect left ventricular hypertrophy (LVH) in some cases.

Valvular pulmonic stenosis may manifest after the age of 2 years with dyspnea, easy fatigability, and, in a few cases, cyanosis. A thrill is palpable. A loud, harsh systolic murmur is heard in second, third, and fourth left intercostal spaces.

X-ray shows dilatation of main pulmonary artery and right ventricular enlargement.

Electrocardiography is consistent with RVH.

Cardiomyopathy may manifest with dyspnea plus other signs and symptoms depending on the type (whether dilated, hypertrophic or restrictive).

Chest X-ray, ECG, and echocardiography (Figs. 18.18 and 18.19) are needed to confirm the diagnosis.

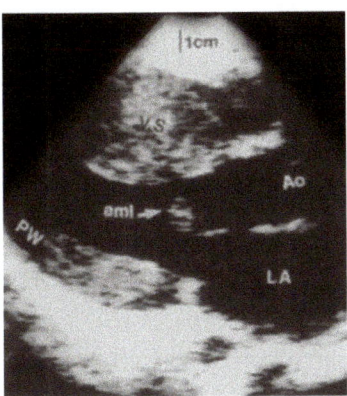

Fig. 18.18: *Hypertrophic cardiomyopathy:* Note that the posterior wall (PW) of the left ventricle is thickened though the interventricular septum (VS) is highly thickened. As a result there is asymmetrical septal hypertrophy. In addition, anterior mitral valve leaflet (AML) shows a systolic anterior motion.

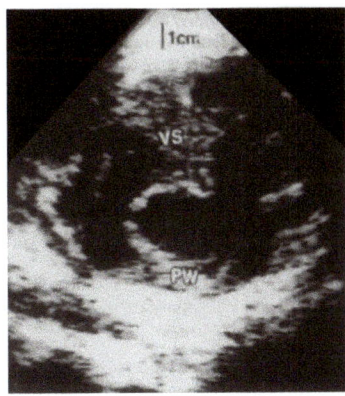

Fig. 18.19: *Hypertrophic cardiomyopathy:* Note the asymmetrical septal hypertrophy in the echocardiography.

Rheumatic Heart Disease

Rheumatic carditis may manifest with dyspnea but the symptom is more often the result of CCF rather than carditis as such.

Rheumatic pericarditis may manifest with dyspnea and chest pain. The former results are from accompanying CCF.

In chronic rheumatic heart disease (mitral stenosis, mitral regurgitation, and aortic regurgitation), dyspnea, palpitations, and easy fatigability may occur.

Intravenous Substance Abuse

Dyspnea may result from intravenous abuse of drugs such as heroin and other opioids via bronchospasm and/or pulmonary edema.

Psychogenic Cause

Hysteria, stress, and tension may cause dyspnea which usually fails to improve with rest. Diagnosis is by exclusion and evidence of psychogenic background of the patient.

Drugs

Salicylates, acetazolamide, aminophylline, nitrofurantoin rifampicin, para-aminosalicylate sodium (PAS), isonex, penicillin, streptomycin, sulfas, methotrexate, cyclophosphamide, vincristine, imipramine, etc.

FURTHER READING

1. Bhat B, Serane VT. Hyaline membrane disease (HMD). In: Gupte S (Ed). *Recent Advances in Pediatrics (Special Vol 8: Emergency Pediatrics)*. New Delhi: Jaypee 2001:348-365.
2. El-Baba MF. Dyspnea. In: Adam HM, Foy JM (Eds). *Signs and Symptoms in Pediatrics*. Illinois: American Academy of Pediatrics 2015:235-246.
3. Green M. *Pediatric Diagnosis*, 6th edn. Philadelphia: Saunders 1998.
4. Louglin GM, Eigen H. *Respiratory Disease in Children: Diagnosis and Management*. Baltimore: Williams and Wilkins 1994.
5. Monton S, Arul KS. Neonatal respiratory distress syndrome. *Lancet* 2006;307:1878-1879.
6. Smith NP, Jesudason EC, Featherstone NC, et al. Recent advances in congenital diaphragmatic hernia. *Arch Dis Child* 2005;90:426-428.

CHAPTER 19

Dysuria

BACKGROUND

The term, *dysuria*, refers to discomfort, burning or pain during micturition. It may be primary or secondary. In primary dysuria (the predominant), the etiologic factors are confined to the urinary tract per se. In secondary dysuria, discomfort occurs because of involvement of the urinary tract in some systemic diseases.

HISTORY

History must be determined if other symptoms related to the urinary tract are present. Is there accompanying frequency, urgency or incontinence? Is the amount passed excessive or scanty? Is there any hematuria? Is there any pruritus ani or itching about the external genitals? Any history of passage of threadworms? How is the urinary stream: forceful or dribbling? Is the child febrile? Does he suffer from any systemic disease? Has he been on such drugs as sulfonamides?

PHYSICAL EXAMINATION

Physical examination must include local, genital, and perineal regions' inspection. Perianal rash with obvious marks from itching points to infection with *Enterobius vermicularis*. Perineal irritation from a diaper rash may be responsible for painful urination. Soreness of vulva is responsible for dysuria in many instances. Congenital anomalies such as meatal stenosis, urethral valves, etc. may also cause this symptom.

Never miss watching the child as and when he passes urine. Because of real dysuria, the child may deliberately withhold urine. An infant may cry on passing urine. If hematuria coexists, diaper may be stained with bloody urine.

INVESTIGATIONS

- Routine urine examination, including microscopy
- Urine culture
- Radiology
  - Plain abdominal film
  - Ultrasonography
  - Cystourethrogram.

IMPORTANT DIFFERENTIALS

Physiologic Dysuria

Concentrated urine as a result of inadequate intake of fluids in hot months, or febrile conditions may cause dysuria.

Urinary Tract Infection

Besides dysuria, described by the child as burning, difficult, painful or hot urination, manifestation may include urgency, frequency, dribbling, foul-smelling urine, enuresis or daytime incontinence of recent onset, fever, anorexia, abdominal pain, irritability, and vomiting. Mucous membrane of external genitalia may be inflamed. Hematuria, jaundice, and a picture of sepsis may occur.

A positive urine culture is essential for establishing the diagnosis. Just pyuria is not a sufficient evidence of urinary tract infection (UTI) to warrant chemotherapy.

Urinary Lithiasis

Irritative symptoms of dysuria along with urgency and frequency may be encountered in calculus lodged in the distal ureter. In case of the calculus in the urethra, dysuria, and difficulty in voiding may occur.

Acute Glomerulonephritis

Dysuria may occasionally be a symptom of acute glomerulonephritis. The onset is usually abrupt. Following pharyngitis or impetigo, the child develops gross hematuria, periorbital edema, abdominal pain, general malaise and irritability, fever, oliguria, and hypertension. Characteristic urinary findings are a gross hematuria and mixture of casts (mostly red cell and granular). With the clinical recovery, gross hematuria disappears, in about a week. But, microscopic hematuria may persist for 4–8 weeks.

Local Factors Involving Urethra, etc.

Anterior urethritis may result from a nonspecific infection, gonorrhea, irritation by a wet diaper, local injury (say accidental, intentional as in battered baby syndrome, or iatrogenic), an extension of balanitis (inflammation of glans), or posthitis (inflammation of prepuce), severe vulvitis, urethral carbuncle, or *Enterobius vermicularis*. Symptoms include dysuria and postvoiding spotty urethral bleeding.

Prostatitis, occurring mostly in adolescents, may cause dysuria together with frequency and urgency of micturition, fever, purulent discharge per urethra, and perineal or low backache. Rectal examination reveals an enlarged and tender prostate. It may result from gonococcal and other microorganisms.

Meatal stenosis, resulting from perimeatal inflammation (diaper rash) or ulceration following circumcision, may cause dysuria, terminal hematuria or urinary spotting. Inspection shows a narrow-looking meatal orifice and, more importantly, a urinary stream that is typically needle-like and dorsally deflected.

Urethral valves, hyperplastic folds of tissue located mostly in posterior urethra, are usually symptomatic in male neonates, infants, and toddlers. Manifestations include dysuria, weak dribbling urinary stream, distended bladder hematuria, urinary tract infection, azotemia, and hydronephrosis or hydroureter. Voiding cystourethrogram clinches the diagnosis.

Drugs

Sulfas, isonex, chlordiazepoxide, imipramine, amitriptyline, etc.

FURTHER READING

1. Goilan B, Kaskel FJ. Dysuria. In: Adam HM, Foy JM (Eds). *Signs and Symptoms in Pediatrics*. Illinois: American Academy of Pediatrics 2015.
2. Herz D, Weiser A, Colette T, et al. Dysfunctional elimination syndrome as an etiology of idiopathic urethritis in childhood. *J Urol* 2005;173:2132-2137.
3. Lande A. *The Child with Dysuria*. Philadelphia: Academicia 2007.
4. Nicoletta JA, Lande MB. Medical evaluation and treatment of urolithiasis. *Pediatr Clin North Am* 2006;53:479-491.

CHAPTER 20

Edema

BACKGROUND

The term, *edema*, denotes an increase in the extravascular component of the extracellular fluid volume. Before clinically recognizable edema becomes apparent, a considerable rise in the extravascular component occurs, resulting in an appreciable weight gain.

Two major forms of edema are generally recognized: "localized" and "generalized". The gross generalized edema is often termed as "anasarca". Examples of localized edema include ascites, hydrothorax (which may be secondary to a systemic disease), excessive crying, conjunctivitis, insect bite, Milroy's disease, etc. Examples of generalized edema include kwashiorkor, nephrotic syndrome, cirrhosis of liver, congestive cardiac failure (CCF), etc.

An edematous arm may be the result of arm presentation or its isolated exposure in cold environment.

Edema over feet and legs ever since birth is usually due to Milroy's disease, or Turner's syndrome.

Box 20.1 lists important causes of edema.

BOX 20.1: Etiology of edema.

Generalized edema
- Renal disease
  - Nephrotic syndrome
  - Acute glomerulonephritis
  - Urinary tract infection
- Liver disease
  - Liver failure
  - Cirrhosis
- Heart disease
  - Congestive cardiac failure
  - Pericardial effusion
- Malnutrition
  - Kwashiorkor
  - Anemia with hypoproteinemia

Localized edema
- Angioneurotic edema
- Thrombophlebitis
- Snake bite
- Angiotensin-converting enzyme (ACE) inhibitor-induced edema
- Cold injury to an exposed part
- Allergic reaction
- Excessive crying
- Conjunctivitis/blepharitis
- Genetic/chromosomal disorders: Turner's syndrome, Milroy's disease, etc.

HISTORY

The patient's history is important in the formulation of a differential diagnosis. In case of generalized edema of the newborn, specific questioning should include information on blood group incompatibility (hemolytic disease of the newborn). Any suggestion of CCF (as manifested by dyspnea, cyanosis, etc. besides edema), fulminant infection, cold injury, overhydration/hypernatremia or maternal diabetes?

After the neonatal period, history should aim at specifically excluding malnutrition (both primary and secondary), renal disease, CCF, and liver disease as the most potent causes of generalized edema. Also, is there any history of allergy to aspirin or some other agent? Any history of subcutaneous bleeding with abdominal pain or arthritis (anaphylactoid purpura)? Has there been excessive intake of sodium or fluid? Any predisposition to sodium retention (steroids)? Has the patient been recently started on treatment for diabetes mellitus?

In localized edema, specific questioning depends upon the site affected. For instance, edema of the face must elicit such information as excessive crying, excessive rubbing of the eyes, conjunctivitis, blepharitis, allergy to eye drops or some other agents, "congress" grass (parthenium), acute sinusitis, dental abscess, orbital cellulitis or cavernous sinus thrombosis. Is there any accompanying facial palsy with furrowed tongue (Melkersson's syndrome)?

Table 20.1 lists the significance of some important observations in the history.

PHYSICAL EXAMINATION

Table 20.2 lists significance of some important clinical findings. Box 20.2 provides the clinical diagnostic aids in case of systemic examination.

TABLE 20.1: Significance of some important observations in history.

Observation	Significance
Mode of onset	Sudden (<72 hours)—acute glomerulonephritis, allergic reaction, etc.
Site and evolution	• Legs → Face → Ascites (cardiac) • Ascites → Legs → Face (hepatic) • Face → Legs → Ascites (renal) acute edema of face and neck—SVC obstruction
Timing	• Increase in morning—hypoproteinemia • Increase in evening—congestive cardiac failure
Exposure	Medications, food preservatives, allergic reaction, etc.
Nutritional history	Low protein intake—PEM
Past/allergic history	• Sore throat and joint pain—rheumatic carditis • Neonatal umbilical vein sepsis or umbilical vein catheterization—portal hypertension • Chronic illnesses (persistent/chronic diarrhea)—PEM • Milk intolerance—cow's milk protein hypersensitivity • Wheat sensitivity—celiac disease

(SVC: superior vena cava; PEM: protein-energy malnutrition)

TABLE 20.2: Significance of important clinical findings.

Findings	Significance
Tachycardia, prolonged	Cardiac diseases
Hypertension	Acute glomerulonephritis
Tachypnea	Pulmonary edema
Raised JVP	Congestive cardiac failure
Altered consciousness disoriented	Hepatic encephalopathy, hypertensive encephalopathy (renal), etc.
Asterixis	Hepatic encephalopathy
Pallor	Anemia, malnutrition, etc.
Icterus, spider angioma, and other stigmata	Chronic hepatic diseases
Cyanosis and clubbing	Congenital heart disease
Flag sign, Bitot's spot, stomatitis, muscle wasting, dehydration, hypothermia, etc.	Malnutrition
Abnormal anthropometry	Malnutrition

(JVP: jugular venous pressure)

BOX 20.2: Clinical diagnostic aids in systemic examination.

- Gallop, tachycardia, tachypnea, inspiratory crackles, hepatomegaly: Heart disease
- Pericardial rub, pulsus paradoxus, muffled heart sounds, jugular venous distention: Pericardial effusion
- Hepatosplenomegaly and ascites: Hepatic cause (if no icterus: exclude portal vein thrombosis)
- Hepatomegaly (fatty liver): Malnutrition

INVESTIGATIONS

General Investigations

- Urine dipstick and microscopy
  - Proteinuria, casts, and hematuria are indicative of renal disease
- Renal function test and electrolytes
  - Raised serum urea and creatinine are indicative of renal disease
  - Hyperkalemia, hypokalemia, hyperphosphatemia, hypocalcemia
- Complete blood count and peripheral blood smear
  - Normochromic normocytic anemia suggests chronic disease
  - Hypochromic microcytic anemia suggests iron deficiency from occult gastrointestinal bleeding, i.e. cow's milk allergy
  - Megaloblastic anemia suggests vitamin B_{12} and folate deficiency from small bowel disease
  - Eosinophilia suggests angioedema or protein losing enteropathy
- Liver function test (LFT)
  - Hypoalbuminemia in the absence of circulatory overload suggests hypoproteinemic states
  - Hyperbilirubinemia and transaminitis suggests liver disease
- Chest X-ray and electrocardiogram
  - Cardiomegaly with prominent perihilar vascular marking and left ventricular hypertrophy confirms intravascular fluid overload
  - ST elevation with T wave inversion (pericarditis)
  - Electrocardiography (ECG) can provide clue to other causes of heart failure.

Specific Investigations

Depending upon the most likely cause:
- *Cardiac cause*: Echocardiography
- *Nephrotic syndrome*: 24-hour urine protein, urine protein to creatinine ratio, fasting lipids, screen for secondary causes, e.g. systemic lupus erythematosus (SLE), hepatitis B, etc.

- *Nephritic syndrome*: Serum complements, screen for secondary causes, e.g. streptococcal infection, SLE, immunoglobulin A (IgA) nephropathy, etc.
- *Chronic liver disease*: Screen for underlying cause, assess complication, e.g. hyperammonemia, coagulopathy, etc.
- *Cow's milk allergy*: FAST test for cow milk IgE, patch test, jejunal biopsy, etc.
- *Gluten hypersensitivity*: Anti-gliadin IgG/IgA, anti-endomysial IgA, jejunal biopsy, etc.
- *Malnutrition*: Blood glucose, septic screening, stool and urine for parasites and germs, electrolytes, Ca, pH and ALP, serum proteins, chest X-ray (CXR) and Mantoux test, exclude human immunodeficiency virus (HIV) and malabsorption.

DIFFERENTIALS

Generalized Edema

Generalized Edema in Newborn

Hemolytic disease of newborn: In the severest form of Rhesus (Rh) hemolytic disease, *hydrops fetalis*, the baby is remarkably edematous with effusion in serous cavities and massive hepatosplenomegaly. The baby is usually born preterm and may die shortly after birth as a result of severe anemia and CCF. In case of death in utero, the baby is macerated. The placenta is invariably large and edematous.

Alpha-thalassemia may present as fatal hydrops fetalis or hemoglobin H disease in which only Bart hemoglobin and hemoglobin H are present.

Congestive cardiac failure: Infrequently, generalized edema involving the feet, legs, sacrum, and eyelids may be a sign of CCF in the newborn. The accompanying manifestations include tachypnea, irritability, feeding difficulty, poor weight gain, weak cry, tachycardia, hepatomegaly, cardiomegaly, and gallop rhythm. A common finding is pneumonitis with or without collapse of a part of the lung. A clinical assessment of jugular venous pressure (JVP) is rather difficult because of the shortness of the neck and difficulty in securing a relaxed state in case of newborns.

Even in the absence of a murmur, the probability of newborn's CCF being secondary to congenital heart disease should be seriously considered.

Cold injury: Neonatal cold injury occurs most often in low birth weight infants as a result of exposure to freezing cold, or following a resuscitation procedure or a cold snap.

Clinical features include a low body temperature (30–35°C or even less), cold skin (color may, however, remain pink giving an erroneous impression of good health), lethargy, refusal to accept feed, oliguria, and bradycardia. Over areas of edema, skin may become hard and fixed to the underlying structures. The so-called sclerema may be confused with scleredema.

Complications of cold injury include hypoglycemia, acidosis and hemorrhagic manifestations, such as massive pulmonary hemorrhage.

Electrolyte imbalance: Overhydration, excessive administration of sodium through oral or intravenous rehydration therapy or concentrated milk formula, and inadequate excretion of sodium by immature kidneys in preterm newborns may be accompanied by clinically detectable edema.

Hypokalemia also is likely to cause edema in association with other manifestations such as muscular weakness.

Excess solute load as a result of high protein formula may also be responsible for clinical edema, more so in a preterm infant.

Hypoallergenic formula in cystic fibrosis may result in edema in neonatal period.

Nutritional edema: Anemia with hypoproteinemia, idiopathic hypoproteinemia, and vitamin E deficiency may manifest with neonatal edema. Whereas idiopathic hypoproteinemia occurs in term infants, the remaining two conditions usually are encountered in preterm infants.

Renal edema: In congenital nephrosis, the newborn may present with hypoproteinemia and edema. Two major types (infantile microcytic disease—Finnish type and membranous nephropathy of congenital syphilis) are recognized.

Remaining causes include congenital toxoplasmosis, congenital rubella, nail-patella syndrome, etc.

Maternal diabetes: The newborn of a diabetic mother is usually remarkably heavy, plump, full-faced, plethoric, and covered with lot of vernix caseosa. He is prone to develop hypoglycemia, hypocalcemia, idiopathic respiratory distress syndrome (hyaline membrane disease), hyperbilirubinemia, renal and adrenal vein thrombosis, and polycythemia. Incidence of congenital malformations is high.

Generalized Edema after Neonatal Period

Nutritional disorders: Gross protein-energy malnutrition (PEM) in the form of kwashiorkor is by and large the most common nutritional disorder causing generalized edema in children, usually between the ages of 1 year and 4 years (Fig. 20.1).

The fundamental nutritional inadequacy is primarily of proteins though energy deficiency and deficiencies of several vitamins and minerals also coexist. The essential features of the disease are growth retardation as evidenced by significantly low weight and height for age, gross muscle wasting with retention of some subcutaneous fat, mental apathy and edema (at least over pretibial region) with serum albumin less than 2.5 g%. The variable (nonessential) features include dermatosis, diarrhea, hepatomegaly, superimposed infections, hair changes, and vitamin and mineral deficiencies. Marasmic-kwashiorkor refers to the state in which the child has gross wasting of muscles as well as subcutaneous fat (in short he looks marasmic), and also has developed edema.

Conditions such as celiac disease, cystic fibrosis, endemic tropical sprue, tuberculosis, hookworm disease, and protein-losing enteropathy may cause secondary malnutrition and hypoproteinemic edema.

Renal disorders: Nephrotic syndrome, no matter whether it is idiopathic or secondary to conditions such as chronic glomerulonephritis, diabetes mellitus, renal vein thrombosis, SLE, malignant hypertension, amyloidosis, plasmodium malarial infection HIV, HB or drug toxicity, is characterized by massive edema, gross albuminuria and hypercholesterolemia.

The onset is usually insidious. A previously well child begins to gain weight over a period of days to weeks. This may be accompanied by periorbital puffiness. In due course, he presents with massive generalized edema involving the face, extremities (Figs. 20.2A and B), trunk, abdomen, and genitalia, especially marked scrotal edema almost resembling hydrocele. Hydrothorax and massive ascites may cause respiratory embarrassment. Edema of gut epithelium may result in diarrhea. Some hepatomegaly is usual. Blood pressure usually remains within normal range.

Acute nephritis is characterized by acute onset of fever, edema (most marked over face), and smoky or frankly bloody urine. Oliguria and hypertension are usually present. Occasionally, the child may present with hypertensive encephalopathy. Acute renal shutdown and CCF are other serious complications. Preceding these manifestations by 1–2 weeks is a streptococcal (beta-hemolytic type 12) infection of throat or skin. Urinalysis reveals few to numerous red cells, many granular casts and mild-to-moderate albuminuria.

Remember that edema of acute nephritis is due to impaired function of the capillary wall. It, therefore, does not follow the hydrostatic pressure and does not accumulate in the dependent parts. Its characteristic sites are face, pretibial region, and ankles.

Cardiovascular disorders: Congestive cardiac failure may at times manifest with generalized edema. Remaining evidence of CCF in the form of dyspnea, basal crepitations, and hepatomegaly should be looked for. Raised JVP is certainly an important finding but it may be quite difficult to detect it in infants.

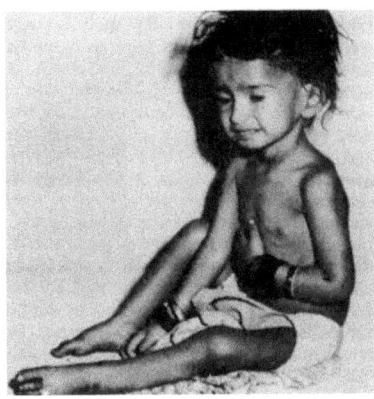

Fig. 20.1: *Kwashiorkor*: Note the pedal edema, listlessness, muscle wasting with retention of some subcutaneous adiposity, and growth retardation (weight 8.5 kg, height 72 cm) in this 2-year-old girl.

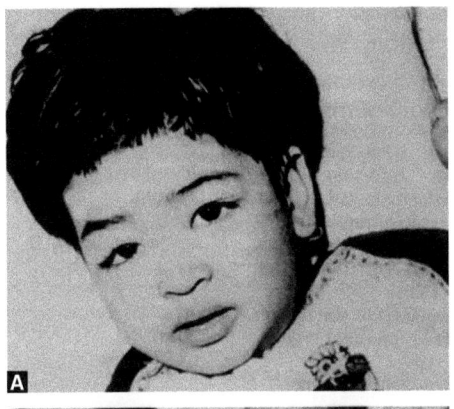

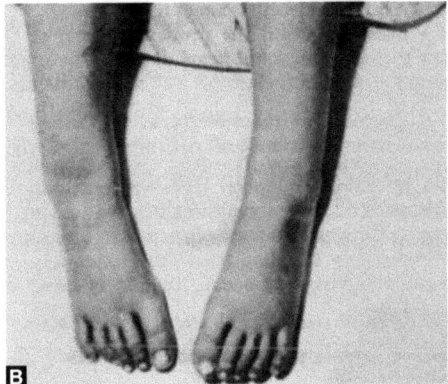

Figs. 20.2A and B: *Nephrotic syndrome*: Note the periorbital puffiness and pedal edema. Urinalysis showed gross proteinuria serum albuminuria was 2 g% and cholesterol 218 mg%.

You must ascertain the probable cause of CCF. The causes include congenital heart disease, rheumatic carditis, viral carditis, fibroelastosis, and severe anemia.

Liver disorders: Ascites, jaundice, and hepatosplenomegaly characterize edema of Indian childhood cirrhosis, particularly in the second stage. Liver is typically firm with a sharp leafy margin. Superficial abdominal veins are quite prominent.

Remaining Causes of Generalized Edema after Neonatal Period

Beginning of treatment of diabetes mellitus, overhydration and hypernatremia, aspirin sensitivity, etc.

Localized Edema in the Newborn

Head

Caput succedaneum is an edematous swelling, as a result of serosanginous collection from pressure over the presenting part between the pericranium and scalp tissue. It is present at birth, crosses the suture-line and disappears within a few hours to a day or so. It should not be confused with cephalhematoma in which swelling results from collection of blood between skull bone and overlying pericranium. It is, therefore, limited by suture lines. Regression takes a few weeks.

Face

Excessive crying, infections such as conjunctivitis or boils, and drugs (say sensitivity to eye drops) may be responsible for edema of face and eyelids.

Limbs

Edema of an arm may well be due to arm presentation or exposure of the arm to low temperature. It may last for several hours.

Non-pitting or pitting edema, often unilateral, present over legs ever since birth is in all probability Milroy's disease (Fig. 20.3). It is predominantly lymphatic.

A characteristic edema of the dorsum of hand and feet in association with loose skin folds at the nape is a feature of gonadal dysgenesis, also termed as Turner's syndrome. Other manifestations of this 45,"X" disorder at birth includes a significantly low birth weight and low crown-heel length.

Genitalia

Edema involving genitalia is a common finding in newborns. It is physiological and disappears without any intervention.

Some newborns develop a transient edema of scrotum. It may well be allergic in origin (say, sensitivity to detergents employed for washing the nappies), or due to insect bite or superficial cellulitis accompanying a pustule or abrasion. The edema and erythema tend to spread beyond the scrotum into the groin and perineum. As a rule, the manifestations are unilateral. This condition is accompanied by eosinophilia and usually responds to an antihistaminic agent like cetirizine. This poorly understood entity has been termed as "idiopathic scrotal edema".

Abdominal Wall

Edema of abdominal wall may accompany peritonitis, necrotizing enterocolitis, and appendicitis in newborn. Edema in the last-named situation is localized to the right flank. At times, there is an associated erythema. Remaining manifestations include abdominal distention, irritability, vomiting, and pyuria.

Localized Edema after the Neonatal Period

Excessive crying, excessive rubbing of the eyes, conjunctivitis, blepharitis, and sensitivity to eye drops or certain other drugs are common causes of edema about the eye.

Angioneurotic edema or Quincke edema results from an immune deficiency or secondary to a number of allergens including agents such as tartrazine (coloring matter in foods and drugs), disodium cromoglycate, demeclocycline, and clonidine.

Face edema as a part of drug reaction may also occur in case of aspirin, cotrimoxazole, penicillin, nitrofurantoin, chlordiazepoxide, cephaloridine, amitriptyline, clonazepam, ethosuximide, imipramine, primidone, troxidone, and vitamin A toxicity.

Infections and inflammations such as boils, sinusitis, dental abscess, orbital cellulitis, chronic lymphangitis, resection of regional lymph nodes, filariasis, etc. are well-known causes of localized edema (Fig. 20.4).

Mumps may be accompanied by edema over the manubrium (sternal edema) and upper chest wall as a result of lymphatic obstruction. It manifests approximately 5 days after the appearance of parotid swelling and lasts for almost an equal period.

Epidemic dropsy: Infrequently, edema may result from adverse effect of a toxic substance. In epidemic dropsy which caused panic in Delhi and several other States of

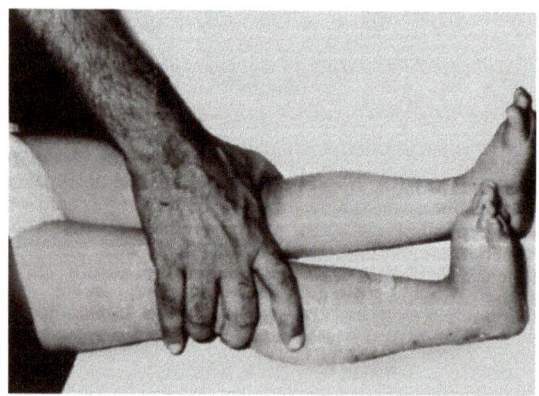

Fig. 20.3: *Milroy's disease*: The non-pitting edema in this child was present ever since birth.

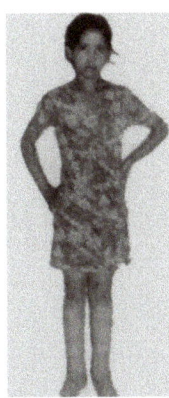

Fig. 20.4: *Lymphedema precox*: Note the lower extremity edema in a 12-year-old girl without any obvious cause, even on usual investigations. This condition of progressive lymphedema is usually encountered in females between 10 years and 25 years of age.

India in August–September 1998, consumption of an oil (usually mustard oil) adulterated with argemone oil was the etiologic factor. The adulterant acts through a toxic alkaloid, sanguinarine, and interferes with oxidation of pyruvic acid that accumulates in blood. The seeds of the wild *Argemone mexicana* (the so-called "prickly poppy") very much resemble the mustard seeds. The former has a tendency to grow in the thick of the latter. The intermixing of the two types of seeds, therefore, is understandable. In addition to its being accidental, it may also be done deliberately by unscrupulous elements.

Manifestations of epidemic dropsy include development of an acute noninflammatory swelling in both legs, nausea and vomiting, diarrhea, dyspnea, and CCF. A small number of subjects may develop glaucoma. Mortality in severe disease is high.

Diagnosis is primarily clinical and by exclusion of other causes of the clinical picture seen in dropsy. Two laboratory tests are available for establishing the diagnosis namely:

Nitric acid test: It consists of adding nitric acid to a suspected sample. If argemone is present in at least 0.25% proportion, the sample will turn brown to orange-red.

Paper chromatography: It is the most sensitive and dependable parameter, gives positive result when mustard or some other oil contains as low as 0.001% of argemone.

Treatment of dropsy is by and large symptomatic and supportive.

FURTHER READING

1. EpoMedicine. Approach to a child with edema Available at: http://epomedicine.com/clinical-medicine/approach-to-a-child-with-edema. Accessed on: 21 July 2019.
2. Lande A, Brook EA, Whitehead C. *The Child with Edema*. Philadelphia: Academicia 2005.
3. Levy PA. Edema. In: Adam HM, Foy JM (Eds). *Signs and Symptoms in Pediatrics*. Illinois: American Academy of Pediatrics 2015:255-262.
4. Turchin A, Seifter JL, Seely EW. Clinical problem-solving: Mind the gap. *N Engl J Med* 2003;349:1465-1469.

CHAPTER 21

Encopresis

BACKGROUND

Encopresis, also termed *fecal soiling or incontinence*, means involuntary passage of feces in the clothing repeatedly. Until the age of 4–5 years, it may well be a developmental variation. Thereafter, it is considered indicative of a disorder such as severe chronic constipation, mental retardation, neurologic defects such as progressive degenerative disease, or anal and rectal abnormalities.

HISTORY

History should seek information whether fecal incontinence is of recent onset or it has been like that since long as a part of unsuccessful toilet training. What is its frequency? Is there any relationship with time of the day? Is the child constipated? Is the constipated stool accompanied by streaks of blood? Is constipation indeed painful? Is the child mentally normal? Any neurologic disease he is known to suffer from?

PHYSICAL EXAMINATION

Clinical examination should focus on psychological, developmental and neurological evaluation. Rectal examination is imperative to check for impacted stool by inserting a lubricated gloved finger into child's rectum while pressing on his or her abdomen with the other hand.

A psychological evaluation for emotional issues is important.

INVESTIGATIONS

Usually, no investigations are needed.

An abdominal X-ray may be helpful in estimating the magnitude of fecal impaction.

IMPORTANT DIFFERENTIALS

Chronic Constipation

In severe chronic constipation, associated with fecal impaction or painful defecation, the mother may complain that the child simply soils or that he has diarrhea with soiling. In actuality, the so-called "diarrhea" is the liquid fecal matter that spills around the edges of a solid fecal mass situated either in the rectum or low in the colon. Rectum is found to be full of large fecal lumps.

This type of encopresis (the so-called "overflow" type) is responsible for a vast majority of the cases encountered in pediatric practice. For some unexplained reasons, it occurs dominantly in boys.

Emotional Disturbance

In some children, such emotional disturbances as separation from parents (usually the mother), starting school, or arrival of a younger sibling, may manifest with fecal soiling. There is evidence that these children seldom have had right bowel training. In fact, they rarely, if ever, have controlled the bowel.

Encopresis in these children reflects uncontrolled anger and defiance at the subconscious level.

The offensive odor from the child makes him a target of rebuke and scorn at home as well as at school. Naturally, his social relationship as also school performance and attendance suffer considerably.

Mental Retardation

Adequate bowel control needs normal anatomical relationships, an intact voluntary and involuntary nervous system, and consciousness of the urge to defecate.

Since all these requirements may not be met within many mentally retarded children, encopresis is a common observation in them.

Neurological Defects

Fecal soiling may well be an important manifestation of such neurological abnormalities as degenerative diseases, meningomyelocele, lipoma of the spinal cord, tumors of the spinal cord and trauma to the spinal cord. In such lesions, the urge to defecate is simply absent.

Local Defects

Absence of external and internal sphincter mechanisms may be responsible for encopresis in a small proportion of cases.

FURTHER READING

1. Chong SK. Gastrointestinal problems in the handicapped child. *Opin Pediatr* 2001;13:441-446.
2. Field DJ, Isaacs D, Stroobant J. Enuresis and encoporesis. In: Stroobant J (Ed). *Tutorials in Pediatric Differential Diagnosis.* New York: Churchill Livingstone 1989;1989:164-170.
3. Mayo Clinic. Encopresis. Available at: http://www.mayoclinic.org/diseases-conditions/encopresis/home/ovc-20253388. Accessed on: 21 July 2019.
4. Mikkelsen EJ. Enuresis and encopresis: ten years of progress. *J Am Acad Child Adolesc Psychiatr* 2001;40:1146-1452.

CHAPTER 22

Enuresis

BACKGROUND

The term, *enuresis*, usually denotes occurrence of involuntary voiding of urine into bed or clothes at or after the age of 5 years (age at which volitional bladder control should have been established). According to Diagnostic and Statistical Manual of Mental Disorders-5 (DSM-5), even such voluntary (intentional) voiding should also be considered enuresis (Box 22.1).

INTRODUCTION

Enuresis may be diurnal or nocturnal. In the former, lack of bladder control occurs during waking hours. It should not be considered abnormal if it occurs less than twice a week. During the first several years after being toilet trained, some children occasionally wet themselves while awake since they remain preoccupied with play and postpone emptying the bladder. Nocturnal diuresis is relatively more common and often a cause of considerable anxiety to the parents.

Enuresis may also be primary or secondary. *Primary enuresis* means that the child has never been able to have control over voiding during night. This is also termed "persistent enuresis". *Secondary or regressive enuresis* means that wetting occurs after the child has attained the normal bladder control. Whereas persistent enuresis is often the result of poor toilet training, the most important cause of regressive enuresis is a precipitating stressful situation like parental quarrelsomeness, arrival of a sibling, or a family tragedy. Organic pathology is found in only a small proportion of cases in both types of enuresis.

HISTORY

History should include a detailed interview with the parents as well as the enuretic child to find out the natural history of the problem, and possible etiologic or at least precipitating emotional factors. Obtain information about child's fluid intake and urinary output. Is there any history of associated fever or dysuria? Any worm infestation?

PHYSICAL EXAMINATION

Physical examination should particularly exclude presence of neurological and spinal abnormalities. The possibility of chronically distended abdomen should be evaluated by abdominal and rectal examination after the child has voided. It is advisable to watch the child for force and quality of urinary stream during the act of micturition.

INVESTIGATIONS

Most children need no investigations, except for the routine urine, stool and hemogram.

In a limited number of cases where organic pathology is suspected, urine culture, an X-ray of lumbosacral spine, ultrasonography, voiding cystourethrogram, urodynamic studies or test(s) dictated by the merits of the case may be carried out.

DIFFERENTIALS

Primary (Persistent) Enuresis

Poor Toilet Training

Mismanagement of toilet training, especially when the child is about the stage of maturation that enables him to control micturition, can delay the acquisition of control, causing

---

BOX 22.1: DSM-5 criteria for enuresis.

- Repeated voiding of urine into bed or clothes (whether involuntary or intentional).
- Behavior must be clinically significant as manifested by either a frequency of twice a week for at least three consecutive months or the presence of clinically significant distress or impairment in social, academic (occupational), or other important areas of functioning.
- Chronological age is at least 5 years of age (or equivalent developmental level).
- The behavior is not due exclusively to the direct physiological effect of a substance [such as a diuretic, antipsychotic or selective serotonin reuptake inhibitors (SSRI)] or to incontinence uncured as a result of polyuria or during loss of consciousness.
- These symptoms must not be due to a general loss of consciousness.

enuresis. Over enthusiastic parents make a significant error in far-too-early "potting", compelling the child to sit on pottie for too long and smacking him for not using the pottie.

Familial

In some families, enuresis occurs as a familial trait. There is delay in the maturation of the relevant components of the CNS. Hence, children are late in attaining bladder control. Undoubtedly, additional psychological overlay may complicate the problem.

Anatomical Defects

Such anatomical anomalies as bladder-neck or urethral obstruction, ectopic ureter entering the vagina, diverticulum of the anterior urethra, sacral agenesis, etc. may infrequently be responsible for primary enuresis.

Mental Retardation

Just like delay in walking and talking, a mentally subnormal is likely to acquire bladder control significantly late. Understandably, this is related to the delayed maturation of the nervous system.

Emotional Deprivation

An emotionally deprived child, particularly if he is brought up in an orthodox type of institution, is likely to suffer from delayed acquisition of bladder control.

Secondary (Regressive) Enuresis

Psychological

Secondary enuresis is most often a manifestation of family conflict and maladjustment, e.g. too strict parents, rejection, sibling rivalry, quarrelsomeness between the parents, problems at school, acute anxiety, etc.

Worm Infestation

Heavy threadworm infestation (enterobiasis or oxyuriasis) is frequently associated with enuresis. Eradication of the infestation leads to regression in frequency of enuresis and in some even full recovery from it.

Metabolic Disorders

Enuresis may well be the first manifestation of diabetes mellitus or diabetes insipidus in a child who had till recently been dry. The child with diabetes mellitus may also suffer from such additional manifestations as excessive thirst (polydypsia), polyuria, excessive hunger (polyphagia), weight loss, general weakness, tiredness and bodily pains. Fainting attacks due to spontaneous hypoglycemia, vulvitis, abdominal pain, nausea and vomiting, irritability and deterioration in school performance.

In diabetes insipidus, enuresis is accompanied by polydipsia and polypuria.

Neurogenic Bladder

Such congenital conditions as meningomyelocele, lipomeningocele, sacral agenesis, or other spinal abnormalities may cause neurogenic bladder and resultant enuresis. In addition, cerebral palsy, CNS tumors, repair of imperforate anus or excision of sacrococcygeal teratoma may lead to abnormal innervation of bladder and sphincters, resulting in urinary incontinence.

Urinary Tract Infection

Urinary tract infection is an important cause of secondary enuresis, especially when it is accompanied by fever and dysuria. Besides urinalysis, it is advisable to do the urine culture.

FURTHER READING

1. Field DJ, Isaacs D, Stroobant J. Enuresis and encoporesis. In: Stroobant J (Ed). *Tutorials in Pediatric Differential Diagnosis*. New York: Churchill Livingstone 1989:164-170.
2. Glazener CM, Evans JH, Peto RV. Alarm interventions for nocturnal enuresis in children. *Cochrane Database Syst Rev* 2005(2): CD002911.
3. Kalia A. Enuresis. In: Gupte S, Srivastava RN, Kalia A (Eds). *Recent Advances in Pediatrics (Special Vol 15: Pediatric Nephrology)*. New Delhi: Jaypee 2005:171-202.
4. Mikkelson EJ. Enuresis and encopresis: ten years of progress. *J Am Acad Child Adolesc Psychiatr* 2001;40:1146-1152.
5. Sharma M, Singh T, Hans G, et al. Developmental, behavioral and psychiatric disorders. In: Gupte S (Ed): *The Short Textbook of Pediatrics*, 13th edn. New Delhi: Jaypee 2020.

CHAPTER 23

Epistaxis

BACKGROUND

Epistaxis, also called *nosebleeds* or nasal bleeding, is a common symptom after the first year and up to puberty, causing considerable anxiety to the sufferer as well as the parents. In our experience, it occurs in 10% of children. In a vast majority of the cases, blood loss is small. Of course, it appeals quite large to the parents. Moreover, the episode is frequently transient, stopping spontaneously or after application of little pressure.

Irrespective of the basic cause of bleeding, the fact remains that the site of epistaxis usually is the anteroinferior part of the cartilaginous nasal septum which has a rich vascular plexus (Kiesselbach's plexus, area or triangle the anastomotic site for a number of terminal arterioles, 0.5 cm within the nose and above the nasal floor) followed by the mucosa lining the anterior portion of the turbinates. Notably, even in such bleeding disorders as leukemias, purpuras or hemophilia, this is the usual location of epistaxis.

HISTORY

In clinical history-taking, it is vital to determine if there has been any sort of physical injury to the nose with special reference to nose picking. Is the patient a habitual nose picker? Any history of foreign body, overexposure to solar radiation, allergic rhinitis, upper respiratory catarrh, pertussis, cystic fibrosis, etc.? Enquire if the subject is suffering from such diseases as uremia, hypertension, or liver disorder. A child who manifests epistaxis along with throbbing headache may well be suffering from hypertension. Any relationship with menses?

When you encounter epistaxis in association with bleeding from one or more additional sites, remember to exclude blood dyscrasias like leukemias.

A careful search for a bleeding disorder in family members (say, in maternal uncles in case of hemophilia A) points to a genetically determined etiology.

PHYSICAL EXAMINATION

The most important part of physical examination is detailed and careful examination of the nose for deformity, a bleeding point, a telangiectasia spot over Kiesselbach's area, congestion or pallor of mucosa, foreign body, polyp, ulceration, etc. Is there any evidence of sinusitis in the form of local sinus tenderness and/or purulent discharge oozing out of the sinus opening in the nose. Look for purpuric lesions over skin or active bleeding from other sites. What is the blood pressure? Any organomegaly, particularly with reference to liver, spleen and lymph glands?

Direct visualization with a good directed light source, a nasal speculum, and nasal suction should be sufficient in most patients.

INVESTIGATIONS

Generally speaking, investigations are neither needed nor helpful for first-time nosebleeds or infrequent recurrences secondary to nose picking/injury to the nose. However, they are recommended if major bleeding is present or if a coagulopathy is suspected.

- Complete blood count (CBP), hematocrit and type and cross-match in persistent heavy bleeding.
- CBP with differential in recurrent epistaxis from a platelet disorder or neoplasia.
- Bleeding time if suspicion of a bleeding disorder is present.
- International normalized ratio (INR)/prothrombin time (PT) if the patient is taking warfarin or if liver disease is suspected.
- Activated partial thromboplastin time (aPTT) is necessary.
- CT scan, MRI or both may be indicated to evaluate the surgical anatomy and to determine the presence and extent of rhinosinusitis, foreign bodies, and neoplasms.
- Nasopharyngoscopy if a tumor is suspected.

IMPORTANT DIFFERENTIALS

Trauma

Nose picking is the most common cause of epistaxis in childhood. The location of trauma is usually the anterior portion of the nasal septum, about the Kiesselbach's area. The bleeding spot can frequently be inspected after cleaning the area of the clots. A careful examination may reveal presence of dried blood under the patient's fingernails. This kind of nosebleed is termed epistaxis digitorum.

Nasal trauma, say from other causes like a hard blow over the nose, may cause laceration of the mucosa, deformity and fracture in association with epistaxis.

Basal skull fracture may manifest as epistaxis with CSF rhinorrhea.

Foreign Body

As and when recurrent epistaxis accompanies unilateral nasal obstruction, foul discharge, particularly in a child with older sibling who is in the habit of inserting nuts, beads, crayons, plastic pieces or similar objects into the patient's nose during play, a foreign body must be suspected. A careful examination usually enables visualization of the foreign body.

Solar Radiation

Though this factor as a cause of epistaxis has generally been neglected in the western literature, there is little doubt that it is an important and common cause of recurrent epistaxis in India and other tropical countries.

Solar radiation induces sudden nosebleed in individuals with very thin-walled anastomotic vessels over the Kiesselbach's area.

Nasal Polyposis

Recurrent epistaxis in association with manifestations of nasal obstruction, including mouth breathing, hyposmia, postnasal drip, persistent cold and sneezing should arouse suspicion of nasal polyposis. Visualization of pedunculated hypertrophied edematous nasal mucosa confirms the diagnosis.

Incidence of nasal polyposis is particularly high in cystic fibrosis.

Upper Respiratory Infection/Allergy

Such states as adenoidal hypertrophy/adenitis, allergic rhinitis, atrophic rhinitis, hypertrophic rhinitis, sinusitis, etc. may be accompanied by epistaxis.

In nasal diphtheria, besides blood-stained and mucopurulent discharge, the anterior nares show excoriation. Whereas in acute form toxemic symptoms are dominant, a grayish-white membrane is the hallmark of chronic form.

Physical and Emotional Stress and Strain

Violent exertion, vigorous blowing, sneezing, paroxysmal and forceful cough as in pertussis or cystic fibrosis, excitement, etc. are also known to foster nosebleeds.

Congenital Vascular Defect

Rendu-Osler-Weber disease, which usually manifests with epistaxis, is characterized by presence of telangiectasia on nasal mucosa (septum and turbinates) as also on oral mucosa, on skin and under fingernails. Family history is usually positive for epistaxis/telangiectasia. The cause of bleeding is increased capillary fragility. There is no defect/deficiency of platelets or coagulation factors.

Systemic Diseases

Hypertension, uremia, cirrhosis of liver, rheumatic fever, acute nephritis, anemia, enteric fever, measles, etc. may well be complicated by epistaxis.

Bleeding Disorders

In leukemias, purpuras, hemophilia, Von Willebrand disease and DIC, epistaxis may be the presenting features. Remaining features of these bleeding disorders aided by specific investigations help to reach the precise diagnosis.

Remaining Causes of Epistaxis

Tuberculosis, syphilis, leprosy, fungal infections, tumors, puberty, high altitude, scurvy, vitamin K deficiency, sickle-cell disease, brucellosis, prolonged use of phenylephrine nasal drops, juvenile angiofibroma of the nasopharynx, lymphoepithelioma, etc.

FURTHER READING

1. Makura ZG, Porter GC, McCormick MS. Pediatric epistaxis: Alder Hey experience. *J Laryngol Otol* 2002;116:903-906.
2. Malbury PE. Recurrent epistaxis. *Pediatric Rev* 1991;12:213-216.
3. Medscape. Epistaxis workup. Available at: http://emedicine.medscape.com/article/863220-workup#c9. Accessed on: 21st July 2019.
4. Wurman LH. Epistaxis. In: Gates GA (Ed). *Current Therapy in Otolaryngology—Head and Neck Surgery*, 5th edn. St Louis: Mosby 1994:354-359.

CHAPTER 24

Floppy Baby Syndrome

BACKGROUND

The term, *floppy baby syndrome*, denotes flabby muscles in an infant. A large number of conditions may be hidden behind this symptom complex, ranging from the benign congenital hypotonia through Down syndrome to Werdnig-Hoffmann disease (Box 24.1).

HISTORY

Interrogation must clarify if the floppiness has been there ever since birth or it occurred later. Is it stationary, improving or progressing? Any feeding problem, respiratory difficulty, lethargy, hoarseness, prolongation of physiologic icterus, or anemia unresponsive to usual therapy? Is there any mental and/or developmental retardation? Any history of birth trauma or asphyxia? Any seizures? Any suggestion of a preceding illness? Has any other sibling or family member suffered from such an illness? Did the mother experience absence or reduction of fetal movements in utero? Is she suffering from myasthenia gravis?

PHYSICAL EXAMINATION

Physical examination must, in first place, confirm if the baby is indeed floppy with remarkable hypotonia of all his muscles, especially skeletal muscles. Observations on ventral suspension (Figs. 24.1A and B) and on "pull-to-sit" provide good idea about hypotonia. What is the state of affairs regarding tendon reflexes? Any sensory involvement? Any mental or developmental retardation and its extent? Any involvement of tongue, jaw, and face muscles? Are extraocular muscles or sphincters spared? Any respiratory muscle involvement? Are there any facial features which may be compatible with Down syndrome or cretinism? Is he obese? Is he grossly malnourished? Any evidence of rickets or scurvy?

INVESTIGATIONS

An etiology diagnosed is reached in half of the cases through good history and physical examination. Rest of the cases

BOX 24.1: Causes of floppy baby syndrome.

- *Benign:* Congenital hypotonia
- *Chromosomal disorders:* Down syndrome, trisomies 13–15
- *Neurological disorders:* Atonic cerebral palsy, poliomyelitis, glycogen storage disease, cerebral lipidosis, congenital myopathy, myasthenia gravis, polyneuritis, polymyositis (dermatomyositis), Werdnig-Hoffmann disease's, Prader-Willi syndrome
- *Endocrinopathy:* Congenital hypothyroidism
- *Nutritional:* Advanced PEM, rickets, scurvy
- *Miscellaneous disorders:* Acrodynia, Ehlers-Danlos syndrome, infant botulism, kernicterus.

(PEM: protein-energy malnutrition)

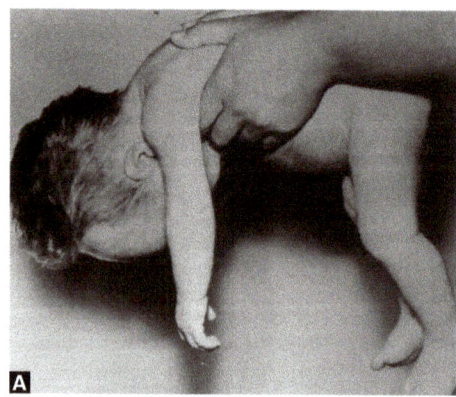
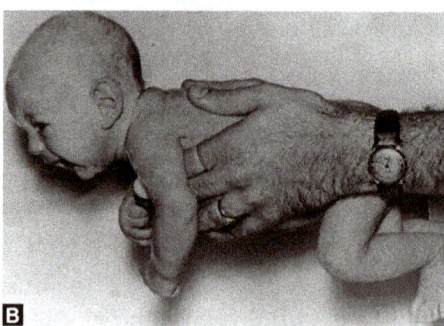

Figs. 24.1A and B: Floppy baby. (A) Note the remarkable hypotonia (weakness) of limbs, trunk, and neck on ventral suspension; and (B) The normal response in a healthy infant.

need investigations to establish the diagnosis. Of course the choice of tests is guided by the merits of each case.

Central Etiology

- Neuroimaging
  - Ultrasound scan in the first instance.
  - Magnetic resonance imaging (MRI) may be indicated if a structural abnormality of brain development is suspected and to exclude other abnormalities [say, evidence of hypoxic-ischemic encephalopathy (HIE)]
- *Electroencephalogram (EEG)*: Good for prognostic information as to brain function, useful clinically if seizures are suspected
- *Genetics review*: If dysmorphic features, consider molecular karyotype and DNA methylation studies or fluorescent in-situ hybridization (FISH) for Prader-Willi syndrome (if indicated)
- Congenital infection screen
- Metabolic workup.

Peripheral Etiology

- Molecular genetics
- Creatine kinase
- Nerve conduction studies
- Muscle biopsy.

IMPORTANT DIFFERENTIALS

Benign Congenital Hypotonia

This condition, familial in some instances, is characterized by presence of gross hypotonia and delayed motor development. The infant's muscles are soft and flabby, allowing remarkable range of movements. Some tendon reflexes are elicitable whereas others are absent. Spontaneous movements are prominent. Intellectual development is always normal.

The disease may take one of the three courses. First—it may remain stationary and nonprogressive. Second—some children may develop contractures though joints always remain hypermobile. Third—most subjects recover fully by the age of 8–10 years.

Spinal Muscular Atrophy

Spinal muscular atrophy (SMA) may be of four types:
1. Spinal muscular atrophy type I (acute infantile SMA, Werdnig-Hoffman disease) (Fig. 24.2)
2. Spinal muscular atrophy type II (chronic infantile SMA)
3. Spinal muscular atrophy type III (chronic juvenile SMA)
4. Spinal muscular atrophy type IV (adult SMA).

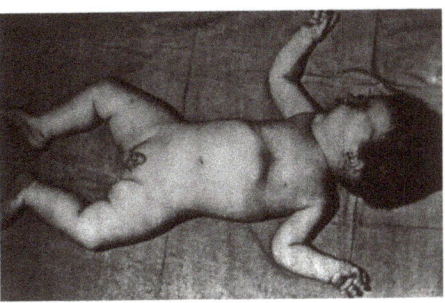

Fig. 24.2: Spinal muscular atrophy (SMA) type I (Werdnig–Hoffmann disease). Note the characteristic posture (the so-called frog-leg posture) of lower limbs and external rotation at the shoulders together with chest retraction.

Werdnig-Hoffmann disease, also called *spinal muscular atrophy* (type I), an autosomal recessive disorder, is characterized by a positive family history, absence or reduction of fetal movements in utero, and manifestations occurring before the age of 2 years and, frequently, right at birth.

Classically, gross hypotonia with areflexia manifests early in infancy. The legs assume the so-called "frog leg position" with abduction at hips and flexion at knees. Intercostal and bulbar muscles are involved whereas diaphragm is more or less spared, resulting in characteristic paradoxical respiration with inward movement of the chest on inspiration. Fasciculations or fibrillations are visible in the tongue which may also show atrophy. The mental development, on the contrary, is remarkably normal. The infant tends to be obese in initial stages.

In a large majority of the cases, the disease progresses rapidly, proving fatal during infancy *per se*. The cause of death is neurologic involvement of muscles of thorax, respiratory failure, aspiration of food and/or fulminant infection. The survivors, infrequently reaching adolescence and, rarely, adulthood, are in a completely helpless state.

The diagnosis is mainly clinical. Muscle biopsy shows classical features of denervation atrophy with large patches of small atrophic fibers with residual muscle fibers with or somewhat enlarged diameter.

Myasthenia Gravis

This disorder, occurring secondary to an autoimmune reaction against acetylcholine receptors, may be responsible for floppiness in the newborn. Two types are recognized:
1. *First type:* Transient neonatal myasthenia gravis which the baby acquires from the mother with established, mild or even unrecognized disease. The infant is floppy and weak with poor feeding, feeble cry, feeble respiratory effort, lots of oral secretions, and ptosis. However, he appears alert with normal deep tendon reflexes. Response to edrophonium/neostigmine

(intramuscular) is excellent. Even without therapy, many infants show spontaneous recovery within 3–4 weeks.
2. *Second type:* Persistent neonatal myasthenia gravis occurs without any evidence of the disease in the mother. Chances of occurrence of the condition in other sibling(s) are high. Besides manifestations of the transient form, the eyelids and extraocular muscles are severely affected. It is likely to persist throughout life.

Cerebral Palsy

Two forms of nonprogressive central motor deficit dating to events in prenatal, natal or perinatal period (most often cerebral anoxia) are accompanied by floppiness.

Atonic diplegia is characterized by hypotonia, motor disability, and, usually, severe mental retardation. Tendon reflexes are easily elicitable. These may well be rather brisk. As the child grows, some degree of spasticity develops.

Congenital cerebellar ataxia, a rare form of cerebral palsy, is characterized by hypotonia, hypoactive tendon reflexes, and later, gait ataxia with intention tremors. Slight mental retardation and nystagmus may develop.

Congenital Hypothyroidism

The hypothyroid infant often attracts attention in the neonatal period only because of hypotonia, lethargy, sluggishness, hoarse cry, feeding difficulty, oversleeping, persistent jaundice, persistent constipation, abdominal distention with umbilical hernia, cold, rough, dry and thickened skin, a thickened protruding tongue, very large posterior fontanel, and anemia that respond poorly to hematinics. The infant is usually large and heavy at birth.

The classical features of congenital hypothyroidism usually take a few weeks (8–12) to develop. The facies are characteristic a large tongue protruding from large open mouth with thick lips, puffy eyelids, depressed nasal bridge, pseudohypertelorism, and wrinkled forehead with sparse eyebrows and the hairline reaching very low over it (Fig. 24.3).

Neck is short and there is often a pad of supraclavicular fat. Scalp hair is scanty, rough, dry, and brittle. Skin is rough, thick, dry, and cold. Anterior fontanel and coronal sutures are often widely open. Voice is hoarse. Dentition is delayed. Floppiness is virtually a rule. Abdomen is often distended and an umbilical hernia of variable size is present. Hands are broad with short fingers. Constipation, not responding to courses of laxatives and changes in feeding regimes, is usual.

Also, mental retardation and physical and growth retardation invariably coexist. The upper/lower segments ratio may continue to be infantile, i.e. 1.7:1.

The diagnosis may be confirmed by X-ray studies for bone age and epiphyseal dysgenesis, elevated serum cholesterol, low serum alkaline phosphatase, low protein-bound iodine (PBI), low radioactive iodine (^{131}I), high plasma thyroid-stimulating hormone (TSH), and most importantly, low T_3 and T_4.

Down Syndrome

Like congenital hypothyroidism, it is not difficult to make diagnosis of Down syndrome, the 21 trisomy, in a floppy infant because of the classical stigmata, including obvious features and mental retardation.

Apparently, the infant is a cheerful idiot with microcephaly, low hairline, and short neck (Figs. 24.4A and B). Facial features include upward slant of the eyes, epicanthal folds and, occasionally, Brushfield spots. Nose is

Fig. 24.3: Congenital hypothyroidism—Note the infantile body proportions and characteristic coarse facial features with short neck in this mentally and physically retarded child.

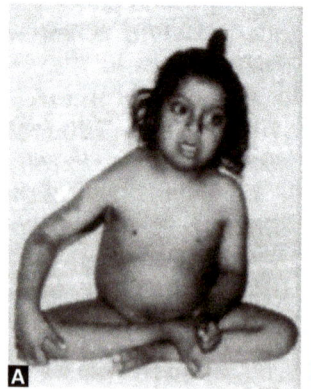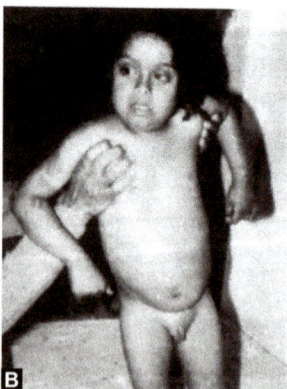

Figs. 24.4A and B: Down syndrome—Note cheerful idiocy, microcephaly, upward slant of eyes, epicanthal folds, depressed bridge of nose, widely apart eyes, and short neck and hypotonia. IQ was just 30. He also had ventricular septal defect (VSD), Simian crease (bilateral), and in curved little finger (bilateral).

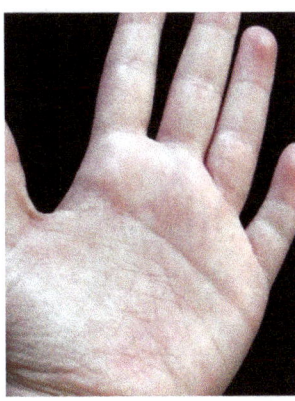

Fig. 24.5: Single palmar crease across the palm.

short with flattened bridge, which, together with epicanthal folds, gives an impression of increased distance between the eyes, the so-called "pseudohypertelorism". Tongue is protruded from small buccal cavity and may be furrowed, the so-called "scrotal tongue". Ears are low-set and may be deformed. High-arched palate and malocclusion of teeth may be present. Hands are short and broad with a single palmar crease, the so-called "Simian crease" and an incurved little finger due to rudimentary middle phalanx (Fig. 24.5). Feet show wide gap between the big and second toes and, at times, a deep crease starting between them and extending on to the sole.

There is a significantly enhanced incidence of congenital heart disease, duodenal atresia, Hirschsprung disease, and leukemia in subjects with Down syndrome.

Prader-Willi Syndrome

Floppiness is an important feature of the multisystem disorder, Prader–Willi syndrome. The remaining features of the syndrome include obesity, hypotonia, hypogonadism, strabismus, and tendency to diabetes mellitus.

Marfan Syndrome

In this congenital disorder of the connective tissues, manifestation in the neonatal period and early infancy may include muscle floppiness, arachnodactyly (spider fingers), and hyperextensibility of the joints. Lenticular subluxation and dilatation of the aorta may also develop early in life.

Drugs

Diazepam, tricyclic antidepressants, kanamycin, colistin sulfalc, cycloserine, ethionamide, gentamicin, nitrofurantoin, neomycin, INH, cyclophosphamide, 6-MP, meprobomate, lead, vincristine, etc.

Remaining Causes of Floppy Baby Syndrome

- *Central nervous system (CNS)*—Kernicterus, chromosomal defects, Lowe (oculocerebrorenal) syndrome, cerebral lipidosis, mucoviscidosis, etc.
- *Spinal cord*—Trauma, epidural abscess, shock phase of transverse myelitis, extensive poliomyelitis, etc.
- *Peripheral nerves*—Guillain-Barré syndrome, extensive diphtheritic paralysis, arsenical neuropathy, familial dysautonomia, congenital sensory neuropathy, etc.
- *Neuromuscular junction*—Infantile botulism.
- *Muscles*—Congenital muscular dystrophy, myotonic dystrophy, Pompe type of glycogen storage disease, central core disease, nemaline myopathy, mitochondrial myopathies, polymyositis, arthrogryposis multiplex congenital, etc.
- *Miscellaneous*—Advanced protein-energy malnutrition, rickets, scurvy, acrodynia, Ehler–Danlos syndrome, cutis laxa, etc.

FURTHER READING

1. Crawford TO. Clinical evaluation of floppy infant. *Pediatric Ann* 1992;21:348-354.
2. Gulati S, Thukral A, Das M. The floppy child: An approach. In: Gupte S (Ed). *Recent Advances in Pediatrics (Special Vol 18: Pediatric Neurology)*. New Delhi: Jaypee 2008:395-421.
3. Gulati S, Singh LR, Gupte S, Chowdhary B. Pediatric neurology. In: Gupte S (Ed). *The Short Textbook of Pediatrics*, 13th edn. New Delhi: Jaypee 2020.
4. Newborn Sevices Clinical Guidelines. Neonatal hypotonia. Available at: www.adhb.govt.nz/newborn/Guidelines/Neurology/Hypotonia.htm Accessed on: 21st July 2019.

CHAPTER 25

Failure to Thrive

BACKGROUND

The term, *failure to thrive (FTT)*, is applied to infants and young children (usually up to the age of 5 years) who show failure of expected weight gain and striking lack of wellbeing. It is a descriptive and not a diagnostic term.

The essential component in FTT is sluggish weight gain compared to the peers of same age and sex.

In practice, one of the following criteria must be met:
- Weight <3rd percentile (some experts consider even <5th percentile),
- A change in the rate of growth crossing two major centiles (say, 75th to 50th) over a period of time.

Slow length/height gain and/or development may accompany FTT.

In a way the term, FTT, is employed for infants and children who fail to gain weight proportional to length or height and may even lose it though there is no superficially apparent cause for it. The anthropometric index used for FTT should be weight for length or height. Empirically, the observation period should be at least 1 month. At best, it is a descriptive and not a diagnostic term. In other words, a thorough clinical, investigative and follow-up evaluation is needed in subjects given this designation.

A "constitutionally light child" with weight below 3rd percentile but showing an appropriate weight gain should not be labeled "FTT" (Fig. 25.1). Figure 25.2 depicts three patterns of FTT:
1. Fall-off in weight gain
2. Static weight
3. Weight loss.

HISTORY

History-taking in this particular situation brings out more important information if it is conducted by different interviewers at different times.

A detailed information on child's dietary intake is crucial. How is his appetite? Does he eat enough and yet is not gaining adequate weight? Or, is it that poor appetite is responsible for a significantly poor intake? Make a rough calculation of his actual calorie and protein intake and assess it in relation to the recommended intake for his age. I often come across 2 or 3-year-old fed only on milk (which means enough of proteins but inadequate calories) and the parents wondering why, in spite of such a nutritious diet, the child is not thriving well.

Is there any history of intestinal parasitosis—direct or indirect? Any chronic diarrhea? Any suggestion of malabsorption? In celiac disease, tropical sprue, etc. not

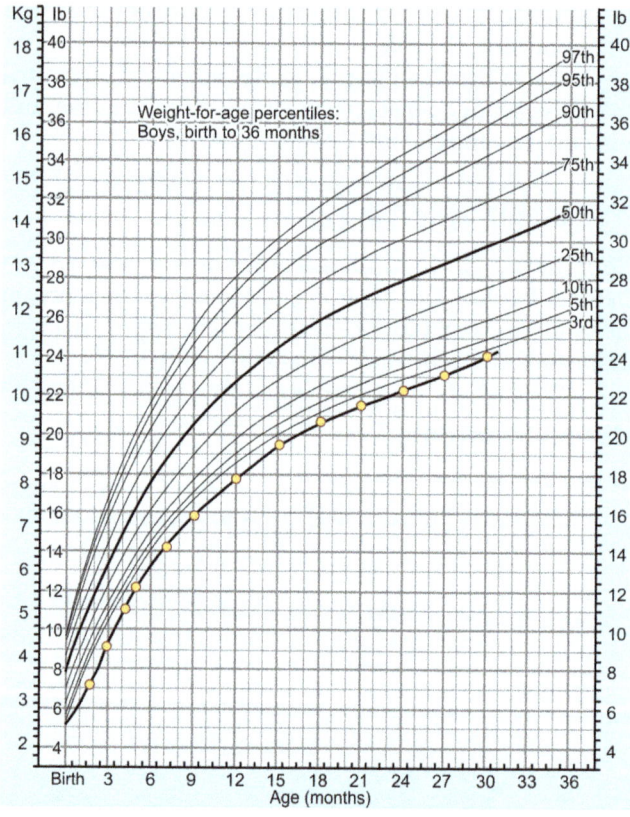

Fig. 25.1: Growth chart showing "constitutionally light child" with weight less than 3rd percentile but weight gain at an appropriate rate. This should not be considered as "failure to thrive (FTT)".

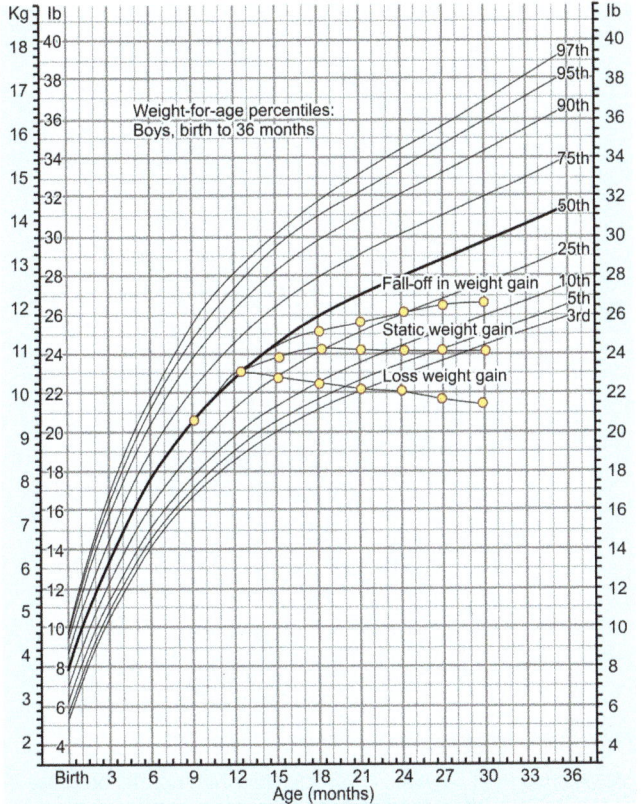

Fig. 25.2: Growth chart showing three patterns of failure to thrive (FTT), i.e. fall-off in weight gain, static weight and weight loss.

only reduced appetite causes reduced intake, whatever is eaten is only poorly absorbed. In cystic fibrosis, appetite is usually voracious. But the ingested food becomes available only in a small proportion for body building because of presence of pancreatogenous steatorrhea.

Any family history of tuberculosis? Failure to thrive may well be the only apparent manifestation of primary complex.

Any physical handicap? At times, physical handicap such as cerebral palsy, partial cleft palate, etc. may be contributing to child's inability to thrive well.

Every effort must be made to trace the adverse factors in child's family environment. Any evidence of maternal deprivation? Is there any suggestion of child abuse and neglect? What is the parent-child conflict precisely, if any?

PHYSICAL EXAMINATION

Physical examination should aim at assessment of the nutritional status and finding the known cause that may be operating in the case under reference. Study of growth chart (Fig. 25.3), if constructed, and a developmental flow sheet assist in identifying the physical or environmental factor(s) responsible for failure to thrive.

In case clinical work-up suggests disturbance in a particular organ system, appropriate screening tests must be carried out. However, before resorting to sophisticated and cumbersome investigations, it is important to carry out meticulous microscopic examinations of stools, at least on three successive days (preferably, on 5 or 6 successive days), treat intestinal parasites if detected in stools, and give a trial of feeding for at least 2 weeks, in the hospital *per se*.

INVESTIGATIONS

Generally speaking, history and physical examination should guide any laboratory or ancillary testing.
- Complete blood picture (CBP) warranted with specific gravity, evidence of infection, renal tubular acidosis
- Stool microscopy for ova and cysts
- Renal function tests: Serum electrolytes, BUN, and creatinine levels
- Liver function tests
- HIV testing if risk factors are noted or if history and examination are at all suggestive
- Sweat chloride test for cystic fibrosis
- Zinc level reported to be low in malnourished infants and children
- Tuberculosis testing
- Malabsorption studies
- Metabolic screening
- Endocrinal screening.

IMPORTANT DIFFERENTIALS

Nutritional Deprivation

In the developing world, this appears to be the most important factor in causation of the syndrome of failure to thrive. Gross deficiency of protein and energy intake, no doubt, clearly leads to overt syndromal states of kwashiorkor and marasmus. In the present context, our concern is the mild-to-moderate deficiency, usually resulting from ignorance about nutritional needs of the child. For instance, slow, chronic borderline dietary inadequacy starting fairly early in life may not cause overt picture of kwashiorkor or marasmus. The child rather slows down in gaining height as well as weight. Seemingly, his weight for height is nearly all right though it is significantly less than expected for actual age. This state is termed nutritional dwarfing. Of course, such a child may develop acute malnutrition on top of existing chronic malnutrition, leading to acute on chronic malnutrition (Fig. 25. 4).

Nutritional dwarfing is a common problem in our settings. But the cases are not as often detected. The condition seems to be a kind of "adaptation" to poor diet (not as grave as to cause frank kwashiorkor or marasmus) over a prolonged period. The affected child is less active and less lively and is more susceptible to diarrheal disease, pneumonia, tuberculosis or other infections prevalent in the region.

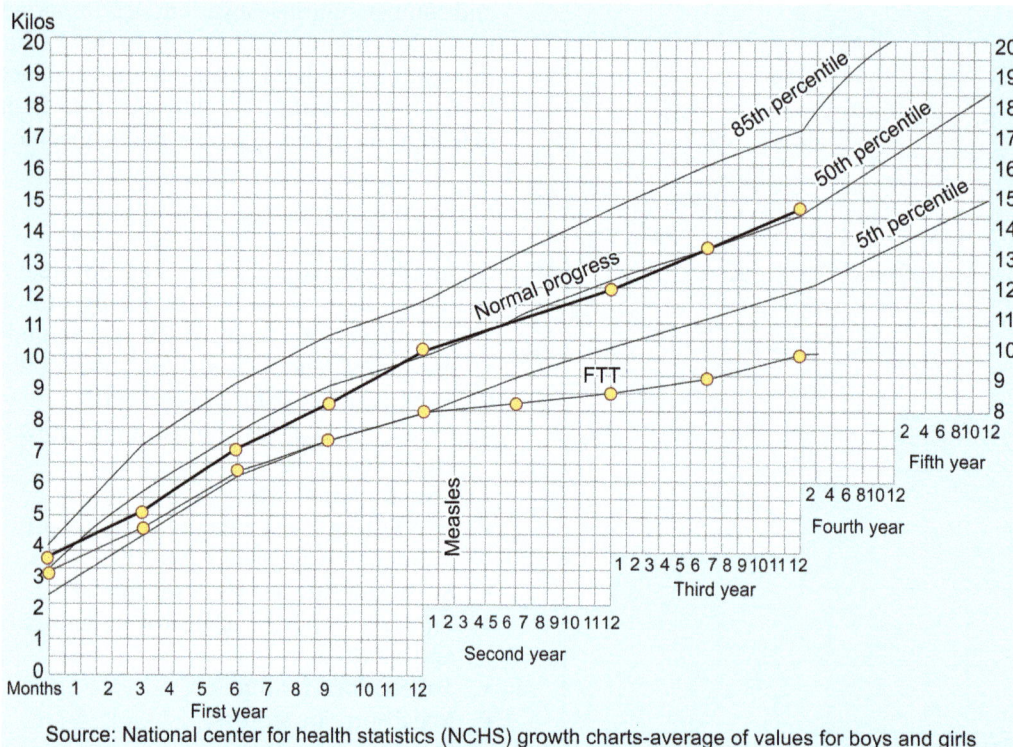

Fig. 25.3: "Road to Health" card showing progress of a child with failure to thrive (FTT) against a healthy child with normal progress in weight gain. Note that the FTT child was doing fine during the first 6 months. Then his progress slowed down, probably secondary to negligible intake of semisolids. An attack of measles at age 15 months further proved a setback. This is reflected in the growth becoming almost flat and falling below 5th percentile.

Over and above protein-energy malnutrition, even vitamin deficiencies diseases, e.g. rickets may cause FTT (Fig. 25.5).

Maternal/Social/Environmental Deprivation

Emotional deprivation resulting from psychosocial circumstances (often not quite obvious) may affect child's intake, absorption or utilization of food considerably. In the affluent countries where primary nutritional deprivation is not much of a problem, this factor is known to be the most common cause of failure to thrive. In fact, some authorities believe that the term, failure to thrive, psychosomatic growth failure, and maternal deprivation syndrome may be considered synonymous. No doubt, emotional deprivation does play considerable role in our infants and children too. Nevertheless, I maintain that nutritional deprivation takes the major share of etiologic factors in failure to thrive in our set-up.

The circumstances of the parents that may contribute to the syndrome include general immaturity of one or both parents, irresponsible/antisocial behavior, drug abuse, economic stress and strain, marital disharmony, dislike of children, low tolerance for stress, single parenthood, etc.

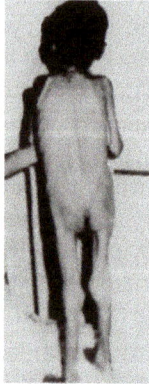

Fig. 25.4: Acute on chronic malnutrition. This 8-year-old boy who had not been thriving well over the years on account of inadequate dietary intake weight 17.5 kg (height 107 cm), suffered further following an episode of acute diarrhea 2 months prior to admission. During this episode, he had been nearly semistarved. His weight on admission was only 13 kg.

Intestinal Parasitosis

Though not a significant factor in the etiology of failure to thrive in the developed regions, intestinal parasitosis

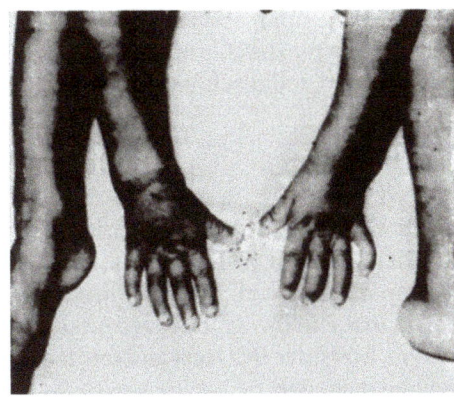

Fig. 25.5: Vitamin D-deficiency rickets in a child with failure to thrive (FTT). Note the remarkable widening of the wrists. The child was plump-looking and yet anemic (hemoglobin 8 g%). Frontal bossing of head, a widely open anterior fontanel and rachitic rosary were also present in this 18-month-old boy. Dietary history revealed that he was on almost entirely bottle feeding, consuming about 1.5–2 kg cow's milk daily.

decidedly occupies pride of place among the leading causes of the syndrome in India and other developing regions because of continued poor personal, water, food and environmental hygiene.

Chronic giardiasis is characterized by, besides failure to thrive, vague upper abdominal pain, recurrent diarrhea (stools are generally steatorrheic and often whitish with lots of undigested material), and nutritional deficiencies. Occasionally, there may be acute dysentery like presentation. Even transient ulcerative colitis has been observed.

Chronic amebiasis is characterized by failure to thrive, chronic diarrhea which may be accompanied by mucus and blood, recurrent abdominal pain and tenesmus. The complications include hepatitis, liver abscess, partial or complete intestinal obstruction, intussusception, perforation of colon, peritonitis, rectal ulcers and fistula and empyema.

Ascariasis is characterized by, in addition to growth failure, abdominal distention and pain, anemia vitamin deficiencies and voracious appetite. Pica, sleeplessness, irritability, urticaria, diarrhea and eosinophilia are encountered in a proportion to the cases. Occasionally, intestinal obstruction may occur. Migration of larvae may cause ascaris pneumonia (Löffler's pneumonia or syndrome), asthma-like manifestations, hepatosplenomegaly, or encephalopathy.

Ancylostomiasis is characterized by progressive anemia, anorexia, pain abdomen and malnutrition. Pica is often present. With the development of severe anemia and hypoproteinemia, the child may have edema which could become massive and generalized (anasarca). Diarrhea alternating with constipation may also be present. Some degree of malabsorption, as a result of histologic as well as functional insult to the small intestinal mucosa, occurs in many cases. The ground itch as a result of larval skin invasion over feet (buttocks in infants) is often mild and unnoticed. Occasionally, it may be seen as an irritant papulovesicular rash or even as cutaneous larva migrans.

Strongyloidiasis, relatively infrequent in India, resembles ancylostomiasis in many a way. Mild itching and urticaria at the site of penetration into the skin, pain abdomen, severe diarrhea, malabsorption, malnutrition and chest manifestations simulating Löffler's syndrome are the chief presenting features.

Trichuriasis, though seen quite infrequently in most parts of India, may well be responsible for failure to thrive in the sufferer. Remaining manifestations include prolonged diarrhea with bloodstreaked stools, right lower abdominal pain, tenesmus, malnutrition with anemia, rectal prolapse, eosinophilia and Charcot-Leyden crystals in stools. In heavy infestation, worms may be seen over surface of prolapsed rectal mucosa.

Oxyuriasis could well be responsible for failure to thrive in some of its sufferers. Of the various manifestation, pruritus ani tops the list. In some girls, vulvovaginitis may be present. Irritability, restlessness, sleep disturbances, behavior problems like bruxism, masturbation and enuresis, abdominal pain, diarrhea and poor appetite are encountered in some cases. Rarely, serious complications like appendicitis and salpingitis may occur.

Tapeworms may contribute to growth failure. In case of *Taenia solium* (pork tapeworm), most often the parents bring the child for 1–2 cm long segments (proglottids) passing in stools or crawling over the perianal area. Growth failure despite voracious appetite, abdominal distention and pain, and recurrent diarrhea may be the presenting manifestations in some.

Cysticercosis may lodge anywhere in the body. Brain involvement, manifesting as calcification in the skull X-ray, may cause convulsions. Calcified nodules may be palpable in the muscles.

Taenia saginata (beef tapeworm) causes manifestations that are similar to those of *Taenia solium*. It is less likely to cause cysticercosis. Absorption of the neurotoxin may, however, cause paresthesia and squint. Calcification may be detected in X-ray skull.

Hymenolepis nana (dwarf tapeworm) causes abdominal pain, loss of appetite, chronic diarrhea and growth failure.

Malabsorption States

Celiac disease (gluten sensitivity or gluten-induced enteropathy), is an abnormal response to the gliadin fraction of gluten present in wheat, rye and barley resulting in villus atrophy and absorptive defect. It manifests a few months after the introduction of gluten-containing foods (often a wheat preparation) in infant's feeding schedule. Chronic diarrhea with large, pale, highly foul-smelling stools which stick to the pan, failure to thrive, anemia and other nutritional deficiencies, abdominal distention, irritability and anorexia are usual presenting features.

In order to confirm the diagnosis, you must establish existence of significant rise in daily stool fat excretion with normal D-xylose absorption, histological abnormality of the small intestinal mucosa in peroral jejunal biopsy, and positive response to gluten-free diet followed by recurrence of the manifestations as also biochemical and histological defect following gluten challenge.

Cystic fibrosis (fibrocystic disease or mucoviscidosis) has only recently been documented in Indian children. It is characterized by such manifestations as chronic/recurrent diarrhea together with recurrent respiratory infections since early infancy, failure to thrive despite exceptionally good appetite, and multiple nutritional deficiencies. Stools are characteristically steatorrheic but may be loose. An obstinate catarrhal cough or "frog in the throat" may be present ever since the first week of life.

Abdominal distention, a palpable liver, clubbing and higher incidence of rectal prolapse and nasal polyposis are other associated findings. A noteworthy finding by the mother is "a line of salt on the forehead after swelling", or "the baby tastes salty when kissed".

Diagnosis is established by demonstrating existence of chemical steatorrhea, a normal D-xylose absorption, poor tryptic activity, and a high sweat chloride.

Endemic tropical sprue is characterized by chronic diarrhea, malabsorption, considerable malnutrition, and anemia typically in a grown-up child. Steatorrhea is usually moderate to severe. Partial or subtotal villus atrophy is present. D-xylose test shows poor intestinal absorption. Schilling's test is invariably abnormal, indicating that the intestinal mucosal atrophy and absorptive defect are not limited to the upper gut but are present in the ileum too.

These subjects do not respond to gluten-free diet or to gluten challenge as is remarkable of celiac disease. However, response to folic acid, tetracyclines, or both is gratifying.

Tuberculosis

Undiagnosed primary complex may be responsible for a good proportion of cases of failure to thrive in developing world, including India. In such instances, failure to thrive may be accompanied by such vague symptoms as malaise, fatigue, weight loss and low grade fever. A recent Mantoux test conversion, a positive BCG test and routine X-ray chest often clinch the diagnosis.

Remaining Causes of Failure to Thrive

Cirrhosis of liver, congenital megacolon, congenital heart disease, rheumatic heart disease, bronchial asthma, bronchiectasis, renal rickets, diabetes mellitus, cleft palate, chronic rumination, cerebral palsy, mental retardation, primordial dwarfism, constitutional dwarfism, AIDS, etc.

FURTHER READING

1. Bodhankar U, Girish M. The child with failure to thrive. In: Gupte S (Ed). *Textbook of Pediatric Nutrition*. New Delhi: Peepee 2011:335-339.
2. Chawla A. Failure to thrive. In: Gupte S (Ed). *Pediatric Gastroenterology, Hepatology and Nutrition*. New Delhi: Peepee 2009:565-571.
3. Gupte S, Gomez EM. Growth disorders. In: Gupte S (Ed). *The Short Textbook of Pediatrics*, 13th edn. New Delhi: Jaypee 2020.
4. Medscape. Failure to thrive workup. [online] Available at http://emedicine.medscape.com/article/915575-workup. Accessed on: 21 July 2019.
5. Racine AD. Failure to thrive. In: Adam HM, Foy JM (Eds). *Signs and Symptoms in Pediatrics*. Illinois: American Academy of Pediatrics 2015:301-315.

CHAPTER 26

Frequency of Micturition

BACKGROUND

The term, *frequency of micturition*, points to an increase in the number of "voids" regarding urination in a day. Whether or not there is an increase in urine volume is immaterial for qualifying to have this designation. As a matter of fact, in a significant proportion of the cases, volume of urine voided is rather smaller than the subject's usual output.

HISTORY

While taking history, it is important to know if the complaint has been there for quite some time with waxing and waning, or the phenomenon is essentially of a very recent onset. Does the subject drink unusually large amounts of fluid and whether the amount of urine produced is very much? Are there any accompanying symptoms such as dysuria, urgency, hematuria, etc.? Is frequency of micturition accompanied by a triad of polyuria, polydipsia, and polyphagia? Or, are polyuria and polydipsia accompanied by anorexia rather than polyphagia?

PHYSICAL EXAMINATION

Physical examination should specifically exclude presence of periorbital puffiness and edema, pyrexia, hypertension, palpable bladder, and hydronephrosis.

INVESTIGATIONS

- Urinary tract infection (UTI)
- Urinalysis, including microscopy for pus cells and culture
- Urine microscopy
- Urine culture
- Imaging studies in
  - age < 2 years
  - recurrent UTI
  - Chronic bacterial prostatitis (CBP) in chronic UTI.

Diabetes mellitus
- Urine examination for sugar and acetone by Benedict test/Diastix and ferric chloride and Rothera's test/Ketodiastix, respectively
- Fasting blood sugar above 126 mg/dL (fasting) is a diagnostic test. A level between 100 mg/dL and 126 mg/dL is strongly suggestive
- Postprandial blood sugar
- Random blood sugar more than 200 mg/dL is strongly suggestive
- Glucose tolerance test is indicated in doubtful cases—in 2 hours more than 200 mg/dL is diagnostic
- Glycated hemoglobin (HBA1c) test—6–6.4%, prediabetic; 6.5% and above, diabetes.

Diabetes insipidus
- Twenty-four-hour urine output
- Urine specific gravity
- Three-hour water deprivation
- Radioimmunoassay for vasopressin level in blood.

IMPORTANT DIFFERENTIALS

Unusually Large Fluid Intake

When a child consumes unusually large amounts of fluids, he is bound to have frequency of micturition. He also produces large volume of urine. Otherwise, he is fine.

Cystitis

Urinary tract infection, particularly when there is cystitis, may manifest as frequency of micturition together with urgency, dysuria, dribbling, nocturnal enuresis, fever, irritability, anorexia, abdominal pain, vomiting, jaundice, and hematuria. A word of caution—avoid counting totally on symptoms for diagnosis of UTI; you must have laboratory confirmation of the diagnosis before starting the therapy.

Diabetes Insipidus

Frequency of urination with polyuria may be indicative of diabetes insipidus, a chronic disorder that, in a vast majority, occurs from a defect of the neurohypophyseal system. More precisely called as vasopressin-sensitive diabetes insipidus, the condition is characterized by an inability to concentrate urine, polyuria of 5–20 L/day and corresponding polydipsia. Frequency and polyuria may disturb sleep. Polydipsia may be severe enough to force the patient to resort to drinking his own urine at times. Restriction of free fluid intake may lead to severe dehydration, dyselectrolytemia, and weight loss.

The causes of damage to neurohypophysis include craniopharyngioma, optic gliomas, and other tumors, histiocytic infiltration, reticuloendotheliosis, leukemia, encephalitis, tuberculosis, sarcoidosis, actinomycosis, and operative procedures or trauma about the base of the skull. The genetic forms of the disease (autosomal dominant and X-linked recessive) are also known.

Investigations reveal 24-hour urine output as high as 4–10 liters (or even more), the specific gravity varying between 1,000 and 1,005 and the osmolality 50–200 mOsm/kg water. The 3-hour water deprivation may cause rise in plasma osmolality though the urine osmolality remains less than that of the plasma. Administration of vasopressin raises urine osmolality. Radioimmunoassay, showing vasopressin plasma level under 0.5 pg/mL, is a highly sensitive and more dependable test.

Diabetes Mellitus

Frequency of micturition may accompany the classical manifestations of diabetes mellitus such as polydipsia, polyuria and polyphagia, weight loss, general weakness, tiredness, and body pains. Fainting episodes due to spontaneous hypoglycemia, vulvitis, pain abdomen, nausea and vomiting, irritability and deterioration in school performance may also occur.

For confirmation of the diagnosis, you must carry certain investigations. First, urine examination for sugar and acetone by Benedict test/Diastix and ferric chloride and Rothera's test/Keto-diastix, respectively. Secondly, blood sugar above 126 mg/dL (fasting) is a diagnostic test. A level of 100–126 is strongly suggestive. Thirdly, glucose tolerance test is indicated in doubtful cases.

Posterior Urethral Valves

In this condition, the child may suffer from frequency since he nearly always has a feeling of unsatisfactory emptying. The amount of urine passed each and every time is naturally quite small. The child may also suffer from dribbling and hematuria. Often, the urinary bladder is palpable, so are the kidneys due to hydronephrosis.

Attention-seeking Device

The toddlers, upset for want of adequate parental security, may behave as though they have frequency of micturition to seek attention. The child, virtually every few minutes, demands to pass urine. The mother suddenly gets startled, may drop whatever she is holding, and then rushes the child to the washbasin or his potty.

Drugs

Demeclocycline, carbamazepine, hypervitaminosis D, antihistamines, fenfluramine, etc.

Remaining Causes of Frequency of Micturition

Pelvic appendicitis, nephritis, meatal stenosis, renal failure, adrenal cortical hyperplasia, etc.

FURTHER READING

1. Bowwer WF, Yip SK, Yeung CK. Dysfunctional elimination symptoms in childhood and adulthood. *J Urol* 2005;174(4 Pt 2):1623-1627.
2. Feldman AS, Bauer SB. Diagnosis and management of dysfunctional voiding. *Curr Opin Pediatr* 2006;18: 139-147.
3. Jain V, Gupte S, Koff AW. Endocrinology. In: Gupte S (Ed). *The Short Textbook of Pediatrics*, 13th edn. New Delhi: Jaypee 2020.

CHAPTER 27

Feeding Problems

BACKGROUND

Infants frequently suffer from preventable feeding problems such as regurgitation, vomiting, sucking and swallowing difficulties, dehydration fever, excessive crying, "3-month colic", change in bowel habit, underfeeding, overfeeding, or bottle addiction. Among the causative factors rank poor mothering characterized by too little feed, too heavy feed, wrong feeding technique, poor respect to bottle hygiene, etc.

HISTORY

History should be addressed to information whether the infant is being breast or bottle fed, or both. Is it demand or time schedule? Is the feeding technique correct? Does the mother meaningfully do burping? In case of artificial feeding, find out if the dilution and hygienic precautions are adhered to as per recommendations. Is the hole of the nipple the adequate one? Does the mother indulge in forced feeding or too inadequate feeding? Is the infant satisfied after feed, i.e. he sleeps after consuming the feed. Has the mother introduced semisolids? How is the mother's own diet? Is she highly strung?

PHYSICAL EXAMINATION

Physical examination should particularly assess the nutritional status of the infant: whether he is normal, overweight or underweight? How is the hydration status? Look for any congenital defects such as cleft lip, cleft palate, or glossoptosis. Any thrush, abdominal distention or tight anal sphincter?

You must always ensure observing the actual act of feeding and the child's subsequent behavior. This is, by and large, the gold standard for establishing the true nature of the feeding problem (Figs. 27.1 and 27.2).

INVESTIGATIONS

No investigations are, as a rule, required.

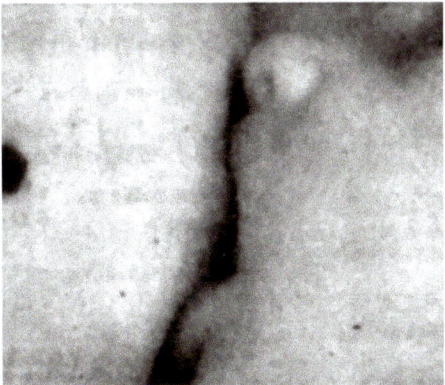

Fig. 27.1: Initiation to breastfeeding shortly after birth with support from the family and the health workers contributes considerably to safeguarding against feeding problems. Note the correct latching (attachment) with most of the areola in infant's mouth, his lower lip everted, chin touching the breast.

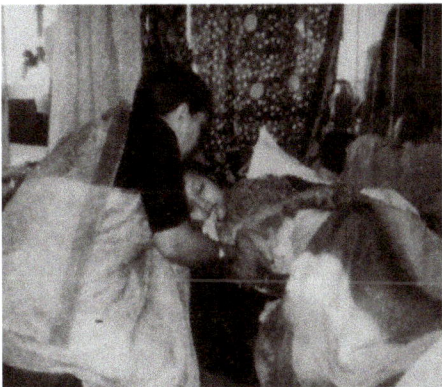

Fig. 27.2: Mothers need to be sufficiently guided about the proper attachment of baby's mouth at the breast. Watching the mother feeding the baby may give you a clue to the baby's feeding problem.

IMPORTANT DIFFERENTIALS

Regurgitation

The phenomenon of bringing up a little of the swallowed feed along with the swallowed air is termed as "regurgitation", "posseting" or "splitting up". In case of some infants, this becomes a habit. They enjoy bringing back some feed and chewing it like a cow chews the cud. This habit, termed as "rumination", is harmless. Nonetheless, this makes the baby somewhat smelly and he runs the risk of aspirating the stuff into the airway. In order that the infant does not inhale any bit of regurgitated milk, he should be placed on his side rather than on the back. This position also interferes with his regurgitation as also rumination.

Since regurgitation results from swallowing excess air by the infant, remedy lies in guiding the mother about the proper technique of feeding.

Vomiting

More complete emptying of stomach by the infant, particularly after some time of feeding, is termed as "vomiting". It may be due to overfeeding, too much of swallowed air, gastroenteritis, gastroesophageal reflux (GER), cow's milk protein intolerance (CMPI), raised intracranial pressure, pyloric stenosis, etc.

In the last named condition, the infant shoots milk halfway across the room (projectile vomiting). Manifestations begin between 2 weeks and 6 weeks of age, typically in a premature first-born male infant.

Sucking and Swallowing Difficulties

During the first few days of birth, some sucking difficulty is expected since this is the period in which both the infant and the mother are endeavoring to master the technique.

Certain mechanical problems, say cleft lip, cleft palate, large tongue, and nasopharyngeal block as in choanal atresia, may interfere with sucking. Local conditions of the breast like cracked nipple, retracted nipple, engorgement or abscess also cause sucking problems.

Prematurity predisposes the infant to sucking and swallowing difficulties. Cardiac or respiratory diseases accompanied by tachypnea, intracranial hemorrhage, and hyperbilirubinemia figure among several causes of feeding difficulties.

Dehydration Fever

Occasionally, on the second, third or fourth day of life, an infant with low intake of fluids or high environmental temperature, say in an incubator, phototherapy unit, or in a bassinet close to a radiator or in the sun, may develop disinclination to feed, fever (38–39°C), restlessness, and drowsiness. In addition, there may be weight loss. Urinary output and frequency of voiding diminishes and the skin loses some of its elasticity. Anterior fontanel may be slightly depressed. What is remarkable is that, despite poor feeding, the infant takes fluid avidly.

This condition, the so-called "dehydration fever", responds dramatically to administration of oral or parenteral fluids and/or lowering the environmental temperature.

Even in an infant with dehydration fever, especially if he appears quite sick, the possibility of local or systemic infection must be considered, more so when he fails to respond within 12–24 hours to the aforesaid suggested measures.

Transient neonatal hyperthermia with feeding disinclination, hot and dry skin, flushing, and apathy followed by stupor, grayish pallor, convulsions, and coma may infrequently occur both in neonates and older infants when they are wrapped in heavy woolens for outdoor cold that does not prevail in their immediate indoor surroundings. This condition may be complicated by hypernatremia, leading to brain damage, sudden infant death syndrome (SIDS), hemorrhagic shock or encephalopathy syndrome.

Excessive Crying

Crying in a neonate is invariably a signal that the infant is hungry or thirsty, he is feeling uncomfortable because of heat or cold, he is wet, or he indeed needs the mother. Repeated crying may begin to get on the mother's nerves. An insecure mother fails to develop the much-needed warm emotional relationship with such an infant. She may indulge in battering. It is not uncommon to hear such a mother shouting: "What can you do with such a rascal? He does not let me relax for a minute".

Irritability of the infant during mother's "periods" is a well-known observation. Whether it is related to fall in the supply of breast milk, mother's irritability, or some substances in the breast milk during menstruation that cause discomfort to the infant remains speculative.

Colic

Some infants begin crying soon after birth, particularly towards the afternoon or evening, and keep doing so till the age of 3 months. The attack begins suddenly. The cry is nearly continuous and loud. The face is flushed or shows circumoral pallor, abdomen is distended and tense, the legs are drawn up over the abdomen, and the hands are clenched. The attack may last for a few hours, terminating with passage of feces or flatus, or when the infant has fully exhausted himself.

The cause of the so-called "3-month colic" or "evening colic" remains elusive. Excessive intestinal activity, borne out by exaggerated bowel sounds, exists during the paroxysm. It has been postulated that, perhaps, events in the household routine (worry, anger, excitement, fear, etc.) cause this problem in infants just as they cause vomiting in older children.

No single treatment consistently gives satisfactory relief. Provision of a stable emotional environment with reassurance to the mother, improvement in feeding technique especially in relation to burping, and identification of possibly allergenic agents in infant's or mother's diet are valuable preventive measures. For relief of the actual attack, holding the infant upright, placing him prone across the mother's lap or hot water bottle, pushing a suppository into the rectum for passage of fecal material, or sedation of the infant may provide variable help. Antispasmodic agents and carminative mixtures are not much effective.

Change in Bowel Habit

- *Constipation:* Infants on artificial feeding, especially if underfed and given inadequate fluids and sugar, may pass stools of very hard consistency that cause good deal of straining and discomfort. As a result, the fear of pain leads to retention. The passage of such a stool on its own or following rectal examination may lead to anal crack or fissure which could also cause constipation. Some infants begin to have spurious diarrhea.

    Most constipated neonates respond to addition of water, some brown sugar, honey or glucose to the feed. Enema, suppository or milk of magnesia should be reserved for unresponsive or severely constipated infants. Liquid paraffin is best avoided since it places the infant at risk for xerophthalmia and lipid pneumonia. Tighter spastic anal sphincters, causing constipation from birth or soon after, usually get corrected by finger dilatation.

    If obstinate constipation is present since birth, cretinism, anal stenosis, and congenital megacolon (Hirschsprung disease) should be suspected.
- *Diarrhea:* In a breastfed infant, stools are naturally soft (not formed) and frequent, the color varying from green-brown to bright yellow. This is, by no means, diarrhea. Nonetheless, when stools are consistently watery, very frequent and foul smelling, the probability of infective etiology must be considered.

    In artificially fed infants, overfeeding, formula that is too concentrated or too high in sugar content, food contamination with pathogenic organisms, etc. may contribute to occurrence of diarrhea.

Underfeeding (Poor Weight Gain)

A highly diluted formula, often due to ignorance on the part of the parents or economic considerations, is a well-known cause of failure to thrive (FTT). Such a baby takes his feed quickly, is restless and crying, and shows poor weight gain, or even an actual loss. Constipation and failure to sleep are common observations. As a result of superimposed gastrointestinal infections, his nutritional status may further deteriorate. Eventually, he may turn into overt malnutrition involving not just energy and proteins but also minerals and vitamins. This is what is termed as "bottle baby disease".

Test weighing, i.e. weighing the infant before and after each feed over 24 hours (using an accurate machine), yields the volume of milk being taken by him. But it may cause undue anxiety to the mother, thereby reducing the milk supply. A recommended alternative is:
- A careful check on baby's weight gain over time
- Behavior between feeds
- Infrequently, outcome of formula supplements.

The management lies in instructing the mother in the art of feeding and correcting the deficiency states in the infant.

Overfeeding (Excessive Weight Gain and Obesity)

Some mothers manage to push into the baby larger amounts of feeds. This sort of overfeeding is a common cause of regurgitation and vomiting as also irritability, excessive crying, and fatty diarrhea. Often, such an infant develops obesity which, at any time in life, is bad.

Bottle Addiction

Some children continue sticking to "bottle feeding" even when they are 2 or 3 years of age. The cause, in actuality, is rooted in mothers' failure to have replaced the bottle by cup and spoon at about 6 months of age or little earlier. Though bottle feeding is seldom good, it is particularly unwise to continue with the bottle after the first-year of life.

Choking

During the first few days of life, history of choking on feeds is relatively common. Usually, the cause is poor feeding technique. If choking persists, GER could be responsible for it. However, anatomical lesions of esophagus, trachea or larynx (say tracheoesophageal fistula, hiatal hernia or laryngeal cleft) should be excluded.

Poor Mothering

Some mothers are sadly lacking in self-confidence and are ignorant about the mother craft, particularly the art of feeding. They are apprehensive, worrying too much. Their nervousness is reflected in the baby. As a result, he becomes more demanding and cries a lot to mother's further annoyance. The resultant unhealthy relationship between the mother and the infant leads to varied feeding and other problems.

FURTHER READING

1. Anand RK, Kumta NB, Kushwaha KP, Gupta A. *The Science of Infant Feeding*. New Delhi: Jaypee 2002.
2. La Leche League International. *The Womanly Art of Breast Feeding*. Franklin Park, Illinois: Leche League International 1976.
3. Tiwari SK, Gupte S, Gomez EM. Infant and young child feeding. In: Gupte S (Ed). *The Short Textbook of Pediatrics*, 13th edn. New Delhi: Jaypee 2020.
4. Writing Committee. *Infant and Young Child Feeding Subspeciality Chapter of the Indian Academy of Pediatrics/Human Milk Banking Association Guidelines*. Mumbai IAP IYCF Subspeciality Chapter 2015.

CHAPTER 28

Gingivostomatitis

BACKGROUND

Gingivostomatitis, meaning inflammatory lesions involving the gums and buccal mucosa, may occur as an isolated entity or secondary to a systemic disease. It causes considerable distress to the child.

HISTORY

While recording the history, make sure if the child is a known case of systemic illnesses such as diabetes mellitus, epilepsy on diphenylhydantoin sodium (phenytoin), or allergy to certain agents. Is he a habitual sufferer from such mouth lesions? Are his teeth in good shape? Any intercurrent illnesses? Any bleeding from sites other than gums, or any other manifestations of scurvy? Is he on any drug(s)?

PHYSICAL EXAMINATION

Physical examination should identify the exact lesion(s) in the mouth, what is the status of the teeth? Is there localized or generalized lymphadenopathy? Is the child a mouth breather?

INVESTIGATIONS

Usually, no investigations are required.

IMPORTANT DIFFERENTIALS

Infections

Herpes gingivostomatitis is a frequent cause of mucosal lesions in the mouth in children of 1-3 years of age. Manifestations such as pain in the mouth, fever, salivation, fetor oris, irritability, and refusal to eat are followed in 1-3 days by appearance of a vesicle which rupture very soon, leaving a residual lesion, 2-10 mm in diameter and covered with a yellow-gray membrane. A true ulcer becomes apparent once the membrane has sloughed. Submaxillary lymphadenitis is present.

Coxsackie stomatitis is characterized by very minute, painful shallow yellowish ulcers most commonly on the posterior buccal and pharyngeal mucosa. Anterior tonsillar pillars are particularly involved.

Vincent angina is characterized by occurrence of necrotic ulcers on tip of papillae, gums, and tonsils in debilitated children. A fetid smell is present. Demonstration of spirochetes in a smear from the lesions confirms the diagnosis.

Cancrum oris, also called noma or gangrenous stomatitis, is caused in hosts with compromised resistance by infection with fusospirochetal and other organisms. A small ulcer grows into a gangrenous area, greenish-black in color, on gums, buccal mucosa, and mucocutaneous junctions. Soon, it slowly spreads to perforate the cheek and denude the jaws.

Oral thrush (moniliasis) appears as irregular white plaques, resembling milk curds, on oral mucosa. The plaques are difficult to remove with a swab and often leave raw, friable bleeding area underneath on strenuous attempt.

Staphylococcal gingivitis occurs usually in children sick from another condition.

Streptococcal gingivitis causes bright red gums.

Hypovitaminosis/Avitaminosis

Riboflavin deficiency manifests as fissuring, cracking, ulceration, and dry scaling of vermilion surface of the lips and angles of the mouth (cheilosis or perleche) together with glossitis. Other manifestations include keratitis, photophobia, conjunctivitis, lacrimation, and remarkable vascularization of corneas. Seborrheic dermatitis is a common accompaniment, so is a normocytic hypochromic anemia with bone marrow hypoplasia.

Niacin deficiency may be responsible for sore tongue and stomatitis. The classical triad of dermatitis, diarrhea, and dementia, the sheet anchor of the disease pellagra, is diagnostic.

Pyridoxine (B_6) deficiency may be responsible for cheilosis, glossitis, and seborrhea. In infancy, more so during the neonatal period, pyridoxine dependency may be the cause for convulsions. In B_6 dependent anemia, red cells are microcytic hypochromic.

Scurvy typically produces bluish-purple spongy swelling of the gums, usually over the upper incisors. Rest of the manifestations include excessive irritability, petechiae, scorbutic rosary, pseudoparalysis, subperiosteal hemorrhages, follicular hyperkeratosis, anemia, and delayed wound healing.

Aphthous Ulcers

Aphthous ulcers, also called "canker sores", these are painful lesions of the oral mucosa, including gingivobuccal groove, tongue, and palate. The ulcers are essentially superficial and consist of highly sensitive "crater" surrounded by erythema. The lesions usually occur singly but, in stress situations, are prone to multiply. They take 1–2 weeks to heal. No scar is left.

Aphthous ulcers, as a rule, occur periodically in a given host. The etiology is essentially not yet known. Viruses, endocrinal factors, obstinate constipation, emotional disturbance, and autoimmune reaction have been incriminated from time-to-time.

Stevens–Johnson Syndrome

This disease causes vesiculobullous lesions in the mouth as well as conjunctivae, nares, anorectal junction, vulvovaginal region, and urethral meatus. An erythematous papular skin rash that involves all the cutaneous surfaces, excepting scalp, is characteristic. The skin rash enlarges by peripheral expansion with a central vesicle. Fever and severe prostration are a rule. Incidence of pulmonary complications is high.

Stevens–Johnson syndrome is believed to be related either to mycoplasma infection or to drugs such as sulfas, anticonvulsants, penicillin, aspirin, rifampicin, quinine or clindamycin.

Fibromatosis Gingivae

This familial condition is characterized by gingival hyperplasia in association with mental deficiency and hypertrichosis. Gum hyperplasia may be so pronounced as to lead to protrusion of lips and displacement of the tongue.

Drugs

Diphenylhydantoin sodium is well known to cause varying degree of gingival hyperplasia which is dose dependent. The gingivitis takes 3–6 months to subside after the drug is withdrawn.

Other drugs that may cause stomatitis include sulfas, actinomycin D, methotrexate, 6-mercaptopurine, vincristine, troxidone, tetracyclines, lincomycin, ethosuximide, griseofulvin, gold salts, and niclosamide.

Local application of aspirin or camphor to oral mucosa may cause chemical burn.

Dental Defects

Dental defects such as carious teeth, malocclusion, or sharp broken edges may cause chronic irritation, resulting in gingival infection and stomatitis.

Chronic Mouth Breathing

The child with chronic mouth breathing, as in case of adenoids or chronic nasal obstruction, is likely to develop dry, friable oral mucosa that begins to bleed easily. The tongue, in particular, becomes furrowed.

FURTHER READING

1. Gritton AL. Pediatric Oral Health. *Pediatr Clin North Am* 2000;47:201-209.
2. Medline Plus. Gingivostomatitis. Available at: medlineplus.gov/ency/article/001052.Htm Accessed on: 21st July 2019.
3. Scully C. Aphthous ulceration. *N Engl J Med* 2006;355: 165-172.
4. Tinanoff N. Common lesions of the oral soft tissues. In: Kleigman RM, St Gems III JW, Blum NJ, et al (Eds). *Nelson Textbook of Pediatrics*, 21st edn. Philadelphia: Elsevier 2020:1539-1540.

CHAPTER 29

Halitosis

BACKGROUND

The term, *halitosis* (Latin halitus means breath) means offensive odor of the breath. Also called *malodorous breath, oral malodor, fetor oris or bad breath*, the symptom is not as uncommon in pediatric practice as the various textbooks and the professional journals would have us believe. In his busy outpatient clinic, the author could find 46 cases over a period of 3 months. Of course, halitosis is only occasionally the chief presenting feature. Most often, the complaint is projected only on specific symptomatic enquiry. The factors considered responsible for the symptom in the assessment are—bad oro-dental hygiene 18%, chronic rhinitis 9%, foreign body in the nose 7%, tonsillitis 6%, diphtheria 1%, bronchiectasis 2%, lung abscess 1.5%, and garlic/onion consumption 2%.

HISTORY

History taking should seek whether it is a chronic or acute complaint. What kind of eating habits does the child command? Does he take care of oro-dental hygiene? Does he take spicy foods, garlic or onion? Any history of sore throat, rhinorrhea, sneezing, sinusitis or foreign body in the nose? Any chronic cough with copious expectoration, particularly having postural relationship? Any dyspepsia or ulcers in the mouth or over the gums? Is there a family history of halitosis of unknown etiology?

PHYSICAL EXAMINATION

Physical examination must in particular aim at excluding oro-dental conditions which may explain halitosis, foreign body in the nose, chronic rhinitis, acute or chronic tonsillitis, diphtheria, etc.

INVESTIGATIONS

Lung abscess and bronchiectasis, once suspected from the history, can convincingly be excluded or confirmed by imaging studies.

Infrequently,
- Throat culture in case of chronic sores
- Blood tests to screen for diabetes or kidney failure
- Endoscopy [esophagogastroduodenoscopy (EGD)]
- X-ray of the abdomen.

IMPORTANT DIFFERENTIALS

Bad Oro-dental Hygiene, etc.

The causes of halitosis secondary to bad oro-dental hygiene include septic tooth, dental canes (which may entrap the food debris), gingivitis, stomatitis, etc. Habitual failure to brush the teeth and wash mouth, particularly after main meals, may also contribute to bad breath.

Chronic Rhinitis

Chronic rhinitis, particularly, atrophic and allergic, may be responsible for halitosis.

In atrophic rhinitis, fetor is often a remarkable feature. Interestingly, it is taken cognizance by the relatives or the examiner. The patient is virtually unaware of it because of anosmia. The remaining manifestations include dryness and obstruction of nose with formation of crusts in nasal cavities. The nostrils are widened and the nose broadened. Nasal mucosa appears congested and atrophic.

Foreign Body in the Nose

Halitosis along with unilateral nasal discharge and obstruction make a strong case for a foreign body such as a piece of food, crayon, plastic, bead, etc. in the nose. In addition, there are manifestations like sneezing, local discomfort, and purulent malodorous or bloody discharge. The foreign body is situated in the beginning anteriorly but is later forced deeper way back in the nose.

Infections

Halitosis may be encountered in some cases of acute or chronic tonsillitis, diphtheria, Vincent's angina, and infectious mononucleosis.

Vincent's angina, caused by usual oral flora and heavy overgrowth of fusiform bacilli and spirochetes in chronically ill and malnourished children, is characterized by remarkable fetid odor, fever, malaise, and oral lesions consisting of gray necrotic membrane and tiny ulcers over tender, congested gingivae.

Bronchiectasis

Halitosis is a prominent feature of bronchiectasis which is characterized by permanent dilatation of the bronchi and bronchioles as a result of obstructions and/or infection, leading to cavitation of bronchial wall and tissue destruction.

The other manifestations of bronchiectasis include persistent or recurrent cough, productive of copious mucopurulent sputum which is foul smelling and has postural relationship. Some fever and recurrent attacks of respiratory infections are frequent. In advanced cases, there may be dyspnea, cyanosis, clubbing, and hemoptysis.

The characteristic auscultatory findings include "localized crepitations" repeatedly found over the involved area.

Diagnosis is confirmed through radiologic examination. X-ray of chest shows increased bronchovascular markings, extending towards the base of the lung. Later areas of cavitation may become apparent. Bronchography, preceded by bronchoscopy, is essential to localize and establish the extent of bronchiectasis.

Lung Abscess

Pulmonary abscess not only produces foul-smelling sputum but frequently halitosis as well. The other symptoms of chronic abscess which usually develop insidiously include fever, persistent cough, and at times, dyspnea and chest pain. Clubbing develops, if the child remains without treatment over a prolonged period.

Chest signs are those of consolidation with bronchial breathing.

X-ray of chest shows characteristic opacities; the cavities may show fluid levels.

Remaining Causes of Halitosis

Intake of onion, garlic, spicy foods, low-fat diet, alcohol, chronic gastrointestinal disease such as dyspepsia, achlorhydria or lowered gastric acidity, esophageal diverticula, cirrhosis, poisoning with lead, mercury, iodide or bismuth. Occasionally, it may be a familial trait. The family members emit an unusual body odor.

FURTHER READING

1. Health Guide. Breathy odor. Available at: www.nytimes.com/health/guides/symptoms/breath-odor/overview.html Accessed on: 21st July 2020.
2. Rosenberg M. The science of bad breath. *Sci Am* 2002; 286:72-79.
3. Rosenberg M, Knaan T, Cohen D. Association among bad breath, body mass index and alcohol intake. *J Dent Res* 2007;86:997-1000.

CHAPTER 30

Headache

BACKGROUND

Headache, a very common symptom in later childhood and adolescence, conventionally means "unpleasant sensations in the region of the cranial vault". Most often, it is benign, reflecting minor tension or fatigue. Only exceptionally does it reflect a serious intracranial disease. The symptom is unusual in infancy and early childhood. When it indeed occurs in this age group, chances of its being an expression of a serious illness are high.

HISTORY

History taking should aim at getting the relevant information that may contribute to reaching the exact diagnosis. When did it start? What is its intensity? What is its quality? Does the patient complain of a particular definable sensation? What is its location? How long does it last? What are the factors that make it worse or better? Does it have a relationship with any biological event(s) or physical environmental changes? Any relationship with head injury in the past? Is there any vomiting, dizziness, visual disturbance, or sweating that accompanies it? Is the patient myopic or having some other visual defect and whether he uses glasses? In adolescent girls, do remember to ask about menses and whether headache precedes the onset of the period every month. In case of headache along with a febrile illness, is there a history of neck stiffness, drowsiness, excessive irritability, etc.? Any associated seizures? Any personality changes and behavioral problems?

PHYSICAL EXAMINATION

A persistent or recurrent headache is a strong indication for carrying out a complete neurologic examination as also for excluding visual defects, sinusitis, and hypertension.

Remember, most pediatric tumors arise either in posterior fossa or suprasellar region. Neurologic examination should, therefore, emphasize tests of coordination (including gait and ocular function), eye movements, visual acuity, field of vision, and optic fundi. A dependable sign of posterior fossa tumor is presence of a head tilt.

INVESTIGATIONS

- X-ray of paranasal sinus (PNS)
- Imaging studies of skull in selected cases
- Electroencephalogram (EEG) in case of accompanying seizure disorder.

IMPORTANT DIFFERENTIALS

Migraine and Other Vascular Headaches

Also termed as hemicrania, this vascular type of headache is due to vasodilatation of cranial vessels, those of scalp in particular. The abnormal vasodilatation and pulsations are supposed to stimulate the pain fibers in the vessel wall. In an overwhelming majority of the patients, a positive family history is present.

Classically, a grown-up child gets an "aura", consisting of zig-zag lines and scintillating scotoma moving gradually across the visual field, diplopia, or transient ataxia, vertigo, hemisensory loss, hemiparesis, or aphasia. Shortly, the aura is followed by throbbing headache (usually unilateral) with nausea or vomiting. The best means of getting rid of the attack is to go for sound sleep. Response to analgesics is poor. Stress is known to increase the frequency of attacks.

Interestingly, more common than the classical form is what is called *partial migraine* in which aura is absent, headache is bilateral and vomiting does not occur.

Fever may also produce a throbbing headache due to peripheral vasodilatation and increased cerebral blood flow. There is ample evidence as to the cause of fever, say acute tonsillitis, malaria, enteric fever, pneumonia, or heat stroke.

Hypertension is another cause of vascular headache. Though, by no means, a common cause, it should always be excluded in children suffering from recurrent headache.

Headache Related to Epilepsy

In grand mal epilepsy, headache may occur as a part of aura or as a postictal event.

In autonomic seizures, headache during the attack *per se*, together with pallor, tachycardia or pupillary dilation, constitutes an important feature.

Headache Secondary to Changes in Intracranial Pressure

The child complaining of morning headache with nausea and vomiting should always arouse suspicion of raised intracranial pressure secondary to brain tumor (Fig. 30.1). Occipital headache is usually a sign of posterior fossa tumor (Fig. 30.2).

In benign intracranial hypertension, irrespective of the cause, there may be an acute onset of headache in association with sixth cranial nerve involvement and papilledema. Loss of consciousness does not occur.

Low cerebrospinal fluid (CSF) pressure headache is a common observation after lumbar puncture. The headache occurs on assuming upright position. On lying down, it disappears.

Tension Headache

Tension headache may occur in adolescents as dull, steady pain which grows as the day advances. After sleep, it is over.

The probable cause appears to be persistent contraction of neck and temporalis muscles, resulting in localized ischemia of these structures.

Headache Related to Psychological Problems

At times, young children (much before they reach adolescence) may also imitate the adults with headache and complain of headache. This age group may also use complaint of headache as an *attention-seeking device,* or as a pretext for not going to school or taking permission from the teacher to return home.

Headache Related to Psychiatric Disease

Unlike intermittent headache in an organic illness, headache in psychiatric illness such as depression is continuously present. Other manifestations of depression include miserable facial expression, anorexia, speech reduced to a sheer whisper, insomnia, and constipation.

Headache Related to Eye Problems

Persistent and prolonged eye strain in a child with myopia, hypermetropia or problems of accommodation and convergence may be responsible for headache though the cause and effect relationship is yet to be confirmed.

Glaucoma is a well-known, though rare, cause of headache. The child with congenital glaucoma has highly hyperemic conjunctivae.

Headache Related to Sinusitis

Infrequently, sinusitis may be accompanied by headache. Other signs and symptoms of sinusitis include continuous purulent nasal discharge or continuous postnasal drip between attacks. Transillumination and radiology help to confirm the diagnosis of sinusitis.

Drugs

Antihistaminics, acetazolamide, amitriptyline, diazepam, chlorpromazine, ephedrine, carbamazepine, vincristine, ethosuximide, ethambutol, troxidone, trimethoprim,

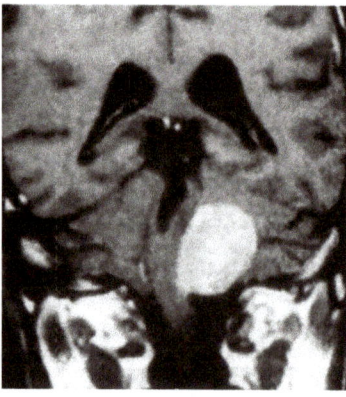

Fig. 30.1: Meningioma—This slow-growing tumor, originating in the arachnoidal space, may present with severe headache defying precise diagnosis on simple evaluation.

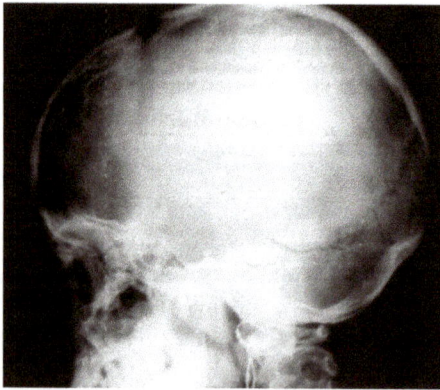

Fig. 30.2: X-ray of skull showing sutural diastasis in intracranial space-occupying lesion (ICSOL) (posterior fossa tumor). The boy was hospitalized for severe intractable headache (occipital).

tetracyclines, thiabendazole, griseofulvin, sulfas, valproate, isoniazid, indomethacin, niclosamide, diphenylhydantoin, nalidixic acid, and nitrofurantoin.

Other Causes of Headache

Otitis media, toothache, lead poisoning, pheochromocytoma, hypoglycemia, hunger, von Recklinghausen's disease, diabetes, leukemia, Sturge–Weber syndrome, basilar impression syndrome, sickle-cell disease, caffeine (caffeine-induced headache), etc.

FURTHER READING

1. Blume HK. Pediatric headache: a review. *Pediatr Rev* 2012;33:562-576.
2. Fuller G, Kaye C. Headaches. *Br Med J* 2007;334:254-256.
3. Greydanus DE, Tsitsika AK, Van Dyke DH, Olson D. Headaches in adolescents. In: Gupte S (Ed). *Recent Advances in Pediatrics (Special Vol 19: Developmental and Behavioral Pediatrics)*. New Delhi: Jaypee 2007:340-352.
4. Mack KJ. What incites new daily persistent headache in children? *Pediatr Neurol* 2004;31:122-125.

CHAPTER 31

Heart Murmurs

BACKGROUND

By definition, *murmurs* are audible sounds arising from the flow of blood through blood vessels, valves or heart chambers evincing turbulence. In children, because of proximation of the heart to the thin chest wall, murmurs are relatively more easily heard. As a rule, narrower the blood vessel or opening, or higher the turbulence of flow, louder is the murmur. Murmurs are usually classified as systolic, diastolic, and continuous.

Systolic murmurs may be ejection, pansystolic or late systolic. An ejection systolic murmur rises to a crescendo in mid-systole. It is, as a rule, coarse. Examples of such murmur are aortic stenosis, aortic coarctation, pulmonary stenosis, and atrial septal defect (ASD). A pansystolic murmur occurs all through systole. It is caused by flow of blood through a septal defect [ventricular septal defect (VSD), or an incompetent mitral or tricuspid valve, mitral incompetence, tricuspid incompetence, or a patent ductus arteriosus (PDA)]. A late systolic murmur is heard well beyond the first sound and stretches to the end of systolic phase (mitral valve prolapse). According to intensity, systolic murmurs are categorized into six grades (Table 31.1).

TABLE 31.1: Six grades of systolic murmurs (Keck's classification).

Grade	Characteristics
1	Faintest, requiring very careful auscultation in noise-free environments (consultant's murmur); innocent
2	Soft though slightly louder; usually innocent
3	Moderately loud without a thrill; may be innocent or organic
4	Loud, accompanied by a thrill; always organic
5	Very loud, accompanied by a thrill, still needs stethoscope in contact with chest; always organic
6	Loudest possible, accompanied by a thrill heard with stethoscope not necessarily in contact with the chest; always organic

Diastolic murmurs may be (i) a high-pitched blowing along the left sternal border, indicating aortic insufficiency or pulmonary valve insufficiency; (ii) early short, lower-pitched protodiastolic along the left mid and upper sternal border, indicating pulmonary valve insufficiency or after repair of pulmonary outflow tract in conditions such as tetralogy of Fallot (TOF); (iii) an early diastolic at the left mid and lower sternal border, indicating ASD or atrial valvular stenosis; (iv) rumbling mid-diastolic at the apex after the third heart sound, indicating large right-to-left shunt or mitral insufficiency; and (v) a long diastolic rumbling murmur at the apex with accentuation at the end of diastole (presystolic), indicating anatomical mitral stenosis.

A continuous murmur (machinery murmur) is a systolic murmur, best heard over the second and third left parasternal spaces, that extends into diastole. It indicates a PDA. It must be differentiated from a pericardial friction rub, as also from a venous hum.

Remember, over 30% children may have a murmur without significant hemodynamic abnormalities. Typically, the so-called "innocent murmur" is heard in the age group 3–7 years, occurs during ejection, is musical and brief, is attenuated in the sitting position, and is intensified by pyrexia, excitement, and exercise. As the child grows, such murmur shows a tendency to be less well heard and may regress fully.

HISTORY

History taking of a child with a murmur (potentially a cardiac case) must focus on cyanosis, squatting, fatigue, orthopnea, nocturnal dyspnea, feeding difficulty or problem, sweating during feeding, and chest pain. Any history of a generalized disorder affecting the heart as well. Any suggestion of a known congenital malformation syndrome, e.g. fetal-alcohol syndrome (ASD, VSD, etc.), VATER association (VSD, TOF, ASD, PDA, etc.), Down syndrome (endocardial cushion defects, VSD, and ASD).

PHYSICAL EXAMINATION

Physical examination must assess the growth and development of the child at the very outset. Presence of cyanosis, clubbing, edema, chest deformity, engorgement of neck veins, tachypnea, and hepatomegaly need to be specially observed. Pulse or cardiac rate and character of pulses provide valuable information. Blood pressure should preferably be recorded in the arms as well as in the legs. For this purpose, flush method is most feasible in restless infants.

Cardiac examination must in particular be very careful, noting the presence of a precordial bulge, substernal thrust, apical heave or a hyperdynamic precordium, thrills (both systolic and diastolic), aortic bruits, etc.

Auscultation of the precordium requires patience, first concentrating on the characteristics of the individual heart sounds and then on the murmurs. An accentuated or loud first heart sound over the mitral area suggests tachycardia, hyperkinetic heart syndrome, hyperthyroidism or mitral stenosis. In mitral regurgitation and myocarditis, the first heart sound over the mitral area is particularly faint. In tricuspid atresia, the first heart sound over the tricuspid area is accentuated or loud. The second sound is split little beyond the peak of inspiration; it closes with expiration. A wide splitting is encountered in pulmonary stenosis, TOF, ASD, total anomalous venous return, and Ebstein's anomaly. A narrow splitting points to pulmonary hypertension. The third sound is best heard with the bell at the apex in mid-diastole, especially if the child assumes a left lateral position. It is of significance in the presence of signs of congestive cardiac failure and tachycardia in which situation it may merge with the fourth sound. The latter, coinciding with atrial contraction, may be heard a little before the first sound in late diastole. The phenomenon of poor compliance of the ventricle with an exaggeration of the normal third sound associated with ventricular filling is termed as "gallop rhythm".

After the heart sounds, attention should be focused on clicks. Aortic systolic clicks, best heard at the left lower sternal border, occur in aortic dilatation as in aortic stenosis, TOF, or truncus arteriosus. Pulmonary ejection clicks, best heard at the left mid-sternal border, occur in pulmonary stenosis. In prolapse of the mitral valve, a mid-systolic click precedes a late systolic murmur at the apex.

Murmurs need to be described as to their timing, intensity, pitch, area of highest intensity, and transmission. Whether a particular murmur is just functional (innocent with no significance) or has a pathological origin (congenital heart disease) must be decided. This may need additional investigations such as electrocardiogram (ECG), X-ray, echocardiography, etc. In certain cases, cardiac catheterization may be required, particularly as a part of preoperative evaluation.

BOX 31.1: Nada's criteria for presence of heart disease.

- Major: Systolic murmur, Grade III or more, always pansystolic
  - Diastolic murmur
  - Cyanosis (primarily central)
  - Congestive cardiac failure
- Minor: Systolic murmur, less than Grade III
  - Abnormal second heart sound
  - Abnormal electrocardiogram (ECG)
  - Abnormal X-ray
  - Abnormal blood pressure.

Note: Heart disease is indicated when one major or two minor criteria are present.

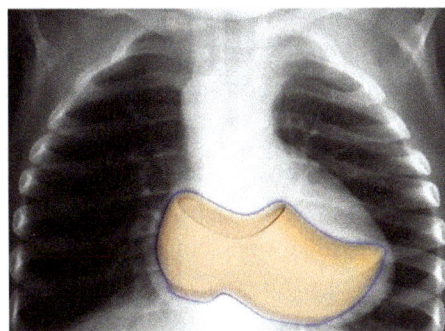

Fig. 31.1: Chest X-ray in tetralogy of Fallot. Note the boot-shaped heart with lifted apex.
Source: Radiographics 2017. Classic imaging signs of congenital cardiovascular disease. [online] RSNA website. Available at: PUBS.RSNA.ORG/DOI/FULL/10.1148/RG.275065148 (Accessed on: 9 January, 2018).

It is of help to apply the time-honored Nada's criteria for presence of heart disease in suspected cases (Box 31.1).

INVESTIGATIONS

- Electrocardiogram is not of much help in children
- Chest X-ray anteroposterior (AP) view (Fig. 31.1)
- Echocardiography is of special value in congenital heart disease
- Cardiac catheterization usually indicated when noninvasive tests are not helpful.

IMPORTANT DIFFERENTIALS

Systolic Murmur

Ejection Systolic Murmur

Aortic stenosis: In this condition, a harsh systolic murmur, usually accompanied by a thrill, is heard in the second intercostal space near the right sternal border. It is radiated to the neck. In young children, this murmur may be best heard on the left rather than the right side. A normally split second sound points to a mild stenosis whereas a single or a faint second sound suggests severe stenosis.

Additional findings include an apical impulse, poorly palpable peripheral pulse and low blood pressure. ECG shows left ventricular hypertrophy.

X-ray shows cardiomegaly with rounding of the left cardiac border as also poststenotic dilatation of the aorta in valvular stenosis, the most common type.

Catheterization and angiography are needed in order to differentiate between different types of aortic stenosis, i.e. whether it is valvular, subvalvular or supravalvular. Notable clinical clues for suspecting supraventricular stenosis are peculiar fades with hypertelorism, prominent forehead, macrostomia, microstomia, microdontia, dental malocclusion, and hypogonadism. The association is termed as Beuren syndrome.

Coarctation of aorta: A left parasternal ejection systolic murmur in the third to fourth intercostal spaces, radiated to the paravertebral area at the back is heard in this condition.

Salient accompanying features include poorly palpable femoral pulses and elevated blood pressure in the upper parts of the body.

Electrocardiogram shows left ventricular hypertrophy.

X-ray shows cardiac enlargement and notching of the ribs.

Pulmonary stenosis: The characteristic murmur is a loud ejection systolic murmur best heard in the second or third left intercostal space. The loudness of the murmur is directly proportional to the severity of stenosis. Second sound is little more widely split and pulmonic sound is faint. Asystolic thrill in the suprasternal notch is usual. A pulmonary ejection click may also be audible in upper left sternal border.

Electrocardiogram shows right ventricular hypertrophy.

X-ray shows mild cardiomegaly with poststenotic dilatation. Catheterization and angiography are essential for differentiating valvular from pulmonary stenosis.

Atrial septal defect: The characteristic murmur in this entity is a soft systolic ejection murmur at the upper left sternal border. An associated soft mid-diastolic murmur at the lower left sternal border is also present. A widely split second sound that does not change with respiration is noteworthy.

Electrocardiogram shows partial right bundle branch block and right axis deviation in the common ostium secundum defect, and left axis deviation and right bundle branch block in ostium primum defect. Signs of biventricular hypertrophy may exist.

X-ray shows cardiomegaly.

Pansystolic Murmur

Ventricular septal defect typically, the murmur is loud pansystolic, best heard down the left sternal border (third, fourth, and fifth interspaces). It is usually accompanied by a thrill. A functional diastolic murmur, due to large blood flow across the mitral valve may also be present. In the presence of pulmonary hypertension, second sound, which is split, becomes accentuated. In such a situation, a pulmonary diastolic murmur may also be found (Graham Steell murmur).

Electrocardiogram shows biventricular hypertrophy in well-established cases, with or without incomplete right bundle branch block. In small defects, it may be normal or show left ventricular hypertrophy.

X-ray is usually normal or shows minimal cardiomegaly with slight increase in pulmonary vascularity. In large VSD, it shows a large left-to-right shunt with enlarged heart (both ventricles and left atrium), enlarged pulmonary artery, and plethoric lung fields (over-vascularity) with or without hilar dance.

Two-dimensional echocardiography shows volume overload of the left ventricle and left atrium and the position and size of the septal defect.

Cardiac catheterization and selective angiography are of much help in locating the exact site of the shunt.

Mitral incompetence: The typical auscultatory finding is a moderately loud, blowing pansystolic murmur at the apex. It may be referred to the left axilla, to the back, or upwards to the left parasternal area. The murmur shows increase in intensity with respiration. The first heart sound is soft or normal but never loud. A soft, low-pitched mid-diastolic murmur at the apex may also be present, ECG shows a wide bifid P wave (P mitrale) along with findings consistent with ventricular hypertrophy.

X-ray shows enlargement of the left ventricle.

Tricuspid incompetence: In this condition, the murmur is pansystolic in the fourth right intercostal space. ECG shows right ventricular enlargement.

X-ray shows right ventricular enlargement.

Diastolic Murmur

Aortic Incompetence

The characteristic murmur is early diastolic. It is blowing in nature and best heard over the pulmonary area with radiation to the mitral and aortic areas. It is advisable to auscultate for this murmur when the patient is leaning forward and during expiration. Sometimes, associated functional mitral stenosis (transitory) may produce mid-diastolic or presystolic murmur, termed as Austin-Flint murmur.

X-ray of chest and ECG confirm presence of right ventricular hypertrophy.

Pulmonary Incompetence

Typically, there is a decrescendo diastolic murmur at the second left intercostal space. X-ray of chest shows right ventricular enlargement and dilated pulmonary vessels. ECG shows right ventricular hypertrophy.

Tricuspid Stenosis

The characteristic murmur in this condition is a diastolic murmur in the third, fourth, and fifth intercostal spaces on the right side.

X-ray of chest shows right atrial dilatation. ECG shows right atrial hypertrophy with tall, wide P waves.

Mitral Stenosis

The characteristic murmur of mitral stenosis is mid-diastolic, filling most of the diastole. It may be presystolic or diastolic with apparent presystolic accentuation. It is usually best heard with the bell of the stethoscope while the patient is lying on the left or soon after some exercise. Its intensity is maximal at the apex and it is low pitched or rumbling. Pulmonary second sound (P_2) is accentuated. Associated pulmonary insufficiency may result in a blowing diastolic murmur down the left sternal border. Association of both mitral stenosis and incompetence, the so called "double mitral", will lead to combined murmurs. Remaining auscultatory findings include a loud first heart sound at the apex and an opening snap.

Continuous Murmur

In PDA, the classical murmur begins immediately after the first heart sound and reaches its peak at the end of the systole. It continues during the most of diastolic phase, gradually disappearing in the later part. This is what has been described as machinery murmur. It is harsh and may be localized to second left intercostal space or transmitted to left clavicle or lower down, i.e. left sternal border. It is usually accompanied by a thrill. There may be paradoxical splitting of the P_2 in PDA.

Associated findings in PDA include a wide pulse pressure, a water-hammer pulse, prominent arterial Corrigan pulsations in the neck, and differential cyanosis. Such a murmur also occurs in:
- Aortopulmonary window, and
- Left-to-right shunt through a small ASD in the presence of mitral valve obstruction.

FURTHER READING

1. Biancaniello T. Innocent murmurs. *Circulation* 2005;111:e20-22.
2. Karunakara BP, Grover A, Gupte S. Pediatric cardiology. In: Gupte S (Ed). *The Short Textbook of Pediatrics*, 13th edn. New Delhi: Jaypee 2020.
3. Keane JF, Lock JE, Fyler DC. *Nadas' Pediatric Cardiology*, 2nd edn. Philadelphia: Elsevier 2006.
4. Pelech AN. The cardiac murmurs: When to refer. *Pediatr Clin North Am* 1998;45:107-122.
5. Tracy C, Walsh CA. Heart murmurs. In: Adam HM, Foy JM (Eds). *Signs and Symptoms in Pediatrics*. Illinois: American Academy of Pediatrics 2015:459-470.

CHAPTER 32

Hematemesis

BACKGROUND

Hematemesis means appearance of blood in vomitus, usually as a result of bleeding from esophagus, stomach or duodenum. Fresh bright-red blood in vomitus is indicative of either quite a proximal origin of bleeding or a massive blood loss. Dark blood, resembling coffee-grounds, is indicative of effect of gastric or intestinal juices.

Common causes of pediatric hematemesis are listed in Box 32.1.

HISTORY

While obtaining history, it must be ascertained at the very outset if what is stated to be blood in vomitus is indeed blood or some food or drink ingested sometimes back. At times, what is thought to be altered blood may turn out to be chocolate. It is a good practice to confirm presence of blood chemically.

What is the amount of blood loss? How often has hematemesis occurred? Any history of bleeding from other sites? Any epistaxis? Any abdominal pain? Any surgery on tonsils? Is there any jaundice?

PHYSICAL EXAMINATION

Physical examination must evaluate if the child is acutely sick. Is he in shock due to massive blood loss? How are the vital signs? Always look for evidence of epistaxis, blood oozing from gums or pharynx, evidence of portal hypertension hemangioma, purpura, telangiectasia, blood dyscrasias, etc.

BOX 32.1: Common causes of pediatric hematemesis.

Neonates
- Blood swallowed during delivery

Children
- Esophagitis
- Gastritis
- Peptic ulcer
- Esophageal/gastric varices.

A simple though often neglected method of demonstrating that bleeding is upper gastrointestinal is passage of a nasogastric tube. However, a negative gastric aspirate does not exclude an upper gastrointestinal source. This is because the bleeding may have stopped or because blood from the duodenum may not be entering the stomach.

INVESTIGATIONS

- Apt's test to confirm presence of blood
- Complete blood picture (CBP) for finding hematologic status
- Endoscopy for esophageal varices
- Liver function test (LFT) for liver function
- Ultrasonography or computed tomography (CT) scan or magnetic resonance imaging (MRI)
- Splenic venoportogram for pinpointing the lesion causing obstruction in the pathway
- Liver biopsy.

IMPORTANT DIFFERENTIALS

Hematemesis in the Newborn

Swallowed Maternal Blood

During delivery, or at the time of breastfeeding, the newborn may swallow maternal blood (from cracked nipple in the latter situation). Such an infant may manifest with hematemesis during the first few days of birth. This may also be accompanied by melena.

That blood in vomitus is indeed that of the mother, which can readily be confirmed by the Apt's test. To 1 mL of vomitus, add 5 mL of tap water and centrifuge or filter the suspension. To the supernatant, add 1 mL of 0.25 N NaOH and mix. On observing for 5 minutes, the color turns brownish-yellow in case of maternal blood and remains pink in case of baby's blood. The principle underlying this test is that fetal hemoglobin is relatively resistant to denaturation by sodium hydroxide, the alkali.

Hemorrhagic Disease of the Newborn

This disorder, representing a deficiency of vitamin K leading to defective coagulation, particularly as a result of prolonged prothrombin time, may manifest with hematemesis. Such signs and symptoms of bleeding in the form of melena or hematochezia are usually present.

The Apt's test comes handy in confirming that the blood in vomitus is indeed that of the infant and not the mother.

Drugs

Drugs such as salicylates, anticoagulants, and diuretics given to the mother during pregnancy.

Remaining Causes of Hematemesis in Newborn

Hemorrhagic gastritis, stress, ulcer, nasogastric tube trauma, hiatal hernia, esophageal or duodenal atresia.

Hematemesis in Later Infancy and Childhood

Hiatal Hernia

This is by far the most common cause of hematemesis (usually blood-streaked vomitus) during infancy. In the most common type, the so-called "sliding variety" (the other being "paraesophageal variety"), the gastroesophageal junction and some of the stomach come to lie within the chest. A gastroesophageal reflux is a common accompaniment and is responsible for many manifestations.

The infant usually presents with vomiting or regurgitation (if blood is present, it is usually in the form of streaks), failure to thrive, and anemia.

Chalasia

Also termed as gastroesophageal reflux, it is characterized by incompetence of the lower esophageal sphincter resulting in exposure of the esophageal epithelium to refluxed gastric contents. Next to hiatal hernia, it is the most frequent cause of hematemesis in infants.

Besides hematemesis, manifestations include anemia, dysphagia, growth failure, and aspiration pneumonia.

Diagnosis is confirmed by barium esophagogram done under fluoroscopic control, and/or, still superior investigation, esophagoscopy.

Swallowed Blood

In childhood, the most common cause of hematemesis is the regurgitation of swallowed blood resulting from epistaxis, acute tonsillitis, tonsillectomy, adenoidectomy, or dental work. Blood streaking of vomitus is usually a result of oozing from gingivae or pharynx in this category of hematemesis.

Peptic Ulceration

Peptic ulceration (duodenal or gastric) is an important though infrequent cause of hematemesis. Such ulceration occurring secondary to infection (Cushing's ulcer), thermal injury (Curling's ulcer), central nervous system (CNS) injury, etc. is often accompanied by copious bleeding in the gastrointestinal tract (GIT). As a matter of fact, acute massive painless bleeding is often the first and the only manifestation of stress ulcers which are responsible for almost 75% of peptic ulceration in the first 5 years of life.

Esophageal Varices

In children above 2 years of age, esophageal varices are perhaps the most common cause of massive hematemesis. Evidence of portal hypertension is available in the form of history of umbilical sepsis, or exchange transfusion by an umbilical vein catheter, together with splenomegaly, prominent superficial abdominal veins, ascites, etc.

Diagnosis is from barium meal studies and esophagoscopy which is a far better tool. Endoscopy is the best method for detecting esophageal varices. Presence of red spots over varices and large size of varices are strong predictors of hemorrhage.

Foreign Body in the Esophagus/Stomach

Sharp-edged foreign bodies such as nail, pin, bone, etc. may ulcerate esophageal or gastric mucosa and can cause hematemesis. Though plain X-ray of neck, chest or abdomen easily detects radiopaque foreign bodies, identification of plastic or glass foreign bodies is often a tedious matter and is facilitated by barium swallow (Fig. 32.1).

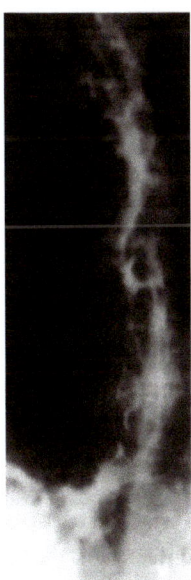

Fig. 32.1: Esophageal varices as seen in a barium swallow X-ray film.

Violent Retching

Severe retching may cause a tear in the esophageal mucosa and submucosa, leading to streaking of vomitus with blood. This is what is known as Mallory-Weiss syndrome. The condition is self-limited, usually responding to a blood transfusion.

Corrosive Esophagitis

Corrosive agents such as hydrochloric acid, sulfuric acid, strong bases, and bleaches, if ingested accidentally, may cause dysphagia and hematemesis. The symptoms clear in 2–4 weeks. An asymptomatic period of weeks or months is followed by esophageal obstruction from formation of strictures, resulting in dysphagia and vomiting.

Blood Dyscrasias

Infrequently, hematemesis may be a presenting symptom in leukemia and consumptive coagulopathy. The diagnosis is reached by high sense of suspicion in the presence of some other features of the diseases and through certain investigations.

Drugs

Salicylates, aminophylline, ferrous sulfate, and boric acid.

Remaining Causes of Hematemesis in Postneonatal Period

Telangiectasia, hemangioma, tumor, intragastric trauma by Ryle's tube, etc.

FURTHER READING

1. Chong SK. Gastrointestinal problems in handicapped child. *Curr Opin Pediatr* 2001;13:441-446.
2. Wyllie R. Major symptoms and signs of digestive tract disorders. In: Kliegman RM, St Geme III JW, Blum NJ, et al (Eds). *Nelson Textbook of Pediatrics*, 21st edn. Philadelphia: Elsevier 2020:1522-1529.

CHAPTER 33

Hematuria

BACKGROUND

Hematuria is the appearance of red blood cells (RBCs) in excess of five per high-power field (HPF) in the sediment of a 10 mL of centrifuged fresh specimen in urine.

Hematuria may be "gross" (macroscopic) or "microscopic". In gross hematuria, the color of urine varies from bright red to dark brown. Whereas bright red urine reflects that the source of blood is in the lower urinary tract, brown or tea-colored urine is suggestive of a renal origin. In microscopic hematuria, the color of urine remains normal and detection of hematuria is only by microscopic examination, or dipstick if available. Note that microscopic hematuria need not essentially be a sign of renal or rest of the urinary tract disorder. It may result from heavy exercise, viral or bacterial respiratory infections, various febrile conditions, gastroenteritis with dehydration, and contamination by red cells from menstrual blood, urethral meatal ulcer, or some other such conditions of the external genitalia. Association of proteinuria and tubular casts with hematuria is nearly always suggestive of a glomerular disorder.

It is of value to identify if hematuria is "total", "initial", or "terminal". Total hematuria is indicative of a lesion above the bladder neck. Initial hematuria points to the source of blood along the urethra. In terminal hematuria, areas last to be emptied of urine—trigone, bladder neck, or prostate—are the source of bleeding. A spotting of blood on the undergarments shows that blood is coming from urethra distal to the sphincteric mechanism.

HISTORY

While recording history, make sure the patient is not taking any drug that is responsible for coloring his urine. Is there accompanying dysuria? Any fever, periorbital edema, and back or abdominal pain? Has there been any recent trauma? Any history of insertion of a foreign body into the urethra. Did the patient have a systemic infection recently? Any preceding suggestion of skin or upper respiratory infection that could be a precursor of acute nephritis? Any bleeding disorder in the patient or family member(s)?

PHYSICAL EXAMINATION

A complete physical examination, including blood pressure determination, is important. Never miss looking for edema. The perineum and urethral meatus need to be thoroughly inspected.

INVESTIGATIONS

- Urinalysis, including microscopy. The presence of red cells in urine must be demonstrated microscopically since red color of urine may well be secondary to hemoglobinuria, myoglobinuria, beeturia, and metabolic products of some drugs or poisons.
- Dip-strip method is currently most commonly used. It has a sensitivity of 100% and a specificity of 99% in detecting one to five RBCs per HPF.
- Urine culture must be performed if a significant number of pus cells are present to determine the causative organism.
- Blood urea nitrogen (BUN) and creatinine.
- Glomerular filtration rate (GFR).
- Coagulation studies.
- *Serological tests*: Complement, antistreptolysin O (ASO).
- Anti-DNase B levels.
- Imaging studies.

IMPORTANT DIFFERENTIALS

Nephropathy

Acute poststreptococcal nephritis: Though now infrequent in European countries, acute nephritis continues to be a common cause of hematuria in tropics and subtropics. This immune-mediated disease typically follows a streptococcal infection (beta-hemolyticus type 12) of throat or skin.

There is acute onset of fever, puffiness of the face, more so around the eyes, and smoky or frankly bloody urine together with, in many cases, vomiting, headache, malaise, and oliguria. Variable degree of hypertension is usual. Acute renal shutdown, congestive cardiac failure (CCF), and hypertensive encephalopathy may occur as complications.

Urine examination reveals, besides few to several red cells, mild-to-moderate albuminuria and many granular casts.

Immunoglobulin A (IgA) nephropathy: Also called as idiopathic recurrent macroscopic hematuria, Bergar's disease, focal proliferative glomerulonephritis, or benign recurrent hematuria; this condition is characterized by episodes of gross hematuria precipitated by mild upper respiratory infection, febrile episodes or, less frequently, strenuous exercise, predominantly in boys after the age of 2 years. The patient may also complain of lethargy, malaise, low backache or abdominal pain. Episodic gross hematuria disappears in 2–4 days though microscopic hematuria may continue over several years. Spontaneous cure occurs in 50% cases.

A renal biopsy is eminently indicated in subjects suspected of this diagnosis, more so in the presence of persistent hematuria.

Systemic lupus erythematosus (SLE) nephropathy: Hematuria secondary to nephritis is an important manifestation of SLE.

Three types are known:
1. Focal proliferative lupus nephritis which is characterized by microscopic hematuria with red cell casts and proteinuria. Generally, the renal involvement is nonprogressive.
2. Diffuse proliferative lupus nephritis which is characterized by, in addition to microscopic or gross hematuria, massive albuminuria, azotemia, hypertension, and edema. In short, the picture is that of nephritic-nephrotic disease. Left unattended, the disease invariably progresses to renal failure.
3. Membranous lupus nephritis which, as a rule, manifests as nephrotic syndrome, may also present with hematuria, hypertension, and slight azotemia. Gradually, renal failure occurs in cases who are not appropriately treated.

Nephritis associated with systemic bacterial infections: In a variety of bacterial infections such as septicemia, coagulase-positive staphylococcal osteomyelitis, infected shunts for hydrocephalus, bacterial endocarditis, and chronic suppuration, hematuria occurs secondary to mixed nephritic-nephrosis. Presence of red cell casts in urine, proteinuria, azotemia, and hypertension are additional findings. The clinical evidence of bacteremia or sepsis (say fever and hepatosplenomegaly) preceding the renal symptoms and signs together with the clinical evidence of the primary predisposing condition helps to reach the diagnosis.

Henoch–Schönlein purpura: Microscopic hematuria or episodic gross hematuria may well occur in children with Henoch–Schönlein purpura having nephritis, usually within 1 month of onset of the syndrome. Clinical features of nephritis are generally, however, overshadowed by the typical rash, and abdominal and/or joint manifestations.

The nephritis associated with Henoch–Schönlein purpura is usually self-limited. It becomes inactive within 6 months of onset. No residual damage, except for minor abnormalities in urine sediment, is usually seen.

Urinary Tract Infection

Slight hematuria may accompany urinary tract infection. The presence of fever with chills, urinary frequency, painful micturition, pain in the loin, vomiting, etc. assists in seriously considering pyelitis as the cause. The characteristic finding in the urine is pyuria. Slight proteinuria may also be present. It is appropriate to do urine culture.

Hemolytic Uremic Syndrome

Hematuria may occur in hemolytic uremic syndrome. This disorder is characterized by the presence of hemolytic anemia secondary to acute renal failure, thrombocytopenia and in most cases, consumptive coagulopathy.

Clinical manifestations are widespread. Onset, usually in children between 6 months and 2 years, is acute but almost always preceded by diarrhea or respiratory infection. Besides the signs and symptoms of bleeding diathesis, hemolysis and nephropathy, involvement of the central nervous system (CNS) may cause progressive drowsiness and seizures.

Nephrotic Syndrome

Transient slight hematuria may be present in some cases of nephrotic syndrome. The characteristic clinical profile of nephrotic syndrome together with demonstration of massive albuminuria and hypercholesterolemia leave little doubt as far as the exact diagnosis is concerned.

Henoch–Schönlein Purpura

Hematuria may well be encountered in Henoch–Schönlein purpura because of vasculitis. Presence of widespread purpuric lesions (especially urticaria-like skin lesions) with involvement of abdominal viscera and/or joints clenches the diagnosis.

Renal Vein Thrombosis

This condition, occurring in high-risk infants (usually newborns), is characterized by sudden onset of hematuria, oliguria, and a lump in a flank with fast deterioration in general condition. Manifestations such as fever, shock, and vomiting are common. In some cases edema and hypertension may occur.

The predisposing factors include maternal diabetes, dehydration, shock, septicemia, severe pyelonephritis, asphyxia, congenital renal anomaly, right-to-left congenital heart shunt, and angiography for congenital heart lesion.

Laboratory findings reveal anemia, leukocytosis, thrombocytopenia, metabolic acidosis and azotemia. Valuable diagnostic information is obtained from intravenous pyelogram (IVP), ultrasonography, and radionuclide studies.

Renal Calculus

Hematuria may be a manifestation of renal calculus which is, of course, less common in childhood than in adulthood. Other symptoms and signs include colicky abdominal pain (usually over the flank), repeated urinary infections, and history of passage of small chunks of the calculus. Infrequently, urethral obstruction may occur.

Renal Tuberculosis

Hematuria, together with persistent sterile pyuria, fever, wasting, dysuria, flank tenderness, and frequency of micturition, usually suggest renal tuberculosis which has a tendency to involve rest of the urinary tract as well.

Radiologic findings may include calyceal cavities, calcification, and stenosis of the excretory tract with dilatation above the stenosis and contraction of the bladder. X-ray of chest to demonstrate primary complex, gastric lavage or sputum for acid-fast bacilli (AFB), and Mantoux/BCG diagnostic test must always be done.

Wilms' Tumor

Hematuria may occur in Wilms' tumor, also called as nephroblastoma. The most important clinical finding in this tumor of embryonal origin is a large unilateral intra-abdominal lump often accompanied by abdominal pain, vomiting or fever. The lump usually does not cross the midline. Hypertension occurs in about half of the cases.

In a small proportion of cases, the tumor may have one of the congenital anomalies such as ambiguous genitalia, undescended testes, hypospadias, duplication of ureter or kidney, horseshoe kidney, aniridia, hemihypertrophy, and Beckwith syndrome.

Diagnosis is confirmed by plain X-ray of abdomen and IVP which shows a large soft tissue opacity displacing the gut in the area of the kidney, and distortion of calyces by a mass within the kidney. X-ray of chest is indicated to detect any metastasis.

Hemorrhagic Cystitis

Gross hematuria may result from acute nonbacterial cystitis, either of viral (adenovirus type 11 and 21) origin or due to chemical irritation of the bladder mucosa by cyclophosphamide.

Foreign Body

It is possible for a child to push a foreign body through the urethra, rarely right into the bladder. This may be responsible for hematuria, dysuria, and urethral obstruction. A foul-smelling purulent discharge is usually present.

Trauma to Perineum

Occasionally, as a part of child abuse and neglect, the mother may cause tear(s) of the perineum, including external urethral opening, leading to contamination of the urine with blood.

Urethritis/Urethral Carbuncle/Meatal Ulceration

Bright-red blood, in small amounts, may be passed in urine. Dysuria and hesitancy are usually present.

Bleeding Diathesis

Blood disorders that cause hematuria include leukemia, purpura, hemophilia, sickle-cell anemia, hemorrhagic disease of the newborn, and consumptive coagulopathy.

Drugs

Anticoagulants, aspirin, methicillin, thorazine, acetazolamide, cyclophosphamide, sulfas, diphenylhydantoin sodium, troxidone, para-amino salicylic acid (PAS), kanamycin, cephalosporins, bacitracin, aminophylline, etc.

Factitious Hematuria

Rarely, a mother may add blood to the child's urine and then report it as hematuria. This condition is termed as Munchausen syndrome by proxy or simply Meadow's syndrome.

The fabricated illness causes unnecessary investigations, hospitalization, and medication. The involved parent frequently has a medical background and is under gross emotional strain.

Remaining Causes of Hematuria

Nail-patella syndrome (hereditary onychoosteodysplasia) scurvy, telangiectasia, etc.

FURTHER READING

1. Gulati S. Hematuria. In: Gupte S (Ed). *Recent Advances in Pediatrics-17*. New Delhi: Jaypee 2007.
2. Gupte S, Shore RM. Nephrology. In: Gupte S (Ed). *The Short Textbook of Pediatrics*, 13th edn. New Delhi: Jaypee 2020: 504-523.

CHAPTER 34

Hemoptysis

BACKGROUND

Hemoptysis, meaning the spitting of blood or bloodstained sputum, is a rather infrequent symptom in pediatric practice. One or two cases in several weeks can be seen. At times, it is indeed hematemesis that is erroneously considered hemoptysis by the parents. In some instances, it is red coloration of the sputum by rifampicin that is confused with hemoptysis, causing undue anxiety to the parents and unnecessary investigations.

HISTORY

History must ascertain whether what is described as hemoptysis is really blood in the sputum or just color of a drug, say rifampicin. If it is indeed blood, is it coming from the lung or is simply secondary to epistaxis, bleeding from the gums, etc.?

Once established to be real hemoptysis, enquiry must attempt at arriving at the cause. Is the sputum entirely blood, or is it streaked or speckled with blood? Is it bright red in color or altered? Any history of chronic or violent cough, foreign body, chest pain, pyrexia, or dyspnea? Is the child a known case of rheumatic heart disease? Any suggestion of tuberculosis in the family? Any bleeding from other sites?

PHYSICAL EXAMINATION

Physical check-up should, in particular, exclude ecchymosis, petechiae, and nasal, pharyngeal or oral lesions. Are there chest findings consistent with bronchiectasis or lobar pneumonia?

INVESTIGATIONS

- Sputum examination
- Mantoux test
- Chest X-ray and imaging studies
- Bronchoscopy
- Pulmonary angiography
- Electrocardiogram (ECG).

IMPORTANT DIFFERENTIALS

Bronchiectasis

Hemoptysis is a feature of advanced bronchiectasis; the disease is characterized by permanent dilatation of the bronchi and bronchioles as a result of obstruction and/or infection followed by cavitation of the bronchial wall and tissue destruction. Along with hemoptysis, the child has dyspnea, cyanosis, and clubbing. This picture is on top of the characteristic persistent or recurrent cough productive of copious, mucopurulent sputum which is foul smelling and has postural relationship. Likewise, patient's breathing also carries bad smell. Some fever and recurrent attacks of respiratory infections are frequent.

The characteristic auscultatory finding is the "localized crepitations" repeatedly found over the affected area. Other signs of collapse-consolidation may also be present.

X-ray of chest reveals increased bronchovascular markings extending towards the base of the lung. In advanced stage, areas of cavitation may become apparent. Bronchoscopy followed by bronchography is essential to localize and establish extent of bronchiectasis.

Foreign Body

An aspirated bronchial foreign body may be responsible for blood-streaked sputum together with cough and metallic taste in case of metallic foreign body. Generally, the foreign body is aspirated into the right lung because of the convenient position of the right bronchus. An enquiry usually reveals that the patient some time ago had a sudden attack of choking and paroxysmal coughing while eating or while handling small objects during play.

The degree of lung involvement depends upon the extent of obstruction caused by the foreign body. An obstructive foreign body may produce obstructive emphysema, obstructive atelectasis or, if either is allowed to remain unattended, chronic pulmonary disease.

Whooping Cough

Rarely, whooping cough may be responsible for slight hemoptysis. Remaining results of forcefulness of the paroxysm include epistaxis, subconjunctival hemorrhages, spinal epidural hemorrhage, melena, tear of frenulum of the tongue, hematoma, rupture of diaphragm, umbilical hernia, inguinal hernia, rectal prolapse, and rupture of alveoli leading to interstitial or subcutaneous emphysema.

Diagnosis of whooping cough is virtually clear in the paroxysmal stage, particularly in the presence of contact with a known case. Leukocytosis with absolute lymphocytosis supports the diagnosis. Recovery of organism on Bordet-Gengou medium confirms the diagnosis.

Remaining Causes of Hemoptysis

Lobar pneumonia, trauma to chest (e.g. broken rib), cystic fibrosis, tuberculosis, mitral stenosis, congestive chest failure (CCF), uremia, pulmonary hemosiderosis, enterogenous cyst, blood dyscrasias, telangiectasia, paragonimiasis, etc.

FURTHER READING

1. Epocrates. Evaluation of hemoptysis. Available at: epocrates.com/diseases/103923/Evaluation-of-hemoptysis/Diagnostic-Tests Accessed on: 23 July 2019.
2. Goodfrey S. Pulmonary hemorrhage/hemoptysis in children. *Pediatr Pulmonol* 2004;37:476-484.

CHAPTER 35

Hepatomegaly

BACKGROUND

Hepatomegaly, meaning actual enlargement (not just palpability of the liver), is a frequent observation in pediatric practice. Quite often, it is detected by the doctor incidentally while examining the child for some other problem.

PHYSICAL EXAMINATION

In order to be sure that it is true hepatomegaly and not sheer apparent hepatomegaly, you must percuss the upper margin of liver. Normally it should be located within 1 cm of the fifth intercostal space in the right midclavicular line. Liver may be pushed down, thereby becoming palpable, though not enlarged, in conditions such as pneumothorax, emphysema, pleural effusion, empyema, and subphrenic abscess. In thoracic deformity, say narrow costal angle, liver may become palpable by over 2 cm though its size remains within normal limits. Relaxation of the abdominal musculature and laxity of the ligaments as in rickets or generalized visceroptosis may also be responsible for apparent hepatomegaly. Remember that in healthy children too, liver may be palpable up to 2.5 cm in infancy and 1–2 cm in later years.

Normal liver span varies from 4.5 cm to 5.0 cm at 1 week of age to 7–8 cm in boys and 6.0–6.5 cm in girls by 12 years of age.

Clinical assessment of hepatomegaly does not end with determination of its size. You must examine the organ for any tenderness, consistency (whether soft or firm), type of border (whether rounded or sharp), type of surface (whether smooth, granular or nodular), and any bruits. You must also carefully examine the abdomen for a palpable spleen, other masses, etc.

Pertinent extrahepatic finding should also be looked for. For example, presence of cataracts in an infant with hepatomegaly may point to the diagnosis of galactosemia, microcephaly to intrauterine infections, neuromuscular abnormality in the form of tremors or flaccidity to lipid storage diseases, and telangiectasia to hereditary hemorrhagic telangiectasia. In later age group, pruritus accompanying hepatomegaly may mean the existence of chronic cholestasis, hemangioma—the hemangiomatosis of the liver, carotenemia—the hypervitaminosis A, Kayser-Fleischer rings, the Wilson's disease, neuromuscular abnormalities again the Wilson's disease, glossitis—the cirrhosis, enlarged kidneys polycystic disease or congenital hepatic fibrosis, and arthritis with erythema nodosum—the liver disease with chronic inflammatory bowel disease.

INVESTIGATIONS

- Abdominal X-ray
- Abdominal imaging: ultrasound (US), computed tomography (CT) scan, magnetic resonance imaging (MRI), etc.
- Ascitic tap
- Liver function test (LFT)
- Splenoportography
- Liver biopsy.

For storage disorders
- Liver/bone marrow biopsy
- Leukocytes showing specific enzyme deficiency.

IMPORTANT DIFFERENTIALS

Hepatomegaly in the Newborn

Congestive Cardiac Failure

Hepatomegaly almost always occurs in congestive cardiac failure which is rather difficult to recognize in newborns. Remaining manifestations may include tachypnea, poor-feeding, excessive sweating, irritability, weak cry, tachycardia, and cardiomegaly. Gallop rhythm is usual. Shortness of the neck and difficulty in securing a relaxed state in the newborn make it rather impracticable to comment on the jugular venous pressure (JVP). Edema, if present, is generalized. Hepatic pulsations may be felt. In longstanding cases, splenomegaly may occur.

Neonatal Hepatitis

In this disorder, liver becomes grossly enlarged, at times filling the whole of the right half of the abdomen. Its consistency is distinctly firm. In one-half of the cases, spleen is moderately enlarged. Accompanying manifestations include jaundice appearing in first week, feeding difficulty, vomiting, anemia, high-colored urine, and intermittent loss of the pigment in stools. Occasionally, there may be thrombocytopenic purpura. The infant appears really sick.

For more details, you may refer to Chapter 39.

Extrahepatic Biliary Atresia

Marked hepatomegaly with firm consistency occurs in extrahepatic biliary atresia only when it has progressed (Fig. 35.1). Accompanying features include persistent jaundice which keeps deepening and lightening alternately, deep-colored urine, clay-colored stools, bronze olive-green skin, splenomegaly, and vitamin deficiencies, especially hemorrhages due to vitamin K deficiency. Unlike the sick-looking infant with neonatal hepatitis, the infant with biliary atresia looks well enough during the neonatal period and for a few months that follow.

Also, see Chapter 39.

Erythroblastosis Fetalis

Both ABO and Rh incompatibility are known to cause hepatomegaly in association with splenomegaly, anemia, and jaundice.

In the severest form of Rh hemolytic disease—hydrops fetalis—infant is usually born preterm with gross edema, effusion in serous cavities, and massive hepatomegaly with splenomegaly. Jaundice is absent at birth.

Also, see Chapter 39.

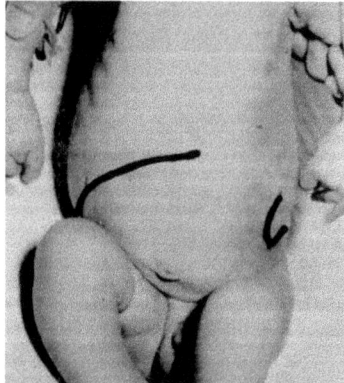

Fig. 35.1: *Extrahepatic biliary atresia*—Besides firm hepatomegaly, the infant had persistent icterus which showed waxing and waning, splenomegaly and vitamin K responsive hemorrhagic tendency.

Intrauterine Infections

Intrauterine infections such as toxoplasmosis, cytomegalic inclusion disease, and rubella, as discussed elsewhere (see Chapter 39), as also congenital syphilis and malaria may be responsible for hepatomegaly in combination with other manifestations such as neonatal jaundice.

In early congenital syphilis, manifestations other than hepatomegaly include snuffles, skin and mucosal lesions such as rhagades, mucus patches, ulcerations and fissures in the mouth and anus, anemia, splenomegaly, jaundice, fever, failure to thrive, lymphadenopathy, and chorioretinitis.

Painful osteochondritis and/or periostitis may cause pseudoparalysis (Parrot paralysis). Meningovascular syphilis may cause manifestations such as permanent brain damage, hydrocephalus, and optic atrophy. Syphilitic nephrosis may be responsible for periorbital puffiness and pedal edema. Serious complications like pneumonia alba and hepatic failure may prove fatal.

Neonatal malaria may be responsible for fever, hepatosplenomegaly, irritability, feeding difficulty and, at times, even seizures.

Septicemia

Hepatomegaly together with jaundice appearing between third and seventh postnatal day, splenomegaly, poor feeding, vomiting, irritability, listlessness, poor activity, abdominal distention, and fever or hypothermia, particularly in the presence of septic umbilicus or aseptic focus elsewhere, strongly suggest the probability of neonatal septicemia.

Also see Chapter 39.

Galactosemia

In this rare autosomal recessive disorder, hepatomegaly occurs fairly early in association with jaundice, poor feeding, vomiting, and fatigue to thrive which follow introduction of milk. Development of splenomegaly takes some more time. Pseudotumor cerebri may occur in some subjects. Delay in withdrawal of milk and its products results in mental retardation and cataracts.

Alpha-1-antitrypsin Deficiency

This defect presents with hepatomegaly and jaundice in neonatal period or in first 3 months of life. Serum alpha-1-antitrypsin level is just 10–20% of the normal. Serum bilirubin, serum glutamic oxaloacetic transaminase (SGOT), serum glutamic pyruvic transaminase (SGPT), and alkaline phosphatase levels are elevated. Pathologically, the characteristic finding is periodic acid-Schiff (PAS) positive diastase-resistant granules restricted to periportal liver cells in the beginning and later spreading to the midzone.

Gangliosidoses (GM1 or Generalized Type)

A severe lipidoses with onset soon after birth, it is characterized by edema, weakness, grotesque facial features, hepatosplenomegaly, hyperacusis, and cherry-red spot of the macula. The disease proves fatal by the second birthday.

Cholesterol Storage Disease

It is characterized by hepatomegaly, dwarfism, persistent blood loss from gastrointestinal tract, chronic anemia, and hyperlipemia. Neurologic manifestations, if present, are minimal. Bone marrow shows foam cells and lamina propria of the intestine shows the lipids. These subjects are prone to atherosclerosis.

Wolman Disease

Also called as primary familial xanthomatosis, an autosomal disorder, it causes storage of lipid in histiocytic foam cells, thereby producing hepatosplenomegaly. Accompanying manifestations include vomiting, diarrhea, abdominal distention, and gross failure to thrive. Bone marrow examination shows a large number of lipoid cells and X-ray of abdomen shows the enlargement and calcification of adrenals.

Hepatomegaly in Later Infancy and Childhood

Infections and Inflammations

Hepatomegaly is a common accompaniment of infections and inflammations such as viral hepatitis, amebic hepatitis/abscess, ascariasis, cholangitis, hydatid disease, tuberculosis, malaria, kala azar, enteric fever, brucellosis, septicemia, infectious mononucleosis, leptospirosis, and histoplasmosis, besides neonatal or intrauterine infections already dealt with in this section.

Viral hepatitis, be it infective, serum, non-A-non-B, or delta and its complication (chronic persistent hepatitis and chronic aggressive hepatitis) is almost always accompanied by liver enlargement.

The onset may be insidious or acute with fever, anorexia, malaise, nausea, vomiting, headache, upper abdominal pain (particularly in the right upper quadrant and/or epigastrium), tender hepatomegaly, constipation/diarrhea, and high-colored urine. This is followed by appearance of jaundice of varying intensity. With appearance of jaundice, fever, and anorexia begin to subside.

About 25% cases have just slight jaundice and abdominal pain. A few may have rapidly fulminant course with hepatocellular failure and hepatic coma. Attempt should be made to delineate whether the child's illness was infective hepatitis (hepatitis A) or serum hepatitis (hepatitis B). In infective hepatitis, incubation period varies from 28 days to 42 days. Gastrointestinal tract is the probable portal of entry, though infrequently hepatitis A virus can gain entry via blood as well. During early stages of the disease, virus can be isolated in blood as well as stools. It continues to pass in stools as long as complete recovery has not occurred (Table 35.1).

In serum hepatitis, incubation period is much longer, 60–150 days. Transmission is nearly always via an apparent parenteral route, e.g. blood transfusion, injection, vaccination, or skin/mucosal abrasion.

Recently, convincing evidence has accumulated for the hepatitis viruses other than A and B. The best-known viruses are hepatitis C, D, and E.

Fulminant hepatitis, or acute yellow atrophy, occurs due to remarkably high virulence of the virus or high host susceptibility as in subjects with immunologic deficiency disease or on immunosuppressant drugs. In one form, the disease proceeds in a rapidly fulminant course with increasing jaundice, ascites shrinking liver, worsening of the laboratory indices, and coma. The other form starts as

TABLE 35.1: Hepatitis A vis-a-vis hepatitis B.

Parameter	Hepatitis A	Hepatitis B
Etiologic agent	RNA virus	DNA virus
Mode of transmission	Feco-oral Parental (occasionally)	Parental Sexual Feco-oral infrequently Skin (child-to-child)
Incubation period	28–42 days	60–150 days
Duration of viremia	3–5 days (transient)	7–8 weeks prolongation
Onset of symptoms	Sudden	Gradual
Duration of acute illness	6–12 weeks	6–12 weeks
Incidence of relapse	5–10%	A carrier state goes on and on
Chronic carrier state	Not at all	90% neonates and up as carriers
Cause of mortality	Acute fulminant hepatitis	Cirrhosis malignancy
Preventive vaccine	Hepatitis A vaccine Havrix	Hepatitis B vaccine, both genetically engineered and plasma-derived available (Engerix B, Shanvac B)

a benign hepatitis. After apparent improvement, the patient suddenly starts worsening in the second week of the disease, eventually ending up in hepatic coma, sepsis, hemorrhage or cardiorespiratory arrest.

Chronic persistent hepatitis is unresolved viral hepatitis characterized by portal inflammation. Liver is enlarged but soft in consistency. The disease runs a slow and benign course.

Chronic active hepatitis is an uncommon sequela of viral hepatitis and is characterized by widespread loss of lobular architecture, portal and periportal inflammation, piecemeal necrosis and active septa. In addition to jaundice, firm hepatomegaly is present (Fig. 35.2). Spleen is usually enlarged. Ascites is present. The course is rapidly progressive and downhill.

Amebic hepatitis causes diffuse liver enlargement, a serious manifestation of disseminated infection, usually accompanying intestinal amebiasis. Liver is palpable and distinctly tender.

Amebic liver abscess is the better defined clinical entity associated with hepatic amebiasis. Manifestations, besides enlarged tender liver, include fever, abdominal pain and distention, and toxemia. Upper border of the liver is at a higher level.

Diagnosis is confirmed by finding *Entamoeba histolytica* in stools (remember that stool examination may be negative for ameba in over half of the cases of documented amebic abscess), elevated and immobile diaphragm on screening, by aspiration of anchovy-sauce (chocolate colored) pus, and by localization of the abscess cavity (usually in the right lobe) through hepatic ultrasonography and isotope scans.

Pyogenic hepatitis/abscess may occur secondary to septicemia, osteomyelitis, infected burns, pyodermas, etc. particularly in children with immunologic defects or on inadequate antibiotic therapy. *Staphylococcus aureus* is the most common causative organism. Abscesses are usually multiple. There is marked toxemia. Liver is enlarged and tender; the upper border too is at a higher level.

Ascariasis, when heavy and chronic, may cause persistent hepatomegaly in tropical children as a result of the continuous transhepatic passage of larvae which is, in any case, normal migration of larvae. That ascariasis indeed is responsible for hepatomegaly which is purely conjunctural. There is no direct proof to this effect.

Hydatid disease involving the liver is rare in childhood. It gives rise to a smooth rounded swelling with hydatid fremitus and fluctuation. Diagnosis in suspected cases is made by Casoni test, X-ray, and ultrasonic studies and, finally, by exploratory laparotomy.

Tuberculosis may cause hepatomegaly by isolated or disseminated hematogenous spread. For establishing the diagnosis, it is important to identify the primary lesion in the lungs or elsewhere. A liver biopsy may reveal tuberculous granulomatous lesion of the liver.

Malaria, particularly when chronic, may be responsible for significant enlargement of liver. More than hepatomegaly, the child demonstrates enlargement of spleen (Fig. 35.3). There are also accompanying anemia and malnutrition. Interestingly, in the cases of repeated attacks, temperature is often normal though, at times, low-grade fever occurs.

Kala azar is an important cause of slow enlargement of liver in endemic areas. Accompanying manifestations include persistent fever (mild-to-moderate) with rapid enlargement of spleen in just 2 weeks' time, malnutrition, pigmentation of skin, and sparse, falling, and brittle scalp hair. Appetite remains good. Diagnosis is made by serologic tests like aldehyde (formal gel) test and Chopra's antimony test, complement fixation test which is positive in 90% of the cases in third week after onset, and blood and bone marrow smear for *Leishmania donovani* (LD) bodies.

Enteric fever may cause hepatomegaly though most often it is the spleen which becomes palpable. Accompanying features include fever (not necessarily

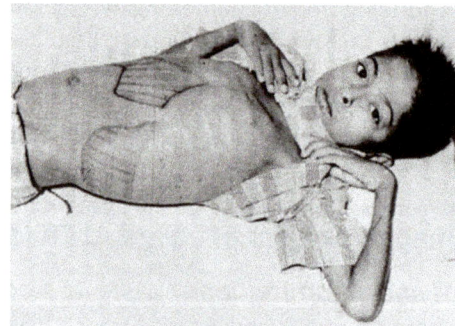

Fig. 35.2: *Chronic active hepatitis*—In addition to the findings of a firm hepatomegaly and splenomegaly, the patient had icterus and ascites.

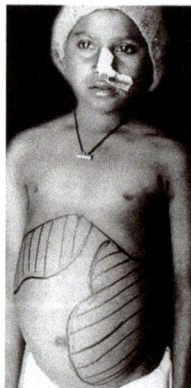

Fig. 35.3: *Chronic malaria*—Note the hepatomegaly with massive splenomegaly in this 12-year-old child with anemia, malnutrition, and low-grade fever.

of step-ladder pattern), marked malaise, anorexia, headache, vomiting and abdominal distention, and pain. Some cloudiness of consciousness is invariably present. Diarrhea occurs more often than constipation. Abdomen has a characteristic doughy feel. Eosinopenia or complete absence of eosinophils is a reliable finding. Leukopenia with relative lymphocytosis, described as an important feature of enteric fever, is most often absent in children. Widal test showing "0" antibody titer of 1 in 250 or more is quite suggestive though a rising titer over a period of 7–10 days is of greater value. Blood and bone marrow culture for *Salmonella typhi* is the most reliable diagnostic measure under ideal conditions.

Brucellosis may be responsible for hepatomegaly in association with splenomegaly and cervical and axillary lymphadenopathy. Remaining manifestations include prodromal symptoms like easy fatigability, weakness, headache, myalgia, constipation, and anorexia, followed by high fever with chills and diaphoresis, epistaxis, abdominal pain, cough, and weight loss. Diagnosis is established by Brucella agglutination test which shows liters over 1 in 160 in acute illness.

Septicemia, implying that bacteremia is severe enough to make the patient critically ill, may be responsible for hepatomegaly with multisystem involvement. It should be suspected in the presence of unexplained fever, involvement of quite a few systems/organs and serious state of the subject, particularly when septic focuses such as pneumonia, osteomyelitis, abscess, endocarditis, etc. are apparent.

Infectious mononucleosis, caused by the Epstein–Barr virus of the herpes group, may lead to hepatomegaly in one third of cases. Accompanying signs include splenomegaly and lymphadenopathy, particularly in the posterior cervical region. The symptoms include malaise, fever, sore throat, headache, nausea or vomiting. At the junction of hard and soft palate, petechiae may be seen. Peripheral blood shows atypical lymphocytes. Heterophilic antibody response is positive.

Acquired immunodeficiency syndrome (AIDS) is beginning to emerge as a noteworthy cause of hepatomegaly. Additional manifestations vary with the type of AIDS. In case of infants born to mothers with risk factors, these include small-for-dates, failure to thrive, microcephaly, splenomegaly, lymphadenopathy, chronic interstitial pneumonia (pneumocystis carinii in particular), recurrent otitis media, chronic sinopulmonary infection, oral candidiasis, chronic diarrhea, and chronic parotid swelling. In case of transfusion-associated AIDS, these include interstitial pneumonia, Kaposi sarcoma, chronic lymphadenopathy, recurrent pyrexia, splenomegaly, night sweats, weight loss, chronic diarrhea, and evidence of other viral infections such as Epstein–Barr virus, hepatitis B or cytomegalovirus.

For diagnosis of pediatric AIDS, presence of a risk factor with demonstration of polyclonal hypergammaglobulinemia, T-cell immunodeficiency, and evidence of infection with human immunodeficiency virus (HIV) are considered sufficient.

World Health Organization has suggested clear-cut criteria for clinical diagnosis of AIDS in developing countries (Box 35.1).

Leptospirosis (icteric type or Weil's disease) has dominant hepatic manifestations in the form of hepatomegaly, right upper quadrant abdominal pain, hyperbilirubinemia (both direct and indirect), and raised serum levels of liver enzymes. Renal manifestations include hematuria, proteinuria, casts, azotemia, and oliguria or anuria. Hemorrhagic and cardiovascular phenomena occur uncommonly. Initial symptoms include fever, shaking chills, myalgia, headache, nausea, vomiting, malaise, dehydration, and prostration. Diagnosis is made by identification of Leptospira in infected tissue or body fluid, and by serologic testing.

Disseminated histoplasmosis, an acute illness particularly of immunosuppressant subjects, is characterized by hepatosplenomegaly, diffuse lymphadenopathy, and pneumonia. Associated manifestations include nausea, vomiting, abdominal pain, and diarrhea. The patient is critically ill with dyspnea. In untreated subjects, respiratory failure, bleeding from various sites as a result of disseminated intravascular coagulation or septicemia may prove fatal.

Hematogenous Diseases

Thalassemia major has hepatosplenomegaly (spleen far bigger than liver) as an important finding. Remaining features include progressive hemolytic anemia with icterus, and growth retardation. Lymphadenopathy, skin

---

BOX 35.1: World Health Organization (WHO) criteria for diagnosing pediatric acquired immunodeficiency syndrome (AIDS) in developing countries.

Major criteria
- Weight loss/abnormally slow weight gain for age
- Chronic diarrhea for over 1 month
- Prolonged/intermittent pyrexia for over 1 month

Minor criteria
- Generalized lymphadenopathy
- Oropharyngeal candidiasis
- Recurrent common bacterial infections
- Persistent cough for over 1 month
- Generalized dermatitis
- Confirmed human immunodeficiency virus (HIV) infection in the mother.

Note: The presence of two major and two minor criteria provided that other known causes of immunodeficiency are not existing is diagnostic of AIDS.

pigmentation, hypogonadism, and recurrent respiratory infections are common. The so-called thalassemic facies are characterized by frontal bossing, depressed nasal bridge, and prominent maxilla exposing maloccluded teeth.

Investigations reveal hemoglobin in the range of 4–9 g% with peripheral blood film showing microcytic-hypochromic erythropoiesis, anisocytosis, poikilocytosis, moderate basophilic stippling, nucleated and fragmented red cells (the so-called target cells), large number of normoblasts and reticulocytosis.

Bone marrow reveals erythroid hyperplasia which is responsible for widening of the medulla and thinning of the cortex of the bones.

Osmotic fragility test reveals a reduced fragility. In other words, there is resistance to hemolysis in highly diluted (hypotonic) solution.

Fetal hemoglobin is always over 40% and usually over 70% during the early years of life.

Radiologic picture is remarkable with findings such as thinning of the cortex, widening of the medulla and coarsening of trabeculations in the long bones, metacarpals, and metatarsals. X-ray of skull shows overgrowth of the maxilla with opacification of the sinuses. The diploic spaces are widened with prominent vertical trabeculae (striations) and atrophy of the outer table. The vertical striations are termed as hair-on-end appearance.

Sickle-cell anemia, an inherited defect of hemoglobin S limited almost to black races (it is rare in most parts of India), may have mild-to-moderate hepatomegaly in association with slight icterus, anemia, fever, headache, arthritis, osteopathy of metacarpals, and phalanges in particular, skin ulceration, nocturnal enuresis, growth retardation, and folic acid deficiency. Splenomegaly, though significant in early years, regresses in older children (autosplenectomy). The child is prone to repeated bacterial infections and anesthetic complications.

Three types of crises worsen patient's condition, namely hemolytic, vaso-occlusive, and aplastic. Laboratory data show severe microcytic–hypochromic anemia with hemoglobin usually less than 8 g% (average 6–8 g%), irreversible sickled cells, poikilocytosis and target cells. Reticulocyte count varies between 5% and 15%. Nucleated red cells and Howell–Jolly bodies are usually present.

Bone marrow is markedly hyperplastic, electrophoresis reveals that 50–100% hemoglobin is of S type and that fetal hemoglobin level is elevated.

X-ray studies show expanded marrow spaces and osteoporosis.

Nutritional Problems

Soft, smooth, round-bordered, nontender enlargement of the liver which may, at times, reach as low down as the umbilicus, is a common observation in edematous type of protein-energy malnutrition, kwashiorkor. It is ascribed to fatty infiltration and is reversible. The essential features of kwashiorkor include: (i) growth retardation as evidenced by low weight and low height, (ii) marked muscle wasting with retention of some subcutaneous fat, (iii) psychomotor change in the form of listless inertness, and (iv) hypoalbuminemic edema at least over the pretibial region, provided that it is not due to congestive cardiac failure, liver disease, kidney disease or any non-nutritional cause. The variable features of kwashiorkor include hair changes, dermatosis, gastrointestinal upset, mineral and vitamin deficiencies, hepatomegaly, and superadded infections and infestations.

Parenteral hyperalimentation may occasionally be accompanied by hepatomegaly which is reversible.

Vascular/Congestive Hepatomegaly

Congestive cardiac failure, even at a fairly early stage, causes enlargement of the liver, its magnitude depending upon the severity of the failure. Accompanying signs include dyspnea, raised JVP, bilateral basal crepitations, and slight generalized edema.

Constrictive pericarditis, occurring months or years after the primary disease (say tuberculous pericarditis, purulent pericarditis, viral pericarditis, trauma, neoplastic invasion of the pericardium, etc.), may cause hepatomegaly and ascites out of proportion to other manifestations. Remaining findings suggesting constriction include distention of neck veins, narrow pulses, quiet precordium, distant heart sounds, pericardial friction rub, and pulsus paradoxus.

Veno-occlusive disease of the liver, supposed to be caused by some hepatotoxins in the bush-tea, is a leading cause of hepatomegaly in West Indian peasant children. Three stages are recognized. The initial acute phase is characterized by acute onset of abdominal discomfort, smooth, firm, nontender hepatomegaly (often massive), and ascites. This is followed by subacute phase which is characterized by persistent hepatomegaly with or without splenomegaly. Often, the child is symptom free. The chronic phase is characterized by cirrhosis with occurrence of repeated hematemesis, presence of an audible continuous venous hum, the Cruveilhier–Baumgarten sign, over the abdomen or lower thorax, hepatic failure, and cholemia.

Storage Diseases

Reye's syndrome is always accompanied by an enlarged fatty liver. In a typical case, there is sudden onset of profound disturbances of sensorium (to the extent of coma), vomiting, and convulsions. Hypoglycemia, hepatomegaly, and hepatic dysfunction are the other prominent manifestations. Jaundice which makes a special note is, as a rule, conspicuous by its absence. Dyselectrolytemia or bleeding diathesis may occur. Complications include pneumonia, respiratory failure, cerebral problems, cardiac arrhythmias, and diabetes insipidus. Clinical spectrum varies from relatively mild to rapidly fatal disease. Mild cases may be missed without liver biopsy.

Investigations show that blood and cerebrospinal fluid (CSF) sugar are consistently low. While SGOT, SGPT, and lactate dehydrogenase (LDH) are significantly raised, serum bilirubin and alkaline phosphatase are either normal or only marginally elevated. Prothrombin time is prolonged. Blood ammonia is elevated in most and urea nitrogen in few cases. Metabolic acidosis and respiratory alkalosis may coexist in the same subject.

Liver biopsy shows diffuse microvesicular steatosis with absence of glycogen and slightest inflammatory changes.

Electroencephalography (EEG) changes consist of predominantly slow wave activity.

Glycogen storage disease, type I (Von Gierke' disease), due to deficiency of the enzyme, glucose-6-phosphatase, is characterized by massive hepatomegaly together with doll-face, stunted growth ketonuria, hyperuricemia, bleeding tendency, and hypoglycemic convulsions. Gout may complicate the clinical picture after puberty.

Diagnosis is confirmed by liver biopsy which shows increased fat and glycogen and absence of glucose-6-phosphatase enzyme.

Gaucher's disease, an autosomal recessive type of lipidosis caused by deficiency of the enzyme, beta-glucosidase, in brain, liver, spleen, bone marrow, and other organs, is characterized by rapidly progressive visceral enlargement, including hepatomegaly, and mental retardation (infantile type) or rapid development of hepatosplenomegaly without brain involvement (juvenile type).

Diagnosis is made by demonstrating typical cells, the so-called Gaucher's cells, in the marrow or splenic puncture.

Niemann-Pick disease, an autosomal recessive type of lipidosis caused by absence of the enzyme, sphingomyelinase, is characterized by mental retardation, hepatosplenomegaly, lymphadenopathy, weight loss, and abdominal distention. A cherry-red spot may be seen in every third child with this disease in the region of macula. Anemia, usually moderate, is invariably present. Death usually occurs in infancy.

Diagnosis is by demonstration of Niemann-Pick cell in blood, marrow or splenic puncture. X-ray may show miliary tuberculosis-like picture.

Galactosemia, causes hepatomegaly early enough along with feeding difficulty, vomiting, failure to thrive, jaundice, and hypoglycemic convulsions as a rule as soon as milk feed is given to the infant. With progression of the disease in later infancy, hepatomegaly shows further increase. Along with this, splenomegaly also appears. If treatment is delayed and the child survives, cataracts and gross mental retardation follow in due course of time. Damage to the kidneys may cause albuminuria and aminoaciduria.

Investigations demonstrate galactosemia, hypoglycemia, and galactosuria. Erythrocytes show increased level of galctose-1-phosphate.

Gargoylism, type 1 mucopolysaccharidosis or Hurler's syndrome, is characterized by hepatosplenomegaly together with grotesque facies, mental retardation, dwarfism, corneal cloudiness, umbilical hernia, and kyphosis.

Diagnosis is usually clinical. Radiologically, elongated sella turcica, shortened vertebral bodies with concave anterior and superior surfaces and thickening of the tubular bones and metacarpals with tapering of ends lend support to the clinical impression.

Urine Shows Large Amounts of Chondroitin Sulfate

Hemosiderosis, meaning iron storage in excess in various organs, may be responsible for hepatomegaly eventually ending up as cirrhosis, together with slate or bronze pigmentation of the skin, diabetes mellitus, and respiratory manifestations. Both primary (increased gastrointestinal absorption of iron) and secondary (repeated blood transfusions as in thalassemia major) forms occur.

Amyloidosis, meaning extracellular deposition of a proteinaceous material, may cause massive liver and splenic enlargement. Yet, there may be no symptoms other than abdominal discomfort. LFTs remain either absolutely normal or these are only minimally affected. Rectal biopsy assists in reaching the diagnosis.

Xanthomatosis, though rare in pediatric practice, may be responsible for hepatomegaly as also involvement of many other organs/systems.

Cystic fibrosis, a disorder of the exocrine glands, particularly the pancreas, may cause biliary cirrhosis in 2-3% of patients. Manifestations include hepatomegaly, jaundice, ascites, hematemesis from esophageal varices and evidence of hypersplenism. In the second decade of life, the child may develop biliary colic from cholelithiasis.

Cystinosis, characterized by accumulation of cystine in various tissues, especially reticuloendothelial system, may be responsible for hepatomegaly in addition to other manifestations like splenomegaly, lymphadenopathy, aminoaciduria, photophobia, etc.

Diabetes mellitus is known to cause enlargement of the liver in longstanding cases. The cause of hepatomegaly is fatty infiltration.

Wilson's disease, an autosomal recessive disorder of copper metabolism, is characterized by the triad of neurologic abnormalities, Kayser-Fleischer rings, and cirrhosis. Hepatomegaly, due to excessive accumulation of copper, is the earliest manifestation. This is followed by splenomegaly, jaundice, and anorexia. Edema, ascites or gastrointestinal bleeding occurs sooner or later. The disease may resemble chronic active hepatitis or, infrequently, even viral hepatitis or cirrhosis.

The most reliable diagnostic criterion is liver tissue copper content exceeding 400 μg/g dry weight.

Malignant Diseases

Leukemia causes some degree of hepatomegaly in almost 80% of the patients, usually in association with splenomegaly, petechiae of mucous membrane, bleeding, progressive anemia, fever, bone pain/tenderness or arthralgia. Diagnosis in a suspected case is made by demonstrating leukemic blast cells in the blood and bone marrow smear.

Lymphomas, both Hodgkin and non-Hodgkin, may eventually involve the liver and other organs, causing organomegaly.

Neuroblastoma may, through hematogenous spread, involve the liver, resulting in hepatomegaly. Additional common findings include a firm, irregular, and nontender upper abdominal swelling which becomes big enough to cross the midline. Hemorrhage in the tumor mass causes significant anemia. Involvement of marrow may cause pancytopenia which leads to further pallor, petechiae, and ecchymosis. Involvement of bones may cause bony tenderness and pain. The remaining features include skin nodules, raised intracranial pressure, fever, lethargy, anorexia, and chronic diarrhea.

Wilms' tumor, if it metastasizes to liver, may cause enlarged nodular liver. Accompanying manifestations include a huge upper abdominal mass which usually does not cross the midline, abdominal pain, vomiting, fever, and hypertension. Hepatoblastoma, occurring nearly always under the age of 3 years, causes massive hepatomegaly with abdominal enlargement (Fig. 35.4). A proportion to the cases (around 20%) has abdominal pain, anorexia, and weight loss. Vomiting and jaundice occur less frequently. Occasionally, virilization may occur.

Liver function tests are usually within normal limits. Alpha-fetoprotein levels in blood and urinary excretion of cystathionine are, however, elevated in a majority of the subjects.

X-ray of abdomen may show calcification in the enlarged liver in approximately 30% of cases.

Miscellaneous Conditions

Indian childhood cirrhosis, irrespective of whether it is of the dominant insidious onset type or the acute onset type, is characterized by the presence of progressive hepatomegaly.

The insidious onset type has three arbitrary stages. First stage is the stage of vague manifestations with liver that is palpable by 3–5 cm. The liver border is typically sharp and leafy and its consistency is firm (Fig. 35.5). Additional manifestations include abdominal distension, anorexia or voracious appetite, lassitude, irritability, slight fever, constipation or diarrhea with clay-colored sticky and formed stools, and growth failure.

Second stage is characterized by further increase in the liver size and its firmness, appearance of a clear-cut jaundice and dominance of the clinical picture by portal hypertension in the form of splenomegaly, ascites, hematemesis, anemia, prominent superficial abdominal veins, and thrombocytopenia.

Third or the terminal stage is characterized by massive hepatosplenomegaly, ascites, protuberant abdomen, prominent superficial abdominal veins, deep jaundice, apathy, emaciation, and evidence of progressive hepatocellular failure.

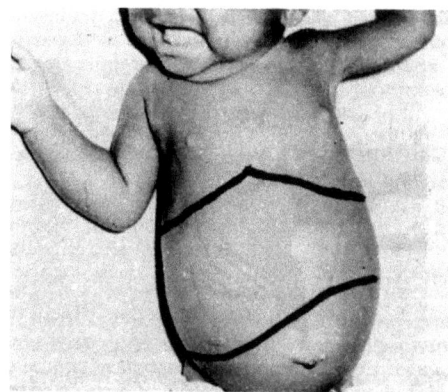

Fig. 35.4: *Hepatoblastoma*—Note the massive hepatomegaly. Abdominal radiograph revealed calcification in the enlarged liver.

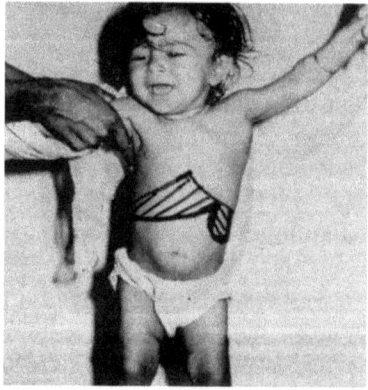

Fig. 35.5: *Indian childhood cirrhosis*—This 10-month-old child presented with moderate icterus, hepatosplenomegaly (very firm liver with a sharp, leafy border, and minima) ascites (stage II). In a matter of couple of days, he developed severe hepatocellular failure, thereby entering stage III.

In the acute onset disease, the infant has sudden onset of jaundice, fever, clay-colored stools, and hepatomegaly. He finally dies in hepatic coma.

Congenital cysts may occasionally be the cause of hepatomegaly in association with portal hypertension and congenital polycystic kidney disease. Diagnosis is by strong suspicion and exclusion. Finally, exploratory laparotomy may have to be resorted to.

Hemangioma of the liver may be responsible for an enlarged liver. Additional symptoms include jaundice, vomiting, diarrhea, and abdominal protuberance. Occasionally, congestive cardiac failure (from arteriovenous fistula), hemolysis, thrombocytopenia, hypofibrogenemia, and refractory anemia may occur.

X-ray of abdomen shows enlarged liver and, at times, calcification in the hemangioma.

Systemic lupus erythematosus (SLE) may be responsible for hepatomegaly together with splenomegaly. Additional common manifestations include prolonged irregular fever with remissions of variable duration, joint or muscle pains, malaise, weight loss, and a characteristic erythematous rash resembling the wings of a butterfly (butterfly rash) over the bridge of the nose and cheeks. Rash may also appear on fingers and palms, soles, palate, and buccal mucosa. Alopecia may also occur.

Diagnosis is made by demonstrating the LE phenomenon and antinuclear antibodies (ANA).

Hepatotoxic drugs are known to produce toxic hepatitis but it is only occasionally that hepatomegaly occurs.

FURTHER READING

1. Balisttreri WF. Pediatric hepatomegaly: A half century of progress. *Clin Liver Dis* 2000;4:191-210.
2. Thapa BR, Kumar M. Liver abscess. In: Gupte S (Ed). *Recent Advances in Peditrics-14*. New Delhi: Jaypee 2004:110-118.

CHAPTER 36

Hoarseness

BACKGROUND

Hoarseness, occurring at all ages including neonatal period, is a frequent problem encountered in pediatric practice. Fortunately, most often it is of benign etiology and resolves in a short span of time.

HISTORY

In the history, ask about the precise duration of hoarseness. How did it start? Was the onset gradual or sudden? Did it follow prolonged crying? Or, did it result after incessant shouting by an older child? Any history of trauma to the larynx as a part of birth injury, or, during the postnatal period, as a result of fall against a hard object or intubation? Any suggestion that the infant is suffering from floppiness which may point to the diagnosis of cretinism, myasthenia gravis or Werdnig-Hoffmann disease?

Is the child quite lethargic, having feeding problems, tendency to hypothermia, and delayed milestones (cretinism)?

Any pyrexia which may suggest infection of the larynx? Any history of foreign body?

PHYSICAL EXAMINATION

Physical examination must include laryngoscopy in case of hoarseness not resolving in a week to 10 days time frame.

INVESTIGATIONS

Flexible laryngoscopy is the most important specific test that should be done in chronic hoarseness.

Tests to exclude GER should also be considered.

IMPORTANT DIFFERENTIALS

Trauma to the Larynx

Birth trauma may cause dislocation of cricothyroid or cricoarytenoid articulations, leading to hoarseness along with, at times, wheeze and fluttering sounds. Another mechanism by which birth trauma may produce hoarseness is through recurrent laryngeal nerve paralysis during forceps delivery. Involvement of only one cord is accompanied by little stridor. However, when both the cords are involved, the child also becomes dyspneic on top of hoarseness and stridor.

Postnatal trauma may result from fall against a hard object, prolonged intubation and high tracheostomy. The resultant injury may be penetrating or nonpenetrating, the latter being deceptive.

Trauma from acute overuse of voice as in excessive crying, screaming or shouting, is a common cause of transient hoarseness. With elimination of the stress and, perhaps, following vocal rest, the voice reverts to normal. In case of chronic hoarseness in singers and screamers, vocal nodules may be detected.

Trauma from heavy cigarette smoking in a teenager may be responsible for hoarseness.

Foreign Body

Laryngeal foreign body hoarseness, croupy cough, and aphonia are the major and most frequent manifestations of a foreign body in the larynx. A combination of obstruction and inflammation may cause dyspnea with wheeze and cyanosis, and hemoptysis.

Tracheal foreign body: A tracheal foreign body may also cause hoarseness, cough, dyspnea, and cyanosis. The most characteristic signs are, however, audible slap and palpable thud because of momentary expiratory impaction at the subglottic level, and asthmatoid wheeze.

Bronchial foreign body: A bronchial foreign body may produce hoarseness and all other manifestations of a laryngeal or tracheal foreign body. Depending on the degree of obstruction, it may remain symptom free, cause only some wheeze, or produce obstructive emphysema or atelectasis. If obstructive emphysema or atelectasis is allowed to persist, the outcome eventually may be chronic bronchopulmonary disease.

Congenital Laryngeal Anomalies

Laryngeal webs cause asphyxiation, respiratory distress, severe stridor, and weak and hoarse cry when the obstruction is complete or almost complete.

Congenital laryngeal stridor is characterized by noisy, crowing respiratory sounds, stridor, hoarseness or aphonia, dyspnea, feeding difficulty, and poor weight gain. The stridor and other symptoms slowly disappear with growth and development of the airway.

Acute Laryngitis

Acute non-diphtheretic laryngitis (infectious croup), almost always viral in etiology, is characterized by a peculiar brassy or croupy cough, usually accompanied by inspiratory stridor, hoarseness, and varying degree of respiratory distress. Four types are recognized:

1. *Acute epiglottitis:* A life-threatening, rapidly progressive infection of the epiglottis and the surrounding structures; it is characterized by sudden onset of high fever, hoarseness, drooling, moderate-to-severe respiratory distress, and stridor during early hours of the night.
2. *Acute infectious laryngitis:* It is characterized by an upper respiratory infection with cough, sore throat, and croup. Hoarseness, dyspnea, and stridor appear in severe cases.
3. *Acute laryngotracheobronchitis*: This is the most common form of croup. An upper respiratory infection is followed in few days by brassy cough, inspiratory stridor, and dyspnea. With progression of the infection lower down, expiratory phase also becomes labored, the child appearing restless and frightened. There may be high fever.
4. *Acute spasmodic laryngitis:* This resembles acute tracheolaryngobronchitis, except that signs of apparent infection are absent. A highly strung child is predisposed to it.

Acute diphtheretic laryngitis is characterized by noisy breathing, progressive stridor, hoarseness, and dry cough. The severity of dyspnea depends upon the extent of obstruction caused by the membrane.

Weakness of Laryngeal Muscles

Generalized muscular weakness as in cretinism, myasthenia gravis, and Werdnig–Hoffmann disease may cause hoarseness.

Cretinism in the newborn may, in fact, be suspected from hoarse cry, in association with hypotonia, lethargy, sluggishness, feeding difficulty, persistent jaundice, oversleeping, persistent constipation, abdominal distension with umbilical hernia, cold, rough, dry and thickened skin, a large protruding tongue, an unusually large anterior fontanel, and anemia showing poor response to hematinics. It takes another few weeks for the classical features, especially the facies, and mental and growth retardation to manifest. With this the voice becomes typically hoarse.

In order to confirm the diagnosis, the investigations needed include radiologic studies for stunted bone age, and epiphyseal dysgenesis, serum cholesterol which is raised, serum alkaline phosphatase, FBI, and radioactive iodine (^{131}I) which are low, and plasma thyroid-stimulating hormone (TSH) which is raised. Most important parameters are T_3 and T_4 which are distinctly reduced.

Myasthenia gravis, resulting from an autoimmune reaction to acetylcholine receptors, may cause hoarseness. In the transient type, which the baby acquires from the mother, the manifestations, other than hoarse, feeble cry, include floppiness, feeding difficulty, feeble respiratory effort, profuse oral secretions, and ptosis though the baby appears alert with normal tendon reflexes. Spontaneous recovery may occur in many within 2–4 weeks. Excellent response to edrophonium or neostigmine is a rule. In the persistent type, which is likely to continue throughout life, eyelids and extraocular muscles are severely involved. Rest of the manifestations are those of the transient type. In this type, there is no evidence of the disease in the mother.

Werdnig–Hoffmann disease or infantile spinal muscular atrophy, an autosomal recessive disorder, may be responsible for a weak, hoarse cry in association with gross floppiness, areflexia, fasciculations or fibrillations in the tongue, neurologic involvement of intercostal and bulbar muscles and normal IQ. Respiratory failure, aspiration or a fulminant infection often proves fatal. The family history is often positive. The mother gives history of absence or reduction of fetal movements in utero.

Remaining Causes of Hoarseness

Laryngismus stridulus, chronic granulomatous disease, vincristine, etc.

FURTHER READING

1. Gupte S. The child with hoarseness. *Eur Bull Pediatr Med* 2002;4:34-39.
2. Green M. Speech. In: *Pediatric Diagnosis*, 6th edn. Philadelphia: Saunders 1998:56-59.
3. Pediatric Ear, Nose and Throat Specialist. Hoarseness. Available at: pediatric-ent.com/hoarseness. Accessed on: 23 July 2019.

CHAPTER 37

Involuntary Movements

BACKGROUND

The term, *involuntary movements*, applies to unintended movements which occur usually on attempt to carry out a skilled motor act to maintain a given posture, and are usually absent during complete relaxation (rest), more so during sleep. Principally, involuntary movements occur from involvement of basal ganglia, cerebellum or extrapyramidal system.

HISTORY

How did the involuntary movements start: Acute or slow process? Any preceding event immediately or in the past, say sore throat, joint pains, anxiety-related episode(s). Any other illness child has been suffering from?

PHYSICAL EXAMINATION

The foremost in physical examination is carefully observing the movements in the patient and provisionally categorizing them in the known type(s). At times, there may be more than one type of movements in a given child. Once it is done, further evaluation should address the following:
- Positive phenomena such as aberrant positions and movements over and above the dominant movement.
- Occult (latent) phenomena in the form of associated aberrant postures and rigidity demonstrated on special testing maneuvers.
- Negative phenomena such as failure to do expected maneuvers such as initiating an action.

IMPORTANT DIFFERENTIALS

Tremors

Tremors are regular or irregular, repetitive, rapid movements occurring usually in distal extremities.

Physiologic tremors may occur in normal children and cause no anxiety, provided that a meticulous central nervous system (CNS) examination reveals no defect.

Mental subnormality may often be accompanied by tremors. Acute anxiety usually causes fine and rapid tremors. Infrequently, however, these may be coarse and irregular.

Thyrotoxicosis is characterized by fine tremors of the fingers if the arm is extended. Other manifestations of thyrotoxicosis (Graves' disease) include emotional disturbances accompanied by motor hyperactivity, irritability, restlessness, voracious appetite with poor or no weight gain, enlarged thyroid, exophthalmos, excessive sweating, palpitations, dyspnea, and cardiomegaly. T_3 and T_4 levels are usually increased.

Hepatolenticular degeneration or Wilson's disease is accompanied by rather proximal tremors of the outstretched arms and wrists ("wing-beating" tremor) in association with dysarthria and dystonia at an advanced stage. Non-neurologic manifestations of the disease, which occur rather early include hepatomegaly, splenomegaly, jaundice, anorexia, edema and ascites, gastrointestinal hemorrhage, and hemolytic crisis. Kayser–Fleischer rings are seen in 75% of cases. Serum copper and ceruloplasmin levels are reduced. Liver tissue copper content exceeding 400 mcg/g dry weight is the most reliable parameter for diagnosis of Wilson's disease.

Benign essential tremors are somewhat coarse and irregular. They occur in distal muscles and become worse in awkward postures such as the outstretched fingers held pointing at each other in front of the nose. They occur as a benign hereditary trait. Interestingly, they subside during movements.

Intention tremors, a sign of cerebellar lesion, are present only during movement and become more marked on approaching to the target. In an infant, these can be elicited by inducing him to reach out for a bright object, say a toy.

Hysterical tremors are characterized by involuntary movements of a limb or the whole body which become worse as the examiner attempts to control them. The problem is encountered in older children and adolescents. History may be of considerable help since such a patient is described as having had a variety of bizarre symptoms and signs earlier too.

Maternal drug addiction may be responsible for tremors in the newborns and infants. The drugs blamed include alcohol, phenothiazine, diazepam, heroin, and diphenhydramine. In the so-called "fetoalcohol syndrome", many other manifestations occur. These include intrauterine and postnatal growth retardation, microcephaly, mental retardation, ptosis, microphthalmia, and short palpebral fissures. Frequent accompaniments include maxillary hypoplasia, congenital heart disease, hemangioma, abnormal external genitalia, abnormal palmar creases, and anomalies of bones and joints.

Drugs given to the child, and possibly responsible for tremors, include phenothiazines, aminophylline, and terbutaline.

Poisoning with thallium may cause tremors. Solvent sniffing is also on record to cause tremors.

Infantile tremor syndrome, a disorder seen almost exclusively in Indian infants and young children and of obscure etiology, is characterized by tremors, anemia, and regression of milestones. Tremors are generalized though most pronounced in distal parts of limbs, especially upper limbs, head, face, and tongue (Figs. 37.1 and 37.2). Even trunk may be involved. Some infants produce tremulous cry like that of a lamb. They keep tossing their head from side to side with saliva drooling from mouth, and have dull, expressionless look. Mental and motor development is impaired in all. As a rule, tremors disappear during sleep in most cases. In others, their intensity remarkably diminishes. Remaining manifestations include hypotonia, hypochromotrichia with sparse hair, moderate anemia, mental apathy, reticular pigmentation, and superimposed nutritional deficiencies.

Spasmus nutans is characterized by rhythmic jerking movements of the head in the form of intermittent head nodding, usually in the lateral or horizontal direction, together with intermittent nystagmus. The manifestations are noted from the age of 4 months to 12 months and disappear spontaneously by the age of 3 years or 4 years. The movements disappear when the child concentrates on something and during sleep.

Jitteriness or jittery tremors are provoked by external stimuli and stopped by flexing the limb. These may be perfectly normal in a newborn. These have, however, to be differentiated from convulsive movements which are neither significantly provoked by external stimuli nor stopped by flexing the limb.

Choreiform Movements

Choreiform movements are irregular jerking and writhing movements which may vary from mild to violent intensity so as to render carrying acts such as walking virtually impossible. The causes of choreiform movements include rheumatic fever (Sydenham's chorea) and drugs like phenothiazines. Occasionally thyrotoxicosis and systemic lupus erythematosus (SLE) may cause such involuntary movements. In adults, Huntington's chorea and senile chorea are well-known causes of such movements.

Rheumatic chorea, one of the five major manifestations of rheumatic fever, is characterized by repeated involuntary movements of the extremities, face and trunk, and emotional stability. Difficulty in walking and speech results from muscle weakness. The condition may be limited to half of the body, the so-called "hemichorea". Most often, chorea occurs as a solitary manifestation, i.e. without any other evidence of rheumatic activity. Onset may be sudden or insidious. The usual patient is preadolescent or adolescent girl.

The parameters which may help in reaching the diagnosis of rheumatic chorea include—(1) finger-nose test, (2) buttoning the clothes test, (3) dinner-fork position of the outstretched hands, (4) pronation of forearm when hands are raised above the head, (5) "Bag of worms" sign, i.e. tongue making peculiar movements when protruded out, (6) "Milkmaid" sign, (7) audible "click" during speech, (8) clumsiness or inability in writing, (9) counting the digits, (10) ataxia, (11) sustained, "hung-up" or double knee jerk, and (12) brisk deep tendon reflexes.

Mild chorea may be confused with tics. A dependable distinguishing feature is that tics are stereotyped sudden movements that are seen in the same group of muscles against chorea in which one does not know which group of muscle is to show movement next. Also, tics can be

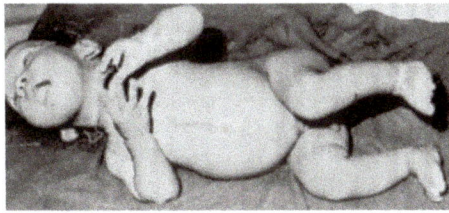

Fig. 37.1: *Infantile tremor syndrome*—Note the tremors, hair changes, chubby appearance despite malnutrition, vacant look, and the reticular pigmentation. The infant was anemic with a hemoglobin of 7 g/dL, the peripheral smear and bone marrow being consistent with dimorphic anemia.

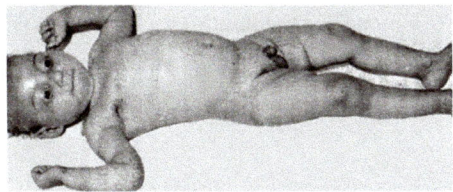

Fig. 37.2: *Infantile tremor syndrome*—Another infant with classical features, precipitated by onset of an episode of lower respiratory tract infection.

voluntarily controlled for a while which is unlikely in case of choreiform movements.

Tics

Also termed as *habit spasm*, tics are fast repetitive movements that are frequently stereotyped but alterable at will. They occur most often in school-going children and are usually a reflection of home conflict, emotional disturbance, maladjustment, and other factors contributing to insecurity. Generally, they are an "outlet" for the pent up anger and worrisomeness following control of aggression from the parents or teacher. Various types of tics include twitching the face, blinking the eyes, shoulder shrugging, gaping (inappropriate mouth opening), tongue sniffing, etc.

A rare type of tic in which extensive and varied bodily movement, including head jerking, is accompanied by vocalization (say barking, hissing originating, etc.) is called Tourette syndrome (also, Gilles de la Tourette syndrome).

Drugs blamed for causing tics include amphetamine.

Athetosis

Athetotic movements, also called as "choreoathetosis", are slow writhing movements, generally more remarkable in distal muscles, consisting of alternating supination–pronation and flexin-extension of the extremity. The movements tend to disappear during sleep. Athetosis, when very severe, may have involvement of axial muscles and trunk so much and so that the subject is hardly in a position to stand. This situation, dystonia musculorum deformans, or torsion dystonia or spasm, occurs in 5–10-year-old. The overall picture is that of a young child with hypertonia of calf muscles resulting in inversion and adduction of the foot, followed by adduction and fixed flexion of hip together with lordosis, torticollis, and writhing movements as if the child is twisting something.

Athetosis, particularly when bilateral, occurs usually in degenerative diseases of the basal ganglia, especially Wilson's disease, Huntington chorea, etc.

Drugs blamed for athetosis, particularly dystonia, include phenothiazines, metoclopramide, haloperidol, and amitriptyline.

Seizure

See Chapter 12.

Myoclonus

These are shock-like, arrhythmic twitches. Myoclonic jerks may occur with voluntary movement (action myoclonus) or as a result of a stimulus (startle or reflex myoclonus). These are not suppressible and are often associated with CNS pathology, hypoxic damage (e.g. during cardiac arrest), neurodegenerative disorders, and encephalopathy.

Drug-induced Involuntary Movements

Usually, acute hyperkinetic drug reactions are in the form of generalized dystonia in children. The causative drugs nclude phenytoin, carbamazepine, lithium, and cimetidine. Such drugs as amphetamines, methylphenidate and cocaine cause tics, chopreiform movements and stereotyped behaviors.

Psychogenic Involuntary Movements

Psychogenic movement disorders may mimic any of the conditions described above. Affected patients, often female, suffer from conversion disorder, malingering, or factitious disorders. Diagnosis is by exclusion, i.e failure to find any organic disease. Clinical features favoring a psychogenic cause are listed in Box 37.1.

BOX 37.1: Features favoring a psychogenic involuntary movements.
- Acute onset.
- Movement patterns not in keeping with the known movement disorder.
- Movements often increasing with attention.
- Following distractibility (performing another task), movements often decrease.
- Tremors of upper extremity are usually psychogenic.
- Variation in tremor frequency is consistent with a psychogenic cause.
- Movements are invariably psychogenic when the patient is asked to tap with one hand and the other hand's tremor entrains with the tapping.

FURTHER READING

1. Cardoso E, Seppi K, Mair KJ, et al. Seminars on chorea. *Lancet Neurol* 2006;5:589-602.
2. Johnston MV. Movement disorders. In: Kliegman RM, St Geme III JW, Blum NJ, et al (Eds). *Nelson Textbook of Pediatrics*, 21st edn. Philadelphia: Elsevier 2020:2488-2493.
3. Tarsy D, Simon DK. Dystonia. *N Engl J Med* 2006;355:818-829.

CHAPTER 38

Irritability

BACKGROUND

Irritability—to be exact, excessive irritability—means exaggerated reaction to a stimulus so that the child demonstrates excessive crying and fretfulness and fails to be calmed down by accepted means such as being held, fed, played with or changed the nappy.

HISTORY

While questioning the parents, find out if the mother had been taking drugs such as narcotics during pregnancy. Is he beginning to erupt teeth? Is he on any drug, say phenobarbital? Is he febrile? Is he vomiting? Did he sleep well? Any cough, ear discharge, drooling, diarrhea or constipation? Any suggestion of colic? Any history of food intolerance? Does he have pruritus, especially in the presence of pinworm infestation?

PHYSICAL EXAMINATION

Physical examination should, in particular, exclude central nervous system (CNS) infection, otitis media, urinary tract infection, pneumonia, and gastroenteritis. Make a special note of the "cry" (Table 38.1).

INVESTIGATIONS

Usually, no investigations are helpful. In serious infections such as meningitis, it is important to do lumbar puncture and carry out biochemical examination of cerebrospinal fluid (CSF). In sepsis, a blood culture is mandatory.

IMPORTANT DIFFERENTIALS

Narcotic Withdrawal Syndrome

Excessive irritability may occur in babies born to mothers addicted to narcotics a few days after birth. Such an infant is usually small-for-dates or preterm. He has excessive drooling, diarrhea or constipation. He coughs and sneezes frequently. He is very irritable and tremulous.

Serious Infections

Undue irritability in the neonatal period should be considered indicative of meningitis or septicemia, unless, of course, an obvious cause is found out. Other manifestations may include high-pitched and shrill cry, fever or hypothermia, feeding difficulty, and lethargy alternating with excessive crying. Seizures may occur though meningeal signs may be absent. A raised anterior fontanel helps, so does the finding of a septic focus such as umbilical sepsis (Fig. 38.1).

Other infections that may contribute to irritability include otitis media, urinary tract infection, pneumonia, and gastroenteritis.

TABLE 38.1: "Cry" as a clue to diagnosis.

Nature of cry	Likely state
Normal	Hunger Wind Soiling of nappies Loneliness
High-pitched shrill	Cerebral irritation Meningitis Hydrocephalus Kernicterus
Hoarse, croaky gruff Cat-like mewing Bleating, lamblike	Hypothyroidism (cretinism) Cri duchat syndrome Cornelia de Lange syndrome Infantile tremor syndrome
Crowing	Laryngeal conditions like laryngomalacia
Weak	Amyotonia congenita Gross malnutrition
Grunting Whimper	Pneumonia Critically sick child

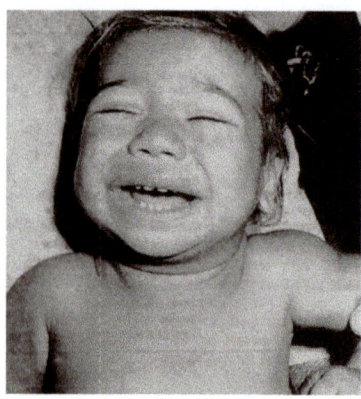

Fig. 38.1: Excessive crying and irritability in a child whose cerebrospinal fluid (CSF) turned out to be consistent with pyogenic meningitis. His cry was characteristically high-pitched and shrill.

Teething

Sharp edge of a tooth cutting through the gums may be responsible for undue irritability. On inspection, gums appear red and swollen and there is excessive drooling.

Colic

Paroxysmal irritability may be related to colic. The condition occurs usually early in infancy and is characterized by recurrent acute abdominal pain. The infant gives shrill cry, sweats profusely, and draws his legs to the chest.

Insecurity

A child, otherwise hale and hearty, may react to want of love, punishment or undue strictness and authoritarianism by throwing tantrums of incessant irritability.

Food Intolerance

Irritability is an important manifestation of gluten-induced enteropathy (gluten-sensitivity or celiac disease). Other manifestations include chronic diarrhea with large pale, highly foul-smelling stools which stick to the pain, growth failure, nutritional deficiencies, abdominal distention, and anorexia. The disease manifests a few months after the introduction of gluten-containing foods, say a wheat preparation, in the infant's diet. Investigations show steatorrhea, D-xylose malabsorption, and varying degree of villus atrophy. Response to withdrawal of gluten from diet is gratifying. Gluten challenge leads to reappearance of the clinical, functional, and histological abnormalities.

Phenylketonuria (PKU), though very rare in our setting, is an important cause of excessive irritability. Other manifestations include vomiting, anorexia, excessive sweating, eczema, blond hair, and blue eyes. Convulsions, mental retardation with hyperactive personality, and erratic behavior become obvious as the child grows. The diagnosis in this familial autosomal recessive disorder due to deficiency of enzyme, phenylalanine hydroxylase, is confirmed by demonstrating serum phenylalanine level exceeding 1.5 mg% and by ferric chloride test or Phenistix paper strips showing excess of phenylalanine and its metabolites.

Hypoglycemia

A school-going child in the habit of reaching home in bad temper is very likely to show gratifying response to a hearty meal. The obvious cause is hypoglycemia.

Pink Disease (Acrodynia)

Excessive irritability is an important feature of pink disease resulting from mercury poisoning. Other manifestations include pinkness of hands and feet, constant crying, photophobia, and undue sweating.

Drugs

Phenobarbital, primidone, ethionamide, cycloserine, hyoscine, cyclopentolate, fenfluramine, aminophylline, acetazolamide, thyroxine, imipramine, troxidone, ephedrine, amphetamine, clonazepam, antihistamines, etc.

FURTHER READING

1. Gupte S. The child who cries and cries. In: Gupte S (Ed). *Speaking of Child Care*, 3rd edn. New Delhi: Sterling 2007.
2. Green M. Irritability; excessive crying. In: *Pediatric Diagnosis*, 6th edn. Philadelphia: Saunders 1998:356-358.
3. King D, Hafeez W. Irritability and fussiness. In: Adam HM, Foy JM (Eds). *Signs and Symptoms in Pediatrics*. Illinois: American Academy of Pediatrics 2015:569-580.
4. Poole SR. The infant with acute unexplained excessive crying. *Pediatrics* 1991;88:450-455.

CHAPTER 39

Jaundice

BACKGROUND

The term, *jaundice* or *icterus*, denotes yellowness of the scleral conjunctiva and skin due to hyperbilirubinemia. Yellow coloration of the skin caused by caroteinemia, due to ingestion by the child or the lactating mother of excess of carrots and other green vegetables, or associated with hypothyroidism, nephrotic syndrome, and diabetes mellitus, should not be confused with true jaundice. Excessive consumption of tomatoes, tomato juice, and commercial infant foods treated with the coloring matter in them (lycopene) may also impart to the skin an orange or reddish-yellow color. This condition is called lycopenemia. Yellow staining may also occur from certain drugs such as mepacrine. Note that there is no rise in the serum bilirubin level in all these situations. In the postmaturity and placental dysfunction syndrome, baby's skin may have a yellow tinge because of the meconium staining.

Jaundice in the newborn is a common observation being encountered in about 75% of the babies. Undoubtedly in vast majority it is physiologic, resulting from insufficiency of the liver enzymes to deal with the bilirubin liberated following normal hemolysis. In our experience, based on a prospective study of over 300 hospitalized cases, the relative frequency of various etiologic factors is as follows—physiologic 47%, ABO incompatibility 16%, Rh incompatibility 12%, septicemia/intrauterine infections 10%, neonatal hepatitis 2%, biliary atresia 2%, glucose-6-phosphate dehydrogenase (G6PD) deficiency 2%, breast milk 1%, cretinism 2%, galactosemia 1%, large cephalhematoma 2%, and undiagnosed/idiopathic hyperbilirubinemia 3%. Quite a few other conditions are stated as causing neonatal jaundice, but their incidence is certainly exceedingly low in Indian settings.

HISTORY

In recording history in case of neonatal jaundice, it is important to enquire about the time of onset of jaundice. For instance, jaundice appearing right at birth or during the very first day of birth is invariably due to blood group in compatibility, intrauterine infections or G6PD deficiency. Jaundice first noticed on second or third day is usually physiologic.

Enquire whether jaundice is decreasing or increasing in intensity. What is the infant's general condition whether healthy, having feeding difficulty, fever, rash, seizures or any other abnormal movements? Any history of excessive crying or drowsiness? Is there any pus discharge from the umbilicus? Is there any evidence of bleeding from any site? What is the type of feeding—breast or bottle?

Also, enquire about the maternal and family history with special reference to maternal infection (during pregnancy), drugs taken during pregnancy or labor, previous sibling(s) affected by jaundice or liver disease, and any family history of jaundice or anemia. What is the ethnic group of parents and ancestors?

PHYSICAL EXAMINATION

Physical examination of the newborn presenting with jaundice must assess the severity of jaundice in daylight. Sclera is not easily available for examination in the newborn because of the photophobia. Clinically, one has got to, therefore, count on skin (Fig. 39.1). The touch of jaundice appears relatively early on face, nasolabial folds, and tip of nose. At times, even marked jaundice may not be detected unless skin is blanched with a finger, preferring a flat area like forehead. This is observed in infants with red or pink skin. The dark-skinned infant may present difficulties. It is advisable to have a look at the hard palate of such babies. As a rough guide, you may refer to Table 39.1.

Also, assess the gestational age, activity, and general condition of the baby. Is the umbilicus healthy or septic? Is there any evidence of hemorrhage, petechiae, etc.? Any congenital malformation? Any neurologic finding? What is the size of liver and spleen? Is the baby significantly anemic? Any cephalhematoma? What is the color of urine and stools?

Jaundice in the later infancy and childhood has altogether different etiology. Viral hepatitis is the most commonly encountered entity in this age group.

History must seek information whether the onset has been insidious with vague symptoms or acute with fever, anorexia, vomiting, right upper quadrant abdominal pain, and high-colored urine. Any history of abdominal distention and lump(s) in abdomen? Is the child becoming progressively anemic? Any history of intake of hepatotoxic drugs? Any symptoms of urinary tract infection? Has the child lost considerable weight? Any delay/regression in milestones? Any restlessness, confusion or change in sensorium? Any flopping tremors?

Find out if there have been cases of jaundice in the family or neighborhood. Did the parents lose earlier a child or two as a result of liver problem? Did the patient get exposed to a case of acute jaundice some weeks ago? Did he have some kind of injection, drip or blood transfusion in the last 3 months or 4 months?

A detailed dietary enquiry must explore history of early introduction of feeds contaminated with copper from copper and/or brass utensils.

Physical check-up should ascertain the extent of jaundice. Does the child have hepatosplenomegaly? What is the liver consistency surface and border like? Is there any evidence of portal hypertension in the form of caput medusae, ascites, esophageal varices, etc.? How is the state of consciousness? Is the child heading for hepatic coma?

JAUNDICE IN THE NEWBORN

Box 39.1 lists etiology of neonatal jaundice according to the age of onset. Causes of unconjugated hyperbilirubinemia are given in Box 39.2.

First Day

Blood group incompatibility, ABO incompatibility or ABO hemolytic disease is by far the most common

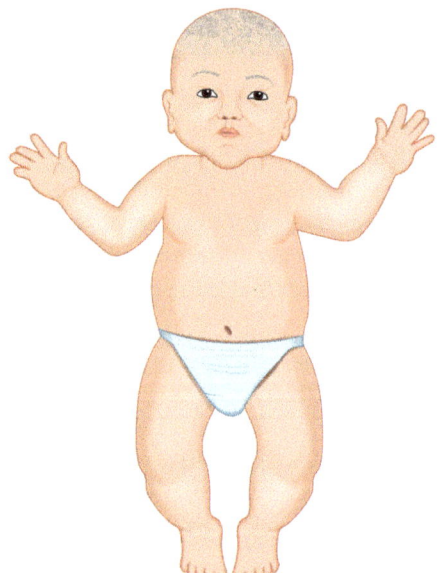

Fig. 39.1: *Neonatal jaundice*—Dermal zones are a good guide for magnitude of hyperbilirubinemia.

TABLE 39.1: Clinical examination as a clue to level of serum bilirubin in the jaundiced neonate as per Krammer's guidelines.

Body surface jaundiced on blanching	Approximate serum bilirubin
Face	5 mg/dL
Chest and upper abdomen	10 mg/dL
Lower abdomen	12 mg/dL
Legs	15 mg/dL
Soles and palms	>15 mg/dL

BOX 39.1: Important causes of neonatal jaundice based on the age of onset.

First day
- Rh and ABO incompatibilities (hemolytic disease of the newborn)
- Intrauterine infections like toxoplasmosis and cytomegalic inclusion disease
- Glucose-6-phosphate dehydrogenase (G6PD) deficiency
- Hereditary spherocytosis
- Drug administration to mother (vitamin K, sulfisoxazole, salicylates, etc.)
- Homozygous alpha-thalassemia

Second and third days
- Physiologic
- Hyperbilirubinemia of newborn
- Birth asphyxia
- Cephalhematoma
- Acidosis
- Hypothermia
- Hypoglycemia
- Drugs
- Familial nonhemolytic icterus as in Crigler-Najjar disease, Gilbert disease, Dubin-Johnson syndrome

Fourth to seventh days
- Septicemia
- Syphilis
- Toxoplasmosis
- Cytomegalic inclusion disease
- Extrahepatic atresia of bile duct
- Breast-milk jaundice

After first week
- Septicemia
- Extrahepatic atresia of bile duct
- Hereditary spherocytosis
- Neonatal hepatitis
- Drug-induced hemolytic anemia
- Galactosemia
- Persistent jaundice during first month
- Inspissated bile syndrome
- Cretinism
- Congenital hypertrophic pyloric stenosis.

BOX 39.2: Causes of unconjugated hyperbilirubinemia.

- Physiologic
- Pathologic
- Increased production of bilirubin
  - *Hemolytic disease of the newborn:* Rh isoimmunization, ABO incompatibility, minor blood group incompatibility
  - Hereditary spherocytosis
  - *Nonspherocytic hemolytic anemia:* Glucose-6-phosphate dehydrogenase (G6PD) deficiency, pyruvate kinase deficiency, alpha-thalassemia
  - *Acquired hemolysis disorders:* Vitamin K3-induced hemolysis, microangiopathies
  - Septicemia
  - *Increased enterohepatic circulation:* Intestinal obstruction, congenital hypertrophic pyloric stenosis, meconium ileus, paralytic ileus, Hirschsprung's disease
- Decreased clearance of bilirubin
  - *Inborn errors of metabolism:* Familial nonhemolytic jaundice (Crigler-Najjar syndrome) types I and II, Gilbert disease
  - *Medications:* Vitamin K3
  - *Hormones:* Breast-milk jaundice, hypothyroidism, hypopituitarism.

form of incompatibility and the most common cause of neonatal jaundice. The most common type involves group "O" mother and group "A" or "B" infant though other incompatibilities also occur. Jaundice is usually mild and nonobstructive. In the presence of adverse/predisposing factors such as prematurity, hypoxia, infection, acidosis, hypoglycemia, hypothermia, and cephalhematoma, its intensity (as measured by bilirubin level in blood) may assume critical level.

Accompanying manifestations may include mild anemia and hepatosplenomegaly that is seldom gross.

Diagnosis is supported by demonstration of reticulocytosis, microspherocytosis, and high fragility of red cells. In differentiating from spherocytosis, remember that in the latter condition one parent and, sometime, a sibling are affected. Moreover, mother's serum does not contain immune anti-A or anti-B bodies except by coincidence. High titer of immunoglobulin G (IgG) hemolysis in maternal blood against infant's blood strongly favors the diagnosis of ABO incompatibility. Also, indirect Coombs test is generally positive and direct Coombs test is negative. Acetylcholinesterase activity of cells is normal or only marginally low.

The Rh incompatibility or hemolytic disease must always be excluded if severe jaundice appears on the first day of birth. The problem arises when an Rh-negative mother carries Rh-positive baby. The first baby is usually not affected unless, of course the mother had an earlier abortion or blood transfusion with Rh-positive blood.

- Hydrops fetalis is the severest form of the disease. The infant is born preterm with gross edema and effusion in serious cavities and massive hepatosplenomegaly. There is history of placenta having been large and edematous.
- Icterus gravis is relatively less severe form of the disease and occurs when hemolysis in utero is not very intense. Deep jaundice appears during the first 12–24 hours. Progressive anemia and hepatosplenomegaly are invariably present. Some affected babies may have purpura. Incidence of kernicterus is high. Those who manage to survive are often left with crippling sequelae.
- Congenital hemolytic anemia is the mildest and also the rarest form of Rh hemolytic disease. Jaundice, if present, is slight. Anemia and hepatosplenomegaly are often detected towards the end of the first week or later.

Diagnosis, if not already made antenatally (remember that in case of ABO incompatibility, antenatal diagnosis is not yet possible), has got to be made immediately after birth if serious consequences are to be prevented. The foremost investigation is to demonstrate that the mother is Rh negative whereas the infant is Rh positive. Occasionally, an Rh-positive infant may type as Rh negative because of the "blocking antibodies". If possible, father's Rh group should also be determined. Secondly, direct Coombs test on infant's red cells is positive and anti-Rh titer of mother is high. Remaining investigations show high serum bilirubin (indirect or unconjugated), reticulocytosis, anemia, anti-Rh agglutinins, and hypoglycemia.

Intrauterine infections: Toxoplasmosis, cytomegalic inclusion disease, and rubella are the leading intrauterine infections that may cause jaundice on the first day or any time during the neonatal period. The infection occurs antenatally by the passage of organisms across the placenta.

Jaundice in the newborn with congenital toxoplasmosis is accompanied by manifestations such as maculopapular rash, pyrexia, poor feeding, hepatosplenomegaly, lymphadenopathy, microphthalmia, microcephaly/hydrocephalus, seizures, chorioretinitis, and cerebral calcification, singly or in some combination.

Congenital rubella may cause jaundice in a proportion to the newborns on the first day, the incidence being much less than that in the case of toxoplasmosis. The remaining manifestations of the disease include congenital heart disease, hepatosplenomegaly, low birth weight, thrombocytopenia, interstitial pneumonia, cataracts, retinopathy, bone lesions, lethargy, irritability, bulging anterior fontanel, and disturbances of tone.

Neonatal jaundice is seen in relatively higher frequency in cytomegalic inclusion disease, also called as cytomegalovirus (CMV) infection than that in the toxoplasmosis and rubella. The remaining manifestations include hepatosplenomegaly, petechial rash, microcephaly, chorioretinitis, and cerebral calcification.

Glucose-6-phosphate dehydrogenase deficiency: Jaundice from this X-linked recessive disorder that has emerged as a leading cause of neonatal jaundice, especially among the

Mediterranean, African, Chinese, and Indian stock, may occur right at birth or any time postnatally. It may be severe enough to warrant resort to exchange blood transfusion to guard against risk of brain damage. The enzymatic deficiency causes failure on the part of the red cells to utilize glucose. The cell membrane suffers and hemolysis follows. In order that significant hemolysis occurs some offending agent (usually a drug such as primaquine, vitamin K, sulfa, chloramphenicol, salicylate, etc. but not uncommonly adverse factors such as hypothermia, hypoglycemia, hypoxia, acidosis, infection, etc.) is needed to trigger off the process. Majority of the newborns are born preterm.

Second or Third Day

Physiologic jaundice: In full-term infants, insufficiency of the liver enzymes to deal with the bilirubin liberated as a result of normal hemolysis may lead to appearance of jaundice on second (at the end) or third day of life. It is usually mild and disappears by 7–10th postnatal day due to the maturation of the liver function (Fig. 39.2). Occasionally, however, serum bilirubin may exceed 12 mg% and jaundice may take 10–14 days to disappear.

In preterm infants, jaundice is relatively deeper (sometime serum bilirubin may be as high as 15 mg%) and takes more days to disappear. Also termed as jaundice of immaturity, it results from the same mechanism as in the full-term infant. As a rule, it appears also on second or third day. It may not reach its peak until the sixth or seventh day.

What needs further emphasis (even at the cost of repetition) is that physiologic jaundice does not make the baby sick and inactive. The liver and spleen are not enlarged. Umbilicus is healthy. The urine and stools are normal in color. If the clinical picture is different from this description, the diagnosis needs revision. You may have to do any certain investigations to arrive at the precise etiology. Important factors that have adverse effect on physiologic jaundice include prematurity (excessive and prolonged immaturity of the liver cells to produce the enzyme, glucuronyl transferase), birth asphyxia, acidosis, hypoglycemia, hypothermia, cephalhematoma, intrauterine

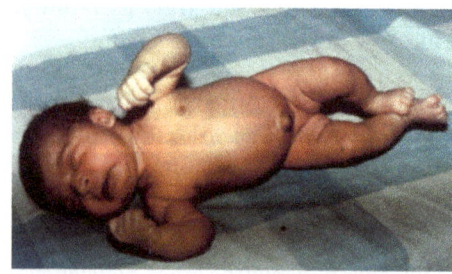

Fig. 39.2: *Neonatal jaundice*—Note that the physiologic jaundice, first noticed on third day, is in the process of regressing in this 8-day-old baby.

or acquired infection, cretinism, possibly breast-milk, and drugs such as vitamin K, novobiocin, kanamycin, furazolidone, nitrofurantoin, sulfas, chloramphenicol, gentamicin, salicylates, steroids, contraceptive pill, etc.

Hyperbilirubinemia of the newborn: The term is applied to those preterm infants whose physiologic jaundice becomes considerably exaggerated so much and so that the infant is at a risk to develop kernicterus from neurotoxicity of unconjugated bilirubin. The primary problem appears to be a deficiency or inactivity of the enzyme, glucuronyl transferase, and not the excess load of bilirubin for excretion.

Familial nonhemolytic jaundice: In rare disorders, Crigler–Najjar syndrome, Dubin–Johnson syndrome, Gilbert's disease, and Rotor's syndrome, there is inability of the liver cells to excrete conjugated bilirubin, resulting in bile in the urine. Familial glucuronyl transferase inhibition/inactivity/deficiency operates as the fundamental cause in all of them.

Fourth to Seventh Day

Septicemia: Jaundice appearing after the third day and until the seventh day strongly suggests septicemia as the probable cause. Besides jaundice, the infant may have poor feeding, vomiting, lethargy, irritability, fever or hypothermia, abdominal distension, hepatosplenomegaly, and respiratory distress. Neonatal reflexes are sluggish often, unhealthy umbilicus or there is evidence of septic focus elsewhere. Incidence of meningitis as a complication is high. Development of scleroma is a bad prognostic sign.

Blood culture is important to establish the diagnosis as also for guidance in therapy. In a large majority of the cases, *Escherichia coli* and *group B Streptococcus* are responsible for the disease. The remaining organisms include *Staphylococcus aureus, Enterococcus, Klebsiella, Enterobacter sp, Pseudomonas, Proteus sp, Listeria monocytogenes,* and anaerobic organisms.

Recently, quite a few studies have registered rising incidence of *Klebsiella aeruginosa* in the etiology of neonatal septicemia. During 1980–1985, it emerged as the dominant causative agent at the Postgraduate Institute of Medical Education and Research, Chandigarh. In subsequent years, similar reports have appeared from many other centers.

Breast-milk jaundice: Infrequently (1 in 200 breastfeed term infants), significant unconjugated hyperbilirubinemia (causing jaundice, that leads to no pathologic problem such as kernicterus) described to breastfeeding may occur between fourth to seventh postnatal day. Its cause is not clear. Of course, it could possibly result from presence of 5 beta-pregnane-3 alpha, 20 beta-diol, and nonesterified long-chain fatty acids in the milk of some of these mothers, leading to competitively inhibited glucuronyl transferase activity. In other instances, lipase in milk may be responsible for jaundice. Another simple explanation is that relative dehydration which is common in the first few days may account for some of the cases.

The kind of jaundice shows its peak in the third week and then gradually disappears.

Though discontinuation of breastfeeding is known to rapidly lower the serum bilirubin level, there is no need to stop breastfeeding even temporarily unless the level reaches a critical point.

Large cephalhematoma: This otherwise benign, self-limited condition characterized by a nonpulsatile swelling, usually over the parietal or occipital region, that neither crosses the suture line nor increases in size on crying, may be large enough to cause massive overloading of the liver with bilirubin. If the liver fails to conjugate this excess bilirubin jaundice may occur. At times, jaundice may be severe enough to warrant aspiration of the cephalhematoma.

Intrauterine infections: Between fourth day and seventh day too, intrauterine infections, say syphilis, toxoplasmosis, and cytomegalic inclusion disease, may cause jaundice.

Neonatal hepatitis: Jaundice due to neonatal hepatitis is usually first noted in the first week (in a large majority about the seventh day) but may appear at any time during the first month and even up to 3 months.

In almost 70% cases, no specific cause can be found. Hence, the term idiopathic neonatal hepatitis has been suggested for this category of cases. The term, neonatal hepatitis syndrome implies that a group of disease entities, predominantly viruses, may cause a similar clinical picture. The causes include—(1) viruses—hepatitis B, herpes simplex, rubella, cytomegalovirus, coxsackie B, adenovirus, (2) bacteria—septicemia, urinary tract infection, syphilis, (3) protozoa—toxoplasmosis, (4) metabolic—galactosemia, alpha-l-antitrypsin deficiency, cystic fibrosis, Rotor's syndrome, Niemann–Pick disease, and (5) chromosomal—Turner's syndrome, trisomy 13–15, 16–18, and 21.

Idiopathic neonatal hepatitis, also termed as giant cell hepatitis, occurs twice as frequently in boys as in girls. It may occur in two or three infants of the same family. The incidence in premature babies is higher. Jaundice appearing in the first week or later may be the only complaint, or there may be accompanying manifestations like poor feeding, anemia, vomiting, high-colored urine, intermittent loss of pigment from stools, and hepatosplenomegaly. Liver is grossly enlarged and has firm consistency. Spleen is only moderately enlarged and that too in only half of the cases. Occasionally, thrombocytopenic purpura may occur.

Investigations show high serum hyperbilirubinemia (mostly conjugated), high serum glutamic-pyruvic transaminase (SGPT), high alkaline phosphatase, and slightly prolonged prothrombin time. Rose-Bengal excretion in stools exceeds 15%. Australia antigen may be positive.

Liver biopsy shows multinucleated giant cells with complete loss of normal pattern of hepatic lobules and increased fibrous tissue around necrotic liver cells as also in portal tracts. Extrahepatic bile ducts are normal unless, of course, the disease has advanced considerably.

Contrary to the belief until recently, steroid therapy is of nonproven value. Complete recovery occurs in 75% of the subjects within a year without any specific treatment. The remaining 25% progresses to chronic liver disease.

Extrahepatic biliary atresia: This obliterative disorder of the extrahepatic bile ducts is the most frequent cause of persistent jaundice that is first noticed about the seventh postnatal day. Quite often, jaundice appears to be a continuation of the physiologic jaundice of the newborn. It is mild to begin with but slowly and progressively it becomes severe. Jaundice seemingly deepens and lightens alternately. Urine is heavily bile-stained. Despite absence of bile in stools, the latter may not become typically clay-colored and putty-like early enough. It is said that, in early neonatal life, jaundiced intestinal epithelium may be sloughed off and added to the bulk of the stool, thereby not letting the latter appear clay-colored. With progression of the disease, skin becomes bronze, olive-green in color. Hepatosplenomegaly and vitamin deficiencies (hemorrhages due to vitamin K deficiency) may occur.

Main differential diagnosis is from neonatal hepatitis (Table 39.2). An important diagnostic measure is the Rose-Bengal test which shows less than 10% fecal excretion of ^{131}I and ^{132}I as against over 15% in case of neonatal hepatitis.

TABLE 39.2: Neonatal hepatitis versus biliary atresia

Feature	Neonatal hepatitis	Biliary atresia
Sex	Predominantly in males	Predominantly in females
Jaundice	Peak, moderate, mild	Mild, moderate, severe
Activity	Normal or slow	Normal
Hepatosplenomegaly	Early	Late
Liver function tests	Grossly abnormal (except alkaline phosphatase, which is only marginally high)	Slightly abnormal (except alkaline phosphatase which is considerably high)
Rose-Bengal test	Over 15%	Under 10%
Liver biopsy	Giant cells	Dilatation and hyperplasia of bile canaliculi
Cholangiogram	Normal	Reveals block
Australia antigen	May be positive	Negative

Liver biopsy should be done in each and every case. Important findings include bile duct and ductular proliferation, hypertrophic changes in hepatic artery branches, bile plugs in dilated ducts, fibrosis, inflammatory changes, and giant cell transformation.

In instances where no single test or battery of tests has conclusively differentiated the biliary atresia from neonatal hepatitis, you may resort to operative cholangiography before 8 weeks of age to demonstrate the patency or obliteration of bile ducts.

After First Week

Septicemia

- Neonatal hepatitis
- Extrahepatic biliary atresia
- Breast-milk jaundice.

Congenital or hereditary spherocytosis: Also called as congenital acholuric jaundice, this disease, occurring usually in people of North European origin, may occasionally present in neonatal period with jaundice and anemia. The spleen is enlarged in some cases. Rarely, hyperbilirubinemia may be severe enough to warrant exchange transfusion because of the serious risk of kernicterus. Investigations show reduced hemoglobin, reticulocytosis, erythroblastemia, increased fragility of red cells, microspherocytes, raised indirect serum bilirubin, and urobilinogenuria.

Drug-induced hemolytic anemia: This occurs in congenital deficiencies of the enzymes G6PD, glutathione, synthetase, reductase or peroxidase. The commonly encountered drugs in causing hemolytic anemia thereby icterus include overdose of vitamin K, sulfas or camphor.

Persistent Jaundice during First Month

- Intrauterine infections
- Neonatal hepatitis
- Extrahepatic biliary atresia
- Familial nonhemolytic jaundice

Inspissated bile syndrome: In this rare condition, persistent jaundice in association with considerable rise in direct as well as indirect serum bilirubin occurs in infants with hemolytic disease, particularly if they have had intrauterine or exchange transfusion. The jaundice regresses within a few weeks or months. No sequelae are left.

Congenital hypothyroidism: Unusual prolongation of the physiologic jaundice may be the earliest sign of cretinism. The cause is delayed maturation of the enzyme, glucuronyl transferase. The infant is considerably heavier at birth than normal newborns and may also have feeding difficulties, sluggishness, respiratory problems, somnolence, obstinate constipation, refractory anemia, cold and mottled skin, umbilical hernia, widely open fontanels, and edema of genitalia and extremities.

Radiology shows retardation in bone age. For instance, the lower femoral center, normally present at birth, is usually absent. T_3, T_4, and TSH (thyroid-stimulating hormone) assays are important to establish the diagnosis.

Galactosemia: In this rare autosomal recessive disorder, due to absence of the enzyme, galactose-l-phosphate-uridyltransferase, which is responsible for converting galactose to glucose, galactose accumulates in blood and tissues.

No sooner does the infant take milk than he develops manifestations which include, besides jaundice, poor feeding, vomiting, and failure to thrive. Hypoglycemic convulsions may occur. Hepatomegaly is usually present though development of splenomegaly takes some time. Pseudotumor cerebri may accompany the clinical picture.

Delay in absolute withdrawal of milk and its products may cause cataracts and mental retardation.

JAUNDICE IN LATER INFANCY AND CHILDHOOD

Viral Hepatitis

This is by and large the most common cause of jaundice in children beyond 1 year of age. Over and above jaundice, the child has anorexia, nausea, vomiting, abdominal discomfort, usually in the upper right and middle quadrant because of tender liver. Often, there is a fatty food intolerance.

Cirrhosis of Liver

A large number of diseases such as atresia of the bile duct, neonatal hepatitis that has failed to clear, cystic fibrosis, Wilson disease, galactosemia, glycogen-storage disease, syphilis, and schistosomiasis may cause cirrhosis. In India, over 90% cases of childhood cirrhosis are accounted by what has been designated as Indian childhood cirrhosis (ICC). Its counterpart in West Indies is known as Jamaican cirrhosis or veno-occlusive disease of the liver.

Indian childhood cirrhosis—a familial disease of unknown etiology (though contamination of feeds with copper appears to be the most likely cause), occurs predominantly in male children, 1–5 years of age, from middle-class families, usually having vegetarian dietary background.

The common form, insidious onset disease, is arbitrarily divided into three stages:
1. First stage consists of sheer vague manifestations. Liver is enlarged by 3–5 cm and has a firm feel with sharp, leafy border. Abdominal distension, anorexia or voracious appetite, lassitude, irritability, slight fever, constipation/

diarrhea with clay-colored, sticky, formed stools, and growth failure may be present.
2. Second stage is characterized by further exaggeration of the manifestations of the second stage. Liver size is increased and liver feels firmer now. Definite jaundice is evident. In addition, manifestations of portal hypertension dominate the picture. These include splenomegaly, ascites, hematemesis, anemia, prominent superficial abdominal venous network, and thrombocytopenia.
3. Third stage, the terminal phase, is characterized by apathy, emaciation, deep jaundice, protuberant abdomen with prominent superficial veins, and ascites. Liver is, as a rule, grossly enlarged but may be shrunk in an occasional case. Spleen is usually considerably enlarged and hard. In addition, there usually exist manifestations of hepatocellular failure. Restlessness and confusion may eventually pass on to frank hepatic in which case flopping tremors of the arms are observed. The child dies at this stage either from hepatocellular failure per se or intercurrent infections.

Total duration of illness varies between 6 months and 3 years.

In the relatively less common form, acute onset disease, the condition suddenly manifests with jaundice, fever, clay-colored stools, and hepatomegaly. All this may have rapid downhill course, the child may finally be dying in hepatic coma. Some cases become asymptomatic for a variable period and then again have reappearance of the manifestations which behave like ICC of insidious onset.

Toxic Hepatitis

Drugs and agents causing hepatitis and thus jaundice include ampicillin, cephalexin, chloramphenicol, cotrimoxazole, erythromycine stolate, ethambutol, kanamycin, nalidixic acid, neomycin, oleandomycin, sulfas, streptomycin, rifampicin, vincristine, acetazolamide, amitriptyline, vancomycin, tetracyclines, para-aminosalicylic acid (PAS), penicillin, phenacetin, paracetamol, anabolic steroids, amphetamine, testosterone, chloroquine, quinine, thiouracil, troxidone, carbamazepine, clonidine, ethionamide, ethosuximide, phenothiazines, diphenylhydantoin, novobiocin, ibuprofen, haloperidol, griseofulvin, lincomycin, methotrexate, nitrofurantoin, pyrazinamide, solvent sniffing.

Hemolysis

Jaundice resulting from hemolysis is characterized by normal-colored stools (not clay-colored) and normal urine (not high-colored).

Thalassemia major also called as Cooley's anemia or Mediterranean anemia, starts manifesting at about 3 months of age with progressive pallor, growth failure, jaundice of varying degree, and hepatosplenomegaly. Recurrent respiratory infections are common. Lymphadenopathy may be present. Physical retardation of growth may be accompanied by hypogonadism. Facial appearance is characteristic with frontal bossing, prominent maxilla (exposing the teeth), depressed bridge of nose, and malocclusion of teeth. The appearance is termed thalassemic or hemolytic facies. Increased pigmentation of skin due to high level or melanin in epithelium and hemosiderin in dermis may be observed.

Blood picture shows a microcytic–hypochromic anemia (usually hemoglobin between 4 g% and 9 g% range), anisocytosis, poikilocytosis, moderate basophilic stippling, nucleated and fragmented erythrocytes, target cells, large number of normoblasts and reticulocytosis.
- Bone marrow shows erythroid hyperplasia
- Osmotic fragility test reveals a reduced fragility
- Fetal hemoglobin measured by electrophoresis exceeds 40% of the total
- Radiologic picture is characteristic.

Sickle-cell anemia, relatively infrequent in most parts of India, is caused by the presence of all the body hemoglobin in the form of Hb-S. Slight jaundice invariably accompanies progressive anemia with fever, headache, arthritis, osteopathy of metacarpals and phalanges in particular, skin ulceration, nocturnal enuresis, growth retardation, and folic acid deficiency. Splenomegaly occurs in early years but, as the disease progresses, spleen shrinks the so-called autosplenectomy. Incidence of superadded bacterial infections and anesthetic complications is high. Hemolytic, vaso-occlusive and aplastic crises may occur.

Besides usual evidence of hemolysis in the blood picture, an added characteristic finding is the "sickle-shaped" red cells.

Electrophoretic pattern shows 50–100% hemoglobin as Hb-S and increased level of Hb-F.

Congenital or hereditary spherocytosis, also called as congenital acholuric jaundice, is uncommon in India. When it manifests in postnatal period, jaundice is slight. Anemia is, however, variable from family to family. Spleen is invariably enlarged. Incidence of aplastic crises is high. Pigmentary gallstones occur usually in later childhood or adolescence.

Besides evidence of hemolysis, one must demonstrate basic defect of the red cells by osmotic fragility studies.

Autoimmune hemolytic anemia, idiopathic or secondary to drugs such as penicillin, cephalosporins, phenacetin, quinidine, alpha-methyldopa, etc. lymphoma, systemic lupus erythematosus (SLE) or immunodeficiency, occur in two patterns.
1. Acute transient type, occurring usually in infants and young children, follows an infection with manifestations such as

pallor, jaundice, prostration, fever, and hemoglobinuria. Splenomegaly is present. Complete cure occurs following prolonged steroid therapy.
2. Chronic prolonged type is characterized by anemia and slight jaundice on top of a systemic disease. Hemolysis goes on and on for quite a few months or years. Response to steroids is not quite gratifying.

Investigations show considerable spherocytosis, polychromasia, remarkable reticulocytosis, leukocytosis and, occasionally thrombocytopenia. The association of autoimmune hemolytic anemia with warm antibodies and immune thrombocytopenic purpura is termed as Evans syndrome. Direct Coombs test is strongly positive. Free antibodies, active at 37°C (warm antibodies) and belonging to IgG class may be detected in some cases.

Autoimmune hemolytic anemia with cold antibodies may occur as cold agglutinin disease in association with viral infections, infectious mononucleosis or mycoplasma pneumonia, or paroxysmal cold hemoglobinuria often in association with syphilis. Jaundice and anemia are found universally in these subjects.

FURTHER READING

1. Bezerra JA, Balistreri WF. Cholestatic syndromes of infancy and childhood. *Semin Gastrointest Dis* 2001;12:54-65.
2. Green M. Jaundice. In: *Pediatric Diagnosis*, 6th edn. Philadelphia: Saunders 1998:260-267.
3. Hutington JE. *Pediatric Jaundice*. 3rd edn. London: Smith & Smith 2017.
4. Pan DH, Rivas Y. Jaundice. In: Adam HM, Foy JM (Eds). *Signs and Symptoms in Pediatrics*. Illinois: American Academy of Pediatrics 2015:581-596.
5. Rosenthal R, Sinatra F. Jaundice in infancy. *Pediatr Rev* 1989;11:79-86.

CHAPTER 40

Joint Pain

BACKGROUND

Joint pain is a common complaint in pediatric practice. It is encountered in approximately 10% of the children seen in the outpatients' wing. The incidence reached at in a study from South India is 6.5%, from Mumbai 11.2%, and from Kolkata 9%.

The terms, *arthritis* and *arthralgia*, need clarification. Arthritis denotes inflammation of a joint manifested by pain, heat, redness, and swelling. Arthralgia means simply pain in the joint, implying absence of inflammation. When we use the term arthralgia, the pointer is towards a definite pathological condition of the joint of some etiology. Whether it is a manifestation of local or systemic illness—obvious or yet to be determined—is altogether a different matter.

HISTORY

During symptomatic enquiry, ask if the pain is in a single joint or number of joints. If only one joint is involved, ask if there has been a history of trauma to the joint. Is the joint visibly swollen? Any limitation of movements? Any increase in pain on weight-bearing or movements? Any fever and other signs of toxemia suggesting local sepsis? Any history of bleeding disorder, say hemophilia? Any complaint of bleeding, spongy, gums, excessive irritability, and malnutrition (scurvy)?

In case of pain involving multiple joints, find out if the pain is simply arthralgia or arthritis. Is the joint involvement migratory (also termed as fleeting or flitting)? Whether the large weight-bearing or small joints are involved? Any fever or other systemic manifestations? Any preceding history of sore throat? Any suggestions of septicemia or some such illness? Any history of drug misuse? Is the patient a known case of sickle-cell anemia, ulcerative colitis, Henoch-Schönlein purpura, etc.?

PHYSICAL EXAMINATION

Physical examination must seek to clarify if the problem is arthritis or arthralgia, the specific joint(s) involved, status of the cardiovascular system (any carditis with or without congestive cardiac failure?), signs pertaining to skin and muscles, organomegaly, etc.

INVESTIGATIONS

- Complete blood picture, including erythrocyte sedimentation rate (ESR)
- C-reactive protein (CRP)
- Antistreptolysin O (ASO) titer
- Electrocardiogram (ECG)
- Echocardiography
- Rheumatoid factor
- Antinuclear antibodies
- Lupus erythematosus (LE) phenomenon
- Rose–Waaler test
- Synovial fluid
- Synovial biopsy
- Plain-film radiographs.

IMPORTANT DIFFERENTIALS

Trauma

As and when pain is confined to a single joint and there is deformity, swelling, discoloration, restricted mobility, hike in pain on movement or weight-bearing, effusion or hematoma, particularly without general symptoms, you must suspect trauma. The trauma may have caused hemarthrosis, effusion, strained ligaments, sprained muscles, dislocation or fracture.

Pulled elbow or traumatic subluxation of the radial head (nursemaid's elbow, Chassaignac's paralysis), occurring quite commonly in children in 1–4 years age group, results from sudden forceful jerk applied by a parent or a teacher while the child is held by the arm. This causes a tear of annular ligament at its attachment to radius. The ligament gets squeezed in between the radius and the capitellum. The result of this subluxation is that the arm is held in a position of slight flexion at the elbow and pronation at the forearm. The child refuses to move the arm, giving a superficial impression of paralysis. The condition is quite painful.

Septic Arthritis

Septic arthritis is also called as suppurative arthritis, the condition occurs most frequently in first year of life following skin or upper respiratory infection. The most common etiologic organism is *Staphylococcus*, irrespective of the age group. The other bacteria include *Haemophilus influenzae* (type B), *Streptococcus, Pneumococcus, Meningococcus, Gram-negative enteric bacteria* such as *Salmonella, Yersinia, Brucella*, etc. In sexually active adolescents, gonococcal arthritis may occur. Large joints are usually involved.

Clinical picture is characterized by sudden onset of fever and other systemic manifestations together with painful, tender local swelling. The local temperature is raised and there is erythema. Mobility of the joint is considerably limited. More often the joint involved is a large one. Limp may be the first and often the only presenting feature initially in some instances.

The joint fluid obtained by arthrocentesis is, as a rule, purulent, showing remarkable rise in white blood cell (WBC), reduced glucose, and positive Gram-stain.

Cultures of joint fluid as well as blood are strongly recommended for confirming the diagnosis.

Viral Arthritis

Arthritis accompanying viral infections (mumps, rubella, chickenpox, influenza, hepatitis B, infectious mononucleosis, etc.), occurring usually in 1–4 years age group, affects more or less large joints. Basically, it is a sort of monoarticular synovitis. Often there is a confusion in its differential diagnosis from arthritis of acute rheumatic fever. Remember that, typically, viral arthritis, runs a mild course of around a week, recurrence is a rarity in its case, and rheumatoid factors remain negative.

Tuberculous Arthritis

The joints that may be involved in tuberculosis include wrist joint, hip joint, knee joint, ankle joint, and spine.

In tuberculosis of the wrist joint, the characteristic picture includes appearance of a doughy swelling over the dorsum, a puffy palmar surface, slightly flexed hands with restricted movements of the fingers, and, later, appearance of sinuses usually over the dorsal aspect.

Tuberculosis of the hip is by far the most common form of tuberculous arthritis. The frank joint involvement follows the initial lesion in the femoral epiphysis, greater trochanter or, infrequently, synovial membrane. The earliest symptom is an intermittent slight limp with pain which is usually referred to the knee or medial aspect of thigh. In due course of time, the thigh is flexed, adducted, and medially rotated. Movements become restricted in all directions. An obvious swelling appears, showing gradual increase in size. An abscess may discharge anteriorly or in other directions.

Tuberculosis of the knee is rather infrequent and is more of a sort of synovitis than involvement of the bone. Besides general features of tuberculosis, including muscular wasting, there appears a white swelling (skin continues to be white and puffy) with local heat and tenderness. With progression of the disease process, the joint is deformed in the so-called "triple displacement" position (flexion, posterior subluxation, and lateral rotation of tibia) due to spasm of the hamstring muscles.

Tuberculosis of the ankle is predominant involvement of the synovial membrane rather than the bone. It is characterized by a swelling around the malleoli, pain, wasting of calf muscles, impaired joint movements, and the joint kept in a position of plantar-flexion to avoid weight-bearing. Later, abscess formation may manifest in the form of sinuses.

Tuberculosis of the spine, also called as Pott spine, is characterized by local and referred pain according to the affected nerve root, rigidity resulting in all movements and deformity. The patient, usually a grown-up child or adolescent, may avoid bending to catch hold of something on the floor. He may walk unduly carefully on toes, keeping the body quite stiff. Often, the subject likes lying on his abdomen or in the mother's lap. In case of cervical involvement, the child has torticollis and he supports his head by his hand or holds stiffly. Thoracic involvement causes kyphosis with gibbus with or without scoliosis. Cervical and upper thoracic involvement is likely to cause paraplegia. A cold abscess may extend to cause retropharyngeal abscess, rupture into the pleura, penetrate to the scapula, gravitate to point above the Poupart ligament, or result in a psoas abscess.

Needless to say, in each and every case of suspected tuberculous arthritis, the diagnosis should be established by conducting investigations such as tuberculin (Mantoux)/BCG diagnostic test, gastric lavage/sputum for acid-fast bacilli (AFB), and X-ray of chest as well as X-ray of the affected part(s).

Osteomyelitis Close to the Joint

Osteomyelitis quite near a joint may give an impression of a swelling involving the joint per se. This may well be confused with septic arthritis. Unlike the case in osteomyelitis, it is virtually impossible to mobilize the joint in septic arthritis without causing considerable pain. Secondly, septic arthritis may be differentiated from osteomyelitis by aspiration of the joint.

Rheumatic Fever

The joint pains of rheumatic fever may be in the form of polyarthritis or just arthralgia.

The polyarthritis, typically tends to be flitting and is manifested by pain and limitation of active movements or by tenderness, redness or swelling of two or more joints, usually the large and most distal and most proximal ones. The other major criteria (Jones-revised) are carditis, chorea, subcutaneous nodules (Figs. 40.1A to C), and erythema marginatum.

Arthralgia alone without objective evidence of joint involvement is not a major manifestation of rheumatic fever. It is a minor criterion, the other minor criteria being fever, previous rheumatic fever or rheumatic heart disease, raised ESR, leukocytosis or presence of CRP, and prolonged P-R interval in the ECG.

All this may be additionally reinforced by supporting evidence of preceding streptococcal infection: history of sore throat or scarlet fever, positive throat culture for group A streptococci, increased ASO titer or other streptococcal antibodies.

The presence of two major criteria or one major and two minor criteria is essential for labeling a case as rheumatic fever.

These criteria, in practice, serve well to minimize the chances of overdiagnosis and underdiagnosis. Nevertheless, an occasional case of rheumatic fever may not satisfy these diagnostic criteria. Likewise, at times, a child suffering from fever accompanied by pains in the extremities of some other etiology may satisfy the criteria. The point the author emphasizes and re-emphasizes is that the Jones criteria must only be regarded as a "guideline". These are, by no means, a substitute for the clinician's valued overall evaluation based on wisdom and judgment.

Juvenile Idiopathic Arthritis

In this collagen disorder, usually having its onset at 2–5 years and occurring more often in girls than in boys, the arthritis involves both small and large joints, including fingers and toes (proximal interphalangeal joints), wrist, temporomandibular joints, ankles, knees, hips, and cervical spine. Joints are little swollen, tender, and warm. Their mobility is reduced and they are kept in flexed position. A single joint may be involved (monoarticular or pauciarticular form) in which case it is most likely ankle or knee, or several joints may be involved (polyarticular form) (Fig. 40.2). In due course (1–3 months), contractures may occur. A noteworthy development is the spindle-shaped

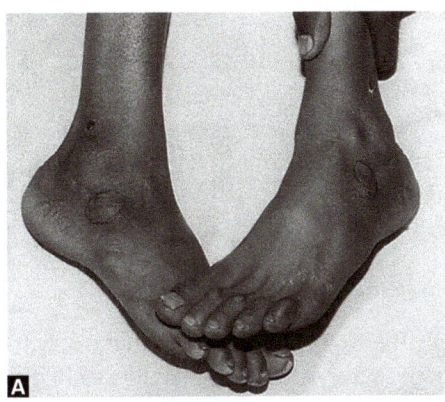
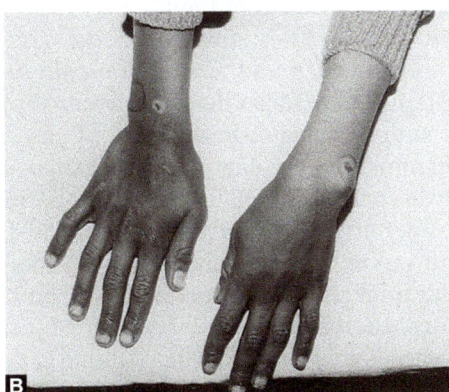
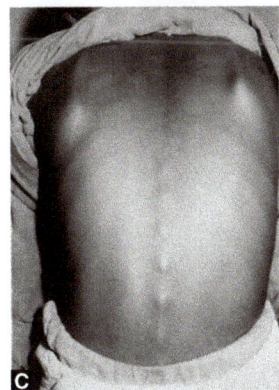

Figs. 40.1A to C: Rheumatic fever—(A and B) Note the subcutaneous firm nodules, about 1 cm in diameter along the extensor surfaces of tendons close to bony prominences and (C) overspinous process of lumbar vertebrae.

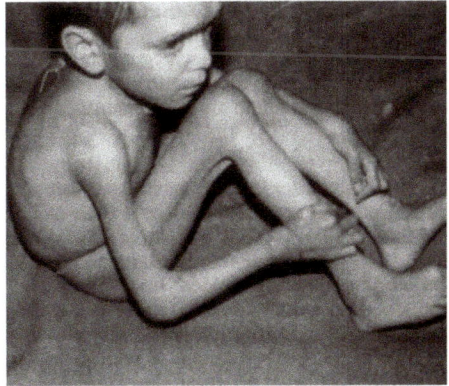

Fig. 40.2: Juvenile rheumatic arthritis (polyarticular)—Note the involvement of several joints (both small and large) with contractures and spindle-shaped fingers and muscle wasting around the affected joints.

fingers with smooth, shiny overlying skin. Early morning stiffness and wasting of muscles around the affected joint are classical.

The accompanying manifestations include prolonged fever (in approximately 10% cases it may precede by several weeks) with a morbilliform transitory rash (mainly over the trunk), muscle aches, weight loss, subcutaneous nodules, hepatosplenomegaly, lymphadenopathy, iridocyclitis, pericarditis, myocarditis, pneumonia, and pleurisy.

Erythrocyte sedimentation rate, if raised, is seldom over 40 mm (first hour) unlike in rheumatic fever. ASO titer is usually negative. CRP is, as a rule, absent.

Systemic Lupus Erythematosus

Joint pain (usually just arthralgia) is a common manifestation of this multisystem collagen disorder. The accompanying manifestations include prolonged irregular fever with remissions of variable duration, muscle pains, malaise, weight loss, and a characteristic erythematous rash over malar area and bridge of the nose (butterfly rash) which appears to be photosensitive (Fig. 40.3). The rash, at times, appears on fingers and palms, soles, palate, and buccal mucosa. Alopecia may also occur.

The disease does not spare any organ, renal involvement being particularly very common in childhood form. Hepatosplenomegaly, generalized lymphadenopathy, thrombocytopenia, neurologic manifestations (including pseudotumor cerebri), pericarditis, pleural effusion, pulmonary infiltration, abdominal pain, vomiting, and diarrhea may occur.

Diagnosis is confirmed by demonstrating typical lupus erythematosus (LE) cell and antinuclear antibodies (ANA), the latter being more sensitive.

Serum Sickness

Arthralgia and/or arthritis is an important manifestation of serum sickness, a systemic immunologic disorder characterized by allergic reaction following the administration of a foreign antigenic material a week or two earlier. The examples of etiologic antigenic material include penicillin, human gamma globulin for diphtheria and tetanus, antitoxins for treatment of rabies, and antilymphocyte serum employed for immunosuppression in transplantation procedures.

The most frequent manifestation is generalized urticaria. The other manifestations include intense pruritus, edema (especially around face and neck), fever, lymphadenopathy, myalgia, and arthralgia and/or arthritis involving multiple joints.

The reaction is self-limited. The patient may suffer from complications such as Guillain-Barré syndrome, peripheral neuritis involving C, and C components of brachial plexus, carditis and nephritis.

Henoch–Schönlein Purpura

Arthritis is encountered in over 60% cases of this syndrome, also termed as anaphylactoid purpura. The involved joints—usually large ones like knees and ankles—are swollen, tender, and painful on passive movements. If effusion is present, which usually is the case, the joint fluid is serous with leukocytosis.

The remaining manifestations of this disease of unknown etiology [preceding upper respiratory tract infection (URI), allergy or drug sensitivity is often blamed as playing a role] include a variety of skin lesions (usually urticaria, petechiae, purpura or ecchymosis) appearing in crops, colicky abdominal pain and azotemia, oliguria, and hypertension.

Quite often, arthritis and purpura may be the only presenting features. This form of disease has excellent prognosis, recovery occurring in a few days. Recurrences are a feature of serious cases.

Investigations are essentially normal. Their importance lies in excluding hemorrhagic diathesis, etc.

Hemarthrosis

In hemophilia, an X-linked recessive disorder due to deficiency of factor 8 (antihemophilic factor) occurring exclusively in males, a minor trauma may cause bleeding into a joint such as knee, ankle or elbow. The affected joint becomes swollen and tender with pain on passive movements. In earlier stages the blood within the joint gets absorbed in due course. Repeated attacks may, however, cause inflammation and degenerative changes, the joint eventually becoming immobile, the so-called "fixed joint".

Radiology shows initially distention of the joint cavity and synovitis. Later, the changes include areas of synovial thickening, demineralization, erosion, and contracture. Increased vascularization of joint space results in accelerated bone growth, resulting in premature appearance of ossification centers. A complete destruction of articular surface and formation of juxta-articular cysts may also occur.

To confirm the diagnosis of hemophilia, a normal bleeding time and a prolonged clotting time together with deficiency of factor 8 in specific factor assay need to be demonstrated.

Sickle Cell Anemia

Joint pains resulting from vaso-occlusive crises are a common observation in this disease characterized by severe, chronic hemolytic anemia due to replacement of the normal hemoglobin with hemoglobin S. The initial manifestation in infancy is in the form of so-called hand-foot syndrome in which sickle-cell dactylitis leads to symmetrical, painful swelling of the hands and feet. In older subjects, large joints and surrounding parts become involved. The modus operandi for causing bone and joint changes is through infarction which may develop spontaneously or is precipitated by infection.

The remaining manifestations include progressive anemia with slight icterus, fever, headache, ulceration of the skin overlying the lower limbs, nocturnal enuresis, growth retardation, and folic acid deficiency. Spleen is enlarged in the very young but undergoes regression as also cessation of functioning following recurrent thrombosis in the subsequent years. This is termed as "autosplenectomy".

Diagnosis is established by electrophoresis which shows that 50-100% of hemoglobin is S and that proportion of hemoglobin F is increased.

Acute Leukemia

Arthralgia may occasionally be the first complaint leading to the diagnosis of acute leukemia, particularly in the presence of anemia, reticulocytopenia/absence of reticulocytes, or thrombocytopenia.

The author has noticed a couple of cases presenting as rheumatic fever with joint pains migrating from one joint to another and high ASO titer turning out to be those of acute lymphoblastic leukemia (ALL) on bone marrow examination.

Psoriasis

Arthritis is seen infrequently in this uncommon condition in childhood, occurring predominantly in girls. Arthritis may precede or follow the skin lesions which consists of erythematous papules. The papules tend to coalesce and form plaques with sharply demarcated but irregular margins. Finally silvery scales develop which leave pinpoint bleeding on removal. Nail involvement is frequent. The common sites for skin lesions are scalp, knees, elbows, umbilicus, and genitalia.

Psoriatic arthritis may begin in one or more joints. The involvement is usually asymmetrical. Distal interphalangeal joints (unlike the proximal interphalangeal joints in rheumatoid arthritis) are involved in over 50% of the cases. In a few cases, sacroiliitis and subsequently losing spondylitis may occur.

Gut Arthropathy

Arthritis may occur in a significant proportion of the children suffering from inflammatory bowel disease (say ulcerative colitis, Crohn's disease), affecting a few large peripheral joints in a pauciarticular way. In the usual variety, arthritis varies in intensity with activity of the underlying bowel disease. Joint destruction and permanent deformity do not occur. In the uncommon variety, ankylosing spondylitis may cause permanent deformity and disability, even though the underlying bowel disease is under control.

Arthritis may also occur in cystic fibrosis of pancreas.

Reiter Disease

Arthritis, sterile urethritis, and ocular inflammation constitute the triad of symptom-complex of Reiter disease which is strongly associated with HLA B27 and may follow infections with *Yersinia enterocolitica*, *Shigella* or *Chlamydia*, or a sexual exposure in adolescents.

The accompanying manifestations may include varied types of skin rash and gastroenteritis.

Reactive Arthritis

A sterile arthritis may follow gut infection such as with *Yersinia enterocolitica*, *Shigella* or *Salmonella*. Only a few peripheral joints in a pauciarticular fashion are involved. In a small proportion of the cases, the disorder is associated with HLA B27.

The prognosis is good. Most cases have only transient disease. In some, chronic spondyloarthropathy may result.

Ankylosing Spondylitis

This disease of young and middle-aged adults may begin in childhood, usually in boys over 8 years of age. Manifestations include stiffness and pain in the low back, hips, and thighs with or without arthritis of peripheral joints. Heel pain is a common observation. The joints are swollen, warm, and tender.

Accompanying manifestations may include low-grade fever, easy fatigability, loss of appetite, and growth retardation. Iridocyclitis occurs in 25% cases at some stage.

Frequently, there is a positive family history for such arthritis or acute iridocyclitis.

Ankylosing spondylitis is often confused with pauciarticular juvenile rheumatoid arthritis. The points that favor the former include—(1) predilection for males, (2) positive family history, (3) characteristic involvement of hip and dorsolumbar joints, (4) high incidence of iridocyclitis, (5) rarity of rheumatoid factor, (6) extreme rarity of subcutaneous nodules, and (7) occurrence, though extremely rarely, of aortitis, resulting in aortic insufficiency.

Drugs

Phenobarbital, carbamazepine, isoniazid, rifampicin, ethambutol, chlordiazepoxide, cimetidine, penicillin, corticosteroid withdrawal after prolonged administration, animal sera, say tetanus or diphtheria antitoxin.

Remaining Causes of Joint Pain

Attention-seeking device, juvenile gout (both primary and secondary), foreign body ("rose-thorn arthritis"), dermatomyositis, scleroderma, periarteritis nodosa, sarcoidosis, brucellosis, syphilis, rubella, infectious mononucleosis, tumors, etc.

FURTHER READING

1. Ayoub EM, Majeed HA. Poststreptococcal reactive arthritis. *Curr Opin Rheumatol* 2000;12:306-310.
2. Miller ML. Evaluation of suspected rheumatic disease. In: Kliegman RM, St Geme III JW, Blum NJ, at al (Eds). *Nelson Textbook of Pediatrics*, 21st edn. Philadelphia: Elsevier 2020:995-997.
3. Olson JC. Juvenile idiopathic arthritis: An update. *Wisc Med J* 2003;102:45-50.
4. Petty RE, Tingle AJ. Arthritis and viral infection. *J Pediatr* 1988;113:948-949.
5. Ravelli A, Martini A. Juvenile idiopathic arthritis. *Lancet* 2007;369:767-778.
6. Siegel DM, Marston B. Joint pain. In: Adam HM, Foy JM (Eds). Signs and Symptoms in Pediatrics. Illinois: American Academy of Pediatrics 2015:597-606.

CHAPTER 41

Large Head

BACKGROUND

Large head is not an uncommon complaint put forward by the parents in our busy outpatients' wings. Often, parents, are unaware of it and somewhat surprised when the doctor questions them about it. On 3 very busy outpatient department (OPD) days in a week, at least 8 out of the 200 and odd patients were noticed with unduly large head. The breakup of these eight cases according to the clinical diagnosis was as follows—two with congenital hydrocephalus (1 progressive, 1 arrested), one with acquired hydrocephalus (postmeningitic), two with vitamin D-deficiency rickets, one with space-occupying lesion (SOL), one with achondroplasia, and one familial.

The term, *macrocephaly*, refers to a head circumference that is more than 2 SD above the mean for age, sex, and gestation. Severe macrocephaly means the head circumference is more than 3 SD of the mean. Box 41.1 lists the important causes of macrocephaly.

BOX 41.1: Important causes of macrocephaly.

- Megalencephaly
  - *Familial:* A benign condition with normal body size and neurodevelopment
  - *Syndrome-associated:* Neurocutaneous syndromes (Von-Recklinghausen, tuberous sclerosis, Sturge-Weber syndrome), fragile X syndrome, Sotos syndrome (cerebral gigantism), GM2 gangliosidosis (Tay-Sachs disease, Sandhoff disease)
  - *Leukodystrophies:* Megalencephalic leukoencephalopathy
  - *Lysosomal storage diseases:* Gangliosidosis (Tay-Sachs disease), mucopolysaccharidosis, gangliosidosis
  - *Raised intracranial pressure (ICP):* Hydrocephalus, hypovitaminosis/hypervitaminosis A, pseudotumor cerebri, galactosemia, lead toxicity
  - *Enlarged vascular compartment:* Arteriovenous (A-V) malformation, intracerebral hemorrhage (ICH) (intraventricular, subdural, epidural, subarachnoid, etc.)
  - *Intravascular:* Bleeding into subdural, epidural, subarachnoid, and intraventricular spaces
  - *Diseases related to bony compartment:* Rickets, osteogenesis imperfecta, achondroplasia, osteopetrosis, cleidocranial dysostosis, hyperphosphatasia
  - *Bone marrow expansion:* Thalassemia major
  - *Intracranial space-occupying lesions (ICSOL):* Tumor, abscess, cyst, etc.

HISTORY

While eliciting history in a case of large head, find out if the size has been large right since birth or it occurred later. Is it still fast increasing? Or, is it arrested now? Did it follow a central nervous system (CNS) illness, say meningitis? Any history of seizures, projectile vomiting, persistent headache, behavior problems, etc.? Any congenital defect, such as talipes or meningocele, the parents are aware of? Any familial tendency to have a large head?

PHYSICAL EXAMINATION

Physical examination should, in the first instance, confirm if the head size is indeed unusually large in relation to the body size, weight, and age. At times, head enlargement may be more apparent than real as in intrauterine growth restriction/retardation (IUGR) infants. Serial measurements may be required in doubtful cases. Just because the size is rapidly increasing it is of no reason to label the observation as hydrocephalus. In infants, we do expect a rapid increase (Box 41.2). What is really important is that this increase is

BOX 41.2: Causes of large head due to hydrocephalus.

- Noncommunicating (obstructive)
  - Aqueduct stenosis/atresia
    - Sporadic
    - Familial
  - Fourth ventricle obstruction
    - Dandy-Walker anomaly
    - Arachnoiditis
  - Obstruction from mass lesion
    - Neoplasm
    - Cyst
    - Hematoma
    - Aneurysmal enlargement of vein of Galen*
    - Aneurysm
- Communicating
  - Arnold-Chiari (AC) malformation
  - Encephalitis
  - Meningeal adhesions
  - Choroid plexus papilloma.

*Vein of Galen, named after the Greek physician Galen, is the other sementic for great cerebral vein. It is a short trunk formed by the union of two internal cerebral veins and the basal veins of Rosenthal.

quite out of proportion to the corresponding increase in the body size.

Note the shape of the head. A large protruding occiput points to Dandy-Walker cyst. An asymmetrical head is typical of unilateral obstruction at the level of foramen of Monro.

Transillumination shows the whole calvarium as "brilliant" if cerebral matter is absent or is extremely thinned down. Focal or generalized areas of abnormal transparency may be seen in porencephalic or other cysts and subdural effusion.

A complete neurologic examination is a must, particularly for signs of meningeal irritation. Is the anterior fontanel bulging? Are the sutures widely separated? Is there any meningocele, meningomyelocele or talipes equinovarus? What are the body measurements like? Any suggestion of rickets, achondroplasia, gigantism, etc.?

INVESTIGATIONS

A skull X-ray, computed tomography (CT) scan, ultrasound (US), or magnetic resonance imaging (MRI) are helpful depending on the merit of the case.

IMPORTANT DIFFERENTIALS

Hydrocephalus

Congenital hydrocephalus, a common cause of unusually large head right at birth or becoming apparent in the first few months of life, may be associated with Arnold-Chiari malformation in which case the infant also has spina bifida and meningomyelocele (Fig. 41.1), Dandy-Walker anomaly (Figs. 41.2A and B), malformation or stenotic lesions of aqueduct cerebri, or malformations of arachnoid villi.

Clinical picture is classical with a large head, wide and bulging anterior fontanel, open sutures, protruding forehead, and dilated prominent scalp veins (Fig. 41.3). The sunset sign, i.e. visible sclera above the iris, is characteristic. The crackpot sign, also called Macewen sign, elicited by percussing the skull, may be positive. Transillumination is positive. The mental faculty and other neurological manifestations vary with the causative and associated factor(s).

Arrested hydrocephalus is the term applied when there is no further progression in head size (Fig. 41.4).

Acquired hydrocephalus, another common cause of unusually large head before the suture closure has

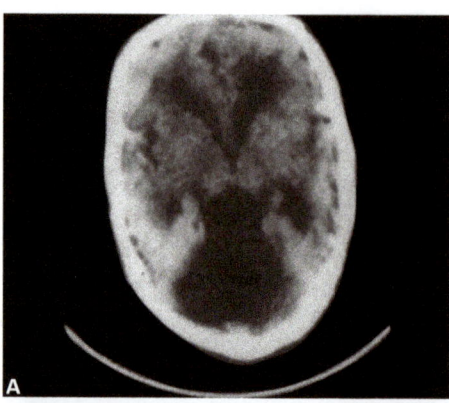
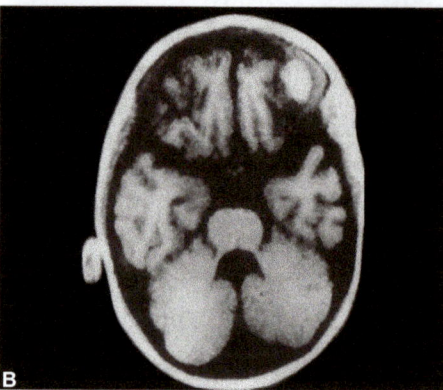

Figs. 41.2A and B: Computed tomography scan showing Dandy-Walker cyst consisting of a cystic expansion of the fourth ventricle in the posterior fossa. The patient usually presents with rapidly increasing hydrocephalus with prominent occiput and evidence of long-tract signs, cerebellar ataxia, and delayed developmental and motor as well as cognitive milestones.

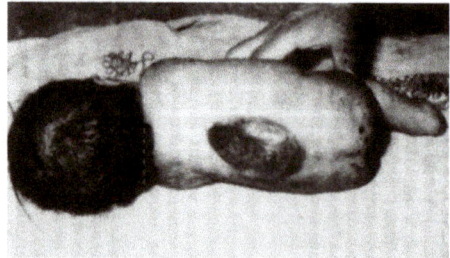

Fig. 41.1: *Meningomyelocele* in association with Arnold-Chiari malformation causing hydrocephalus.

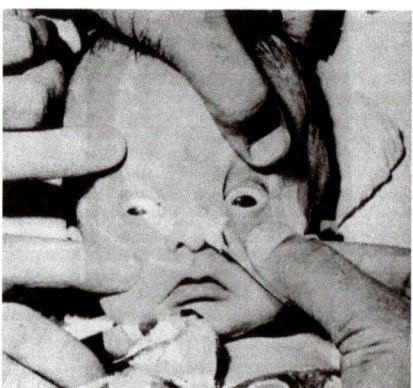

Fig. 41.3: *Congenital hydrocephalus*—Also note the presence of microphthalmia, more marked on right side, as also corneal opacities.

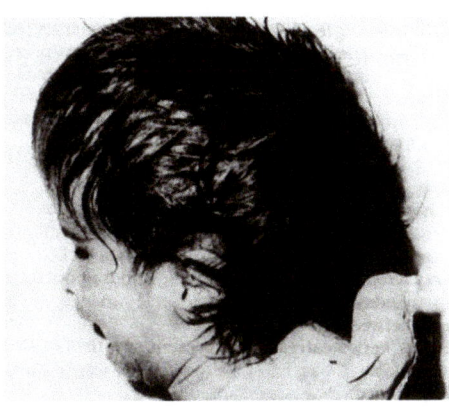

Fig. 41.4: *Arrested hydrocephalus*-The child presented in second stage of tuberculous meningitis. Response to treatment was good.

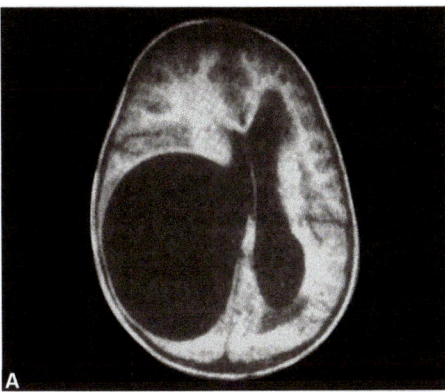
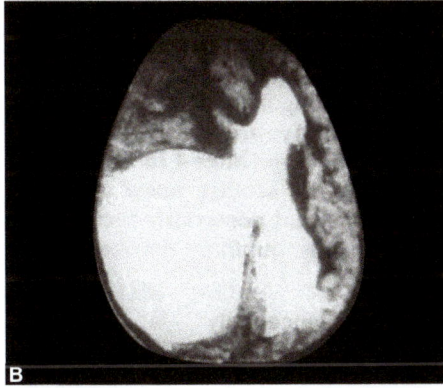

Figs. 41.5A and B: Magnetic resonance imaging (MRI), T1 and T2 weighted axial images, showing a large spherical cystic mass in the right parietotemporal region (hydatid cyst) causing hydrocephalus (acquired). Note the compression and midline shift of the right lateral ventricle and third ventricle.

occurred, may result from inflammatory disorders like meningitis and encephalitis, birth trauma, head injury, intracranial hemorrhage, and space-occupying lesions like tuberculoma, subdural hematoma/abscess, hydatid cyst (Figs. 41.5A and B) or glioma.

Clinical features are those of the raised intracranial pressure described earlier plus those related to the etiologic condition.

Vitamin D Deficiency: Rickets

Macrocephaly with flattening of vertex (box head) may well be associated with nutritional rickets. Accompanying signs in relation to head include frontal and parietal bossing, delayed closure of fontanels, craniotabes [a peculiar softening of occipital and posterior parietal bones which "give in" like a ping-pong (table tennis) ball under pressure from thumb].

The remaining features of rickets include rachitic rosary, pigeon-chest deformity, Harrison's sulcus (a groove along the insertion of diaphragm into the ribs), flaring of lower ribs, widening of wrists, knock knee (genu valgum), bow legs (genu varum), poor muscle tone, potbelly, visceroptosis, and delayed dentition and milestones.

Diagnostic investigations show raised alkaline phosphatase (except in malnourished children), low serum phosphorus, and normal serum calcium. Reduction in serum 25-hydroxy-vitamin D level is a sensitive and reliable index of rickets even in malnourished children.

X-ray of wrist shows cupping, fraying, and fragmentation of the lower ends of radius and ulna. There is an increase in the distance between the epiphyseal centers and the shafts of the long bones. Periosteal reaction is present, so is the prominence of trabeculae.

Cerebral Gigantism (Sotos Syndrome)

Macrocrania is an important feature of this rare disorder characterized by rapid growth, not because of raised growth hormones level but as a result of pathologic cerebral defect.

Accompanying features include birth weight and length above 90th percentile, jumping to over 97th percentile by 1-year of age, prominent forehead, acromegalic facies, large hands and feet, clumsiness, mental subnormality and antimongoloid slant of the eyes.

Remember that excessive growth does not continue throughout life. It stops after 4–5 years of age.

X-ray studies show a large skull, a high orbital roof, somewhat posteriorly inclined sella turcica, and an increased interpupillary distance (hypertelorism).

Megalencephaly

Unusually large head in this rare disorder results from excessive growth of brain during infancy. There is delay in the developmental milestones. There is no evidence of raised intracranial pressure.

Excessive growth of brain occurs in achondroplasia, Hurler's syndrome, Tay–Sachs disease, and metachromatic leukodystrophy.

Hydrancephaly

In this rare condition, there is congenital absence of cerebral hemispheres. Instead, there is a huge fluid-filled cavity. Brainstem and basal ganglia are well formed.

At birth, the infant appears normal except for the increased head size and lack of visual following. He demonstrates no further voluntary motor and mental development. Convulsions may occur.

Diagnosis is made by transillumination of the skull in a darkened room.

Gangliosidosis

Tay–Sachs disease, also called as infantile cerebromacular degeneration, is the most common of the five recognized illnesses under this heading. It is characterized by mental apathy, progressive loss of acquired motor functions, exaggerated startle response, spasticity with hyperreflexia, decerebrate rigidity, poor feeding, wasting, and abnormally large head. Convulsions (grand mal, tonic or myoclonic) may occur. The most glaring finding is a cherry-red spot of macula bright red area in the region of fovea surrounded by a grayish-white rim.

FURTHER READING

1. Chheda D, Hajiani N, Deep A. Approach to a child with large head. In: Gupte S (Ed). *Recent Advances in Pediatrics (Special Vol 18: Pediatric Neurology)*. New Delhi: Jaypee 2008:94-101.
2. Fenichel JM. *Clinical Pediatric Neurology: A Signs and Symptoms Approach*. Philadelphia: Saunders 2001:353-370.
3. Purugganam OH. Macrocephaly. In: Adam HM, Foy JM (Eds). *Signs and Symptoms in Pediatrics*. Illinois: American Academy of Pediatrics 2015:649-656.

CHAPTER 42

Limping

BACKGROUND

The term, *limping*, means to walk lamely or unevenly as when one hip, leg or foot is stiff or hurt. Though majority of the cases of limp in pediatric practice are minor and transient, the problem often causes considerable anxiety to the parents as long as it continues to trouble the child.

This common problem may be caused by a lesion (as minor as trauma from a protruding nail in the shoe, or as serious as paresis) anywhere in the weight-bearing structure-complex consisting chiefly of spine, hips, knees, ankles, and feet. Often the lesion may be inapparent. Infrequently, the complaint may be projected as an attention-seeking device. Whereas a painful (antalgic) limping is usually secondary to injury, infection or pathologic fracture, Trendelenburg limping is predominantly due to congenital, developmental or neuromuscular/musculoskeletal disorder [polio, cerebral: Palsy, myopathy, developmental dysplasia of the hip (DDH)]. Earlier termed congenital dislocation of the hip.

HISTORY

A thorough history and physical examination are central to early identification of the cause of limp.

While recording history, you must put considerable efforts to elicit the particular activity that may have caused limp. Was there a trauma: a fall, a pull, or a blow? Any preceding or accompanying fever? Any joint pain? Is the limp on way to recovery, going downhill or showing no change? Is the child aware of any problem with the shoes? Does the shoe pinch or it has a nail or strap buckle that troubles the child? Is the child suffering from some myopathy, tuberculosis, congenital defect, etc.?

PHYSICAL EXAMINATION

Physical examination must include observation of the child, while he limps, by the physician. Attempt should be made to determine its cause in the spine, hip, knee, ankle, feet,

BOX 42.1: Grading of muscle power.

Grade 0: No contraction at all
Grade 1: Just trace contraction (flicker)
Grade 2: Active movements (gravity eliminated)
Grade 3: Active movements (against gravity)
Grade 4: Active movements (against gravity and some resistance)
Grade 5: Active movements (against full resistance).

bones or soft tissues. Do not forget to look for asymmetry in the size of the legs. Is there any inguinal lymphadenitis? Is there any painful boil? You must also examine shoes for undue tightness, a protruding nail, or a bad buckle. Does the foot show any corn, wart, blisters, paronychia, or ingrowing toenail?

A good musculoskeletal examination, including grading of muscle power, is important. Box 42.1 gives the popular system of grading the muscle power.

INVESTIGATIONS

Based on the most probable diagnoses suggested by the history and physical examination, the appropriate use of laboratory tests and imaging studies can help confirm the diagnosis.
- Radiology of the suspected joint: Plain X-ray film, ultrasound, computed tomography (CT) scan, bone scan, etc.
- Arthrocentesis in septic arthritis
- Erythrocyte sedimentation rate (ESR), C-reactive protein, etc.
- Creatinine phosphokinase (CPK)
- Muscle biopsy.

IMPORTANT DIFFERENTIALS

Joints or Bones

Hips

Developmental dysplasia of the hip: A missed and untreated congenital dislocation of the hip may be responsible for a limp and delayed walking. A close examination of such a child shows asymmetry of the thigh, gluteal and knee creases, inability to abduct the hip fully, shortness of the affected leg, reduced spontaneous movements, and a bulge of the femoral head.

A good screening test (Ortolani sign) consists in abducting the hip passively. A clicking sound is heard from the hip at the end of the maneuver. It results from the jerking of the subluxated head as it reduces back into the acetabulum.

The Barlow maneuver is better than Ortolani maneuver. Here, the pelvis is stabilized with one hand, followed by adduction of the opposite hip and application of a posterior force. A dislocatable hip is readily appreciated.

Diagnosis is confirmed by X-ray of the hip joint and/or ultrasonography. An anteroposterior X-ray view usually reveals superior and lateral displacements of the femoral head from the shallow acetabulum.

Congenital coxa vara: In this disorder of unknown etiology, usually encountered after 2–3 years of age, physical findings simulate a dislocated hip. The basic defect is that the femoral neck makes less than 135° angle with the shaft. Left unattended, varus deformity shows worsening.

Septic arthritis: Suppuration is the most important cause of painful hip and limp in infants and toddlers. Involvement of hip may be direct extension of osteomyelitis of the femoral neck or a blood-borne infection.

For confirmation of the diagnosis, X-ray of hip, showing lateral displacement of the femoral head as also the fat close to the capsule due to fluid accumulation, is of considerable value. Aspiration of thick pus from the joint further establishes the diagnosis. If osteomyelitis coexists, increased bone uptake is demonstrated by a bone scan.

Toxic or transient synovitis: This disorder of toddlers and children may be responsible for painful hip and limp which responds to as simple a treatment as bed rest. The cause is not clear. Frequently, it is preceded by a viral upper respiratory infection a few days to 2 weeks earlier. All signs of inflammation of the joint are observed. The bacterial infection is, however, not responsible for the condition.

Tuberculosis of the hip: An intermittent slight limp with pain, occurring when the subject first gets out of bed and after exercise, is usually the first manifestation of tuberculosis of the hip. Pain is usually referred to the knee or medial aspect of the thigh. Limp and pain may show remission for days or weeks. With progressive destruction of the joint following absorption of the femoral head and neck, the thigh assumes a position of flexion, adduction, and medial (earlier it is lateral) rotation.

Perthes disease: Also termed as Legg-Calve-Perthes disease, this condition of a vascular necrosis of the head of the femur usually occurs in 5–9 years age group and is an important cause of pain and limp. It may be very difficult to differentiate it from tuberculosis of the hip and transient synovitis of the hip in early stages. It is of value to remember that, unlike in tuberculosis, in Perthes disease we have limitation of only abduction and internal rotation.

In the X-ray, head of the femur shows flatting, fragmentation, and condensation and is dense and not lucent. The joint space is widened. Tie involvement does not extend beyond femoral capital epiphysis and metaphysis. In tuberculosis, acetabulum may also be involved, the joint space is narrow and the head of femur appears lucent.

Slipped capital femoral epiphysis: Also called as adolescent coxa vara, this disorder occurs in fatty adolescent boys between 10 years and 14 years of age, usually following trauma. The symptoms include limp with little pain and limited movements of abduction and internal rotation and free or exaggerated abduction and external rotation. The subject's gait is dipping on the affected side (waddling in case of bilateral involvement) and tends to stand with the leg adducted and externally rotated.

X-ray (lateral film) shows displacement of the upper epiphysis of the femur downwards and backwards, neck-shaft angle reduced to a varying extent from the normal 150° in childhood and neck of the femur pushed up and externally rotated so much and so that the lesser trochanter becomes quite prominent.

Traumatic avulsion of muscles: Occasionally, an adolescent may overdo his physical exercise and have the origin or insertion of muscle-pulled, usually along with the apophysis. Thus, hamstring muscles may be pulled off the ischial tuberosity, iliopsoas off the lesser trochanter, sartorius off the anterior superior iliac supine, and rectus femoris off the anterior inferior supine. The symptoms include a limp and pain.

Knees

Knee problems are relatively less often responsible for limp in the infants and young children. In adolescents and preadolescents, knee is a common site for conditions that cause limp.

The knee disorders causing limp include septic arthritis, tuberculosis, rheumatoid arthritis, osteochondritis, trauma, popliteal cyst, and Osgood-Schlatter disease.

Osteochondritis: In this disorder of unknown etiology, avascular necrosis occurs in a small chunk of the bone under the articular cartilage of the knee, usually over the lateral aspect of the medial condyle of the femur. The fragment and the nearby articular cartilage may occasionally break off and float freely in the joint.

Popliteal cysts: Also termed as Baker's cysts, these are found usually posteriorly at the origin of the medial head of the gastrocnemius or semitendinosus muscle, and, rarely, in childhood, as posterior herniations of the knee joint.

Osgood–Schlatter disease: In this disorder, anterior tibial tubercle becomes prominent and tender, resulting in pain and swelling with limp as and when there is excessive activity of the quadriceps.

Ankles

Limp as a result of involvement of ankle joint may occur in septic arthritis, tuberculosis, rheumatoid arthritis, or trauma.

Feet

The major causes of limp due to problem with the foot include ill-fitting shoes, shoes with protruding nail or bad buckle, all painful conditions such as thorn-prick, warts, corns, blister, paronychia, ingrowing toenail, injuries, and congenital defects like talipes, etc.

Spine

The lesions include tuberculosis, sciatica, lumbago, and congenital defects.

Neuromuscular Frame

Poliomyelitis

This condition should always be considered if limp follows a short febrile illness, especially if the latter is accompanied by muscle pain and tenderness. Limp may also be a feature of postpolio residual paresis (Fig. 42.1).

Acute Hemiplegia

In acute infantile hemiplegia to be more exact acute hemiplegia of childhood, irrespective whether it is symptomatic or idiopathic, the onset is sudden with unilateral (occasionally bilateral) convulsions. In between episodes of convulsions, the affected side is flaccid. Unconsciousness, fever, and vomiting may be present. Attention to hemiplegia is often drawn only on recovery of consciousness and cessation of convulsions. In some cases, hemiplegia may occur suddenly without any convulsions and little or no change in consciousness. In carotid artery thrombosis, transient episodes of weakness may be observed.

In 50–75% of the patients, hemiparesis is left as a long-term sequelae. The patient invariably gains enough power to walk but he certainly limps. The arm shows relatively far less recovery, remaining almost useless. Accompanying sequelae include epilepsy and mental subnormality.

Hemihypertrophy

In this congenital disorder, one side of the body is larger than the other. The hypertrophy is usually of the whole one side, including face, tongue, teeth, and genitalia (Figs. 42.2A and B). Associated with it may be malformations like hemangioma, nevi, polydactyly, cryptorchidism, hypospadias, tumors, and calcification of adrenals. With

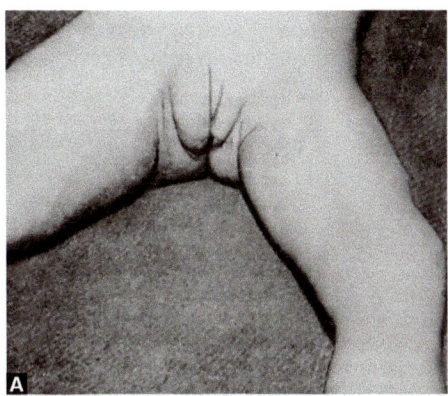

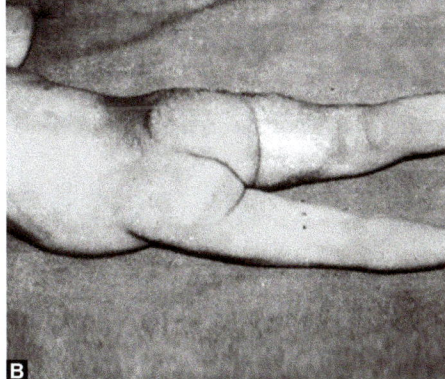

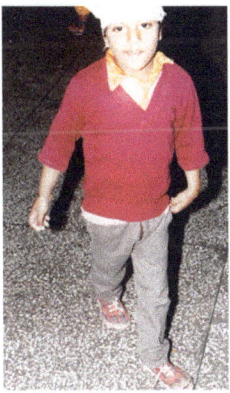

Fig. 42.1: Trendelenburg limping in a child with postpolio residual paresis (PPRP).

Figs. 42.2A and B: *Hemihypertrophy*—Note that right side of the body is impressively larger than the left. Hypertrophy of even labia majora is striking. Also, note the presence of hairy nevus on the affected side.

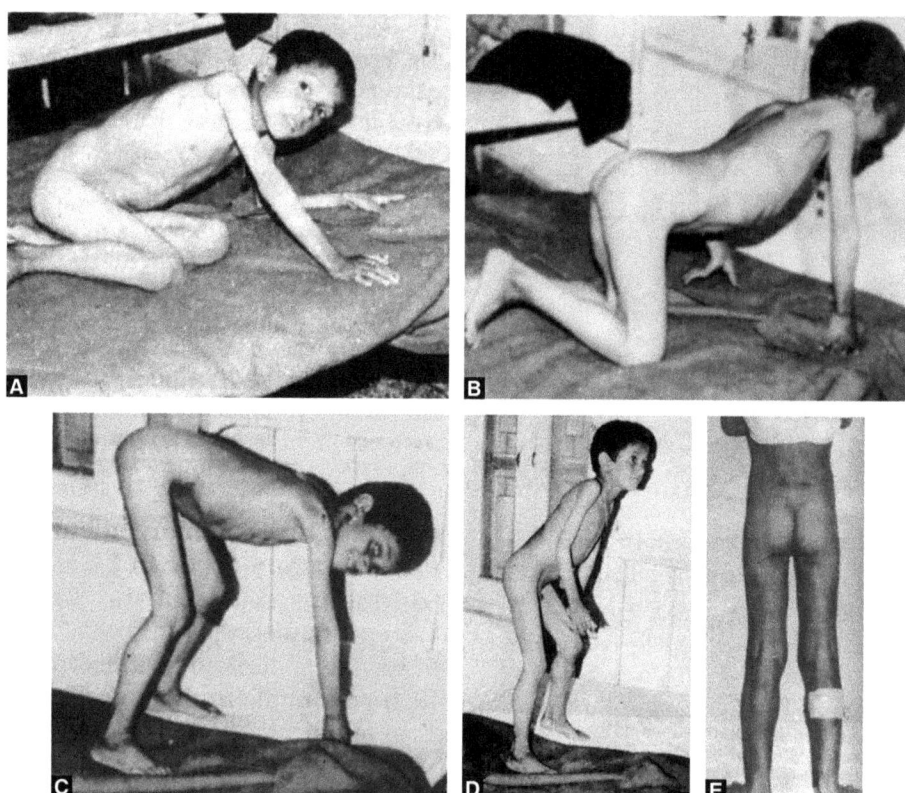

Figs. 42.3A to E: *Pseudohypertrophy muscular dystrophy (Duchenne muscular dystrophy)*—Note the Gower's sign (using the hands to climb up the legs in order to assume an upright position) as also remarkable hypertrophy of the calf girth.

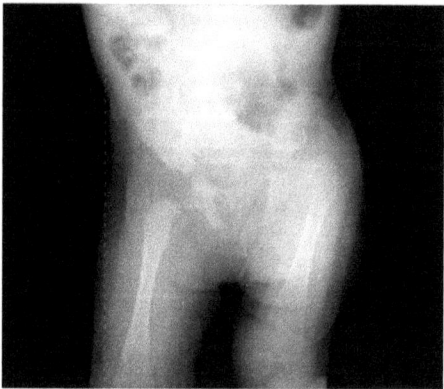

Fig. 42.4: Congenital dislocation (dysplasia) of hip (left).

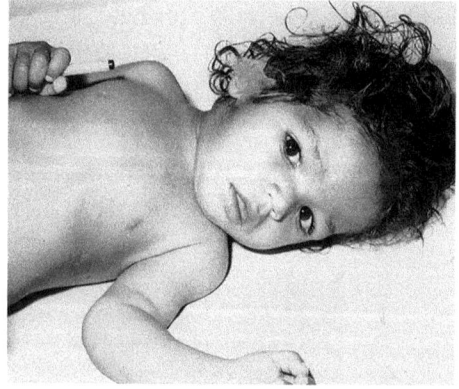

Fig. 42.5: *Myotonic muscular dystrophy*—Note the inverted V-shaped upper lip, facial weakness, thin cheeks, and poor muscle mass in temporal fossae in this infant with high-arched palate. As the child grew gradually muscle weakness of distal distribution became more apparent. At 12 years of age, he needed bracing for stabilizing the ankles. He was going to school though his school performance was subnormal on account of low IQ (75) and cognitive impairment.

gain in age, differences between the two sides become less conspicuous.

Pseudohypertrophy

Muscular dystrophy: Also termed as Duchenne muscular dystrophy or simply Duchenne myopathy, the earliest manifestation of this condition may be a limp, difficulty in walking or standing, or other activities involving the muscles of the pelvis. A waddling gait may be noticed. As the disease assumes a classical picture, the subject shows a characteristic manner of rising from the bed to an upright position. He makes successive attempts as though to climb up his own thighs. This is called as Gower's sign (Figs. 42.3A to E and 42.4). Lordosis and forwardly thrust tummy are outstanding when the child stands upright. Pseudohypertrophy, especially of the calf muscles, is striking. Tendon reflexes are sluggish or absent; ankle reflex is an exception. Cardiac enlargement, persistent tachycardia, and cardiac failure occur in 50–80% of the cases sometimes during the course of the disease. About 33% have mental subnormality.

This disorder having X-linked inheritance usually manifests before fifth year of life and generally proves fatal in the second decade of life.

Myotonic Muscular Dystrophy

This autosomal dominant disease may cause gait difficulty around preschool years. It is characterized by inverted V-shaped upper lip, thin cheeks, scalloped, concave temporalis muscles (*see* Fig. 42.5), high-arched palate, and wasting and weakness of distal muscles (in contrast to proximal distribution in other myopathies).

Besides cognitive dysfunction, speech, cardiac, endocrinal, and immunologic abnormalities may occur. Cataracts are frequent.

Remaining Causes of Limp

Inguinal lymphadenitis, scurvy, cerebral palsy, psychologic, hysteria, polymyositis, leg length inequality, tumors, leukemia, etc.

FURTHER READING

1. Healthline. Septic arthritis. Available at: www.healthline.com/health/septicarthritis#overview1. Accessed on: 24 July 2019.
2. Herring JA. The limping child. In: *Tachdjiasn's Pediatric Orthiopedics*, 3rd edn. Philadelphia: Saunders 2002:83-94.
3. Hensinger RN. Limp. *Pediatr Clin North Am* 1986;33:1355-364.
4. MacEwan GO, Dehne R. The limping child. *Pediatr Rev* 1991;12:266-274.

CHAPTER 43

Lethargy

BACKGROUND

The term, *lethargy*, denotes disinclination to get back to activity. According to the dictionary, it means drowsiness (Greek, lethargos means drowsiness). Just because the child exhausted himself on account of one or the other reasons resulting in lethargy is not important from medical point of view. The role of the physician comes in picture only when it is a prolonged lethargy spread over considerable time and without preceding exertion.

Lethargy may manifest as fatigue, excessive sleepiness (somnolence), mental sluggishness or low activity.

HISTORY

History taking should determine the normal activity and sleep patterns of the child. Any suggestion of his being sick prior to onset of lethargy? Has he been febrile? Is he a patient of seizure disorder? Is he on some drugs, especially narcotics (therapeutic or self-medication)? Does he suffer from vague bodily pains? How has been his school performance—in studies, sports, and other activities? Has he failed in some test? Has he not been able to complete his homework regularly? Is he psychologically upset over some happening or his relationship with peers and teachers?

PHYSICAL EXAMINATION

Physical examination must make a thorough search for signs of infection (including occult infection), such as urinary tract infection, pharyngitis, septic tooth or cellulites. Look for signs of central nervous system (CNS) involvement. It is indeed important to conduct psychological evaluation in the absence of positive physical sign.

INVESTIGATIONS

Clinical impression arrived at following a good clinical workup, which sets the stage for planning investigations.
- Complete blood picture (CBP), including erythrocyte sedimentation rate (ESR)
- Peripheral film for malarial parasite
- C-reactive protein (CRP)
- Lumbar puncture
- Urinalysis
- Stool examination for ova and cysts
- Serum ferritin
- Blood sugar
- Thyroid panel
- Celiac panel.

IMPORTANT DIFFERENTIALS

Infections (including Low-grade Infection)

An infection, even without significant manifestations, is the most common cause of pathological lethargy.

Over and above lethargy, high fever is usually accompanied by symptoms such as prostration, diaphoresis, flushing, and muscle pains.

In case of certain infections (say meningitis, sepsis, etc.), body temperature may not show significant rise. In fact, it may well be lower than normal (hypothermia). In case of meningitis, evidence of meningeal irritation in the form of neck stiffness and positive Kerning's and Brudzinski's signs, seizures, vomiting, etc. may be present. In sepsis, poor feeding, irritability or sluggishness, tachypnea, tachycardia and diarrhea may be encountered.

Infectious mononucleosis may cause lethargy, low-grade fever, generalized adenopathy, periorbital edema, pharyngitis, and splenomegaly.

Anemia

Chronic anemia often leads to some sort of adaptation. But that is only up to a point. In addition to lethargy, the child may suffer from easy fatigability and low blood pressure (usually orthostatic).

Postictal Stage

Following an attack of seizures, the child is likely to sleep, become drowsy or lethargic.

Chronic Fatigue Syndrome

This state, usually seen in adolescence and generally supposed to be caused by a virus (such as Ebstein–Barr), is characterized by lethargy, chronic fatigue, and deterioration in work or school performance, daily activities, exercise tolerance, and interpersonal relationship.

Physical examination usually shows nothing significant.

Diagnosis is mainly being exclusion. A psychological evaluation is important.

Remaining Causes of Lethargy

Obesity, sleeplessness, puberty, hypoglycemia, drugs, Addison's disease, teenage pregnancy, etc.

FURTHER READING

1. Australian Family Physician. Fatigue: A rational approach to investigations. Available at: www.racgp.org.au/afp/2014/july/fatigue. Accessed on: 24 July 2019.
2. Gupte S. Chronic fatigue syndrome (chronic mononucleosis, chronic Epstein-Barr virus infection, immune dysfunction syndrome). In: Gupte S (Ed). *The Short Textbook of Pediatrics*, 13th edn. New Delhi: Jaypee 2020.
3. Hospital Care for Children. Child presenting with lethargy, unconsciousness or convulsion. Available at: http://www.ichrc.org/chapter-153-child-presenting-lethargy-unconsciousness-or-convulsions. Accessed on: 24 July 2019.
4. Magnusson MR. Chronic fatigue syndrome. In: Kliegman RM, St Geme III JW, Blum NJ, et al (Eds). *Nelson Textbook of Pediatrics*, 21st edn. Philadelphia: Elsevier 2020:1093-1096.

CHAPTER 44

Lymphadenopathy

BACKGROUND

The term, *lymphadenopathy*, refers to enlargement of lymph nodes irrespective of its etiology. It is quite a common problem in day-to-day pediatric practice, often baffling the parents, may the attending physician as well. Not infrequently, cumbersome investigations may be required to reach the precise diagnosis of lymphadenopathy which occurs in response to a wide range of infectious, inflammatory, neoplastic, and immunologic conditions as also drugs (Figs. 44.1 and 44.2).

HISTORY

Symptomatic enquiry in a given case must delineate whether the glandular enlargement is localized to a particular region only or is generalized, and whether the duration of such enlargement is short or prolonged. In the event of involvement of several groups of glands, find out which group was the first to be affected? Is the involved region painful? Does the patient suffer from fever? Does the patient have any sore throat, or did he suffer from it recently? Any suggestion of impetigo, particularly infected seborrhea of scalp? Any abrasion or inflammation in the drainage area? Any rash? Any symptoms of mediastinal compression due to concurrent involvement of mediastinal lymph nodes? Any suggestion of crampy abdominal pain?

Also, ask about BCG vaccine having been given in the recent past for prophylactic or diagnostic purposes in case of persistent axillary lymphadenitis.

Is there a history of progressive loss of weight over a prolonged period (tuberculosis) or in the recent past (neoplastic process)?

Never forget to enquire about past history of tuberculosis, including exposure to a tuberculous patient in the family or the neighborhood.

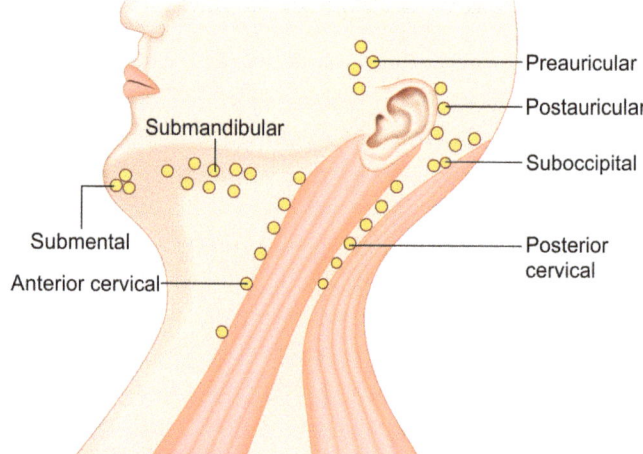

Fig. 44.1: Lymph glands (nodes) of the neck.

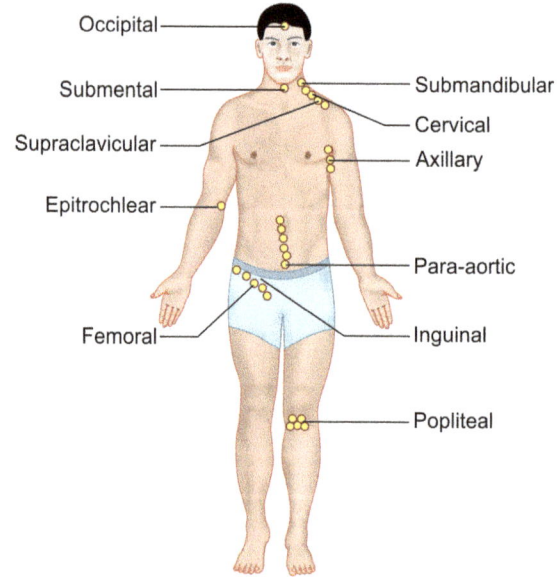

Fig. 44.2: Major groups of lymph glands.

PHYSICAL EXAMINATION

Physical examination should confirm the anatomical group(s) of lymph nodes involved. Note if the overlying skin shows signs of inflammation, abscess formation, ulceration, etc. Ascertain if the nodes are tender, soft, robbery, firm or shotty hard, and whether these are discrete or matted. Are these fixed to the surrounding structures? Look for primary focus in the drainage area. Identify pressure effects like venous engorgement of bead and neck, dyspnea, cyanosis, etc. in case of suspected lymphoma. Do not miss examining spleen, liver, mesenteric nodes, lungs, etc. In suspected syphilis, it would be important to look for syphilitic stigmata.

INVESTIGATIONS

- Complete blood picture (CBP)
- Erythrocyte sedimentation rate (ESR)
- C-reactive protein (CRP)
- Serum lactate dehydrogenase (LDH)
- Tuberculin test
- Chest X-ray
- Biopsy.

IMPORTANT DIFFERENTIALS

Infections/Inflammations

Acute

Acute lymphadenitis (localized) is characterized by swollen, tender, and fixed nodes with hot, red, and brawny overlying skin. The acute inflammatory process in the nodes follows passage of the bacteria, toxins, and other byproducts of acute inflammation from the primary site, say cellulitis or some other infection.

Examples of this kind of lymphadenitis include acute cervical lymphadenitis secondary to acute tonsillitis or pharyngitis and inguinal lymphadenitis resulting from an infection of the lower limb. Mesenteric lymphadenitis may be secondary to some inapparent infection and may be responsible for crampy abdominal pain, at times mimicking acute appendicitis. Yet another example relates to mediastinal lymphadenitis secondary to pulmonary tuberculosis in which case the subject may complain of pressure or obstructive symptoms and cough.

Usually, acute lymphadenitis subsides with regression of the primary condition. Occasionally, however, it may suppurate. In this situation of abscess formation, fluctuation in the center and pitting at the periphery on pressure can be easily elicited. Abscess is a strong indication for needle aspiration or surgical drainage.

Acute lymphadenitis (generalized) occurs in acute infections such as infectious mononucleosis, rubella, measles, enteric fever, and infected eczema.

In infectious mononucleosis (glandular fever), lymphadenopathy is quite a characteristic feature, particularly that of the posterior cervical and epitrochlear group. The remaining features of the full-blown disease, caused by Epstein–Barr (E-B) virus of the herpes group, include malaise, fever, sore throat, hepatosplenomegaly, atypical lymphocytes in the peripheral blood, and a heterophile antibody response. Occurrence of petechiae at the junction of soft and hard palate is frequent. A maculopapular rash occurs in only a small proportion of the cases. However, 80% of the subjects treated with ampicillin develop it for some unknown reason. Edema of the eyelids may occur in a few cases.

Cytomegalovirus infection (acquired form, which usually occurs in grown-up children and adolescents) may be responsible for cervical or other regional lymphadenopathy in addition to sore throat, anorexia, headache, myalgia, abdominal pain, excessive tiredness, excessive sleepiness, and fever with chills. Hepatosplenomegaly is usual. Just as in infectious mononucleosis, ampicillin administration causes a maculopapular rash.

Lymphadenopathy associated with rubella (German measles, 3-day measles) becomes evident at least 24 hours before the rash appears. In a proportion of the cases, it may manifest a week or more earlier. This is by far the only known condition that produces tender massive enlargement of retroauricular, posterior cervical, and postoccipital nodes. The constitutional symptoms are mild. The rash resembles that of measles but is so slight that it is more often than not missed. Just before the onset of rash an exanthem in the form of discrete rose spots on the soft palate may appear.

Measles, so well-known for its classical rash and for causing considerable morbidity in our settings, characteristically causes enlargement of the lymph nodes at the angle of the jaw and in the posterior cervical region. In some instances, mesenteric lymphadenitis, causing crampy abdominal pain, may occur.

In enteric fever, generalized lymphadenitis, including mesenteric involvement, though not a prominent feature, may occur. Manifestations such as prolonged fever, malaise, lethargy, headache, myalgia, abdominal pain, diarrhea/constipation, anorexia, abdominal tenderness, cloudiness of consciousness, and splenomegaly should help in suspecting enteric fever and confirming the diagnosis through Widal's test and blood culture.

Acute brucellosis, primarily a disease of animals but transmissible to man, may be responsible for axillary and cervical lymphadenopathy together with hepatosplenomegaly. Symptoms include a prodromal phase of weakness, myalgia, anorexia, body pains, and constipation, followed by evening pyrexia, often with chills, diaphoresis, abdominal pain, cough, weight loss, and epistaxis.

Infected generalized eczema is an important, though somewhat neglected cause of generalized tender lymphadenitis.

Tularemia, an uncommon disease of children exposed to the causative bacteria, *Francisella tularensis*, may be responsible for development of lymphadenitis as such (glandular form), with ulcerated lesions of skin and/or oral mucosa (ulceroglandular form) or with severe conjunctivitis (oculoglandular form). Accompanying manifestations include myalgia, arthralgia, fever, chills, vomiting, headache, diaphoresis, a generalized maculopapular rash, anemia, and photophobia.

Acquired toxoplasmosis may be responsible for generalized lymphadenopathy, particularly that of posterior cervical region. The nodes are firm and tender. Shortly, they become nontender. There is no suppuration. Accompanying manifestations may include fever, malaise, myalgia, maculopapular rash, hepatomegaly, encephalitis, pneumonia, myocarditis, and, rarely, chorioretinitis.

Chronic

Chronic lymphadenitis is frequently associated with hyperplasia of the nodes.

Infections

Tuberculosis is by far the most common cause of regional lymphadenitis of prolonged duration. It affects most often the upper deep cervical nodes followed by mesenteric nodes. The lymphadenopathy is usually bilateral and occurs by hematogenous spread from the initial infection within 6 months. The nodes are initially firm, nontender, and discrete (Fig. 44.3). In due course, they become somewhat matted together, adhere to the overlying skin and finally caseate, resulting in the formation of cold abscess. The cold abscess bursts through sinuses or ulceration of the skin, which shows no evidence of healing for a long time. This is termed as scrofuloderma (Fig. 44.4).

Since quite a few nontuberculous conditions, say chronic septic lymphadenitis, fungal disease, brucellosis, or lymphoreticular malignancy, may resemble chronic lymphadenitis of tuberculous etiology, accurate diagnosis may need lymph node biopsy, fine needle aspiration cytology (FNAC), and culture of the material thus obtained.

Chronic septic lymphadenitis may closely mimic tuberculous lymphadenitis in its early stages. There is moderate enlargement of the nodes with tenderness and, in some instances, matting. Septic tooth, tonsillitis, pharyngitis, scalp infection, etc. are responsible for majority of such cases of cervical lymphadenopathy. In case of involvement of the inguinal region, unattended cuts, wounds, abrasions, boils, etc. in the lower limbs contribute to this condition.

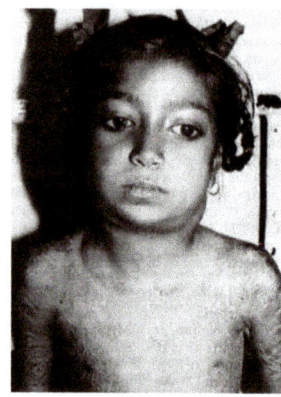

Fig. 44.3: *Tuberculous lymphadenitis*—Note massive bilateral cervical lymphadenopathy which was firm, nontender, and more or less discrete (tendency for some matting had set in). Fine needle aspiration cytology (FNAC) confirmed the diagnosis. Also, note the associated ichthyosis (secondary).

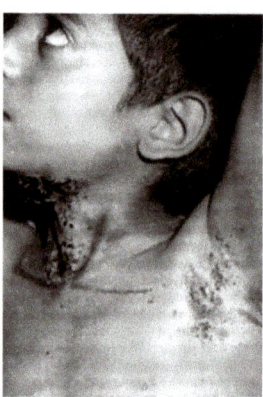

Fig. 44.4: *Scrofuloderma*—Note the skin lesions (sloughing, ulceration, and sinuses) from underlying caseous lymph glands. At times, it may need to be differentiated from pyogenic lymphadenitis, actinomycosis or sporotrichosis.

Syphilis (acquired) is an important cause of chronic lymphadenitis. In primary syphilis, the so-called "chancre" is often accompanied by lymphadenopathy which is characteristically painless, firm, shotty, discrete, and nonsuppurative. In secondary syphilis which manifests 6–8 weeks after the primary chancre, generalized lymphadenopathy occurs. The remaining clinical manifestations include low-grade fever, sore throat, malaise, weight loss, arthralgia, and cutaneous lesions such as eruptions and condylomata.

Chronic brucellosis may present with lymphadenopathy together with manifestations resulting from localization of the organisms in various organs, e.g. hepatitis, endocarditis, osteomyelitis, epididymitis, cholecystitis, myelitis, and encephalitis. A skin rash may occur. Symptoms include prolonged pyrexia, anorexia, myalgia, arthralgia, sweating, easy fatigability, nervousness, and depressive/psychotic episodes.

Filarial lymphadenitis involves the inguinal region. It is nearly always a problem of the males. The nodes are painful, tender, discrete, and swollen. There is simultaneous swelling of the spermatic cord and/or scrotum. Diagnosis is by demonstration of massive eosinophilia and microfilariae in blood drawn at night when the number of parasites in circulation is expected to be highest.

Tropical eosinophilia, supposedly an allergic response to filarial infection, may be accompanied by adenopathy, wheezy bronchitis, and very high eosinophil count.

Lymphogranuloma inguinale, occurring from an infected adult, is a sexually transmitted disease. It is characterized by inguinal lymphadenitis (usually unilateral) developing in 1-4 weeks following the appearance of the primary lesion— usually an erosion, pustule or papule over the glans, prepuce, shaft, scrotum, or coronal sulcus. The lymph nodes, initially firm and tender, become fixed to one another and the skin in due course. Eventually, they suppurate and rupture through a chronic sinus tract in the edematous skin. Resolution takes several months. Recurrences are frequent.

Diagnosis is established by isolation of the etiologic organism related to the virus, *Chlamydia trachomatis* forms infected lymph nodes and an increase in complement fixing antibody and/or micro-immunofluorescent testing.

Benign lymphoreticulosis (cat scratch disease or fever, felinosis), probably caused by a Chlamydia-like microorganism, is characterized by self-limited suppurative lymphadenitis developing 2 weeks after the primary skin lesion at the site of cat scratch. Axillary and epitrochlear nodes are the most often involved followed by those of head and neck, and the lower limbs. The involved nodes, usually superficial, are tender and as big as 10 cm in diameter. Constitutional symptoms include low-grade fever, malaise, easy fatigability, anorexia, etc.

Diagnosis is confirmed by a positive Hanger-Rose test and characteristic histopathologic changes in the involved lymph nodes.

The tender lymphadenitis takes about 2 months to regress.

Sarcoidosis is characterized by chronic generalized involvement of lymph nodes, particularly hilar and paratracheal lymphadenopathy, fever, weight loss, abdominal pain, and anorexia. In this chronic granulomatous disease (CGD) with multisystem involvement, lung is the most often involved organ.

Histopathologic examination of the biopsied lymph node or some other tissue is the most valuable diagnostic parameter. Acquired immunodeficiency syndrome (AIDS) is discussed earlier.

Immunologic Disorders

Chronic granulomatous disease, a neutrophil defect, is characterized by generalized lymphadenopathy in association with granulomatous lesions in skin, liver, lungs, spleen, and bones. Superimposed infections occur by bacteria which normally are of low virulence, and fungi. Cellular and antibody responses are essentially normal.

The real defect lies in the bactericidal activity of the neutrophils due to failure to the latter to generate microbial oxygen products. It can be detected in vitro by the nitroblue tetrazolium (NBT) test. Normally almost 90% of leukocytes reduce the dye to a purple-black compound. In this disease, hardly 10% or even less are able to do so.

The disease is usually X-linked recessive. Males are affected whereas females are purely carriers.

Kawasaki's disease (mucocutaneous lymph node syndrome) is characterized by prolonged fever, stomatitis, conjunctivitis, erythema, and desquamation over palms and soles, erythema multiforme, and lymphadenopathy. Associated with these may be arthralgia/arthritis, myocarditis/pericarditis, aseptic meningitis, hepatitis, pyuria or proteinuria. Coronary vasculitis has also been reported.

Juvenile rheumatoid arthritis of systemic-onset type is characterized by prominent extra-articular manifestations, including generalized lymphadenopathy, high fever, rheumatoid rash, hepatosplenomegaly, pleuritis, and pericarditis.

A high proportion of the patients with polyarticular type may also have lymphadenopathy together with low-grade fever, malaise, irritability, anorexia, anemia, and hepatosplenomegaly.

Serum sickness, a systemic immunologic disorder that follows administration of a foreign antigenic material, may manifest lymphadenopathy as one of the signs. The most important and the most common finding is generalized urticaria.

Neoplastic/Malignant Diseases

Acute leukemias especially acute lymphocytic leukemia (ALL), may present with prominent generalized lymphadenopathy, usually in association with hepatosplenomegaly, petechiae or mucous membrane bleeding, significant anemia, fever, bone pain/tenderness, or arthralgia.

Diagnosis is by demonstration of leukemic lymphoblasts in the blood smear, and bone marrow which invariably shows complete replacement by leukemic lymphoblasts.

Hodgkin's lymphoma is characterized by painless enlargement of lymph nodes (usually unilateral cervical to begin with) is the most frequent presenting feature. The involved nodes are usually matted, firm or robbery, nontender, and mobile. With progression of the disease process, deeper glands may also be involved. They may cause symptoms by compressing the adjacent structures, e.g. chronic pertussis-like cough and respiratory distress.

The disease may involve any organ(s) in addition to lymph nodes, causing corresponding manifestations.

General symptoms of the disease include fever, anorexia, weight loss, night sweats, and pruritus.

The most important investigation is histopathologic study of biopsy material from the involved lymph node.

Non-Hodgkin lymphoma mostly arises in the head and neck regions as a painless cervical or supraclavicular lymphadenopathy. So rapid is the growth that within a matter of 1–3 weeks, the nodes may assume enormous size. Though the nodes are, to begin with, firm, nontender, and discrete, they become confluent as the disease progresses.

Another common site of lymph node involvement is the mediastinum in which the child presents with signs and symptoms of mediastinal compression.

Yet another frequent site of involvement of the nodes is the ileocecal region. The common mode of presentation in such a case is with abdominal lump, intestinal obstruction or intussusception.

Drugs

Diphenylhydantoin, troxidone, carbamazepine, BCG, iron-dextran complex, cephaloridine, meprobamate, p-aminosalicylic acid (PAS), primidone, phenylbutazone, sulfadimidine, etc.

FURTHER READING

1. Nield LS, Kamat D. Lymphadenopathy in children: When and how to evaluate. *Clin Pediatr (Phila)* 2004;43:25-33.
2. Twist CJ, Link MP. Assessment of lymphadenopathy in children. *Pediatr Clin North Am* 2002;49:1009-1025.
3. Weinberg GA, Segel GB, Hall CB. Lymphadenopathy. In: Adam HM, Foy JM (Eds). *Signs and Symptoms in Pediatrics*. Illinois: American Academy of Pediatrics 2014:637-648.

CHAPTER 45

Mass in Abdomen

BACKGROUND

Abdominal mass, lump or swelling is a commonly encountered problem in pediatric practice. Inadequacy of clinical work-up often leads to unnecessary and cumbersome investigations in arriving at its precise diagnosis.

HISTORY

In a given case, ask when the lump was first noticed, provided that the attendants or the patient are indeed aware of it? Is it present since birth? Else, is it of short duration or has been there for quite some time? Did it follow some trauma, or develop spontaneously? Is it growing rapidly or slowly, or regressing? Is it painful and whether pain is localized or referred? Did the pain precede the lump or follow it? What is the stated site of the lump—whether superficial or within the abdomen and roughly in which region? In case of a superficial swelling, any secondary changes such as ulceration, sinus formation, fungation, or softening?

Do not miss asking if the subject is febrile, losing weight, developing considerable pallor or having swellings elsewhere as well. Is the bleeding from anywhere? Any history of jaundice? Any history of ascariasis?

PHYSICAL EXAMINATION

Physical examination must ascertain whether the swelling is in the abdominal wall (parietal) or intra-abdominal, what its exact anatomic position is, whether it is in connection with a particular organ (say liver, spleen, kidney, gut, or lymph nodes) and whether it is inflammatory or a growth.

To decide whether the lump is parietal or intra-abdominal, ask the patient to make his abdominal muscles taut by raising the shoulders with arms folded over the chest while he lies down on the bed. Abdominal muscles can also be made taut by raising the extended legs from the bed, or by trying to blow out with the nose and the mouth covered with something or simply kept closed. A parietal swelling becomes more prominent whereas an intra-abdominal one just disappears or becomes less apparent on any of these maneuvers. The observation that the swelling moves with respiration vertically also favors its intra-abdominal location.

Ascertain the position of the lump in relation to the standard anatomic regions of the abdomen (Fig. 45.1). To recapitulate the division, let us draw two imaginary horizontal and vertical lines. The upper horizontal line runs midway the umbilicus and xiphisternum, the lower at the level of the iliac tubercles. The vertical line passes on either side through the midpoint between anterior superior iliac spine and symphysis pubis. The three regions in the upper quadrant, thus formed, are right hypochondrium, epigastrium, and left hypochondrium. In the middle quadrant, the three regions are right lumbar, umbilical, and left lumbar. The lower-most quadrant consists of right iliac, hypogastric, and left iliac regions. Thus, in total there are nine regions.

In case of intra-abdominal lump, you must try to sort out its relationship with liver, spleen, kidney, gallbladder,

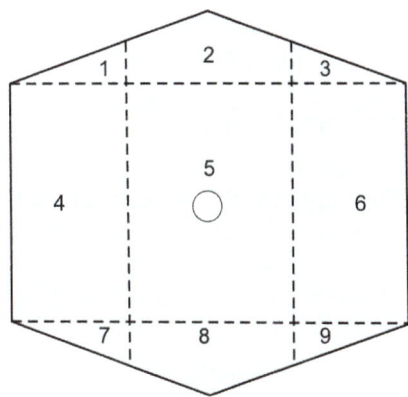

Fig. 45.1: *Anatomical topography of the abdomen*—Region 1 represents right hypochondrium; 2, epigastrium; 3, left hypochondrium; 4, right lumbar; 5, umbilical; 6, left lumbar; 7, right iliac; 8, hypogastrium; 9, left iliac.

stomach, gut, mesentery, etc. Is there any ascites or other evidence of portal hypertension?

Never, forget examining the hernial sites and for undescended testes.

INVESTIGATIONS

- Blood tests
  - Complete blood picture (CBP)
  - Retics
  - Malarial parasite
  - Blood culture
  - Alpha-1-fetoprotein
- Abdominal X-ray
- *Abdominal imaging*: Ultrasonography, computed tomography (CT) scan, magnetic resonance imaging (MRI), etc.
- Biopsy
- Endoscopy
- Endoscopic retrograde cholangiopancreatography (ERCP).

IMPORTANT DIFFERENTIALS

Parietal Lump

Right and Left Hypochondria

In addition to boils, carbuncles, abscesses, lipoma, angioma or neurofibroma, a parietal lump in any of the hypochondria may be an abscess secondary to cold abscess related to canes of the spine or ribs, or to liver or subphrenic abscess.

Epigastrium

Besides the conditions that are described in connection with the hypochondria, a well-built adolescent indulging in strenuous exercise or activity may develop a small rounded lump, about the midline between the umbilicus and the xiphisternum, which causes discomfort, particularly after food. This is called epigastric hernia.

Right and Left Lumbar Regions

The comments given in connection with the hypochondria can be faithfully applied in case of the lumbar regions as well, except that, on rare occasions, a lumbar hernia, may also be responsible for a lump in region.

Umbilical Region

Besides the conditions mentioned in case of hypochondria, umbilical hernia, and hematoma or abscess of the rectus sheath (the former from some trauma) may be responsible for swelling arising from the abdominal wall.

Umbilical hernia is a commonly encountered condition in newborns and infants, occurring as a result of weakness or faulty closure of the umbilical ring. Associated diastasis recti is frequent. The incidence in dark races is several times higher than in the whites. Low-birth-weight infants suffer more often.

The hernia manifests as a soft swelling of variable size that protrudes or becomes more prominent on coughing, crying or straining (Fig. 45.2). It is covered by skin and is easily reducible. It may be found in otherwise normal infants but may well be a part of the manifestations of cretinism or gargoylism.

Two types are recognized. First—"false" in which hernia occurs into the cord itself. It is a persistence of the physiologic state. Second—"true", which is characterized by protrusion through the umbilical cicatrix. In both types, the hernial sac contains omentum or portions of the small intestine.

Spontaneous regression occurs in a large majority of the cases by the age of 18 months.

Umbilical polyp is a rare congenital bright red, firm, and resistant swelling resulting from persistence of all or part of the omphalomesenteric duct or the urachus. It is formed by intestinal or urinary tract mucosa and may intermittently discharge urine or fecal matter in case of a communication with the bladder or the ileum.

Umbilical granuloma, often confused with polyp, is the result of persistence of exuberant granulation tissue at the base of the umbilicus (Fig. 45.3). The area appears pink or reddish with seropurulent secretions. Without cauterization with silver nitrate (often more than once), it usually does not heal.

Congenital omphalocele (exomphalos) refers to herniation of the abdominal contents into the base of the cord, the size of the sac lying outside the abdominal wall depending upon the type of visceral protrusion. Remember,

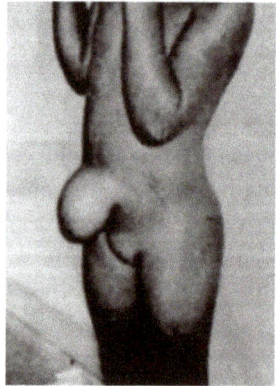

Fig. 45.2: Large umbilical hernia.

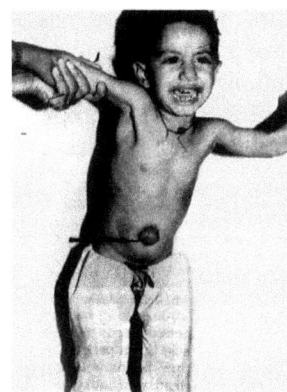

Fig. 45.3: Umbilical granuloma.

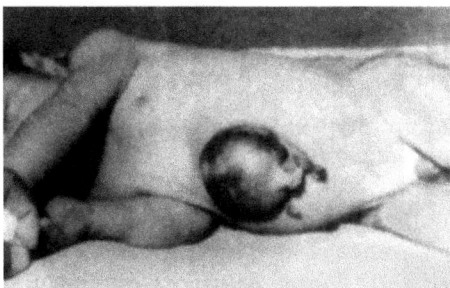

Fig. 45.4: *Exomphalos minor*—Note the protruding umbilical sac of small size without skin covering.

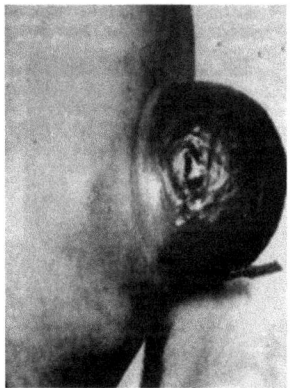

Fig. 45.5: *Exomphalos major*—Note that the thin and translucent sac is not covered by skin unlike the umbilical hernia, which is always covered by skin. Moreover, the defect is over 4 cm in diameter and is accompanied by other abnormalities.

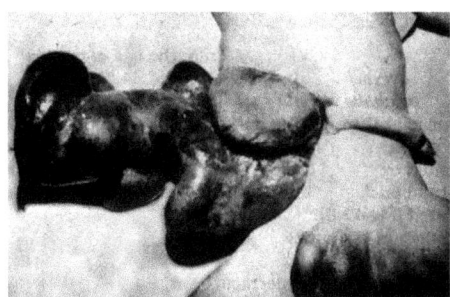

Fig. 45.6: *Gastroschisis*—Note the protrusion of the whole of midgut loop and a part of liver through the defect in the anterior abdominal wall, placed to the right of the umbilicus and separated by a skin bridge.

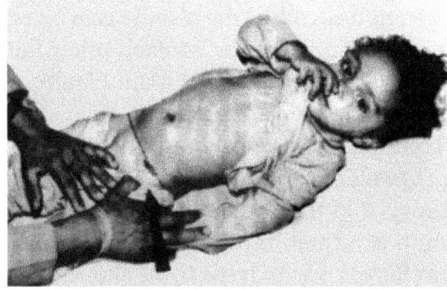

Fig. 45.7: *Inguinal hernia*—The swelling in the groin appeared on crying and reduced spontaneously on relaxing. The "silk glove" sign (feel of a crepitance on rolling thickened spermatic cord between examiner's two fingers) was positive.

in contrast to the umbilical hernia, the sac of omphalocele is never covered by skin (Figs. 45.4 and 45.5).

Gastroschisis refers to small protrusion of whole of the midgut loop through the defect in the anterior abdominal wall, placed usually to the right of the umbilicus and separated by a skin bridge. There is absence of sac. Cord is at normal position. Rarely, whole or part of the liver is also herniated (Fig. 45.6).

Tumors of the umbilicus, though rare, may produce a mass. They include angioma, cysts of urachal or omphalomesenteric remnants, dermoid cyst, enteroteratoma, and myxosarcoma.

Right Iliac Fossa

In addition to the swellings mentioned in connection with the hypochondria, a pyogenic iliac abscess or an appendicular abscess may become parietal by burrowing through the anterior abdominal wall. More important, however, are the inguinal swellings.

Inguinal hernia is characterized by appearance of an intermittent inguinal or inguinoscrotal swelling (rarely involving the labium majus) on crying, coughing vigorously or straining at stools (Fig. 45.7). As a rule, it disappears when the child relaxes in mother's lap or lies down peacefully. Usually, there is no pain due to the swelling. On the other hand, crying thought to be the result of pain is the triggering factor for the swelling.

The observation of an inguinal or inguinoscrotal swelling that is usually right side and reduces spontaneously or on manipulation is virtually diagnostic of inguinal hernia. If the examiner fails to get a chance to observe the swelling even on raising the intra-abdominal pressure, he should roll the thickened spermatic cord on the affected side between his two fingers. He may feel a "crepitance". This is called as "silk glove" sign.

Enlarged lymph nodes, secondary to an inflammatory or other lesion from umbilicus down to the toes, constitute the most important and also the most common cause of swelling in the inguinal region. Most often the swelling is inflammatory, secondary to an acute infective focus in the drainage area. In this case, the nodes become enlarged, tender, and fixed with the overlying skin showing classical signs of acute inflammation. In chronic septic lymphadenitis, the nodes become moderately enlarged with no or little tenderness. In the drainage area, you may find a primary focus, say a septic cut, ulcer, blister, etc. Inguinal lymphadenitis of tuberculous origin is rather infrequent. The enlarged nodes, unless the disease is in an early stage, become matted, i.e. adherent to each other followed by caseation and cold abscess formation. Finally, a more or less nonhealing ulcer or sinus follows.

Undescended testis may be responsible for producing an inguinal swelling (or else in the abdomen, perineum, femoral area, or at the base of the penis over the pubic bone when it is termed ectopic testis). You can ascertain that the swelling is due to testis by its shape, feel, and that typical testicular sensation. The scrotum is empty on the affected side. Moreover, the affected testis is smaller than the normally located testis. In an overwhelming majority of the cases, it is accompanied by inguinal hernia.

Retractile testis may occasionally cause an inguinal swelling. The cause is strong contraction of the cremaster muscle which periodically pulls the testis into the inguinal canal or the inguinal pouch. If this condition is suspected, repeated examinations may be needed.

Psoas abscess, resulting from caries spine or cold abscess, resulting from tuberculosis of hip or sacroiliac joints, may cause a large swelling in the inguinal region. An impulse on coughing, crying or straining on stools occurs in the former. Evidence of a deformity of the spine, hip or sacroiliac joints often clinches the diagnosis.

Causes of inguinal swelling such as femoral hernia, saphena varix, and psoas bursa are virtually seldom seen in childhood.

Left Iliac Fossa

The observations made in connection with the right iliac region are eminently applicable in this region too. However, as is understandable, appendicular abscess is unlikely to push through the abdominal wall on the left side.

Hypogastrium

All that is said in connection with the parietal lumps in the umbilical region holds equally good here as well.

In addition, urachal cyst or persistent urachus, due to failure of closure of the allantoic duct, extending from bladder to the umbilical, may be responsible for a cystic swelling at the umbilical. A clear, light yellow urine-like discharge at the umbilicus continues.

INTRA-ABDOMINAL LUMP

Right Hypochondrium

Liver

Hepatomegaly is a common finding in infancy and childhood. Not always is it of pathologic significance. Quite frequently, liver is palpable in normal, healthy children up to the age of 4 years or 5 years say up to around 2.5 cm in the first 2 years and up to 1 cm from 2 years to 4 years or 5 years. Of course, such a normal liver is soft, smooth, round edged, and nontender.

A large number of conditions may be responsible for organic hepatomegaly, right from infections (such as viral hepatitis) through nutritional disorders (such as kwashiorkor) or essentially malignant states (such as cirrhosis, leukemia or tumors) as follows:

- *Infections/inflammations:* Viral hepatitis, amebic hepatitis/abscess, pyogenic hepatitis/abscess, ascariasis, cholangitis, hydatid disease, tuberculosis, malaria, kala azar, enteric fever, brucellosis, septicemia, neonatal/intrauterine infections like toxoplasmosis, rubella, cytomegalic inclusion disease, syphilis, infectious mononucleosis, leptospirosis, histoplasmosis.
- *Hematogenous diseases:* Congenital hemolytic anemia like thalassemia and sickle-cell anemia, erythroblastosis fetalis, etc.
- *Nutritional problems:* Kwashiorkor, total parenteral alimentation (caloric overload), etc.
- *Vascular/congestive:* Congestive cardiac failure, hepatic vein thrombosis, constrictive pericarditis, veno-occlusive disease of liver, etc.
- *Storage diseases:* Acute-Reye syndrome, chronic-glycogen-storage disease, Gaucher's disease, Niemann-Pick disease, galactosemia, gargoylism, hemosiderosis, amyloidosis, xanthomatosis, cystic fibrosis, cystinosis, diabetes mellitus, Wilson's disease, gangliosidosis, cholesterol storage disease, Wolman's disease, etc.
- *Malignant diseases:* Leukemias, lymphomas, neuroblastoma, Wilms' tumor, gonadal tumors, hepatoblastoma, etc.
- *Miscellaneous:* Cirrhosis (especially Indian childhood cirrhosis), congenital biliary atresia, cysts, alpha-1-antitrypsin deficiency, hemangioma, macroglobulinemia, systemic lupus erythematosus (SLE), drug toxicity, etc.

For details on hepatomegaly, see Chapter 35.

Gallbladder

A palpable tender mass in the right hypochondrium with or without radiation to the right shoulder (just below the scapula) should cause a strong suspicion of cholecystitis, particularly if the patient is an older teenaged girl. Remaining manifestations include fever (with shaking chills in case of cholangitis), jaundice, and, occasionally indigestion, flatulence or food intolerance.

Two types of diseases are known to occur—noncalculus and cholelithiasis. The former is associated with acute systemic infections (say septicemia), enteric fever, giardiasis, ascariasis, leptospirosis, erysipelas, anaerobic diphtheroid infections, Kawasaki disease, gross dehydration, gross protein-energy malnutrition, and neonates with associated amnionitis.

Subphrenic Abscess

Liver, though not actually enlarged, may become palpable due to its depression in subphrenic abscess (on the right side) resulting from an appendiceal or other intra-abdominal suppuration as also from an empyema on rare occasions. A history pointing to some such predisposing conditions can usually be elicited. On local examination, a tender diffuse swelling is found in continuity with the liver. Rarely, you may be able to demonstrate alternate areas of dullness and resonance along the midaxillary line on percussion. Remaining manifestations include hectic rise of temperature with chills, rigors and toxemia.

In order to establish the diagnosis, you must demonstrate elevated diaphragm on right side with gas under it in the X-ray. Screening, in addition, shows that the diaphragm is fixed rather than demonstrating normal up and down movements with respiration.

Aspiration of the pus finally confirms the diagnosis.

Gut

Intussusception: The lump as a result of intussusception is sausage-shaped, somewhat tender and usually located in the right upper quadrant of the abdomen with its long axis directed cephalocaudally. If it increases in size as also firmness under the examining finger during a paroxysm of abdominal pain, the clinical impression is further corroborated. In addition to the lump, rectal examination reveals presence of blood on the examining finger as it is withdrawn. Remaining manifestations include sudden onset of a severe paroxysmal pain, shock-like state, fever, vomiting, and passage of blood and mucus (currant jelly) in stools.

Intestinal tuberculosis: Rarely, a lump formed by ileocecal tuberculosis may get drawn to the right hypochondrium by fibrosis. Barium follow-through shows the "filling defect" along with elevation of the cecum and spasm of the terminal ileum. Diagnosis needs corroboration by Mantoux/BCG test, erythrocyte sedimentation rate (ESR), X-ray chest, and family screening.

Kidney

A kidney swelling is better felt in the loin than anteriorly. Its causes include movable kidney, hydronephrosis or pyonephrosis, tuberculosis, polycystic kidney, renal calculus, Wilms' tumor, neuroblastoma, and perinephric abscess.

Movable kidney is characteristically only slightly enlarged, if at all. Accompanying manifestations may include colicky or dragging pain, and neurasthenia in grown-up children and adolescents who become overconscious that they have such a kidney. In order to establish the diagnosis an intravenous pyelogram (IVP) is needed.

Hydronephrosis produces a lump having general characteristics of a renal swelling, often varying in size with the large passage of urine. It is cystic, fluctuant, and shows positive fluid thrill if large enough in size. Usually, a similar lump is palpable on the left side as well. Until the lump has assumed considerable size, it may remain virtually symptomless. Later, it becomes painful. Hematuria may occur. Fever with chills indicates superimposed infection.

Pyonephrosis produces a clinical picture that closely mimics the one produced by hydronephrosis. In addition, there is hectic rise of temperature, rigors, sweating, toxemia, and leukocytosis.

Renal tuberculosis, a rare cause of lump in the hypochondrium in infancy and childhood, may be accompanied by such manifestations as increased frequency of micturition, pain in the loin, and hematuria. Persistent sterile pyuria is a strong indication for excluding renal tuberculosis. Radiologic findings include calcified tuberculous lesions, calyceal cavities, and dilatation followed by stenosis of the urinary tract. Bladder becomes contracted and small. Typically, there are multiple sites of involvement.

Polycystic kidney may be of two types—infantile form and adult form. In the infantile form, an autosomal recessive disease, the kidney (in fact both kidneys) is enlarged, the whole parenchyma being filled with fusiform or cylindrical cysts. Cysts are found in liver, pancreas, bile duct, and lung as well. Radiology shows radially aligned renal parenchyma opacifications in the shape of streaks, widened calyces, and visible contrast medium in the cortex.

In the adult form (a misnomer because it manifests in childhood as well), an autosomal dominant disease, the subject presents with a renal swelling (rather on the other side also) accompanied by, at times, dragging pain in the loin, hematuria or uremia, and pale urine (of low specific gravity) showing albumin and casts. All through the parenchyma, the kidney shows cysts. Accompanying features may include an intracranial aneurysm. Radiology shows calyces which are elongated and bizarrely distorted with terminal clubbing, making sponge-like appearance.

Renal calculus may occasionally be responsible for an enlarged kidney. Remaining manifestations include colicky abdominal pain, hematuria, recurrent urinary infections, passing of the calculus, and urethral obstruction. X-ray establishes the diagnosis.

Perinephric abscess manifests with diffuse renal swelling, erythema, edema, and tenderness of the flank. The individual is toxic, having pyrexia of unknown origin. The lumbar spine shows scoliosis with the concavity towards the involved side. Movements of the spine to the opposite side are usually painful. There may be limp and fixed flexion of the hip. Radiology shows displacement of the affected kidney and ureter with obliteration of the psoas shadow.

Wilms' tumor, also called as nephroblastoma, may be responsible for a huge painless renal lump in the right upper quadrant. Hematuria is rare. If metastases have occurred, associated symptoms will be seen depending upon the organ(s) involved. Radiology shows a soft tissue opacity displacing the gut in the area normally occupied by the kidney, and distortion of calyces (spider leg deformity).

Adrenals

Neuroblastoma, a malignant tumor arising from adrenal medulla or sympathetic ganglia (so, not a renal growth in actuality) may produce a lump that not only fills the right hypochondrium but also goes down to the left, crossing the midline. The kidney is in reality pushed upward by this mass which is hard and fixed. Remaining manifestations depend upon the extent of the growth. Fever, bone pain, anemia, and weight loss are common. Subcutaneous nodules, adrenal masses with involvement of the bone marrow, hepatomegaly from massive infiltration of the liver, paraplegia, paroxysmal hypertension, and proptosis secondary to retroperitoneal deposits may occur.

Radiology shows displacement of one of the kidneys by a suprarenal mass. Gross skeletal metastases may also be detected.

Urine examination reveals an excessive excretion of catecholamine and/or their metabolites, vanillylmandelic acid (VMA), and cystathionine.

Bone marrow may show secondary deposits, i.e. neuroblasts, which may simulate leukemia.

Epigastrium

Liver and **subphrenic space**: Refer to the details given in connection with the right hypochondrium.

Stomach, duodenum, and gut: Congenital hypertrophic pyloric stenosis, occurring in infants about 3–5 weeks old, may be responsible for epigastric fullness, gastric waves moving from left to right and a palpable olive-shaped lump about the size of the thumb. The classical story is that the infant, usually a first-born male, begins to vomit. Within 30 minutes, vomiting becomes forceful and projectile. He is constantly hungry and fails to thrive. Occasionally, greenish stools (starvation diarrhea), gastric hemorrhage or jaundice may be present. Dehydration, electrolyte imbalance (especially alkalosis, hypokalemia, and hyponatremia), and tetanic spasms may complicate the picture. Barium meal study shows gross narrowing and elongation of pylorus. The stomach is markedly distended, with abnormal retention of barium, and there is increased intensity of peristaltic waves.

Intussusception (though usually its lump is palpable in the right hypochondrium) may cause a lump in the epigastric region in some cases. In the latter situation, its long axis is directed transversely rather than cephalocaudally.

Trichobezoar: Some infants and children, especially if having behavioral problems, may get into the practice of pulling out the head hair and swallow the material. In due course, this chronic practice may lead to collection of a lot of hair in the stomach which becomes palpable as a big lump, the so-called trichobezoar or hairball, particularly after meals. The lump gives a soft crackling feeling when palpated. Symptoms include indigestion, dyspepsia, and epigastric discomfort, more so after meals. Areas of alopecia, secondary to trichotilomania, over head in an emotionally disturbed or mentally retarded child may suggest the diagnosis.

Barium meal study shows a lump outlined by barium.

Intestinal tuberculosis: In hyperplastic tuberculosis, contracted transverse mesocolon may pull the transverse colon to the lower part of the epigastrium, leading to a palpable mass and fullness in the epigastric region.

In tuberculosis, the omentum may get rolled up to form a transverse ridge in the epigastric region. A mass of lymph nodes with adherent intestinal coils may be felt in the epigastrium.

Pancreas

Pseudopancreatic cyst may form a smooth rounded fluctuating lump in the epigastrium. It is a collection of fluid in the lesser sac of the peritoneal cavity. A trauma or inflammation figure among the causes.

Barium meal shows that the lump is situated behind the stomach.

Kidney and Suprarenal

See discussion in connection with the right hypochondrium.

Aorta

A lump in the epigastrium with characteristic expansile pulsation may well be aneurysm of upper part of the abdominal aorta.

Lymph Nodes

Enlarged lymph nodes, of whatsoever etiology, may cause palpable lump in the epigastric region.

Left Hypochondrium

Except for the splenic lump, intra-abdominal mass in this region merits about the same components as given in connection with the right hypochondrium.

A detailed discussion on differential diagnosis of splenomegaly will be found in Chapter 55. A comprehensive list of its causes is as follows:
- *Infections*: Malaria, kala azar, enteric fever, tuberculosis, brucellosis, intrauterine infections, septicemia, infective endocarditis, infectious mononucleosis, histoplasmosis, coma viral fevers, etc.
- *Hematogenous diseases*: Hemolytic anemia, erythroblastosis fetalis, nutritional anemia, hypersplenism, thrombocytopenic purpura, etc.
- *Congestive splenomegaly*: Congestive cardiac failure, cirrhosis, hepatic, portal or splenic vein thrombosis, constrictive pericarditis, etc.
- *Inborn errors of metabolism*: Glycogen storage disease, Gaucher's disease, Niemann–Pick disease, gargoylism, amyloidosis, hemosiderosis, xanthomatosis, cystinosis, cystic fibrosis, etc.
- *Malignant diseases*: Leukemia, lymphosarcoma, Hodgkin's lymphoma, myeloproliferative disorders, etc.
- *Miscellaneous*: Cysts, hemangioma, abscess, SLE, rheumatoid arthritis (Still's disease), osteopetrosis, nutritional recovery syndrome, etc.

Right and Left Lumbar Regions

There is no special comment about the lump in lumbar region, except that it may be either in connection with the kidney or colon, or an extension of a lump in connection with the neighboring structures, say liver, gallbladder, and appendix on the right and spleen on the left.

Umbilical Region

Lump in this region may develop in connection with stomach, gut omentum, pancreas, lymph nodes, kidney, liver, and spleen. In kwashiorkor, hepatomegaly may be huge enough, reaching as low as the umbilicus and even below. Likewise, splenic swelling in tropical splenomegaly syndrome, thalassemia or chronic myeloid leukemia may extend to this region or even lower down.

Right Iliac Fossa

Appendix: Appendicular lump is by and large the most frequent cause of intra-abdominal swelling in the right iliac region. It is tender, firm, irregular, and fixed or little mobile. Inflammatory signs evident over the overlying abdominal wall indicate that the lump is not just a mass of inflamed and swollen appendix wrapped up by omentum, coils of intestine, and lymph but has an element of abscess formation as well.

Leukocytosis is present, particularly in an infant in whom the count may be 20,000/cmm or more.

Gut

Intussusception, as already stated, produces a lump usually in the right hypochondrium and less frequently in the epigastric region. The right iliac fossa is, as a rule, empty. Rarely, however, at an early stage of the disease, a lump may be palpable in the ileocecal region per se.

Roundworm impaction, in children heavily infected with *Ascaris lumbricoides* in the lowermost portion of the ileum, may be responsible for a palpable lump which could easily be confused with an intussusceptum. This possibility should, therefore, be carefully borne in mind in endemic areas.

Amebic colitis may infrequently be responsible for a palpable lump in the right iliac fossa. History of amebic dysentery or diarrhea with demonstration of *Entamoeba histolytica* trophozoites or cysts establishes the diagnosis.

Crohn's disease, also termed as regional ileitis or granulomatous enterocolitis, is a nonspecific inflammatory bowel disease (the other being ulcerative colitis) which may produce a palpable abdominal mass in the iliac fossa in a proportion of the subjects who usually are preadolescents or adolescents. Accompanying manifestations include crampy abdominal pain which shoots up by eating and somewhat subsides after defecation, chronic diarrhea, malnutrition, perianal lesions, aphthous stomatitis, polyarthritis, clubbing, and erythema nodosum.

Diagnosis is established by sigmoidoscopy, rectal biopsy (showing typical granulomas even in the absence of significant segmental involvement on sigmoidoscopy), endoscopy (which defines the limits of colonic lesions), and barium follow-through (which shows irregular mucosa or a "cobbler-stone" pattern, thickened bowel wall, enteric fistulas, and segmental distribution of the lesions).

Lymph Nodes

Lymphadenopathy secondary to conditions such as tuberculosis, filariasis or lymphoma may be responsible for a lump in the right iliac region. Also, see Chapter 44.

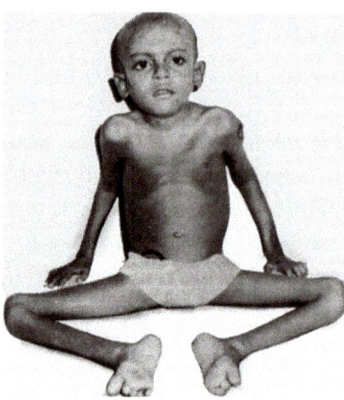

Fig. 45.8: *Iliopsoas abscess*—Note the part of the outline of the mass in the right iliac fossa. Radiologic evidence of caries spine (sacroiliac) was present.

Iliopsoas Sheath

Iliopsoas cold abscess, secondary to caries spine, may cause a lump in the right iliac fossa just above the inguinal ligament and below the inguinal ligament by trickling down from its original site (Fig. 45.8). If the cold abscess fills virtually the whole of right iliac fossa, the primary bony lesion is in all probability tuberculosis of the hip or sacroiliac joint.

Kidney

Movable kidney may be responsible for a palpable lump in the right iliac fossa.

Unascended kidney, may be responsible for a lump in the right iliac fossa (or pelvis), the area where the first rudiment of renal tissue is supposed to appear. IVP must be done in suspected cases.

Gallbladder

Hydrops gallbladder or any condition leading to a massive swelling of the gallbladder may descend down to right iliac fossa where it becomes distinctly palpable, particularly when hepatomegaly accompanies the condition. This is a rare entity.

Testis

Retained testis may rarely become palpable in the right iliac fossa, particularly when it develops a pathology such as malignancy at or after puberty. The lump is fixed, firm, and irregular.

Urinary Bladder

A full distended bladder may assume an enormous size, extending to right iliac fossa as well. It is felt as a tender globular swelling that is dull on percussion and often reaches the umbilicus. When slightly pressed, the child feels a desire to micturate. On micturition, the bladder lump disappears.

Hypogastrium

Except for the swelling produced by a full bladder, it is rather uncommon to have a lump in this region. It may, of course, occur in connection with other structures as well, say small intestine, sigmoid colon, pelvis, etc.

Left Iliac Fossa

The description given for the right iliac fossa is more or less applicable to this region too. Here, rather than gallbladder, a splenic lump may be palpable. Secondly, in place of appendix, here descending colon becomes relevant. Diverticula, congenital anomalies due to persistence of intestinal abnormal tissue in close relation to a part of the alimentary tract, though very rare in childhood (Meckel's diverticulum is an exception), must be mentioned in relation to this region. They may cause mechanical obstruction, and become inflamed (diverticulitis), ulcerated or perforated.

FURTHER READING

1. Golden CB, Feusner JH. Malignant abdominal masses in children: Quick guide to evaluation and diagnosis. *Pediatr Clin North Am* 2002;49:1369-1392.
2. Right Diagnosis. Abdominal masses. Available at: www.rightdiagnosis.com/symptoms/abdominal_mass/tests.htm. Accessed on: 24 July 2019.

CHAPTER 46

Mouth Breathing

BACKGROUND

Mouth breathing is a common observation in pediatric practice. It is responsible for several secondary adverse effects, including dryness of the mouth and lips and their proneness to fissuring and infection.

HISTORY

In a given case, find out if the child mouth breathes just out of habit or he has an obstructive nasal problem. Does he have persistent or recurrent upper respiratory infection? Does he sneeze a lot? Any headache, hyposmia, or postnasal discharge?

PHYSICAL EXAMINATION

Physical examination should, in particular, exclude adenoids, polyp, foreign body, deviated septum, and allergy.

INVESTIGATIONS

In most cases, a good clinical workup suffices. Following investigations may be helpful in difficult situations:
- Enzyme analysis of saliva
- Direct measurement of volatile sulfur compound
- Organoleptic test.

IMPORTANT DIFFERENTIALS

Adenoids

Adenoidal hypertrophy may interfere with the passage of air through the nose, resulting in mouth breathing, especially during sleep when the child lies supine. When gross adenoidal hypertrophy is present, the child develops a tendency to keep the mouth open during day also. Accompanying manifestations may include dryness of the mucous membrane of the mouth and lips, persistent rhinitis, pharyngitis, snoring, nasal voice, offensive breath, impaired taste, bad smell, harassing cough, impaired hearing, and chronic otitis media. Eventually, the child may develop dull expression with open mouth and malocccluded teeth—the so-called adenoid facies. His school performance too suffers.

In a suspected case, digital palpation, indirect visualization with a pharyngeal mirror or fiberoptic bronchoscope, or lateral pharyngeal X-ray may help in clinching the diagnosis.

Choanal Atresia

In bilateral choanal atresia, if the infant is able to mouth breathe, he experiences difficulty when sucking and swallowing. The infant may even become cyanotic on being nursed.

Diagnosis is made by passing firm catheter through each nostril deep into the nasopharynx.

Maternal Medication

A hypertensive mother on reserpine may pass on the drug to the baby and cause nasal obstruction and mouth breathing.

Nasal Allergy

Mouth breathing may accompany nasal allergy, which occurs as a result of changed reactivity of nasal mucosa to a variety of substances. Two types are known—seasonal and perennial. In seasonal allergy, also termed as hay fever or pollinosis, the antigen (allergen) is an inhalant such as pollens of flowers, weeds, trees or grass. In perennial allergy, the allergen may be an inhalant or ingestant like egg white, fish, milk, etc. as also a drug, bacteria or perfume.

Symptoms in either type include, in addition to mouth breathing secondary to nasal obstruction, intense irritation in nose and eyes, sneezing, excessive nasal discharge, and watering of eyes. Local examination reveals that the nasal mucosa is pale/bluish and swollen. Nasal airway is diminished and there is watery nasal discharge. Conjunctiva is congested. There may also be bronchospasm.

Nasal Polyp

Nasal polyposis, meaning a pedunculated, hypertrophied edematous nasal mucosa supposedly due to allergy, infection or both, is an important cause of nasal obstruction and mouth breathing. Accompanying symptoms include persistent cold, sneezing, headache, hyposmia, and postnasal drip.

Foreign Body

A foreign body in the nose (say peas, beans, crayon, beads, buttons, pieces of pencil or plastic, maggots, etc.) produces inflammatory reaction. Nasal obstruction may lead to mouth breathing. Remaining symptoms include a unilateral bloodstained foul-smelling discharge.

Deviated Nasal Septum

Deviated nasal septum (DNS), when gross, may cause unilateral or bilateral nasal obstruction and mouth breathing together with dryness of mouth and pharynx, recurrent attacks of cold, headache and facial pain, epistaxis, cosmetic deformity, anosmia, and local tenderness due to pressure on anterior ethmoidal nerve, the so-called Studer's syndrome.

Mouth Breathing as a Habit

Not infrequently, children (so do adults) get into the habit of mouth breathing without any evidence of nasal obstruction or any reasonable cause.

FURTHER READING

1. Graham CE. *Obstructive Nasal Disease*. New York: Smith and Smith 2001.
2. Motta LJ II, Bachiega JC, Guedes CC, et al. Association between halitosis and mouth breathing in children. *Clinics (Sao Paulo)* 2011;66:939-942.
3. Robinson A. Nasal allergy. *Br Bull Allergy* 2004;7:33-36.

CHAPTER 47

Nystagmus

BACKGROUND

The term, *nystagmus*, means involuntary rapid movements (horizontal, vertical, rotatory, or mixed) of the eyeball, usually causing no or little disturbance to the subject. The most common form of nystagmus seen in pediatric practice is related to visual defects. As many as 22 out of the 40 infants and children with nystagmus seen during the recent months turned out to have one or the other defect of vision as the cause.

HISTORY

History should ascertain whether nystagmus has been there since early infancy or it occurred later. Is it spontaneous, or follows certain stimulus, say when the subject tries to fix at an object placed in an extreme lateral position (end-position nystagmus) or, when the eye attempts at fixing a stationary object while the subject is in a moving vehicle (optokinetic nystagmus)? Does the individual suffer from a visual problem? Is he on antiepileptic drugs, or agents such as aspirin or diphenoxylate hydrochloride? Does the patient have nodding spasm? Any history of associated nausea, vomiting, dizziness, ataxia or tremors?

PHYSICAL EXAMINATION

- Spin the child around for about 30 seconds. Then make him to stare at an object. If he has nystagmus, the eyes will first move slowly in one direction, then move rapidly in the opposite direction.
- Eye-movement recordings
- Neurologic examination.

Physical examination should, in particular, focus on vision and central nervous system (CNS) besides routine examination. Is there any evidence of albinism?

INVESTIGATIONS

Images of the brain, including
- Computerized tomography (CT)
- Magnetic resonance imaging (MRI).

IMPORTANT DIFFERENTIALS

Physiologic Nystagmus

Physiologic types of nystagmus require a stimulus before these occur. In a neonate (after the first week) and an infant, it is an expected finding, provided that the ocular muscles are functioning normally.

Train, railroad or optokinetic nystagmus is characterized by occurrence of rhythmic oscillations of the eyes occurring when an individual, travelling in a moving vehicle, attempts at fixating a nonmoving object.

End-position nystagmus is a nystagmus in the direction of fixating an object that has been placed in an extreme lateral position.

Organic Nystagmus

Visual defects constitute the most common cause of nystagmus. The defects include optic atrophy and astigmatism.

Optic atrophy, characterized by marked pallor of the disk and loss of nerve head substance, at times with enlargement of the disk cup, may be traumatic, inflammatory, degenerative, vascular or neoplastic. The chief causes in pediatric practice are hydrocephalus and space-occupying lesions (intracranial tumors).

Astigmatism, meaning a difference in the refractive power of the corneal meridians mostly due to irregularity in the curvature of the cornea and infrequently due to changes in the lens, manifests with eye strain, headache, fatigue, school failure/indifference, restlessness, and conjunctival hyperemia in addition to nystagmus.

Labyrinthine nystagmus is as, rule, unidirectional, showing horizontal or jerking movements with the eyes at rest. Accompanying symptoms include nausea, vomiting, and dizziness. The most common cause of this vestibular nystagmus is labyrinthitis, which may occur secondary to acute or chronic otitis media.

Congenital nystagmus may occur as congenital pendular nystagmus or congenital jerky nystagmus.

In congenital jerky nystagmus, in some instances familial, the subject shows horizontal jerky oscillations on lateral gaze with eyes at rest. The nystagmus is bilaterally symmetrical. In a particular eye, of course, nystagmus is coarser in one direction of gaze than in the other. Visual acuity and fixation are considerably affected. There always is a point at which nystagmus is least and the vision is the best. Hence, the patient has a strong tendency to adopt a compensatory posturing, turning the head to bring the eyes into the position of minimal nystagmus.

In congenital pendular nystagmus, associations with visual and/or ocular defects (albinism, congenital cataracts, congenital optic atrophy, total color blindness, retrolental fibroplasia, aniridia, achromatopsia, congenital macular defects, high refractory errors, etc.) are very common. Only in a small proportion, it occurs as a dominant or X-linked familial disorder without any evident ocular lesion. This form of nystagmus is characterized by rhythmical to-and-fro movements of the eyeball while the individual is looking forward or attempting to fixate an object.

Spasmus nutans is characterized by nystagmus that is very fine, rapid, horizontal, and pendular. It is nearly always bilateral. When unilateral, one eye is more involved than the other. Remaining components of the disorder, which is benign, self-limiting, and starts within the first 1–2 years of life, are head nodding and torticollis. The components of the disorder, however, may manifest at different times.

Albinism, a defect in the formation of melanin, is usually accompanied by nystagmus, the remaining manifestations depending upon whether it is generalized oculocutaneous type or partial type involving the eyes. Note that impartial type, involving localized areas of skin and hair, nystagmus is absent. The last-named is autosomal dominant.

Oculocutaneous albinism, also called as autosomal recessive albinism, has as many as six variants. In addition to nystagmus, an albino has extremely fair skin, fine silky hair, gray or blue iris, refractory errors with poor visual acuity, strabismus, and photophobia. Fundoscopy reveals that retina is devoid of pigment. Red reflex may be present.

In partial albinism (ocular variety), also called as X-linked albinism, the patient has poor visual acuity, depigmentation of iris and/or retina, photophobia, and nystagmus.

Nystagmus secondary to neurologic disease may occur in cerebellar ataxia, cerebellar tumor or abscess, hydrocephalus, Friedreich's ataxia or infratentorial tumors.

An interesting condition, characterized by rapid jerking of the eyeballs towards each other or into the orbit together with vertical gaze palsy usually secondary to hydrocephalus or pinealoma, is termed as convergent nystagmus or nystagmus retractorius.

Drugs may cause nystagmus through idiosyncrasy, overdose or as side effect. Drug-induced nystagmus is characterized by rhythmic jerking of the eyeball, which is more remarkable on the lateral gaze and by the slow component being towards the midline. The offending agents in this category include diphenylhydantoin sodium and other anticonvulsants, aspirin, diphenoxylate hydrochloride and colistin sulfate.

Nystagmus-simulating Eye Movements

Opsoclonus, occurring secondary to encephalitis or neuroblastoma, is characterized by chaotic movements of the eyeballs in various directions. The movements are nonrhythmic, spontaneous, and multidirectional.

Ocular motor dysmetria, occurring secondary to cerebellar disorder, is characterized by lack of precision in performing movements of refixation. When the individual attempts to look from one point to another, the eyes overshoot or undershoot with several corrective to-and-fro movements.

Flutter, occurring in cerebellar disease, is characterized by intermittent to-and-fro horizontal movements of the eyeballs which may occur spontaneously or on changing fixation.

FURTHER READING

1. American Academy of Ophthalmology. Nystagmus diagnosis. Available at: www.aao.org/eye-health/diseases/nystagmus-diagnosis. Accessed on: 24 July 2019.
2. Strominger M. Nystagmus. In: Nelson LB, Olitsky SE (Eds). *Harley's Pediatric Ophthalmology*, 5th edn. Philadelphia: Lippincott Williams and Wilkins 2005:475-507.

CHAPTER 48

Obesity

BACKGROUND

The term, *obesity*, denotes overweight, as a result of excessive accumulation of fat in the subcutaneous and other tissues. Thus, overweight in which body size is increased from increased lean body mass rather than accumulation of fat is, in reality, not obesity. Understandably, stocky children with large skeletal body frames and higher than the average muscular tissue, are bound to have weight, height, and overall body size that exceeds those of the average child of their age. They need not (in fact, they must not) be considered "obese".

HISTORY

When confronting an obese child, always ask parents if the child has an excessive appetite, and whether he indulges in overeating? It is useful to ask them to prepare a detailed daily intake chart of their child spread over a week's period, and then scan it to get as impression about his dietary intake on an average. Find out about his activities, including participation in sports. Does he watch too-much of television (TV)? Any drug intake (clonazepam, valproate, steroids, etc.). What is the status of his physical activity?

Is there any history of headache, vomiting, visual disturbances or poor school performance? Has the problem followed a serious illness like meningitis or encephalitis?

PHYSICAL EXAMINATION

The best parameter for evaluating obesity is the body mass index (BMI). It correlates well with both subcutaneous and total body fat while, at the same time, allowing a variation in lean body mass.

$$BMI = \frac{Weight\ (kg)}{Height\ (m)^2} = kg/m^2$$

Generally speaking BMI more than 95th percentile or more than 30 kg/m² for age establishes existence of obesity. However, in children, BMI of more than 25 kg/m² should be considered obesity.

Look for distribution of the fat (whether truncal or generalized) and for, any other malformations like polydactyly, syndactyly, hypogonadism, excessive hypotonia, hepatosplenomegaly (glycogenosis I-VG), short extremities and brachymetacarpia, especially of third, fourth, and fifth digits (pseudohypoparathyroidism), hypoplasia of dental enamel, tetany, respiratory distress, cyanosis, etc. had polycythemia.

In case of associated short stature, evaluate the anthropometry in details.

INVESTIGATIONS

- Blood sugar
- Fasting lipid panel for detection of dyslipidemia
- Thyroid function tests
- Serum leptin
- Adrenal function tests for Cushing syndrome
- Karyotyping
- Growth hormone secretion and function tests, when indicated
- Assessment of reproductive hormones (including prolactin), when indicated
- Serum calcium, phosphorus, and parathyroid hormone levels to evaluate for suspected pseudohypoparathyroidism
- *Cranial imaging*: Computed tomography (CT) scan, magnetic resonance imaging (MRI) of the brain with focus on the hypothalamus and pituitary.
- Genetic studies
- Urinary free cortisol, and overnight dexamethasone suppression test.

IMPORTANT DIFFERENTIALS

Exogenous Obesity

Obesity usually becomes evident in the first year of life, at 5–6 years of age and during adolescence. In a large majority of the cases, it is exogenous in etiology, i.e. energy intake exceeds expenditure leading to increased body fat stores. Such a child is overweight, i.e. weight over 20% of expected for height and relatively taller usually with advanced bone age. Facial features are fine with deposition of fat in the mammary regions of boys, giving an appearance of breast enlargement, which often puts the child in an embarrassing situation. Abdomen is pendulous with white or purple striae; even normal-sized external genitalia may remain imbedded in pubic fat and thus appear disproportionately small. Menarche may be somewhat advanced. Puberty occurs rather early, so that eventual height of the obese adolescent turns out to be less than the normal persons. Obesity is more evident in upper arms and thighs. Most of them have genu valgum. Social and psychological disturbances are common.

Endogenous Obesity

Cushing Syndrome

In infancy, manifestations include moon facies (rounded face with prominent cheeks and flushing), double chin, buffalo hump and generalized obesity, signs of masculinization (hypertrichosis over face and trunk, pubic hair, acne, deepening of voice, enlargement of clitoris), growth retardation, fragility despite a robust appearance, hypertension, congestive cardiac failure (CCF), vulnerability to infections, and congenital defects like hemihypertrophy.

In older children, manifestations include obesity, short stature, delayed puberty, purplish striae over abdomen, hips, and thighs, amenorrhea in girls past puberty, headache, weakness, emotional lability, poor school performance, hypertension, and renal stones.

Hypothyroidism

Obesity may occur in some children with congenital or acquired hypothyroidism. The diagnosis becomes obvious from the characteristic clinical profile.

Pseudohypoparathyroidism (Albright's syndrome or Albright's hereditary osteodystrophy): In addition to obesity, the patient has mental retardation, short stature, tetany, lenticular cataracts, brachydactyly with dimpling of the dorsum of the hands, brachymetacarpia, especially of third, fourth, and fifth digits with index finger being occasionally longer than the others, and hypoplasia of the enamel of the teeth. Serum calcium is low, whereas phosphorus and alkaline phosphatases are high.

Hypothalamic Dysfunction

In pituitary diencephalic syndrome, resulting from involvement of the hypothalamus following a central nervous system (CNS) infection, i.e. encephalitis, meningitis, etc., child may have obesity in addition to diabetes insipidus, disturbed temperature regulation, sleep abnormalities, etc.

In Frohlich's syndrome, resulting from damage to hypothalamic center, obesity is characteristically truncal. Additional manifestations are short stature hypogonadism, diabetes insipidus, visual disturbances, headache, seizures, and increased carbohydrate tolerance. The condition is extremely rare.

Polycystic Ovaries (Stein–Leventhal Syndrome)

Obesity is accompanied by hirsutism, secondary amenorrhea, and infertility. A combined rectal and abdominal examination shows palpable ovaries which are considerably enlarged.

Prader-Willi Syndrome

In this condition, obesity develops in association with hypotonia, hypogenitalism, mental retardation, and hyperphagia. Extreme obesity may cause respiratory embarrassment in some of the cases. Such cases may develop cyanosis, somnolence, and, at times, CCF. The so-called "obesity-hypoventilation" state, i.e. Pickwickian syndrome results because chest and diaphragmatic movements become restricted, causing rapid, shallow breathing, and alveolar ventilation reduction with ensuing hypoxemia.

Genetic Syndromes

Laurence-Moon-Biedl Syndrome

The boys with this syndrome have obesity, short stature, mental retardation, polydactyly (hexadactyly or syndactyly), and retinitis pigmentosa.

Turner Syndrome

In this disorder (usual chromosomal pattern 45 XO), obesity may add up to the characteristic features of the condition, say short stature, peripheral edema, lymphedema, extra skin fold, webbing of neck, gonadal dysplasia, renal, and CVS anomalies, etc.

Other Causes of Obesity

Drugs such as steroids and anticonvulsants, like clonazepam and valproate may also cause obesity.

FURTHER READING

1. Aulakh R, Chaudhry GK, Singh T. Obesity. In: Gupte S, Karoly H (Eds). *Pediatric Gastroenterology, Hepatology and Nutrition.* New Delhi: Peepee 2009:572-591.
2. Jain V, Gupte S, Koff AW. Pediatric endocrinology. In: Gupte S (Ed). *The Short Textbook of Pediatrics*, 13th edn. New Delhi: Jaypee 2020:739-760.
3. Prasad R, Singh UK. Obesity. In: Gupte S (Ed). *Recent Advances in Pediatrics (Special Vol 20: Nutrition, Growth & Development).* New Delhi: Jaypee 2009:208-218.

CHAPTER 49

Precocious Puberty

BACKGROUND

The term, *precocious puberty* or *sexual precocity*, denotes development of secondary sex characters before the anticipated age. In subtropical and tropical settings, the age landmark for boys is 10 years and for girls is 8 years. The guideline, is, however, purely arbitrary. Appearance, before the age of 8–10 years, of the following characters should arouse suspicion of this diagnosis: breast enlargement, menarche, excessive enlargement of penis or clitoris, dark and coarse axillary and pubic hair, change in voice, and acne.

Precocious puberty may be true or pseudopuberty. True precocious puberty is always isosexual, implying early appearance of the features of the same sex. Here, both secondary sex characters and maturation of gonads (spermatogenesis or ovulation) occur early enough. Precocious pseudopuberty is characterized by premature appearance of secondary sex characters and rapid somatic growth. The gonads, however, do not mature. Sex characters may be isosexual or heterosexual, the latter implying the appearance of secondary sex characters of the opposite sex.

HISTORY

History taking should pay special attention to the age at which sexual precocity was noticed by the parents. If it occurred right in infancy, chances are that the child has a significant organic problem. Occurrence of precocity in late childhood may mean just the normal variation, say early isosexual development or constitutional precocity.

It is also of value to determine the sibling's development as also parents' height and the age at which they had experienced puberty.

Ascertain if there has been history of head injury, or central nervous system (CNS) infection in the past. Does the infant develop dehydration easily?

PHYSICAL EXAMINATION

Girls

- Most reliable sign of increased estrogen production is breast enlargement. Initially, breast budding may be unilateral or asymmetric. Gradually, the breast diameter increases, the areola darkens and thickens, and the nipple becomes more prominent.
- Distinguishing glandular breast tissue from fat, which can mimic true breast tissue, is essential. Examining the patient while she is in the supine position usually minimizes the chance of misinterpreting fat as true breast enlargement.
- Genital examination may or may not reveal pubic hair. Enlargement of the clitoris indicates significant androgen excess. Vaginal mucosa, which is a deep-red color in prepubertal girls, takes on a moist pastel-pink appearance as estrogen exposure rises.
- Rapid onset of severe acne raises suspicion of an androgen-excess disorder.

Boys

- Earliest sign of central precocious puberty (CPP) is enlargement of the testes, which depends on increased production of follicle-stimulating hormone (FSH); testicular length is more than 2.5 cm or testicular volume (with Prader orchidometer beads) is 4 mL or more. If progressive signs of androgen excess occur in a boy without increased testicular size, consider possible causes of precocious pseudopuberty, including congenital adrenal hyperplasia, familial male precocious puberty, and Leydig cell tumors (a testicular nodule is usually palpable). Human chorionic gonadotropin (hCG) secreting tumors somewhat increase testicular size by stimulating testicular Leydig cell luteinizing hormone (LH) receptors.

- Other signs of puberty (say, penis growth, reddening and thinning of the scrotum, increased pubic hair, etc.) are a consequence of increased testosterone production and occur within 1–2 years after testicular enlargement.
- Pubic hair growth that occurs without penis and testicular enlargement and other signs of increased androgen production (say, premature adrenarche or a mild, nonclassic form of congenital adrenal hyperplasia) rather than true puberty.
- Later signs of puberty include the pubertal growth spurt, acne, voice change, and facial hair.

INVESTIGATIONS

After initial evaluation employing detailed medical history, and physical examination (including anthropometry and pubertal staging), endocrine evaluation should include:
- Measurement of LH, FSH, E2 gonadotropin-releasing hormone (GnRH) stimulation test, etc.
- Pelvic ultrasound for ovaries and uterus
- Measurement of 17 hydroxyprogesterone (17OHP), dehydroepiandrosterone sulfate (DHEAS), plasma insulin, etc.
- Follicle-stimulating hormone and LH
- Cranial magnetic resonance imaging (cMRI)

IMPORTANT DIFFERENTIALS

True Precocious Puberty

Constitutional Precocity

This condition is responsible for 80–90% of the girls and 50% of the boys with precocious puberty. There are no pathologic findings. It is surmised that the hypothalamic mechanism concerned with initiation of puberty gets activated precociously. Whereas the female cases are sporadic, in males the condition may be familial.

Besides precocious development of sex characters, these children, irrespective of the sex, height, weight, and osseous maturation, are advanced though eventually, because of early closer of the ossification centers, the stature turns out to be much less than it would have been normally.

McCune-Albright Syndrome

Also called as polyostotic fibrous dysplasia, this condition is characterized by fibrous dysplasia of the bones, patchy skin pigmentation, and endocrine disturbances in the form of precocious puberty as such or with Cushing syndrome or hyperthyroidism. The endocrine disturbances are now believed to originate not in the hypothalamus but as a result of autonomous hyperfunction of peripheral target glands.

In addition to the manifestations of precocity, such as menarche, the child may develop gigantism and/or acromegaly.

Organic Brain Lesions

Next to constitutional precocity in frequency come the organic brain tumors which are responsible for the condition in 10% of the girls and 40% of the boys. Pinealomas, gliomas, suprasellar teratomas, neurofibromas, astrocytomas, ependymomas, and hypothalamic hamartomas are examples of such tumors.

Any child presenting with true precocious puberty (particularly a boy) in association with hypothalamic manifestations such as diabetes insipidus, hypernatremia, hyperthermia, obesity, wasting, and unnatural crying or laughing must arouse suspicion of an intracranial tumor. Such manifestations as deterioration in mental faculty, seizures, and neurologic signs should also point to this diagnosis.

Hypothyroidism

It is now being increasingly recognized that half of the untreated cases of hypothyroidism may have varying degrees of isosexual development early enough for their osseous development.

Sex maturation usually encountered is breast development in girls and testicular enlargement in boys. Pubic and axillary hair growth is only sparse. Menstrual bleeding is common. Galactorrhea and excessive pigmentation occur in only a small proportion of the cases.

Rare Causes of True Precocious Puberty

Hepatoblastoma, hepatoma, intracranial chorioepithelioma, choriocarcinoma, polyembryoma of the posterior mediastinum, post-CNS infection, hydrocephalus, medicaments, etc.

Precocious Pseudopuberty

Adrenogenital Syndrome

Congenital adrenal hyperplasia, caused by an inborn defect in the biosynthesis of adrenal corticoids, may be responsible for precocious pseudopuberty.

Salt-sparing type is characterized by premature isosexual development, appearing by the age of 6 months or at 4–5 years or later in the male. In case of the female, it results in female pseudohermaphroditism. Right at birth, you may find evidence of masculinization in the form of enlargement of the clitoris and labial fusion. The clitoris may be large enough to look like a penis.

It causes virilization of the external genitalia in females and no genital change in males. Such accompanying manifestations as failure to regain birth weight, progressive weight loss, vomiting, poor feeding, dehydration, dyspnea, and cyanosis in a female with virilization of the external genitalia, therefore, virtually establish the clinical diagnosis.

Virilizing Adrenocortical Tumors

Precocious pseudopuberty in association with hypertension and features of Cushing syndrome suggest the diagnosis of tumors of the adrenal cortex. The fact that these symptoms occur in later life helps to differentiate this entity from the congenital adrenal hyperplasia which begins to manifest right at birth or soon after.

Feminizing Adrenal Tumors

These tumors may cause heterosexual precocious pseudopuberty in boys through excess of estrogen production.

Tumors of the Testes

Functional tumors of the testes are a rare cause of the precocious pseudopuberty in the form of gynecomastia and other signs of puberty. Clinical detection of a testicular tumor in a suspected case helps to diagnose this condition.

FURTHER READING

1. Carel JC, Lahlou N, Roger M, et al. Precocious puberty and statural growth. *Hum Reprod Update* 2004;10:135-147.
2. Medscape. Precocious puberty: Clinical presentation. Available at: medscape.com/article/924002-clinical#b4. Accessed on: 24 July 2019.
3. Neville KA, Walker JL. Precocious puberty is associated with SGA, prematurity, weight gain and obesity. *Arch Dis Child* 2005;90:258-261.
4. Venkataraman P, Sundararaman PG. Precocious puberty. In: Gupte S (Ed). *Recent Advances in Pediatrics (Special Vol 13: Pediatric Endocrinology)*. New Delhi: Jaypee 2004: 202-227.

CHAPTER 50

Purpura

BACKGROUND

The term, *purpura*, is employed to refer to a group of diseases in which small hemorrhages occur in the superficial layers of the skin, leading to areas of purple discoloration.

When purpura takes the shape of minute pinpoint hemorrhages (less than 1 mm diameter) about the small blood vessels, the latter are termed petechiae. When hemorrhages are extensive (over 5 mm diameter) the condition is called ecchymoses. For those between 2 mm and 5 mm, the term purpuric spots is used.

It is customary to designate purpura as thrombocytopenic or nonthrombocytopenic. In thrombocytopenic purpura, hemorrhages are secondary to remarkably reduced platelet count (less than 40,000/cmm). In nonthrombocytopenic purpura, platelet count is within normal limits and the cause of bleeding is either in the small blood vessels or secondary to the qualitative defect in platelet function.

HISTORY

History should include information whether purpura has occurred spontaneously in an otherwise healthy child or in an already ill child. Is there a preceding history of trauma, infection or drug intake? Is there bleeding from other sites, say epistaxis? Any history of previous episodes of purpura? Is there any accompanying joint or abdominal pain?

PHYSICAL EXAMINATION

Physical examination should ascertain the exact location, size, and distribution of the petechiae, purpuric spots, ecchymoses or hematomas (Fig. 50.1).

Changing color of bruise is a good guide to its age. Look for any bleeding from the mucosal sites such as mouth and rectum (Table 50.1). Is there any abnormal bleeding from the venipuncture sites? Any arthritis, evidence of intestinal obstruction (say, intussusception), or urticaria? Any signs of liver disease in the form of hepatosplenomegaly, icterus, liver palms, spider angiomata, or abnormal venous pattern? Any accompanying bony pain or tenderness, lymphadenopathy, or frank bleeding?

Find out if there is any abnormal skin elasticity and hyperextensibility of joints, pointing to inherited connective tissue disease.

It is useful to do Hess or tourniquet test. Mark an area 2.5 cm^2 on the flexor aspect of the forearm. Notice if any purpuric spots are present. Now apply the blood pressure cuff and record the systolic and diastolic pressures. Maintain the pressure between the two readings for 5 minutes. After the cuff is deflated, appearance of more than eight fresh spots in the circumscribed area indicates a positive test. In case numerous petechiae appear before the deadline of 5 minutes, deflate the cuff immediately.

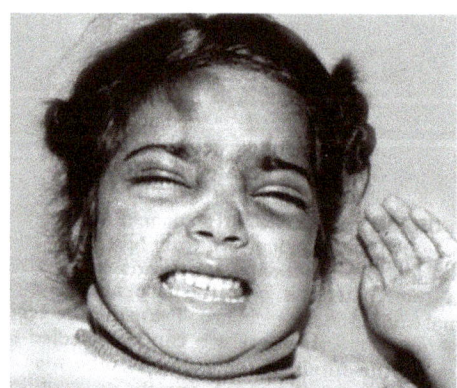

Fig. 50.1: Bruising and hematoma.

TABLE 50.1: Aging of bruises.	
Color	Age (days)
Red blue	1
Dark blue to blue-brown	1–3
Green yellow	7–10
Yellow brown	Over 8
Fading to pink	14–28

INVESTIGATIONS

- Complete blood picture (CBP)
- Bleeding time (BT), clotting time (CT), etc.
- Blood smear to exclude disseminated intravascular coagulation (DIC)
- Prothrombin time (PT)
- Activated partial thromboplastin time (APTT)
- Platelet count
- Mixing study
- Thrombin time.

IMPORTANT DIFFERENTIALS

Purpura in the Newborn

Normal Finding

Occasional petechiae over the face and forehead are the normal findings in the newborn. These may be accompanied by retinal hemorrhages, which can be detected on examination of the fundi. If the infant is otherwise well, this observation causes no anxiety since it disappears without any intervention. The cause appears to be the normal birth trauma.

Maternal Medication during Pregnancy

Drugs such as chloroquine, quinine, anticoagulants, anticonvulsants, salicylates, and thiazide diuretics taken by the mother during pregnancy may be responsible for purpura in the newborn.

Intrauterine Infections

Rubella: Almost one-half of the newborns with congenital rubella suffer from thrombocytopenic purpura. It is usually slight to moderate in intensity and resolved per se during the first month only.

Cytomegalovirus infection: Just like congenital rubella, cytomegalovirus infection too may cause thrombocytopenic purpura. In 50% of the severely affected newborn, the purpuric rash is generalized and tends to disappear in 48–72 hours. It is believed that the cytomegalovirus has a direct adverse effect on the bone marrow.

Toxoplasmosis: Infrequently, congenital toxoplasmosis may cause slight purpuric rash, usually in the form of small petechiae. More often, the rash is of maculopapular type. Remaining manifestations of the disease include fever, poor feeding, hepatosplenomegaly, lymphadenopathy, jaundice, hydrocephalus, microcephaly, microphthalmia, convulsions, cerebral calcification, and chorioretinitis singly or in combination.

Hemolytic Disease of the Newborn

Severe cases of Rh hemolytic disease, hydrops fetalis, may develop petechiae and purpuric spots due to thrombocytopenia and possibly concurrent consumptive coagulopathy.

Septicemia

Advanced fulminant septicemia (especially gram-negative) in the newborn may be accompanied by petechiae. Remaining manifestations of septicemia may include hyperthermia or hypothermia, icterus, feeding difficulty, poor activity, respiratory distress, abdominal distention, vomiting, hepatomegaly, and convulsions. A high index of suspicion in a newborn at risk assists in arriving at the diagnosis.

Immune Neonatal Thrombocytopenia

In one in three newborns of mothers suffering from active idiopathic thrombocytopenic purpura, widespread petechiae may appear within few minutes of birth. There may be evidence of hemorrhage from sites such as brain, kidney, and gastrointestinal tract. The disease is self-limited, taking 2–3 months to disappear.

Thrombocytopenia-absent Radius Syndrome

In this familial disorder (resembling Fanconi pancytopenia, an altogether different entity), severe bleeding manifestations appear on the very first day of life. Associated findings include aplasia of the radii and thumbs and cardiac and renal anomalies. There is absence of megakaryocytes from the bone marrow.

Disseminated Intravascular Coagulation (Consumptive Coagulopathy)

The newborn infant may manifest with petechiae or purpuric spots in a number of pathologic processes including septicemia (especially gram-negative), giant hemangioma, etc. There usually is evidence of bleeding from many sites, leading rapidly to severe anemia. Infarction of large areas of skin and subcutaneous tissue occurs. Investigations show prolongation of prothrombin, partial thromboplastin, and thrombin times, remarkable reduction in platelet count and fragmented burr and helmet-shaped red cells (schizocytes) and fibrin-split products (FSP).

Remaining Causes of Purpura in the Newborn

Congenital leukemia, renal vein thrombosis, generalized herpes, syphilis, galactosemia, etc.

Purpura in Later Infancy and Childhood

Thrombocytopenic Purpura

Immune (idiopathic) thrombocytopenic purpura (ITP): This is by far the most common of the thrombocytopenic purpuras seen in childhood. In the predominant form, acute type, an upper respiratory infection is followed in 1–4 weeks span by sudden onset of bruising, petechiae, and bleeding from the mucosal surfaces such as those of the nose, gums, gut, and urinary tract. There is no evidence of injury. Spleen may become just palpable in only 25% of the cases. After a few days, there is reduction in bleeding due to an improvement in capillary integrity though thrombocytopenia continues to be present. Most subjects completely recover in 6 months. Only a small proportion of cases pass on to the chronic stage.

Chronic type accounts for 10–15% of the cases of childhood ITP. There usually is a prolonged history of bleeding or a bruising tendency. The course is marked by relapses and remissions. Bleeding is, as a rule, less severe because of less severe involvement of the capillaries. Chronic ITP may persist for years at a stretch.

Diagnostic investigations should include tourniquet (Hess) test which is positive, bleeding time which is prolonged, clotting time which is normal, clot retraction which is poor, platelet count which is below 40,000/cmm, and bone marrow which shows normal or increased megakaryocytes. Some megakaryocytes are immatured with deep basophilic cytoplasm. Platelet budding may be scanty.

Drug-induced Thrombocytopenic Purpura

Drugs that may cause immune thrombocytopenic purpura include quinidine, quinine, apronalide, carbenicillin, cephalexin, penicillin, p-aminosalicylic acid (PAS), rifampicin, sulfadimidine, salicylates, indomethacin, phenylbutazone, trimethoprim, tolbutamide, acetazolamide, anticonvulsants, atropine, meprobamate, penicillamine, novobiocin, iodides, methimazole, actinomycin D, chlordiazepoxide, antihistamines, corticosteroids, and digoxin. In each and every instance of thrombocytopenic purpura, a careful search for a drug exposure should be made.

Hemolytic-Uremic Syndrome

This condition is characterized by an acute onset of renal failure, microangiopathic hemolytic anemia, and thrombocytopenic purpura. These features occur several days to weeks after an attack of gastroenteritis, an acute flu-like illness or an upper respiratory infection. The syndrome recurs over periods of several years.

Investigations reveal a gross hemolytic anemia. Reticulocyte count is high. Red cells show fragmented, helmet-shaped, and burr cells. Platelet count falls below 100,000/cmm within the first week of onset. Azotemia and electrolyte imbalance may be present. Serum uric acid and lactate dehydrogenase (LDH) activity are high. Hematuria and proteinuria with red blood cells (RBCs) or granular casts are usually present. Some cases may show paradoxical hypokalemia.

Wiskott-Aldrich Syndrome

This syndrome is characterized by a triad of recurrent infection, eczema, and thrombocytopenic purpura due to an X-linked recessive immunologic defect. Bloody diarrhea, and hemorrhage during the first month of life are the first symptoms. Hepatosplenomegaly develops in due course of time. There is an increased incidence of lymphoreticular malignancy.

Thrombopoietin Deficiency

In this rare disorder, chronic thrombocytopenic purpura results from a deficiency of a megakaryocyte maturation factor that is an integral component of normal plasma.

Kasabach-Merritt Syndrome

A large cavernous hemangioma of the trunk, limbs or abdominal viscera may trap and destroy platelets within its extensive vascular bed, causing severe thrombocytopenia and other evidence of consumptive coagulopathy. Bone marrow shows adequate number of megakaryocytes. Spontaneous recovery may occur.

Nonthrombocytopenic Purpura

Henoch–Schönlein purpura: Also called as anaphylactoid purpura, the condition is perhaps the most common type of purpura seen in pediatric practice. In all probability, it is a collagen disorder characterized by widespread purpuric lesions (particularly urticaria-like skin eruptions) due to angitis with involvement of abdominal viscera and/or joints. Henoch purpura is dominated by signs of acute abdomen. At times, the picture almost mimics that of intestinal obstruction, volvulus intussusception or appendicitis. Schönlein purpura is dominated by signs of arthritis, especially of the knees and ankles. At times, it could be mistaken for rheumatic or rheumatoid arthritis.

Hematologic Investigations Reveal Normal Results

Thrombocytopathic purpura: Also called as thrombasthenia, this condition is characterized by appearance of petechiae and excessive bleeding due to platelets which are normal quantitatively but have defective function.

Purpura Fulminans

This serious condition occurs as a complication of a bacterial or viral infection, usually chickenpox or scarlet fever, during the convalescent phase. Manifestations include acute onset of shock, toxicity, fever, and diffuse symmetrical hemorrhages with overwhelming inflammatory vasculitis and necrosis of skin and subcutaneous tissues, especially over the buttocks and lower limbs. In those who manage to survive, sloughing of large areas of skin and muscle results. Platelet count is usually adequate.

Hereditary Hemorrhagic Telangiectasia

Also termed as Osler–Weber–Rendu disease, this autosomal dominant disease usually causes purpura at puberty. The mucocutaneous lesions are 1–4 mm macules, papules, or spider-like projections made of tortuous telangiectatic vessels. Recurrent epistaxis may occur before skin and mucous membrane lesions become apparent. Bleeding from the lesions may occur spontaneously or following slight trauma. Massive hemorrhage may cause severe anemia.

von Willebrand Disease

This autosomal disorder, also called as pseudohemophilia, is characterized by purpura and disproportionately excessive bleeding following minor trauma. Bleeding time is prolonged, whereas clotting time is normal.

The cause appears to be operation by an unidentified plasma factor that leads to reduced synthesis of clotting factor VII and abnormal platelet adhesiveness. A capillary defect is also described.

Ehlers-Danlos Syndrome

This syndrome is characterized by hyperextensibility of joints, hyperelasticity of skin, remarkable friability of skin and blood vessels and subcutaneous nodules, easy bruising and purpura. Eight distinct forms of the syndrome, which is supposed to be a collagen defect, are recognized.

Meningococcemia

A child presenting with petechiae, purpuric spots or ecchymotic lesions in the presence of meningeal irritation should be regarded as suffering from meningococcemia unless proved otherwise. You should lance the skin lesions and smear the material for gram-negative diplococci. In order to establish the diagnosis, organisms need to be cultured from blood, cerebrospinal fluid (CSF), skin lesions or other locations of infection.

Dengue Hemorrhagic Fever

Purpura is a feature of second stage of dengue hemorrhagic fever (DHF). Classically, hemorrhagic manifestations are usually cutaneous but bleeding may occur from other locations. In the epidemic seen by us in Jammu in the fall and autumn of 1993, gastrointestinal hemorrhage dominated the scene. Box 50.1 presents the clinical picture of DHF and dengue shock syndrome (DSS) in relation to various grades.

The DHF/DSS is believed to be a hypersensitivity response to a repeat attack with a dengue fever virus. According to Halstrea's antibody-dependent immune enhancement theory, prior sensitization with dengue fever virus causes collection of subneutralizing concentrations of antibodies to the virus. Presence of these sensitized antibodies leads to an enhanced replication of the dengue virus. Once T-cells recognize infected monocytes, cytokines are released. These cytokines activate the complement and clotting cascade. What follows is the release of vasoactive mediators, resulting in enhanced capillary permeability. Capillary leakage causes bleeding, shock, and hypoproteinemia.

Diagnosis is by and large clinical. A high index of suspicion, especially during an epidemic, is the cornerstone of diagnosis. Thrombocytopenia, though never severe enough, hemoconcentration and a right-sided pleural effusion are quite characteristic.

For specific confirmation of the diagnosis, virus isolation is ideal. However, since it is quite time-consuming, in practice, demonstration of a four-fold rise in immunoglobulin M (IgM)-antibody titer is considered good enough.

BOX 50.1: Standard grading of dengue hemorrhagic fever (DHF) or dengue shock syndrome (DSS) as recommended by World Health Organization (WHO).

- Grade 1: Fever, nonspecific constitutional manifestations, tourniquet (Hess) test positive
- Grade 2: Grade 1 + spontaneous bleeding (cutaneous or other locations)
- Grade 3: Grades 1 and 2 + circulatory failure (shock) manifested by rapid weak pulse, low blood pressure, low pulse pressure, cold and clammy skin, restlessness
- Grade 4: Profound shock (unrecordable blood pressure and pulse) dominates the scene.

FURTHER READING

1. Blanchatte V. Childhood chronic immune thrombocytopenic purpura (ITP). *Blood Rev* 2002;16:23-26.
2. Montgomery RR. Platelet and blood vessel disorders. In: Kliegmoon RM, St Geme JII JW, Blum NJ, et al (Eds). *Nelson Textbook of Pediatrics*, 21st edn. Philadelphia: Elsevier 2020:2081-2089.
3. Sobti P, Chandra J, Gupte S. Pediatric hematology. In: Gupte S (Ed). *The Short Textbook of Pediatrics*, 13th edn. New Delhi: Jaypee 2020:631-664.

CHAPTER 51

Fever of Unknown Origin

BACKGROUND

Currently, fever of unknown origin (FUO) is defined as a prolonged fever of 3 weeks or more duration without obvious cause on evaluation and simple investigations carried out at outpatient level or after 1 week of evaluation in the hospital.

In etiology, infections continue to dominate the scene with over 60% cases being due to them (Box 51.1). Important causative infection in FUO are typhoid, urinary tract infection (UTI), malaria, and tuberculosis Nevertheless, as the illness becomes more prolonged, their incidence considerably falls down giving space to less common causes such as connective tissue/autoimmune disorders [say rheumatoid arthritis, systemic lupus erythematosus (SLE), Kawasaki disease, etc.] followed by malignancies (say leukemia, lymphomas, etc.).

Occasionally, drug fever (with intense itching), diabetes insipidus, sensory autonomic neuropathies, etc. may be responsible for FUO.

At the outset, make sure that it is not a factitious fever. Diagnostic evaluation revolves around detailed history and physical examination followed by screening tests. With feedback from these, if the need be, further tests and imaging studies may be carried out.

Clinical workup is very important in evaluation of an FUO case. The aim of the whole exercise is to find clues that may point to a specific infection or area of suspicion.

BOX 51.1: Etiology of pyrexia of unknown origin (PUO).

Infectious diseases
- Enteric fever
- Malaria
- Tuberculosis
- Urinary tract infection (UTI)
- Infective endocarditis
- Human immunodeficiency virus (HIV) or acquired immunodeficiency syndrome (AIDS) with opportunistic infection
- Viral hepatitis
- Liver abscess (occult)
- Kala-azar
- Rickettsial fever
- Spirochetal fever
- Brucellosis
- Leptospirosis

Autoimmune disorders
- Juvenile rheumatoid arthritis
- Systemic lupus erythematosus (SLE)
- Kawasaki disease
- Rheumatic fever
- Polyarteritis nodosa
- Inflammatory bowel disease (IBD)

Malignancies
- Leukemia
- Lymphomas
- Wilms tumor
- Neuroblastoma
- Pheochromocytoma
- Histiocytosis (Langerhans cell type)

Miscellaneous
- Drug fever
- Serum sickness
- Diabetes insipidus
- Chronic active hepatitis
- Sickle cell crisis
- Ichthyosis.

HISTORY

History should elicit details about onset and other aspects of fever, e.g. whether continuous, intermittent or remittent; whether tertian, quotidian or quartan; whether accompanied by chills and rigors; accompanying manifestations. Age of the patient needs consideration. Adolescents, in addition to other childhood conditions are more likely to have tuberculosis, inflammatory bowel disease (IBD), autoimmune disease or lymphoma. Likewise, likelihood of a respiratory infection, genitourinary infection, abscess, and osteomyelitis in more than 6-year olds is high.

History of pica may arouse suspicion of visceral larva migrans (*Toxocara canis*) and toxoplasmosis (*Toxoplasma gondii*). History of exposure to wild animals or pets may point to a zoonotic infection. History of use of medication such as atropine eye drops which may be responsible for atropine-induced fever.

Personal History

In the very first instance, as you would appreciate, it is important to establish that the child indeed has pyrexia. How have the parents been recording the temperature? Mouth or rectal temperature is decidedly more reliable than the groin or axilla temperature. The latter site gives a record of the skin temperature, which is considerably influenced by the environmental temperature and whether the child is overclothed or underclothed. Also it is worth remembering that, even in healthy children, temperature recording just following some vigorous activity may give an erroneously high reading of up to 37.7°C (100°F).

Find out the exact length of time the child has been suffering from fever. Is the fever continuous, remittent or intermittent? In continuous fever, the temperature never touches the normal temperature though there may be fluctuation not exceeding 1°C (1.5°F) during the 24 hours. In remittent fever, the daily temperature fluctuation is more than 2°C (3°F). When fever is present only for several hours during the day, the temperature remaining normal rest of the time, it is called intermittent fever. Intermittent fever may be "quotidian" when temperature touches normal daily, "tertian" when it happens so on alternate days, or "quartan" if it happens every 2 days.*

Always enquire about history of medication for fever or preceding it. Antipyretics with or without chemotherapy may alter the true pattern of fever. Drug fever is usually an isolated symptom, the temperature remaining high at a particular level. Usually within 72 hours of its withdrawal, the temperature returns to normal, except in the case of agents such as iodides where fever may take up to a month to resolve. Do not miss asking about the intake of over-the-counter (OTC) agents and topical preparations including eye drops, e.g. atropine-induced fever.

It is important to enquire about the chronologic development of symptoms accompanying fever, preceding acute diarrheal disease, boil or such other infectious illnesses, contact with an individual suffering from tuberculosis, etc. Are there any localizing manifestations that may provide a clue to the organ system which is involved?

PHYSICAL EXAMINATION

A detailed head-to-toe examination at the outset and every day is important to catch any emerging findings as a clue to the causative condition. Make a note of child's overall general activity and nutritional status.

- *Sweating*: Persistent absence of sweating despite high fever should arouse suspicion of dehydration, nephrogenic diabetes insipidus, anhidrotic ectodermal dysplasia, familial dysautonomia, and atropine-induced fever.
- *Eye findings*: A good ophthalmic examination may turn out to be revealing.
  - Petechial hemorrhages suggest infective endocarditis.
  - Uveitis points to juvenile rheumatoid arthritis, SLE, Kawasaki disease, Behcet disease, and vasculitis.
  - Chorioretinitis may suggest toxoplasmosis, cytomegalovirus (CMV), rubella, and syphilis.
  - Proptosis may mean orbital tumor, chloroma, thyrotoxicosis, neuroblastoma secondaries, orbital infection pseudotumor, and Wegener's granulomatosis.
  - Failure of pupillary constriction may point to hypothalamic dysfunction as the cause of FUO.
  - Lack of tears with absent corneal reflex suggests familial dysautonomia.
- *Ear, nose, and throat (ENT) findings*: Tenderness over sinuses or the upper teeth suggests sinusitis.
- *Oral cavity*
  - Recurrent oral candidiasis suggests immune system disorders.
  - Fever blisters point to pneumococcal, streptococcal, malaria, and rickettsial infections and sometime to salmonella and staphylococcal infections.
- Muscle/bone tenderness
  - *Generalized*: Kawasaki disease, dermatomyositis, polyarteritis, trichinosis, mycoplasma or arbovirus infection.
  - *Point tenderness*: Occult osteomyelitis, bone marrow invasion from neoplastic disease.
  - *Tenderness of trapezius*: Subdiaphragmatic abscess.
- *Rectal examination*: It may reveal per rectal adenopathy or deep pelvic abscess, iliac adenitis or pelvic osteomyelitis.
  - *Occult blood*: It may point to ulcerative colitis or granulomatous colitis as the cause of FUO.
- Hyperactive deep tendon reflexes suggest thyrotoxicosis.
- Chills and rigors suggest sepsis, malaria, UTI, abscess, infective endocarditis, brucellosis, rat-bite fever, etc.

Currently, the term, *pyrexia of unknown origin* (PUO), denotes a prolonged fever of 3 weeks or more duration without obvious cause on evaluation and simple investigations carried out at outpatient level or after 1 week of evaluation in the hospital.

---

*Undoubtedly, a core or central temperature reading (mouth or rectal) is the best. In most of the situations a peripheral reading, i.e. axillary is good enough. An inexperienced parent or attendant may cause injury to the child from broken glass. Note that axillary temperature is, as a rule, 0.5°C less than that recorded centrally. Also, note that for recording the mouth temperature, a thermometer must be left *in situ* for at least 2 minutes (preferably 3 minutes), in order to obtain correct reading. The so-called "strip thermometers" (disposable) for use over the forehead are available, but these are usually less accurate.

The problem is one of the common reasons for pediatric consultations and may often prove quite perplexing even with the support of reasonable laboratory facilities. Nevertheless, it needs to be clearly understood that most cases of PUO result from common diseases that may be atypical rather than classic in their presentation. In our as well as others' experience, over 50% of the pediatric subjects with PUO are due to infections.

Physical examination should be thorough with special search for lymphadenopathy, hepatosplenomegaly, and deep in-apparent abscess such as subphrenic or liver abscess. You must make a careful search for skin rashes and petechial hemorrhages in skin, fundi, nail beds, and conjunctiva.

Fever blisters may be a manifestation of pneumococcal, streptococcal, meningococcal, malarial or rickettsial infection. Rarely, they may occur in salmonella or staphylococcal infection.

Repetitive chills and rigors are common in malaria, or septicemia accompanying UTI, infective endocarditis, or localized collection of large amount of pus. Remember, young children may fail to convey their parents, their perception of extraordinary cold chills. Nonetheless, the rigors can be always observed as vigorous shaking movements of the body.

Oral thrush may point to an immunologic disorder.

Congestion of the pharynx suggests salmonellosis, infectious mononucleosis, toxoplasmosis or cytomegalic inclusion disease.

Generalized muscle tenderness may mean arboviral or mycoplasmal infection, dermatomyositis polyarteritis or trichinosis. Localized tenderness over the trapezius muscle may point to a subdiaphragmatic abscess. Point tenderness over a bone may suggest osteomyelitis or a neoplasm invading the marrow.

Absence of sweating in the presence of fever may mean diabetes insipidus, anhidrotic ectodermal dysplasia, exposure to atropine or familial dysautonomia.

Persistent red eye may be a sign of a collagen disorder such as polyarteritis nodosa.

Thyrotoxicosis may be suggested by hyperactive deep tendon reflexes.

Rectal examination may point to iliac adenopathy, pelvic abscess or osteomyelitis.

The presence of occult blood in stools may mean ulcerative colitis as the cause of PUO.

INVESTIGATIONS

- Cerebral perfusion pressure (CPP), including peripheral film for malarial parasite
- Erythrocyte sedimentation rate (ESR)
- C-reactive protein (CRP)
- Urinalysis, including microscopy
- *Cultures*: Blood, urine, stool, etc.
- Epstein-Barr virus (EBV) and CMV serology
- Fecal calprotectin testing in suspected cases of inflammatory bowel disease
- Tuberculin test
- Imaging studies
  - Chest X-ray and paranasal sinus (PNS) X-ray
  - Paranasal sinus ultrasonography
  - Abdominal ultrasonography
  - Skeletal X-ray examination, magnetic resonance imaging (MRI) or a bone scan are indicated if osteomyelitis is suspected.
  - A white blood cell scan, a nuclear medicine procedure, may be beneficial in some cases in order to localize the focus of it.

IMPORTANT DIFFERENTIALS

Infections

Bacterial Infections

Localized bacterial infections: These include walled or closed-off abscesses, UTI, osteomyelitis, sinusitis, chronic mastoiditis, chronic appendicitis, and periappendicitis.

Closed-off abscesses, subphrenic abscess, and liver abscess may be responsible for PUO without any other apparent symptoms and signs. A persistent fever following attack of abdominal pain may mean subphrenic abscess following perforation of appendix. A careful palpation during inspiration and expiration may reveal that liver is palpable and tender though absence of these findings does not necessarily rule out the possibility of subphrenic or liver abscess. An X-ray must be obtained for presence of gas under the diaphragm which too may be raised.

Perinephric abscess as a cause of unexplained fever may cause considerable difficulties in arriving at its diagnosis. It may follow rupture of a renal carbuncle or pyonephrosis into the tissue around the kidney, or a staphylococcal skin infection. The availability of history of trauma preceding it may, therefore, be an important clue. Clinical findings include diffuse swelling, edema, and erythema in the lumbar region, percussion tenderness of the costovertebral angle, and renal tenderness on bimanual examination. Rigors, toxemia, and limp or fixed flexion of the hip on the affected side are likely to be present. Intermittent pyuria is usual. X-ray shows a bulging psoas shadow. Intravenous pyelogram (IVP) shows obliteration of the psoas shadow with displacement of the affected kidney and ureter.

Lung abscess should be suspected if there is history of aspiration of a foreign body or severe coughing episodes of short duration, particularly when accompanied by hemoptysis and production of copious amount of foul smelling or purulent sputum. Areas of bronchial breathing with amphoric breathing are found on auscultation. X-ray of chest shows a cavity (with or without a fluid level) surrounded by alveolar infiltration. A mixture of anaerobic bacteria may be detected in the sputum.

Brain abscess should be suspected in cases of unexplained fever in association with headache, particularly when accompanied by neck stiffness. You must explore history of a focus of infection in the neighborhood (discharging ear, scalp infection, sinusitis, etc.), bronchiectasis or congenital heart disease. Total leukocyte count (TLC) shows polymorphonuclear leukocytosis. ESR is raised. Cerebrospinal fluid (CSF) shows high protein and high white blood cell count with predominance of lymphocytes. You must remember to avoid doing lumbar puncture when intracranial pressure is elevated. Electroencephalograph (EEG), computed tomography (CAT) scan, and radionuclide scan are useful diagnostic tools in reaching the diagnosis.

Pelvic abscess should be expected in the presence of abdominal distention, bladder irritability, and rectal tenesmus with or without the passage of small fecal matter containing mucus. A tender mass may be felt on rectal examination.

Appendiceal abscess is suggested by a tenderness in the right lower quadrant, usually in association with a palpable lump.

Dental abscess may be suggested by a localized swelling and redness with chronically draining fistula.

- *Urinary tract infection:* This is by far the most common cause of pediatric PUO without abnormal findings. The diagnosis is by high index of suspicion. One or two negative urine examinations certainly do not exclude it. Of course, repeated negative tests reduce its possibility. Suprapubic aspiration of urine may be warranted to avoid contamination of the sample.
- *Osteomyelitis:* A low-grade osteomyelitis/ostitis may persist over several weeks before the classical signs become apparent. You must, therefore, make it a habit to palpate all the bones for local tenderness in every child with PUO. Also, look for minor limitation of movements. If tenderness or pain is suspected, an X-ray should be taken.
- *Mastoiditis:* Inflammation of the mastoid air cell system as a complication of otitis media (both acute and chronic) is a frequent cause of obscure pyrexia in children. The patient has earache but he may be able to give expression to it only in the form of incessant crying or pulling at the ear. X-ray reveals a cloudy mastoid.
- *Sinusitis:* At times, protracted sinusitis may remain undetected as a cause of obscure pyrexia over considerable period. A meticulous clinical examination usually brings out the diagnosis which can be confirmed by radiologic examination.
- *Chronic appendicitis and periappendicitis:* Occasionally, these conditions, representing the sequelae of a conservatively managed acute appendicitis, may be responsible for unexplained prolonged pyrexia. Nausea, anorexia or localized pain usually accompanies the clinical picture. Guarding and pain during bimanual rectal and abdominal palpation often suggest the diagnosis. High ESR and leukocytosis with left shift of the white cells—both signs of chronic inflammation—are invariably present.

Generalized bacterial infections: Various generalized bacterial infections are as follows

- *Tuberculosis:* In India and other developing countries, tuberculosis is a leading cause of prolonged pyrexia of obscure origin. Tuberculin (Mantoux) or BCG diagnostic test together with X-ray of chest often help to clinch the diagnosis, particularly if there is history of tuberculosis in the family or close neighborhood. Diagnosis of central nervous system (CNS) tuberculosis needs lumbar puncture as also fundoscopic examination for presence of choroid tubercles.
- *Enteric fever:* Salmonellosis, especially typhoid and paratyphoid fever, is characterized by a soft palpable spleen in association with prolonged pyrexia. Rose spots, so prominently highlighted by the Western books, are seldom seen in patients in the tropics and subtropics.
- *Septicemia*: Low-grade septicemia may cause unexplained prolonged fever without any abnormal physical signs. This sort of situation is encountered usually in gram-negative septicemia in children with impaired immunity. Repeated blood cultures are strongly recommended in such instances.
- *Infective endocarditis*: Obscure pyrexia in a child with congenital or acquired heart disease, particularly with chills, may well be indicative of infective endocarditis. You must look for petechiae, more so under the nails, splenomegaly, and hematuria to clinch the diagnosis.
- *Brucellosis*: Chronic brucellosis is an important, though infrequent, cause of PUO. Complaints such as fatigue, sweating, myalgia, arthralgia, anorexia nervousness, depression, and a rash in the presence of hepatosplenomegaly and lymphadenopathy should arouse suspicion of this diagnosis. Diagnosis is confirmed by brucella agglutination test which shows titers more than 1:160 and isolation of brucella organism by cultures of blood or infected material such as abscess or tissue.
- *Tularemia*: In this uncommon infection, fever is usually accompanied by chills, myalgia, arthralgia, vomiting, headache, anemia, photophobia, maculopapular rash, and diaphoresis. There is also lymphadenitis, ulcerated skin and/or mucosal lesions or conjunctivitis. A history of contact with rabbit, ingestion of rabbit or squirrel

meat, or bite by fly, tick or some other vector should suggest the diagnosis. Diagnostic tests include smear and gram stains of sputum or some other infected material, serum agglutination test, skin testing, and direct culture of the organisms.

- *Yersinial infection*: Occasionally, *Yersinia enterocolitica* or pseudotuberculosis may account for unexplained fever. *Yersinia enterocolitica* causes usually appendicitis-like disease with mesenteric adenitis and terminal ileitis manifesting as severe abdominal pain. Diagnosis is by identification of the organisms in stools, blood culture, and passive hemagglutination tests.

Viral Infections

Viral hepatitis: Anicteric hepatitis may well be responsible for unexplained fever. Anorexia, nausea/vomiting, enlarged, and tender liver. High-colored urine and light-colored stools point to this diagnosis, warranting investigations. Chronic active hepatitis may at the onset manifest with only unexplained fever. Other symptoms, though present, are so minimal that they go unnoticed. You must ascertain if the patient has fluctuating jaundice, fatigue, anorexia, hepatosplenomegaly, gastrointestinal bleeding, arthralgia, edema, colitis, etc.

Serum glutamic oxaloacetic transaminase (SGOT) and serum glutamic pyruvic transaminase (SGPT) are remarkably raised. Hyperbilirubinemia is mild to severe. Prothrombin time is usually prolonged.

Cytomegalic inclusion disease: Acquired cytomegalovirus (CMV) infection may occasionally become responsible for obscure pyrexia in premature newborns and infants (1–2 months old) who are residents for a prolonged period in intensive care unit and those having been given blood transfusions from seropositive donors. The infant manifests a septic look, gray pallor, fast deterioration in respiratory status, hepatosplenomegaly, and atypical lymphocytosis. In immunosuppressed subjects, chorioretinitis may be detected.

Acquired disease in older children presents with sore throat, malaise, myalgia, anorexia, headache, abdominal pain, cervical or other regional lymphadenopathy, hepatosplenomegaly, and excessive sleep. Fever with chills may persist for 2 or more weeks. Liver dysfunction and atypical lymphocytosis are prominent.

Infectious mononucleosis: This disease caused by EBV of the herpes group is characterized by malaise, fever, sore throat, lymphadenopathy, hepatosplenomegaly, atypical lymphocytosis, and a heterophilic antibody response. Clinically, it is very difficult to distinguish it from acquired CMV disease. The latter is heterophil-negative rather than positive.

Acquired immunodeficiency syndrome (AIDS): Prolonged or intermittent pyrexia is an important feature of pediatric AIDS, especially when the human immunodeficiency virus (HIV) infection follows a transfusion. Accompanying lymphadenopathy, failure to thrive, and chronic/recurrent infections like candida in a vulnerable situations, must arouse suspicion of pediatric AIDS.

Parasitic Infections

Malaria: It may present in pediatric practice with obscure fever which is irregular rather than with classical febrile episodes, more so in children less than 5 years of age. Accompanying manifestations may include body pains, headache, nausea, abdominal pain, and splenomegaly. In falciparum malaria, in particular, fever is less classical and may even be continuous. Severe manifestations pertaining to cerebral, respiratory, urinary or gastrointestinal system are usually a feature of falciparum infection. In algid malaria, shock is followed by coma. Repeated attacks of malaria in malnourished children in endemic areas may lead to a very large and firm splenomegaly as an abnormal immune response to the parasite. This condition, a sort of chronic malaria, has been termed as tropical splenomegaly, idiopathic splenomegaly or big spleen disease.

Diagnosis of malaria is confirmed by identifying the parasite in properly stained thick and thin blood smear.

Toxoplasmosis: Acquired toxoplasmosis may present with unexplained fever with or without malaise, myalgia, generalized lymphadenopathy, hepatomegaly, pneumonia, myocarditis, encephalitis, and maculopapular rash. Dye test is the most sensitive and dependable tool for detecting the antibodies of causative organism, *Toxoplasma gondii*, in human sera.

Visceral larva migrans: This parasitic infection, caused by larvae of toxocara species (hence the other name toxocariasis) occurring in preschool children suffering from pica and coming in close contact with dogs and cats, may cause an obscure pyrexia. Remaining manifestations may include wheezy bronchitis, convulsions, hepatomegaly, papular or urticarial skin lesions, lymphadenopathy, and abdominal pain. Eosinophilia is more or less a rule. Chest X-ray shows scattered patchy infiltrates. Enzyme-linked immunosorbent assay (ELISA) is the only dependable diagnostic tool available at present.

Trichinosis: Occasionally, trichinosis may be responsible for unexplained fever. In the presence of periorbital edema, myalgia (most marked in masseters, intercostals, and diaphragm) and eosinophilia, especially if there is history of eating uncooked meat, this possibility must be seriously considered. The diagnosis is established by serologic studies and muscle biopsy.

Rickettsial Infection

Rickettsial diseases, Q fever, and rocky mountain spotted fever, may cause unexplained pyrexia in endemic areas. These are virtually nonexistent in the Indian subcontinent.

Chlamydial Infection

Psittacosis: Also called as ornithosis, this disease is usually characterized by an abrupt onset with fever, sore throat, headache, malaise, myalgia, cough, nausea, vomiting, and mental confusion. Hepatosplenomegaly, carditis, and pneumonia may occur. Fever may persist for 3 weeks or more.

Lymphogranuloma venereum: This disease, caused by an agent related to *Chlamydia trachomatis*, is sexually transmitted and occurs in children from an infected adult. It is a systemic disease and may cause obscure febrile illness together with malaise, anorexia, headache, a pustule or a papule, inguinal lymphadenitis, and terminally, elephantiasis. The diagnosis is confirmed by isolation of the organism from infected lymph nodes.

Fungal Infection

Histoplasmosis: Disseminated histoplasmosis is an important though infrequent cause of PUO. Remaining manifestations include acute lower respiratory infection, nausea, vomiting, abdominal pain, and diarrhea. Diffuse lymphadenopathy and hepatosplenomegaly are invariably present. X-ray of chest shows a diffuse interstitial pneumonia.

Blastomycosis: A child with PUO presenting with any combination of lung, skin, bone or genitourinary disease should arouse suspicion of blastomycosis. Identification of the yeast forms of *Blastomyces dermatitidis* in sputum, abscess or biopsy material and isolation of the organism confirms the diagnosis.

Collagen Disorders

Juvenile Rheumatoid Arthritis

This is an important cause of unexplained pyrexia. Onset of the disease may be with a precipitous (sleepy) fever with chills or episodes of remittent fever lasting for quite a few weeks. Accompanying manifestations may include weight loss, anorexia, excessive sweating, an exanthem, lymphadenopathy, splenomegaly, morning stiffness of affected joints, cyanosis of the adjoining skin, conjunctivitis, and photophobia. Diagnosis is based mainly on clinical evaluation as well as on exclusion of other conditions. Rheumatoid factor is positive in as low as just 5% of the affected children.

Systemic Lupus Erythematosus

This diagnosis must be entertained in cases of obscure pyrexia. Once the typical butterfly rash appears on the face, the diagnosis becomes evident. Remaining manifestations of the disease include hepatosplenomegaly, polyserositis, arthritis, lymphadenopathy, hypertension, albuminuria, thrombocytopenia, abdominal pain, and puncta on palms and fingers.

Diagnosis is established by demonstrating antinuclear antibodies (ANA) which is a more sensitive test than LE preparation.

Dermatomyositis

In this rare disorder, clinical manifestations include fever, muscle tenderness and pain, weight loss, malaise, pseudoparalysis, arthralgia, and an erythematous rash which first develops over the bridge of the nose and around eyes and then anywhere over trunk and limbs. An edematous swelling of the malar area and visible capillaries in the nail bed and gum margin are highly suggestive. Eventually, the affected muscles become firm, atrophic, and contracted. Calcinosis may occur. The face may develop an expressionless appearance, the child hardly being able to open the mouth in hilly areas.

Polyarteritis Nodosa

This rare disorder too can present with obscure fever. Remaining manifestations include weight loss, generalized body pains, abdominal pain, skin eruptions, subcutaneous nodules, hypertension, hematuria, convulsions, paralysis, congestive cardiac failure, and ischemic gangrene of a limb.

Malignancies

Hodgkin Lymphoma

This entity should be suspected in a child with unexplained fever and persistent lymphadenopathy, particularly if an infective/inflammatory process is no longer on the card. Usually, fever is irregular but occasionally it may be characterized by periods of hyperpyrexia followed by afebrile intervals. This is what is called as Pel-Ebstein fever. Accompanying symptoms include anorexia, fatigue, weight loss, night sweats, nonproductive cough or symptoms of mediastinal compression, pruritus, hepatosplenomegaly, anemia, thrombocytopenia, and nephrotic syndrome.

Investigations reveal neutrophilic leukocytosis, lymphopenia, and, in some instances, eosinophilia and monocytosis. ESR is usually elevated. Sternberg-Reed cells may be seen in the marrow. Lymph node biopsy is diagnostic.

Non-Hodgkin Lymphoma

Unexplained fever may be one of the systemic manifestations of non-Hodgkin lymphoma. Rapidly growing painless noninflammatory swelling of lymph nodes, usually in the region of head and neck, or anterior mediastinum is characteristic of the disease. Lymphoma of the abdomen and bone is less frequent. Anemia, thrombocytopenia, neutropenia, weakness, fatigue, weight loss, increased intracranial pressure, and cranial nerve involvement (seventh in particular) are some of its other manifestations. Definitive diagnosis is by biopsy from the available tumor mass.

Leukemia

Occasionally patients with leukemia manifest only prolonged pyrexia spread over quite a few weeks before other manifestations of the disease become apparent. In suspected cases, it is important to do bone marrow.

Histiocytosis

Also termed reticuloendotheliosis and comprising of three diseases (i.e. Hand–Schuller–Christian disease, Letterer–Siwe disease and eosinophilic granuloma), this group of disorders may have its onset in the form of recurrent febrile episodes without any definite pattern. Hepatomegaly, splenomegaly, painless adenopathy, petechiae, ecchymosis, papules or flat infiltration on trunk, in particular, take time to occur. Diagnosis is by demonstration of histiocytes in peripheral blood and bone marrow aspirate, which appears scanty.

Brain Tumor

If despite a reasonable clinical and investigative workup, the cause of PUO is not becoming clear, the possibility of a slowly growing space-occupying lesion of the CNS needs to be entertained. Look for, in particular, signs of raised intracranial pressure and involvement of the cranial nerves.

Wilms Tumor

Wilms tumor also termed as nephroblastoma. This tumor may be responsible for obscure pyrexia in approximately one in five instances of the growth. In a child aged around 3 years, it would be reasonable to suspect this diagnosis when there is large intra-abdominal smooth and firm mass, that does not cross the midline. Additional features include abdominal pain, vomiting, hypertension, and microscopic hematuria. IVP is the most important diagnostic tool for this tumor.

Neuroblastoma

Obscure fever may be a feature of neuroblastoma, both localized and disseminated. There usually is an abdominal mass (nontender, firm, and irregular) which sooner or later crosses the midline, invariably in the upper abdomen. Anemia, body tenderness, petechiae, ecchymoses, skin nodules raised intracranial pressure, chronic diarrhea, and hepatomegaly are some of the remaining manifestations. Raised catecholamine level in urine is diagnostic of the disease.

Drug Fever

All drugs, particularly those listed as follows, could cause obscure fever by pharmacologic action, effect on thermoregulation, immunologic action, local complication, parenteral administration or overdosage:

Aspirin, sulfonamides, rifampicin, acetazolamide, cephalosporins, colistin, erythromycin, nitrofurantoin, isonex, para-amino salicylic acid (PAS), ethambutol, amphetamine, azathioprine, carbamazepine, meprobamate, penicillamine, diphenylhydantoin, potassium iodide, streptokinase, thiouracil, atropine and allied agents, haloperidol, indomethacin, monoaminoxidase inhibitors.

Malingering (Factitious Fever)

Malingering, though infrequent in pediatric practice as a cause of unexplained pyrexia, may at times cause considerable difficulty in tackling the problem. The subject is usually an older child who wishes to bunk school. He manages to cause the thermometer to register incorrectly high reading by rubbing the bulb of the thermometer vigorously against the bedclothes, giving it a dip in a hot drink, placing it in contact with a hot water bottle, or vigorously shaking it while it is inverted. Factitious fever is characterized by high swinging fever usually only when temperature is recorded.

When the caretaker of the child, usually the mother with some medical background, fabricates, falsifies or actually induces symptom or apparent symptom of a disease in the child as a part of child abuse, the phenomenon is termed as Munchausen's syndrome by proxy or Meadow's syndrome. The symptoms may vary from pyrexia through host of gastrointestinal manifestations, rashes, bleeding from various sites, and renal stones to induced apnea that, at times, prove fatal.

When malingering as a cause of unexplained fever is suspected, you must conduct measurements of temperature under close personal observation. Alternatively, you may record temperature of the voided urine immediately to get correct estimate of the body core temperature. Remember, urine temperature, as a role, is about the same as rectal temperature.

Dehydration Fever

Anhidrotic Ectodermal Dysplasia

In this condition, the child may experience episodes of high fever when in a warm environment since he is not able to sweat. The remaining features of this X-linked recessive disorder, include frontal bossing, malar hypoplasia, flat nose, thick everted lips, prominent low-set ears, thin, dry, and hypopigmented skin, absent or sparse eyelashes, and widely spaced peg-shaped teeth.

Diabetes Insipidus

Both nephrogenic and non-nephrogenic diabetes insipidus may cause dehydration and resultant hyperthermia. The former fails to respond to exogenous vasopressin (pitressin) whereas the latter, being a congenital vasopressin-dependent disease, is characterized by an excellent response.

Normal High Temperature

Infrequently, a child, otherwise quite fine, cheerful, and energetic, has a little persistent rise of body temperature or a daily rise up to 38°C (101°F). No abnormality on clinical and investigative check-up is found. A follow-up too reveals that all is well. Such a child should be declared as "normal" and the parents told to stop recording the temperature.

Some parents develop an obsession for recording the rectal temperature every now and then. They do not appreciate that the rectal temperature is a degree higher than that of the mouth and 2° higher than the axillary temperature. They, therefore, start worrying that the child has pyrexia, which he indeed does not have. Often, they lead the doctor also to the garden path. Needless to say, many avoidable investigations are conducted for nothing.

Miscellaneous Causes of Fever of Unknown Etiology

Sarcoidosis, mucocutaneous lymph node disease, ulcerative colitis, Crohn's disease, pancreatitis, familial dysautonomia, Caffey disease, periodic fever, serum sickness, thyrotoxicosis agammaglobulinemia, liver disease [e.g. Indian childhood cirrhosis (ICC)], subdural effusion, sickle-cell anemia, dengue fever, etc.

FURTHER READING

1. Gupte S, Quereshi S. Pyrexia of obscure origin. *Asian Med* 2005;11:111-120.
2. Powell KR. Fever without a focus. In: Kliegman RM, St Geme III JW, Blum NJ, et al (Eds). *Nelson Textbook of Pediatrics*, 21st edn. Philadelphia: Elsevier 2020:1087-1093.

CHAPTER 52

Rash

BACKGROUND

The term *rash* (French: rasche) refers to an eruption of the skin, usually as a result of communicable (contagious) diseases. Also termed, exanthema, it is a shade of red with variation from disease to disease.

HISTORY

While confronting a child presenting with a skin rash, ask parents, if it followed a few days' fever and cold, irritability, malaise, etc. Is it accompanied by intense itching? Is there any history of known allergy to a drug(s)? Has the child been exposed to an index case of a contagious disease such as measles, rubella or chicken pox in the preceding 2–3-week period? Is he on any particular drug currently? Do not miss out on asking about the accompanying problems, which may give clues about the primary disease causing the rash or about its possible complications that may need immediate attention.

PHYSICAL EXAMINATION

During physical examination, make it a point to carefully observe the location and characteristics of the rash, say its exact color, size (diameter as well as height), pattern, secondary changes in the form of crusting, and whether discrete or coalesced (Box 52.1). An indirect evidence of pruritus is presence of signs of scratching.

BOX 52.1: Different forms of skin rash.

- *Macule:* Flat and impalpable
- *Papule:* Raised and circumscribed; palpable
- *Vesicle:* Raised, circumscribed, filled with fluid, under 0.5 cm in diameter
- *Pustules:* Raised lesions filled with purulent exudate (pus)
- *Petechiae:* Flat or raised hemorrhagic, 1–5 mm in diameter, which cannot be blenched by compression
- *Purpura:* Flat or raised hemorrhagic spots 5–10 mm in diameter
- *Ecchymosis:* Large, irregular discolored areas (irregular), blue black (originally), greenish brown or yellow later; resulting from extravasation of blood into skin (even mucous membrane at times); over 10 mm in diameter

General physical examination must also make a note about child's overall condition, sensorium, signs of shock, temperature, state of conjunctiva, appearance of mucous membrane, cervical lymphadenitis, liver and spleen, etc. in particular.

INVESTIGATIONS

Usually, diagnosis is clinical. Investigations are not routinely required.
Laboratory tests may be appropriate in patients in whom the cause is unclear.

- *Complete blood picture (CBP)*: Mild-to-moderate peripheral eosinophilia.
- Viral exanthema, depending on the particular virus involved, may need to be confirmed by serologically demonstrable antibody titres, viral culture, or molecular studies (e.g. polymerase chain reaction).
- Suspected human immunodeficiency virus (HIV) exanthem may screen positive for HIV viral RNA or core antigen.
- Children with more significant clinical disease, including serious bacterial infections, or with extracutaneous findings require a more complete workup.

IMPORTANT DIFFERENTIALS

Rash in the Newborn

Erythema Toxicum

The lesions are characterized by a mixture of erythematous macules and white or yellow papules that appear in first few days, usually first 3 days and may persist until tail end of first fortnight. If a needle is employed to lift the head from a macule and a Gram stain is performed, predominantly eosinophils are seen (Fig. 52.1).

Staphylococcal Skin Infection of the Newborn

The lesions are predominantly vesicles and pustules, though macules may also be seen. At times, differentiation from erythema toxicum becomes rather difficult. In such a situation, a needle needs to be employed to lift the head from a vesicle or a papule. After gram staining, many polymorphs and gram-positive cocci are seen as against eosinophils in erythema toxicum.

Neonatal Varicella

Neonates exposed to maternal varicella may develop varicella (chicken pox), provided that maternal chicken pox has occurred 5 days on either side of delivery. Neonatal varicella is a very serious condition and is a strong indication for administering varicella-zoster immune globulin (VZIG) by intramuscular injection, together with oral acyclovir, 20 mg/kg every 6 hour.

Herpes Simplex

In case of neonatal herpes simplex, herpetic lesions of maternal genetic tract are traceable. The vesicles are fairly large and are not quite opaque, unlike in staphylococcal lesions.

Neonatal Miliaria

Classically, the lesions are very small pustular rashes over nasal bridge, cheeks or chin. The cause is retention of sebum.

Impetigo Neonatorum

The lesions characteristically are small pustules with surrounding red area. More often, the cause is *Staphylococcus aureus* rather than Streptococcal infection.

Other Causes of Neonatal Rash

Congenital rubella (petechial, purpuric, etc.), congenital cytomegalovirus (CMV) (petechial, purpuric, etc.), birth asphyxia, phototherapy, immune thrombocytopenia, etc.

Rash in Infancy and Childhood

Maculopapular Rash

Measles (Fig. 52.2): Measles (rubeola) is characterized by a 3–5-day prodromal phase of catarrhal symptoms, followed by a classical measly rash with the following features:
- Pink or red blotchy irregular erythema (macular) which fades in pressure and quickly darkens and blends into large red patches of varying size and shape. The rash has a tendency to become confluent over upper part of the body; in lower part, it remains rather discrete.
- Face and areas behind the ears are the locations where the rash appears first. It travels lower down to trunk and limbs subsequently.

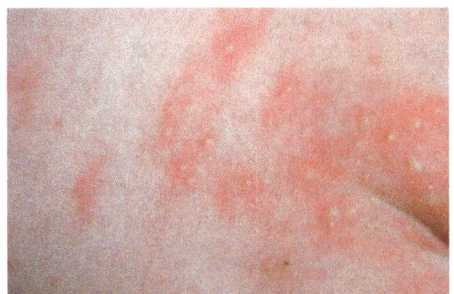

Fig. 52.1: Erythema toxicum. Note the widespread erythematous macules.

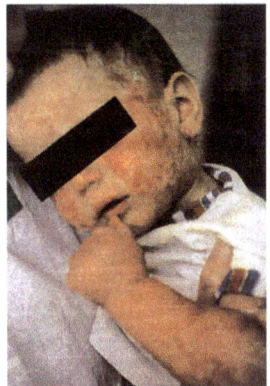

Fig. 52.2: *Measles*—Note the classical red maculopapular rash, displaying tendency for confluence, on the third day.

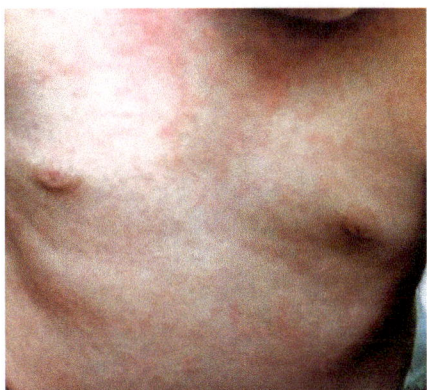

Fig. 52.3: Roseola infantum. Note the macular rash, which is short-lived.

- The rash tends to fade after 3–4 days. Mild itching may accompany it. It disappears in the same order as it appears.
- Finally, there results a fine shedding, i.e. desquamation of the superficial skin of the face followed by that of the trunk and limbs with the exception of hands and feet, leaving behind a light-brown pigmentation.

Roseola infantum (Fig. 52.3): Its pink macular rash usually appears on trunk, neck, and proximal areas of the limbs only. As the rash appears, the fever which is present in the preceding 4 days subsides. Typically, the rash is discrete and lasts for just 24 hours or so as against measles in which it lasts for 4–7 days. The cause is human herpes virus II.

Erythema infectiosum (Fig. 52.4): Also called fifth disease, it is caused by parvovirus B19. Besides a rash, especially over the cheeks, symptoms include low-grade fever, sore throat, headache, abdominal pain, joint pains, and fatigue.

Rubella (German measles, 3-day measles): The pink rash is discrete and mild, appearing and disappearing more rapidly than in measles without any desquamation. There is a significant posterior cervical lymphadenopathy. Prodromal phase too is slight and brief.

Infectious mononucleosis (Fig. 52.5): In infectious mononucleosis (glandular fever), the maculopapular rash often becomes manifest following administration of ampicillin. Accompanying features are fever, generalized lymphadenopathy, and hepatosplenomegaly. The disease, caused by Epstein–Barr virus (EBV) is benign.

Scarlet fever (Fig. 52.6): The dark-red and punctiform rash is most remarkable over neck and major skinfolds. Since the rash spares the area around the mouth, a circumoral pallor is prominent. Desquamation occurs but, unlike in measles, hands and feet are involved. White and red strawberry tongue due to inflammation is characteristic of true scarlet fever.

Typhus: Pinkish red macules are by and large centripetal. Other manifestations include change in sensorium, hypotension, oliguria, and azotemia.

Kawasaki disease (Fig. 52.7): The characteristic rash is in the form of discrete red maculopapules on trunk, feet, around knees, and in the axillary and inguinal skin creases. Desquamation of hands and feet is frequent.

Miliaria rubra (prickly heat, sudamina, heat rash, etc.): The characteristic eruption is a pinhead-sized erythematous papule over the areas where sweat glands are in abundance.

Vesicular Rash

Chicken pox (Fig. 52.8): In chicken pox (varicella), the characteristic eruption appears rapidly following a short

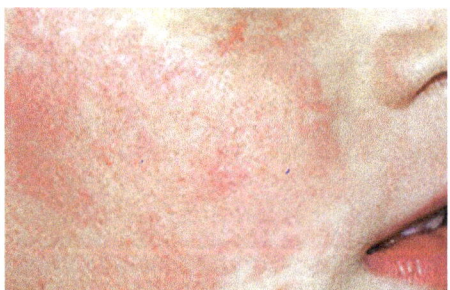

Fig. 52.4: Erythema infectiosum. Note the "slapped cheek rash".

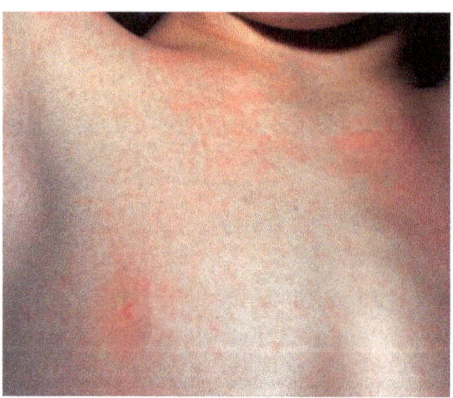

Fig. 52.6: Scarlet fever rash. Note the multiple tiny sandpaper-like bumps in a child with fever, sore throat, and red strawberry tongue.

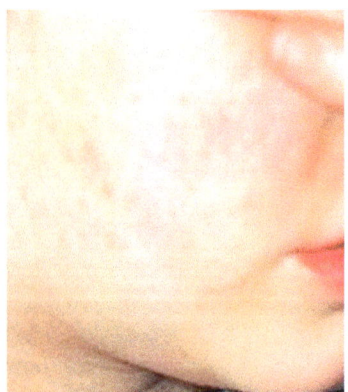

Fig. 52.5: Infectious mononucleosis. Note the maculopapular rash in a girl with fever, lymphadenopathy, and hepatosplenomegaly following ampicillin administration.

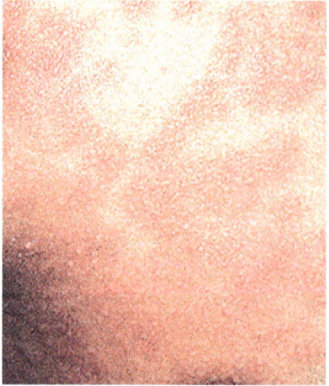

Fig. 52.7: Kawasaki disease. Note the blotchy erythema on the trunk of a child with a week's history of fever, neck lymph nodes swelling, red conjunctiva, strawberry tongue, and peeling of palms or soles.

and mild prodromal phase and is in crops of various stages of development (macules, papules, vesicles, pustules, etc.). The crops are profusely spread over the trunk and proximal limbs. Even buccal mucosa may exhibit some vesicles.

Herpes Zoster

The lesions, resulting from activation of the dormant herpes zoster virus usually in immunocompromised children and adolescents, closely resemble those seen in chicken pox but are restricted to specific dermatomes or cranial nerves and are usually unilateral (Fig. 52.9).

Herpes Simplex-Type I

Typically, the vesicles appear in crops following high fever and irritability over the eczematous skin. Nonetheless, the most frequent presentation of herpes simplex in childhood, is in the form of gingivostomatitis (Fig. 52.10).

Impetigo

Both streptococcal and staphylococcal impetigo are present as red macules, which eventually become vesicles. The small vesicles later burst, leaving behind a honeycomb crust. On removal, the crusts leave a moist raw surface (Fig. 52.11).

Dermatitis herpetiformis (Fig. 52.12): This condition, often associated with celiac disease, i.e. gluten-induced enteropathy, is characterized by appearance of recurrent crops of pruritic papulovesicles over extensor surfaces, including elbows, knees, and buttocks.

Molluscum Contagiosum

Flesh-colored papules with a central dimple initially firm, softer, and more waxy later, 2–5 mm in size are seen over the face, trunk, and limbs, more often in school-going children (Fig. 52.13).

Petechial and Purpuric Rash

Meningococcemia (Fig. 52.14): Petechial or purpuric rash anywhere on the body may well be the first sign of meningococcemia as such or preceded or accompanied by a maculopapular rash. Other signs of septicemia such

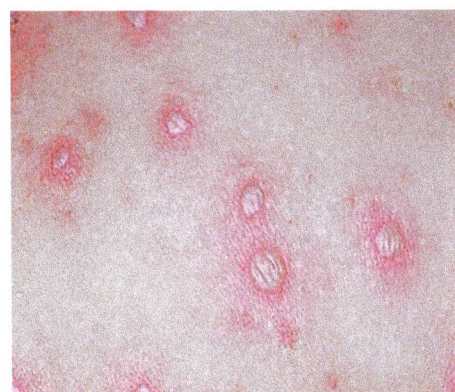

Fig. 52.8: Chicken pox rash. Note the pleomorphic rash over the trunk of a child.

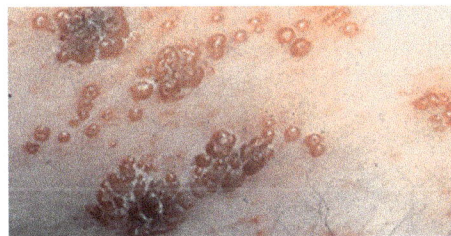

Fig. 52.9: Herpes zoster (shingles). Note the unilateral varicella-like rash along the dermatomes. Pain and burning sensation accompany the rash.

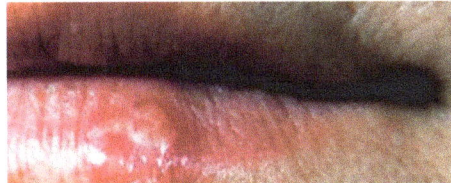

Fig. 52.10: Herpes simplex. Note the lesion over the lower lip.

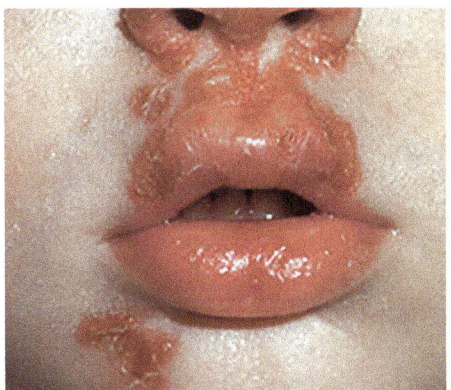

Fig. 52.11: Impetigo.

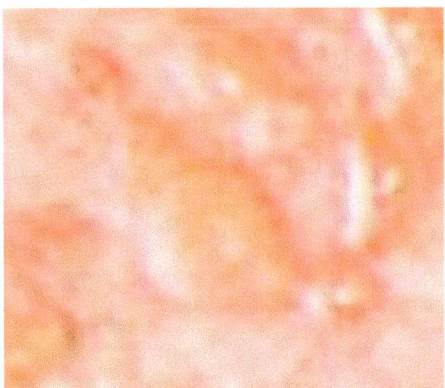

Fig. 52.12: Dermatitis herpetiformis.

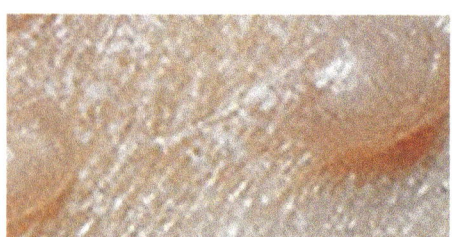

Fig. 52.13: Molloscum contagiosum.

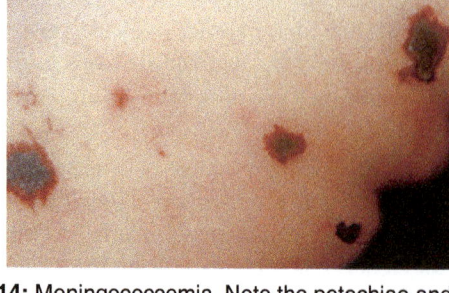

Fig. 52.14: Meningococcemia. Note the petechiae and purpura.

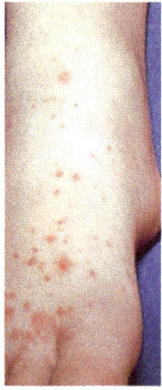

Fig. 52.15: Henoch-Schonlein purpura. Note the petechiae and purpura over the dorsum of the foot and leg.

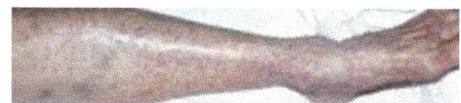

Fig. 52.16: Immune thrombocytopenic purpura (ITP). Note the widespread bruising over the leg.

as meningitis and toxemia are present. Lancing may assist in isolation of the bacteria from the skin lesions.

Occasionally, septicemia resulting from other bacteria, especially *Haemophilus influenzae* may cause similar petechial rash.

Henoch–Schönlein Purpura

In anaphylactoid purpura, as upper respiratory catarrh may be followed by appearance of a maculopapular hemorrhagic rash on buttocks and extensor surfaces of limbs (especially knees and ankles). The lesions, which appear in crops, fade over the next few days, leaving a brownish pigmentation. The cause of purpura in this autoimmune disorder is a type of vasculitis (Fig. 52.15).

Immune (Idiopathic) Thrombocytopenic Purpura

In immune thrombocytopenic purpura (ITP), characterized by severe thrombocytopenia, purpuric rash is often accompanied by frank bleeding from other sites, say epistaxis (Fig. 52.16).

Leukemia

Hemorrhagic rash with evidence of bleeding from other sites, considerable anemia, lymphadenopathy, and hepatosplenomegaly should strongly point to the diagnosis of a blood dyscrasia such as leukemia.

FURTHER READING

1. BMJ Best Practice. Assessment of rash in children. Available at: http://bestpractice.bmj.com/best-practice/monograph/857/diagnosis/step-by-step.html. Accessed on: July 24 2019.
2. Gaur A. Fever with rash. In: Gupte S (Ed). *Recent Advances in Pediatrics-16*. New Delhi: Jaypee 2006:114-132.

CHAPTER 53

Short Stature

BACKGROUND

The term, *short stature*, means length/height
- Less by more than 2 standard deviations (SD) of mean for age and sex
- Below third percentile for age and sex.

Short stature may be primary or secondary. Primary short stature is usually due to an intrinsic defect in the skeletal system as a result of some genetic or prenatal damage [say intrauterine growth retardation (IUGR)]. Here, the potential for normal bone growth is impaired though skeletal age is unaffected. Main effect is on diaphyseal growth. Secondary short stature is characterized by: impairment of bone age and height to the same extent. Here, the potential for reaching the adult height is subjected to availability of suitable treatment. Box 53.1 lists the various causes of PEM.

HISTORY

While obtaining history, confirm child's exact age. Find out specifically if the child was of low birth weight and/or preterm. Has he been suffering from chronic diarrhea, chronic nutritional deprivation, chronic worm infestation or any other chronic/recurrent ailment that may have adversely affected his growth? What about the nature of the parents, siblings, and the grandparents? Is his intellectual development also affected? Get an idea if the secondary sex characters were delayed in one or both parents.

PHYSICAL EXAMINATION

Physical examination with special emphasis on the following measurements, recorded accurately, is of paramount importance:
- *Height/length*: At 2 years and after, height is measured with a stadiometer. This instrument consists of a sliding rigid board mounted at right angles onto a vertical scale. The child stands erect barefoot, making himself as tall as possible without elevating his feet. His head needs to be in the Frankfurt plane, meaning the line passing through outer canthi and external auditory meatuses should be parallel to the ground. The knees need to be straight. All these requirements are met if it is ensured that, while he stands, his occiput, shoulders, buttocks, and heels are in touch with the vertical surface.

BOX 53.1: Causes of short stature based on body proportions.

Proportionate short stature
- Normal variants
  - Constitutional
  - Familial/genetic
- Prenatal origin
  - *Intrauterine growth retardation (IUGR):* Maternal diabetes, toxemias, infections teratogens (alcohol, nicotine, etc.)
  - *Dysmorphic syndromes:* Silver-Russell syndrome
  - *Chromosomal anomalies:* Turner syndrome, Down syndrome, etc.
- Postnatal origin
  - *Nutritional:* Chronic malnutrition spread over a prolonged period
  - Organic diseases
  - *Gastrointestinal:* Malabsorption syndrome in the form of celiac disease, endemic tropical sprue or cystic fibrosis, heavy intestinal parasitism, cirrhosis of liver, congenital megacolon, etc.
  - *Cardiovascular:* Congenital heart disease, rheumatic heart disease, etc.
  - *Respiratory:* Pulmonary tuberculosis, bronchial asthma, bronchiectasis, cystic fibrosis, etc.
  - *Hematologic:* Chronic iron deficiency anemia (IDA), thalassemia, sickle-cell anemia, etc.
  - *Endocrinal:* Pituitary dwarfism, hypothyroidism, hypogonadism, dysmorphic syndromes, precocious puberty, pseudohypoparathyroidism, diabetes mellitus, Cushing syndrome, Laurence-Moon-Biedl syndrome, Frohlich's syndrome, etc.
  - *Renal:* Renal rickets from chronic renal failure and tubular disorders
  - *Chronic infection:* Tuberculosis, malaria, syphilis, heavy parasitic infestation, *Helicobacter pylori* infection, etc.
- *Drug induced:* Prolonged use of anabolic steroids or corticosteroids.
- *Psychosocial:* Emotional deprivation, parental neglect, child abuse and neglect, etc.

Disproportionate short stature
- *Short limbs:* Congenital hypothyroidism, achondroplasia, osteogenesis imperfecta, amelia, rickets*
- *Short trunk:* Mucopolysaccharidosis (Morquio disease), spondyloepiphyseal dysplasia#, mucolipidosis, caries spine, hemivertebrae, rickets*

*Rickets figures in both since it may cause gross deformities (shortening) of trunk and legs.
#Spondyloepiphyseal dysplasia denotes a group of disorders with primary involvement of the vertebrae and epiphyseal centers, resulting in a short-trunk disproportionate dwarfism.
Source: Gupte S, Gomez EM. Growth disorders. In: Gupte S (Ed). *The Short Textbook of Pediatrics*, 12th edition. New Delhi: Jaypee 2016:66-83.

For children under 2 years, supine (recumbent) length rather than standing height (the latter may be less by 2 cm the exact measurement), using an infantometer, is recommended. While making this measurement, it must be ensured that the child's legs are extended fully at hips and knees and the feet are at right angles to the legs. Assistance from a parent or attendant is usually needed for this purpose.

The term, height age, means age at which the child is expected to have the said height.

Height velocity, calculated from at least two accurate readings at least 6 months (but preferably 1 year) apart, is more useful than a single recording of height. A velocity of less than 4 cm/year between 5 years of age and adolescence points to a pathologic state. For younger children, the figure is variable with age, i.e. 15 cm for 0–6 months, 7 cm for 6–12 months, 10 cm for 1–2 years, and 5 cm for 2–5 years.

Body proportions are considered to be the most accurate measure of height, helping in deciding whether short stature is proportionate or disproportionate. Upper segment/lower segment ratio (1:7:1.0 at birth, 1:3:1.0 at 3 years, 1:1 by 7–8 years) is increased in hypothyroidism and achondroplasia (Fig. 53.1). Span (measurement from middle fingertip to middle fingertip) in case of fully outstretched arms and hands is increased (more than height) in spondyloepiphyseal dysplasia and Morquio disease.

It is useful to measure height of parents and siblings. Midparental height, a genetic component, gives the subject's target height. It is denoted by the mean of the heights of father and mother plus 13 in boys. In girls, it is obtained as a mean of the heights of the mother and father minus 13.

- *Weight*: If weight is proportionally less than height, nutritional deprivation must be seriously considered. On the other hand, if weight is nearly normal but height is significantly less, hypothyroidism, growth hormone deficiency, and hypercorticism need to be considered in the differential diagnosis.

The term weight age means the age at which the said weight is expected to be attained.

Pubertal staging is done by Tanner's classification, based on pubic hair, penis, and testes in boys and pubic hair and breast in girls as shown in Tables 53.1 and 53.2.

TABLE 53.1: Pubertal (sex maturity) stages in boys.

SMR	Pubic hair stage	Penis	Testes
1.	None	Preadolescent	Preadolescent
2.	Scanty, long, slightly pigmented	Slight enlargement	Enlarged scrotum, pink, texture altered
3.	Darker, stats to curl, small amount	Longer	Larger
4.	Resembles adult type but less in quantity; coarse, curly	Larger, glans and breadth increase in size	Larger, scrotum dark
5.	Adult distribution, spread to medial surface of thigh	Adult size	Adult size

(SMR: sexual maturity rating)

TABLE 53.2: Pubertal (sex maturity) stages in girls.

SMR	Pubic hair stage	Breasts
1.	Preadolescent	Preadolescent
2.	Sparse, lightly pigmented, straight, medial border of labia	Breast and papilla elevated as small mound; areolar diameter increased
3.	Darker, beginning to curl, increased amount	Breast and areola enlarged; no contour separation
4.	Coarse, curly, abundant but amount less than that in adults	Areola and papilla form secondary mound
5.	Adult feminine triangle, spread to medial surface of thighs	Mature; nipple projects, areola part of general breast contour

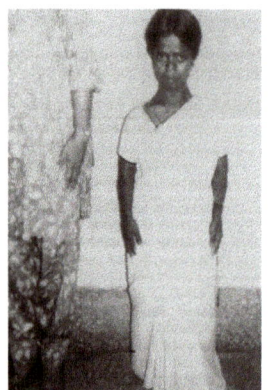

Fig. 53.1: *Achondroplasia*—This 18-year-old girl, standing by the side of a normal adult, had large head with depressed bridge of nose due to midfacial dysplasia and prominent forehead, short height (125 cm), and limb shortening with the hands falling short of reaching the normal level when allowed to hang down by the body sides. The closest differential diagnosis is spondyloepiphyseal dysplasia. Skiagrams are required for differentiation between these two conditions.

Short Stature

Children with delayed puberty and short stature should arouse suspicion of sex chromosomal anomalies such as Turner's syndrome. Here, stature, despite timely onset of puberty, is likely to end up with short stature. In "late maturers", both short stature and delayed onset of puberty coexist. It is noteworthy that these late maturers eventually attain better heights compared to early maturers.

Bone age, assessed through radiologic examination of certain bones and then comparing the appearance and fusion of epiphyseal centers with standard normal radiographs for different ages, is of vital importance. In infancy, knee, wrist, and hand are most useful sites. In later years, elbow, wrist, and hand are suitable (Table 53.3).

TABLE 53.3: Bone age through radiology.

Bones	Average age, at appearance of ossification center	
	Males	Females
Carpal bones		
Capitate	2 months	2 months
Hamate	3 months	2 months
Triangular (triquetral)	30 months	21 months
Lunate	42 months	34 months
Trapezium	67 months	47 months
Trapezoid	69 months	49 months
Scaphoid	66 months	51 months
Pisiform	13 years	10 years
Metacarpal bones		
Second	18 months	12 months
Third	20 months	13 months
Fourth	23 months	15 months
Fifth	26 months	16 months
First	32 months	18 months
Fingers		
Proximal, 3rd finger	16 months	10 months
Proximal, 2nd finger	16 months	11 months
Proximal, 4th finger	17 months	11 months
Distal, 1st finger	19 months	12 months
Proximal, 5th finger	21 months	14 months
Middle, 3rd finger	24 months	15 months
Middle, 4th finger	24 months	15 months
Middle, 2nd finger	26 months	16 months
Distal, 3rd finger	28 months	18 months
Distal, 4th finger	28 months	18 months
Proximal, 1st finger	32 months	20 months
Distal, 5th finger	37 months	23 months
Distal, 2nd finger	37 months	23 months
Middle, 5th finger	39 months	22 months
Sesamoid (adductor pollicis)	152 months	121 months
Contd...		
Shoulder		
Acromion	14 years	12 years
Coracoid	6 years	13 years
Clavicle (medial end)	17 years	17 years
Humerus (head)	3 weeks	3 weeks
Greater tuberosity	3.5 years	3 years
Elbow		
Radius	6 years	3.5 years
Medial condyle	7.5 years	5.5 years
Lateral condyle	6 years	7.5 years
Trochlea	8 years	7.5 years
Capitulum	2 weeks	2 weeks
Ulna	10 months	9 months
Wrists	1.7 years	3.5 years
Radius	1.7 years	3.5 years
Ulna	7.4 years	6.5 years
Hip and knee		
Femur (distal end)	At birth	At birth
Tibia (proximal end)	At birth	At birth
Femur (head)	4 months	4 months
Greater trochanter	24 months	–
Lesser trochanter	12 years	–
Patella	16 years	29 months
Iliac crest	16 years	16 years

Based on the assessment mentioned so far, the following guidelines must be borne in mind:
- If height age falls within 2 years of the chronological age, child needs not to be considered of short stature.
- If height age is less than the chronological age and the bone age is equal to height age, slow growth, meaning constitutional delay, is the likely cause of short stature. Chances are that, such a child will attain his normal height subsequently.
- If the height age is less than the chronological age and the bone age is equal to chronological age, genetic short stature is the diagnosis. Such a child has the short parents and is likely to remain short.
- Bone age less than chronological age should suggest constitutional growth retardation, hypothyroidism, malnutrition, growth, hormone deficiency or chronic systemic diseases as the probable causes of short stature.

INVESTIGATIONS

Level I

- Complete blood picture (CBP)
- Urinalysis
- Stool microscopy for ova and cysts on at least 3 (preferably 5 or 6) successive days

- *Bone age* assessed through radiologic examination of certain bones and then comparing the appearance and fusion of epiphyseal centers with standard normal radiographs for different ages is of considerable value.

In infancy, knee, wrist, and hand, and in later years elbow, wrist, and hand are appropriate sites for bone age determination. Interpretation of bone age in terms of cause of short stature is presented in Box 53.2. With the availability of assessment mentioned so far, the following guidelines are suggested:
- If height age falls within 2 years of the chronological age, the subject needs not to be considered to have short stature.
- If height age is less than the chronological age and the bone age is equal to height age, slow growth—in other words, constitutional delay—is the likely cause of short stature. In this situation, the child attains his target height subsequently.
- If the height age is less than the chronological age and the bone age is equal to chronological age, genetic short stature is the diagnosis. Such a child has short parents and is likely to remain short.
- If bone age is less than the chronological age, one should consider constitutional growth retardation, hypothyroidism, malnutrition, growth hormone deficiency, and chronic systemic disease as the cause of short stature.

Level II: Specific Investigations

Besides radiology and routine investigations, including meticulous stool examination on at least 3 successive days, it should be ascertained if there is a need for intensive workup. The indications for such a workup are listed in Box 53.3. The specific investigations are:
- Karyotyping, especially in girls in order to exclude Turner syndrome
- Thyroid function tests.

BOX 53.2: Interpretation of bone age.

Normal
- Familial

Delayed
- Constitutional
- Hypothyroidism
- Growth hormone deficiency
- Cushing syndrome
- Chronic malnutrition
- Chronic systemic diseases
- Delayed adolescence/puberty
- Turner syndrome
- Noonan syndrome

Advanced
- Genetic and chromosomal disorders (Down syndrome)
- Sexual precocious puberty
- Obesity
- Hyperthyroidism
- Adrenal hyperplasia.

Level III: Sophisticated Tests (Intensive Workup)

Intensive workup is indicated if the diagnosis remains elusive in spite of Levels 1 and 2 workup.
- Imaging studies like ultrasound, computed tomography (CT) scan (pituitary, adrenals, pelvic organs, etc.)
- Somatomedin-C measurement
- Cortisol, luteinizing hormone (LH), follicle stimulating hormone (FSH), prolactin (PRL), testosterone, estrogen levels, etc.
- Malabsorption studies, especially celiac serology
- Renal acidification test
- Urinary aminoacidogram
- Urinary iodine levels.

IMPORTANT DIFFERENTIALS

Genetic (Familial) Short Stature

This is a leading cause of short stature universally. It runs as a familial trait with one or both parents and sibling(s) being short. A noteworthy feature is that bone age is consistent with chronological age. Growth occurs at the genetic potential. Eventually, the child attains a height that is consistent with the midparental height.

Constitutional Short Stature

This is a sheer variant of normal growth and is, therefore, more appropriately termed as constitutional growth delay (Fig. 53.2). Here, bone age is consistent with height age rather than the chronological age—a point in sharp contrast with the observation in genetic short stature. Onset of puberty is delayed. Eventually, however, adult height and sexual maturation are normal.

Persistence of the relatively hypogonadotrophic state of childhood is believed to be responsible for this kind of short stature. Frequently, one or both parents or other close family members have a history of short stature in childhood, delayed puberty and, finally, normal stature.

Classically, a constitutional short child is born with normal weight and length. Growth remains normal for the first 4–12 months. Then, it slows down until 2–3 years of age then it becomes normal but at a relatively lower level of normal (5 cm or little more per year). Puberty too is delayed. Nevertheless, final outcome is satisfactory as normal adult height as well as sexual development is attained.

BOX 53.3: Indications for intensive investigational workup.
- Height > 2SD less than the mean for that age.
- Height velocity <4 cm/year.
- Height centile showing subnormality in relation to family stature (midparental height).
- Inappropriate bone age compared to height age and actual (chronologic) age.
- Characteristic features of an endocrine cause or a syndromal state.

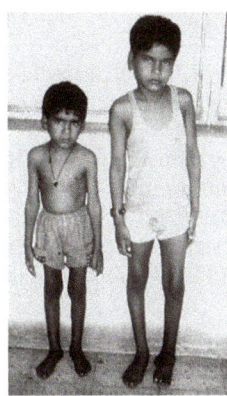

Fig. 53.2: *Short stature*—Note that the height of the 8-year-old child (left) is just 108 cm against 123 cm of the child of about the same age.

Primordial Dwarfism

In this condition, IUGR is responsible for short stature. It is claimed that arrest of the fetal growth early in pregnancy results in reduction in number of cells. As a consequence, growth potential in the postnatal period is diminished. Bone age is normal, corresponding to the chronological age. Usually, prognosis for adult height is poor, particularly in the subjects who are small for gestational age.

Silver–Russell syndrome is characterized by short stature, small triangular facies, frontal bossing, scanty subcutaneous fat, and short and incurved fifth finger with or without hemihypertrophy in a child who had low birth weight for gestational age.

Nutritional Stunting

Chronic malnutrition of long-standing, particularly when it is not gross enough to cause overt kwashiorkor or marasmus, leads to stunting in height as an adaptation response. Bone age is, as a rule, less than the chronological age.

Catch-up growth, though incomplete, is expected in these children once nutritional rehabilitation is satisfactorily achieved.

Emotional Deprivation

Also termed as psychosocial dwarfism, deprivation dwarfism or reversible hyposomatotropism, this condition, perhaps, causes short stature through functional hypopituitarism. These children have perverted appetite, enuresis, encopresis, insomnia, crying spasms, and sudden tantrums. They may be passive or aggressive. History of upset mother—child or family relations provides clue to the diagnosis. Bone age is little delayed or just normal. Body proportions are normal.

Following availability of emotional warmth and security, these children show catch-up growth.

Chronic Visceral Diseases

Most chronic visceral diseases (malabsorption syndrome, congenital heart disease, renal tubular acidosis, chronic renal failure, diabetes mellitus, thalassemia, bronchial asthma, etc.) also chronic infections (tuberculosis, chronic intestinal parasitosis, malaria, kala-azar, syphilis, pyelonephritis, etc.) cause retardation in stature, in fact in total growth as such. Recently, it is being increasingly recognized that short stature may be the solitary manifestation in certain cases of celiac disease. The implication of this observation, particularly in areas where this disease occurs, is significant.

Endocrinopathies

Remarkable delay in bone age is characteristic of short stature accompanying endocrinal disorders.

Growth hormone deficiency should be suspected if the subject's appearance is infantile, bone age is remarkable retarded and the growth velocity is less than 4 cm/year. Diagnosis is confirmed by testing growth hormone levels after provocative stimulation (say exercise, insulin, propranolol, arginine, L-dopa, etc.).

Remember that growth hormone deficiency is an uncommon cause of short stature. It may occur in isolation or in association with other pituitary hormones when the condition is termed as panhypopituitarism.

- *Hypothyroidism:* The clinical profile of a full-blown case is classical so that the condition is easily recognized. What needs to be borne in mind is that hypothyroidism can present with short stature and growth retardation alone. Body proportions remain infantile. Bone age is retarded remarkably. Diagnosis must be confirmed by demonstrating low T_4 and high thyroid-stimulating hormone (TSH) levels.
- *Cushing syndrome*: It may result from exogenous steroid therapy or secondary to a pituitary or adrenal tumor. Despite being overweight, the child has growth retardation, short stature, and delayed epiphyseal maturation. Remaining features of the syndrome such as moon facies, abdominal striae, plethora, hypertension, and reduced glucose tolerance may be present.
- *Diabetes mellitus* is usually accompanied by growth retardation, particularly when it is poorly controlled. There may be history of polyuria, nocturnal enuresis, polydipsia, and polyphagia. Urine and blood sugar clinch the diagnosis.

Skeletal Disorders

In case of disproportionate short stature, chondrodystrophies such as achondroplasia, pseudoachondroplasia, osteogenesis imperfecta, rickets, spondyloepiphyseal dysplasia, caries spine or hemivertebrae must be suspected.

Chromosomal Disorders

Turner's syndrome (XO) must always be considered in the differential diagnosis of short stature in girls. Remaining features of the condition include webbing of neck, edema of lower limbs, widely placed nipples, cubitus valgus, coarctation of aorta, and a short fourth metacarpal as also absence of secondary sex characters.

Noonan's syndrome is just the prototype of Turner's syndrome in boys with the exception that chromosomal count is normal and, in place of coarctation of aorta, pulmonary stenosis with or without atrial septal defect (ASD) is more common.

FURTHER READING

1. Gupte S, Gomez EM. Growth disorders. In: Gupte S (Ed). *The Short Textbook of Pediatrics,* 13th edn. New Delhi: Jaypee 2020.
2. Kaplowitz P. Short stature. In: Adam HM, Foy JM (Eds). *Signs and Symptoms in Pediatrics.* Illinois: American Academy of Pediatrics 2015:819-826.
3. Zargar AH. Short stature. In: Gupte S (Ed). *Recent Advances in Pediatrics (Special Vol: Pediatric Endocrinology).* New Delhi: Jaypee 2003.

CHAPTER 54

Small Head

BACKGROUND

Small head often accounts for pediatric cases presenting to the doctor for elucidation as regards the precise diagnosis.

Microcephaly means head circumference less by 2 standard deviation (SD) for age and sex. When it is less by 3 SD, microcephaly is usually accompanied by mental retardation. Primary microcephaly means the brain size per se is small. Secondary microcephaly means that head size is small because of premature union of skull sutures (craniosynostosis).

HISTORY

History should seek information whether the developmental and mental milestones have been delayed or are within normal limits. Any history of seizures? Are the parents consanguinously related? Do other children in the family and the parents have small heads? Any history of alcoholism in the mother?

PHYSICAL EXAMINATION

Physical examination should first establish if the head size is indeed significantly small in relation to the body size, weight, and age. In doubtful cases, it is important to record serial measurements. Is the shape of the head also abnormal? Are there any characteristic facies and congenital anomalies? In infants and small toddlers, find out if the anterior fontanel is prematurely closed? Is a ridge palpable in the region of the sutures? Any papilledema?

A complete neurologic examination must be undertaken. What is the child's developmental age? What is his intelligence quotient? Look for signs of raised intracranial pressure.

INVESTIGATIONS

Skull roentgenogram is important for diagnosing intrauterine infection or craniosynostosis.

Early diagnosis of microcephaly can be made by fetal ultrasound at the end of the second trimester, around 28 weeks, or in the third trimester of pregnancy.

Usually, diagnosis is made on birth or at a later stage.

IMPORTANT DIFFERENTIALS

Microcephaly

Strictly speaking, the term should be reserved for small size of head (3 SD below the average) as a result of developmental abnormalities and/or destructive processes of the brain, usually during the intrauterine life or early infancy.

The following conditions need to be considered in the differential diagnosis of true microcephaly:
- *Defects in brain development:* Hereditary (recessive) microcephaly, trisomy especially Down syndrome, phenylketonuria, Cornelia de Lange syndrome, Rubinstein-Taybi syndrome, Smith-Lemli-Opitz syndrome, fetal alcohol syndrome, Seckel dwarfism, fetal ionizing radiation exposure, etc.
- *Intrauterine infections*: Rubella, cytomegalovirus infection, toxoplasmosis, syphilis, etc.
- *Natal and postnatal disorders*: Anoxia, gross malnutrition, neonatal herpes virus infection, etc.

Craniosynostosis (Craniostenosis)

Small head secondary to premature closure of the skull sutures, which interfere with proper brain growth, is often accompanied by asymmetry of the head as well. One or more sutures may be involved. Since the stiff skull vault does not allow the brain to grow, a kind of situation resembling raised intracranial pressure results.

Oxycephaly means fusion of coronal and, in some cases, all sutures. The head may be anteroposteriorly flattened and elongated transversely and upwardly. This is called acrocephaly. When all the sutures are fused, head is symmetrically small (Fig. 54.1).

Scaphocephaly results from fusion of the sagittal suture. Skull grows anteroposteriorly and assumes an elongated appearance resembling a boat (Fig. 54.2). This is the most common type of craniosynostosis, accounting for around 50% of the cases (Fig. 54.3).

Plagiocephaly is characterized by asymmetrical skull resulting from asymmetrical fusion of the suture(s).

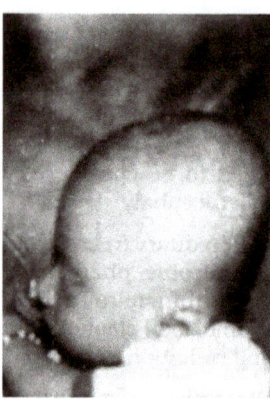

Fig. 54.1: *Microcephaly secondary to craniosynostosis*—Clinically, the ridges over suture lines were palpable and anterior fontanel was prematurely closed.

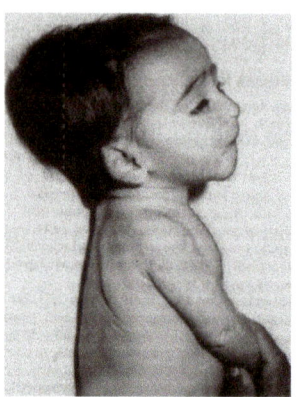

Fig. 54.2: *Scaphocephaly*—Microcephaly secondary to craniosynostosis of the sagittal suture leading to boat-shaped skull (scaphocephaly). Half of the cases of craniosynostosis belong to this category.

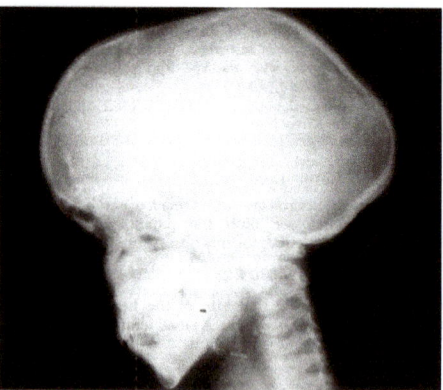

Fig. 54.3: X-ray of a scaphocephalic skull. Note the premature synostosis of sagittal suture.

The symptomatic subjects have manifestations secondary to high intracranial pressure. These include headache, vomiting, proptosis, squint, convulsions, hyperreflexia, hypertonia, and mental retardation.

Physical examination shows typical appearance. The concerned sutures are united and fontanels prematurely closed, or in the process of doing so. There may be signs of neurologic deficit.

Apert syndrome refers to occurrence of craniosynostosis in association with syndactyly. When oxycephaly is accompanied by beaked nose, proptosis, and hypertelorism, the combination is termed as craniofacial dysostosis or Crouzon disease. In Carpenter syndrome, there is acrocephaly, syndactyly in the hands, polydactyly and syndactyly in the feet, and tendency to mental retardation.

Diagnosis is based on characteristic clinical appearance, palpability of a ridge along the involved suture(s), and premature closure of the fontanels. X-ray of skull confirms the closure of suture(s). When craniosynostosis is of severe degree with marked and prolonged rise of intracranial pressure, distinct impressions over the skull vault, the so-called copper or silver-beaten appearance, are seen in the X-ray film.

Familial Small Head

At times, small head without any manifestation of mental retardation or neurologic deficit may occur as a family trait. You must see both the parents in suspected instances, in particular, for this observation.

Small Infant

An often-ignored fact is that size of the head normally is proportionate to the body size. A small infant is expected to have small head whereas a big infant is likely to have a big head.

Normal Variation

Not infrequently, a diagnosis of microcephaly is wrongly made when in fact the head size, though apparently small, falls within the normal range. Some years ago, a family approached the author, complaining that their 1-year-old son's head size was much smaller than that of his cousin aged exactly the same. On examination, it was found that the child in question had a head circumference of 44 cm against the 45 cm of his cousin. Both children were perfectly normal. Both children had average growth and development.

FURTHER READING

1. Kinsman SL, Johnston MV. Microcephaly. In: Kliegman RM, St Geme III JW, Blum NJ, et al (Eds). *Nelson Textbook of Pediatrics*, 21st edn. Philadelphia: Elsevier 2020:2451-2452.
2. World Health Organization. Microcephaly. Available at: http://www.who.int/mediacentre/factsheets/microcephaly/en. Accessed on: 24 July 2019.

CHAPTER 55

Splenomegaly

BACKGROUND

Splenic enlargement ranks only next to hepatomegaly in frequency of occurrence of intra-abdominal lumps in infancy and childhood.

HISTORY

Ask about the onset of the splenic lump: sudden or gradual; recent or since quite sometime? Any febrile illness suggestive of malaria or typhoid?

It is relevant to find out if the child has been developing progressive pallor suggesting anemia which could well be secondary to nutritonal deficiencies, diseases lke thalassemia, sickle cell disease, leukemias, malignancies, etc.

Any hematemesis? This could be the result of esophageal varices in portal hypertension. In this situation, it is advisable to trace history of umbilical sepsis in the neonatal period. Also find out any history of blood transfusions and occurrence of Simlar problem in family member(s).

PHYSICAL EXAMINATION

Like hepatomegaly, this too is more often detected by the examiner than by the patient or attendant himself. Just palpability of this organ means that it has already enlarged by two to three times its normal size. For detection of lesser degrees of enlargement, clinical palpation does not help. You would have to resort to radiography.

In order to palpate the spleen, you should preferably stand on the patient's right side. Then, you should place the flat side of your left hand over the left lateral and posterior part of the chest and the right hand just below the left costal margin. During the inspiratory phase, right hand is insinuated underneath the costal margin to feel the organ. While this is being done, the left hand engages in pressing the chest wall. Spleen is usually felt as a firm mass with smooth rounded borders and a notch. If you fail to feel it this way, the subject may be turned halfway to the right and the maneuver repeated. Make sure that careful and gentle palpation of the relaxed abdomen is conducted if you wish to obtain reliable information about the size of the spleen.

In infants, spleen enlarges vertically downward against its diagonally downward enlargement in children and adults (Fig. 55.1).

A significantly enlarged spleen must be differentiated from other masses in the left hypochondrium, notably the kidney. The points that may help you in establishing that it indeed is spleen are:

- Upper margin of the spleen is concealed by the rib cage and, therefore, cannot be felt underneath the subcostal margin.
- Medial border of the spleen has a characteristic notch.
- In splenic swelling, the overlying bowel is absent.
- Splenic swelling tends to extend towards the umbilicus, which means downward, forward, and inward. Kidney swelling, on the other hand, enlarges forward and vertically downward toward the iliac fossa.
- Splenic swelling moves freely with respiration. Renal swelling does not move with respiration.
- Splenic swelling is palpated from the anterior aspect whereas kidney enlargement is palpable from the posterior aspect or bimanually.

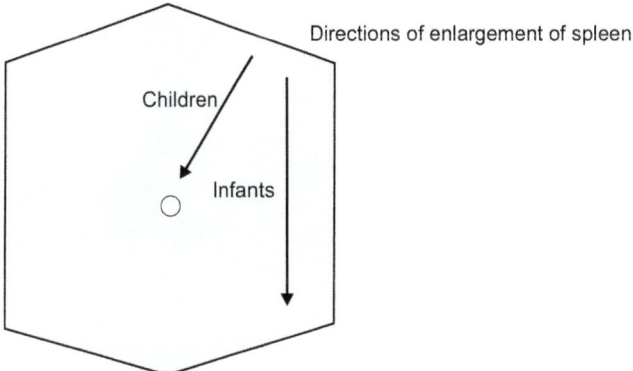

Fig. 55.1: In infants, spleen enlarges vertically downward against its diagonally downward enlargement in children and adults.

- Splenic swelling is not ballotable unlike the kidney swelling.

Slight palpability of spleen is encountered in approximately 5–10% of normal children, especially the neonates.

INVESTIGATIONS

- Complete blood picture (CBP) with differential, platelet count, and peripheral blood smear in suspected sickle cell disease, spherocytosis, and other hereditary hemolytic anemias, leukemias, malaria, kala-azar, etc.
- Imaging for splenic size
- Splenoportography.

IMPORTANT DIFFERENTIALS

Infections

Malaria

This is, perhaps, the most common cause of a large, firm splenic lump in children in areas endemic for malaria (Fig. 55.2). Manifestations other than splenomegaly include classical febrile episodes of irregular fever, body pains, headache, nausea, abdominal pain, and hepatomegaly. Severe manifestations related to central nervous system (CNS), respiratory system, and gastrointestinal tract point to the diagnosis of falciparum malaria. Shock followed by coma is a feature of algid malaria.

In chronic malaria, spleen is quite big and firm. In addition the child is malnourished, anemic, and stunted. In these cases, febrile episodes are either absent or simply nonspecific as in sepsis. The terms, tropical splenomegaly, idiopathic splenomegaly or big spleen disease refer to this condition.

Diagnosis is made by demonstrating the malarial parasite in the thick and thin blood film.

Enteric Fever

Spleen usually becomes palpable in the second week in enteric fever (Fig. 55.3). Remaining manifestations include fever, malaise, anorexia, vomiting, abdominal distention, abdominal pain, headache, diarrhea, sometimes constipation, cloudiness of consciousness, doughy abdomen, and hepatomegaly.

Investigations may reveal eosinopenia, leukopenia with relative lymphocytosis in a proportion of the cases, Widal test with "O" antibody titer of 1 in 250 or more, and *Salmonella typhi* in blood and bone marrow culture.

Tuberculosis

In generalized tuberculosis, splenomegaly may accompany hepatomegaly and other signs of tuberculosis (Fig. 55.4). Attempts must be made to identify the primary lesion in the lungs or elsewhere.

Septicemia

Any child with acute splenomegaly and multisystem involvement, especially when osteomyelitis, an abscess, pneumonia, endocarditis or some septic focus is apparent, must have septicema (severe bacteremia making the patient

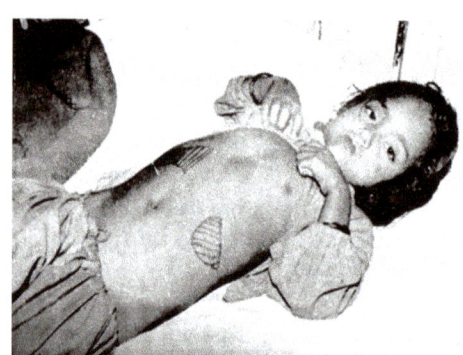

Fig. 55.3: *Enteric fever*—Note the soft modest splenomegaly and slight hepatomegaly. This child presented with 9 days history of pyrexia. Widal test showed a titer of 1 in 320.

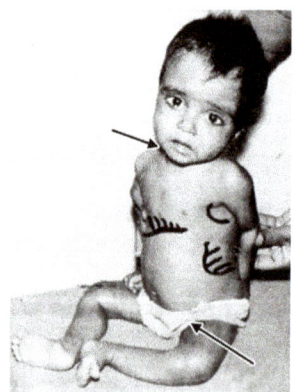

Fig. 55.4: *Generalized tuberculosis*—Note the splenohepatomegaly and generalized lymphadenopathy—cervical (indicated by the arrow), axillary, and inguinal (also indicated by the arrow).

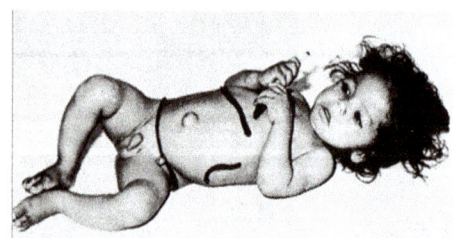

Fig. 55.2: *Malaria*—Note the significant enlargement of spleen which was quite firm as also just palpable liver. Presenting complaint was just episodes of hyperpyrexia of short duration (3 days). Response to chloroquine was dramatic.

critically ill) excluded. A blood culture is mandatory before initiating intensive antibacterial therapy.

Infective Endocarditis

In this condition caused by *Streptococcus viridans*, *Escherichia coli*, *Staphylococcus albus* or other infective agents in subjects with congenital or acquired valvular heart disease, a sort of septicemic stage develops. Clinical features include, besides splenomegaly, low-grade fever, general weakness, malaise, anorexia, and splinter hemorrhages. Splenomegaly, anemia, and clubbing are usually present. Osier nodes may be found in some patients. Microscopic hematuria is invariably present. Leukocytosis is usual. Erythrocyte sedimentation rate (ESR) is high.

Diagnosis is confirmed by positive blood culture, taken every 6 hours for 36 hours, while the patient is yet to be started on appropriate intensive chemotherapy.

Brucellosis

Splenomegaly in brucellosis is accompanied by hepatomegaly, cervical and axillary lymphadenopathy, high fever with chills and diaphoresis, epistaxis, cough, abdominal pain, and weight loss. These manifestations are preceded by prodromal symptoms such as tiredness, weakness, headache, myalgia, constipation, and anorexia.

Diagnosis can be confirmed by brucella agglutination test showing titers over 1 in 60 in acute illness.

Kala-azar

Spleen enlarges quite rapidly in kala-azar. This contrast with the slow enlargement of the liver in this condition. Remaining manifestations include mild-to-moderate persistent pyrexia, skin pigmentation, weight loss despite good dietary intake since the appetite remains good, and scalp hair which become sparse and brittle, leaving areas of alopecia (Fig. 55.5).

Investigations show positive aldehyde (formal gel) test, Chopra antimony test, complement fixation test, and *Leishmania donovani* (LD) bodies in blood and bone marrow smears.

Intrauterine Infections

Toxoplasmosis, rubella, cytomegalovirus, syphilis, and herpes are nearly always accompanied by splenomegaly.

Extended rubella syndrome is characterized by, besides splenomegaly, growth, retardation, congenital heart disease (patent ductus arteriosus), hepatitis with hepatomegaly, thrombocytopenic purpura, deafness, otitis media, pancreatitis, pneumonitis, cerebral diplegia, cleft palate and foot, syndactyly, spina bifida and talipes equinovarus, dental malformations, microphthalmia, buphthalmos, and retinal lesions.

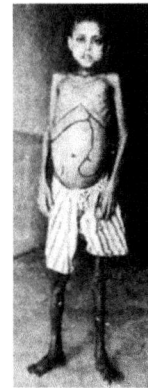

Fig. 55.5: *Kala-azar*—Note the massive splenomegaly (quite out of proportion to hepatomegaly), remarkable wasting, pigmentation, and sparse brittle hair.

Congenital toxoplasmosis is characterized by, besides splenomegaly, poor feeding, maculopapular rash, pyrexia, hepatomegaly, lymphadenopathy, jaundice, hydrocephalus/microcephaly, microphthalmia, seizures, cerebral calcification radiologically, and chorioretinitis.

Cytomegalovirus infection, both congenital and postnatally acquired, is accompanied by splenomegaly. Remaining manifestations of the congenital infection include—jaundice, purpura, hepatomegaly, microcephaly, cerebral calcification, and chorioretinitis. Appearance of a petechial rash in association with splenomegaly on the very first day of birth strongly suggests this condition as the probable diagnosis. Isolate congenital anomalies such as high-arched palate, clubfoot, microcephaly, and deafness may also occur in this disease.

Acquired infection too is accompanied by splenomegaly. Other features include—pyrexia, septic shock, gray pallor, fast deterioration in respiratory status, hepatomegaly, and atypical lymphocytosis in premature newborns and infants 1-2 months of age.

Acquired infection in older children also causes hepatosplenomegaly in addition to sore throat, malaise, myalgia, anorexia, headache, abdominal pain, cervical or other regional lymphadenopathy, pyrexia, excessive sleep, atypical lymphocytosis, and liver dysfunction.

Congenital syphilis (early) may manifest in first 6 weeks of life with snuffles, rhagades, lesions over skin, soles, and palms, mucous patches, ulceration and fissuring in mouth and anus, anemia, hepatosplenomegaly, jaundice, fever, failure to thrive, lymphadenopathy, and chorioretinitis. Painful osteochondritis and/or priostitis may cause pseudoparalysis, the so-called parrot paralysis. Renal, meningovascular, respiratory, and hepatic complications may occur.

Neonatal herpes simplex, usually acquired during passage through the birth canal, may be responsible for splenomegaly in association with hepatomegaly, jaundice, seizures, apneic spells, cyanosis, respiratory distress, bulging anterior fontanel, paralysis opisthotonos, decerebrate rigidity, and coma.

Infectious Mononucleosis

This condition, caused by Epstein–Barr (EB) virus with positive heterophilic antibody response, is an important cause of marked splenomegaly. Remaining manifestations include malaise, pyrexia, sore throat, headache, nausea or vomiting, hepatomegaly, lymphadenopathy, petechiae at the junction of hard and soft palate and atypical lymphocytosis.

Neonatal Hepatitis

In almost half of the infants with neonatal hepatitis, moderate splenic enlargement occurs. Remaining features of this condition include jaundice, poor feeding, vomiting, anemia, high-colored urine, and intermittent loss of pigment in the stools. Liver is grossly enlarged with firm consistency. The differential diagnosis from extrahepatic biliary atresia often poses problem.

For details see Chapter 39 (Jaundice).

Common Viral Infections

Common nonspecific viral infections responsible for producing unexplained pyrexia, body pains, malaise, etc. are often accompanied by splenomegaly. This diagnosis, therefore, should be seriously considered before subjecting the patient to cumbersome investigations.

For details of acquired immunodeficiency syndrome (AIDS) see Chapter 35.

Histoplasmosis

Occurrence of splenomegaly in combination with hepatomegaly, pyrexia, generalized lymphadenopathy, anemia, and leukopenia should arouse suspicion of disseminated histoplasmosis. Histoplasmin skin test is indicated in such a situation.

Hydatid Disease

Rarely, echinococcal infection may produce one or more cysts in the spleen resulting in marked splenomegaly. Similar cysts may be found in lungs, liver, and other organs. Skin test and/or indirect hemagglutination reaction may help in confirming the clinical diagnosis.

Hematogenous Diseases

Anemias

Splenomegaly is an important feature of hemolytic anemia as a result of extramedullary hematopoiesis and hyperplasia of the reticuloendothelial system. It occurs in congenital (thalassemia major, sickle cell disease) as well as acquired hemolytic state (Figs. 55.6 and 55.7).

Splenomegaly occurs also in nutritional anemias due to iron, folate, vitamin B_{12}, or combined deficiency.

Hypersplenism

This state is characterized by an enlarged spleen usually secondary to a large number of causes, depression of one or more cellular elements of blood (anemia, leukopenia, thrombocytopenia, etc.), active formation of these elements in the bone marrow, and correction of the said hematologic abnormalities resulting from splenectomy.

Thrombocytopenic purpura

In approximately 25% children with acute idiopathic thrombocytopenic purpura (ITP), slight splenomegaly may be encountered. Moderate splenomegaly occurs in recurrent or chronic ITP cases.

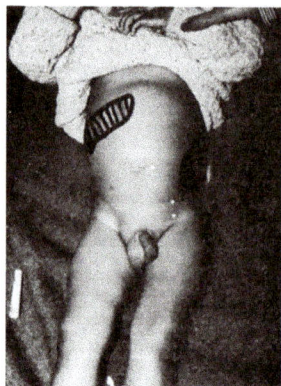

Fig. 55.6: *Thalassemia major*—Note the splenohepatomegaly in the child whose chronic anemia failed to respond to iron therapy. His fetal hemoglobin turned out to be 65%.

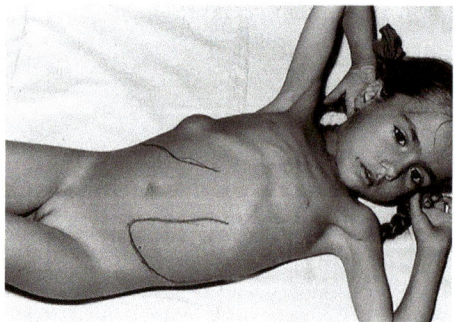

Fig. 55.7: *Splenohepatomegaly* in a 3-year-old girl with sickle cell anemia. Spleen tends to shrink as also cease to function (autosplenectomy) in the subsequent years as a result of repeated thrombosis.

Congestive Splenomegaly

This state may occur secondary to portal or splenic vein obstruction, to intrahepatic disease (cirrhosis, Wilson disease, galactosemia, biliary atresia, cystic fibrosis, alpha-l-antitrypsin deficiency) or to chronic congestive cardiac failure.

Manifestations include splenomegaly, thrombocytopenic hemorrhages, anemia, prominent superficial abdominal veins (collaterals), hemorrhoids/esophageal varices and ascites.

Investigations show abnormal liver function, pancytopenia, active hematopoiesis with abundant megakaryocytes in the marrow and raised portal venous pressure with visualization of the obstructive lesion of splenic and portal veins, on splenoportogram.

Inborn Errors of Metabolism

Splenomegaly is a feature of several inborn errors of metabolism and storage diseases, including glycogen-storage disease, Gaucher disease, Niemann–Pick disease, gargoylism, amyloidosis, hemosiderosis, xanthomatosis, cystinosis, and cystic fibrosis. A reasonable discussion on these conditions is available elsewhere in this book, particularly in Chapter 35, which deals with hepatomegaly.

Malignant Diseases

Splenomegaly occurs in malignant diseases such as leukemias (its size is enormous in chronic myeloid leukemias), Hodgkin lymphoma, non-Hodgkin lymphoma, etc.

Miscellaneous

Splenic Cysts

An asymptomatic smooth lump in the left upper quadrant of abdomen displacing the stomach medially should arouse suspicion of splenic cysts. These cysts may be—(i) epidermoid cysts, or (ii) pseudocysts which follow trauma or infection.

Hemangioma

Rarely, a large hemangioma may be responsible for splenic enlargement. X-ray of abdomen shows an enlarged spleen and, occasionally, calcification in the hemangiomatous growth.

Abscess

Splenic abscess may result as a part of multiple pyemic abscesses or septicemia.

Systemic Lupus Erythematosus

Splenomegaly together with hepatomegaly constitutes an important finding in systemic lupus erythematosus (SLE). The diagnosis needs to be seriously considered in the presence of additional features such as unexplained pyrexia of prolonged duration, butterfly rash over cheeks and bridge of the nose, joint or muscle pains, and weight loss.

Demonstration of LE cell phenomenon or, more importantly, antinuclear antibodies (ANA) establishes the diagnosis.

Still's Disease

In this form of juvenile rheumatoid arthritis (JRA), splenomegaly occurs in association with arthritis/arthralgia and lymphadenopathy. The illness has an acute febrile or systemic onset.

Nutritional Recovery Syndrome

Splenomegaly may occur in a proportion of cases with nutritional recovery syndrome. This syndrome is encountered in grossly malnourished children who are being treated with very high quantity of proteins. Manifestations include increasing hepatomegaly, abdominal distention, ascites, prominent thoracoabdominal venous network, hypertrichosis, parotid swelling, gynecomastia, and eosinophilia. It occurs both in kwashiorkor and marasmus and is supposed to be related to endocrinal disturbances.

Extrahepatic Biliary Atresia

In advanced stage of this condition, marked hepatomegaly is accompanied by splenomegaly. Jaundice keeps deepening and lightening. Vitamin K deficiency may cause hemorrhages. Often, it becomes difficult to differentiate it from neonatal hepatitis.

FURTHER READING

1. Chadburn A. The spleen: Anatomy and anatomic function. *Semin Hematol* 2003;37:13-21.
2. Camitta BM. Splenomegaly. In: Kliegman RM, St Geme JII JW, Blum NJ, et al (Eds). *Nelson Textbook of Pediatrics,* 18th edition. Philadelphia: Saunders 2008:2091.
3. Medscape. Splenomegaly workup. Available at: http://emedicine.medscape.com/article/206208-workup. Accessed on: August 2017.

CHAPTER 56

Stiff Neck

BACKGROUND

Stiff neck is an alarming complaint, calling upon the clinician to use his skill, knowledge, and experience in arriving at its precise diagnosis with judicious use of investigations. The cause may be as simple as a self-limited phenothiazine toxicity, cervical lymphadenitis or viral myalgia involving the sternomastoid muscle, or as serious as meningitis.

HISTORY

In a given case, you must ask about the onset of the complaint. Has it been there for quite some time or it occurred only now or recently? Any history of trauma, fever, muscle pains, sore throat, dysphagia, drugging especially to check vomiting associated with gastroenteritis, convulsions, change in sensorium, odd behavior, etc.? Did it follow lumbar puncture, which may have been done elsewhere before the child reports to you? In neck stiffness of slow, chronic onset in a young child, find out if the parents had all along been aware of a small hard swelling in connection with the sternomastoid muscle ever since the neonatal period or little later.

PHYSICAL EXAMINATION

Clinical examination should, besides other things, be particularly aimed at evaluation of the central nervous system (CNS) status. Cervical lymphadenopathy, tonsillitis, pharyngitis, local findings in connection with the sternomastoid muscles, evidence of trauma, and vertebral anomalies.

INVESTIGATIONS

Imaging

- Plain X-ray—different views
- Computed tomography (CT) scan
- Magnetic resonance imaging (MRI).

Lumbar puncture in case of signs suggestive of meningitis.

IMPORTANT DIFFERENTIALS

Phenothiazine Toxicity

Neck stiffness is a common manifestation of phenothiazine toxicity/idiosyncrasy. Clinical picture is dominated by acute onset of signs and symptoms pertaining to the extrapyramidal system. The characteristic features include, besides torticollis, choreiform movements, muscle rigidity, opisthotonos, marked deviation of the eyes, and oculogyric crisis. Trismus, swallowing difficulties, drooling, tremors, ataxia, and coma occur much less frequently.

Drugs responsible for this self-limited condition include triflupromazine, prochlorperazine, and chlorpromazine. Concomitant administration of chloroquine, amodiaquine, metoclopramide, haloperidol, phenytoin, diazoxide, lithium, reserpine, chlorprothixene as also the presence of dehydration boosts the risk of phenothiazine toxicity, both in frequency and severity. Now it is being increasingly appreciated that some of these drugs—metoclopramide, for instance—may per se cause extrapyramidal manifestations. Several cases as a result of metoclopramide, and occasionally, cases related to chloroquine, haloperidol, and phenytoin have been seen.

Meningitis and Other CNS Infections

Meningitis must always be excluded as a cause of stiff neck. Neck stiffness in this condition (as also in meningism secondary to a host of viral, bacterial, and parasitic infections such as pneumonia, mumps, malaria, etc.) is observed on flexion only and not on lateral movements.

Pyogenic meningitis is characterized by sudden onset of high fever, vomiting, restlessness, irritability, headache, and often convulsions with or without neck stiffness as a leading complaint. The younger the age of the child the lesser the specific manifestations are. In a newborn, for instance, pyogenic meningitis may have insidious onset with meager symptoms like refusal to take feed, fever, and irritability. Some may have convulsions. These, especially in the presence of bulging anterior fontanel, must arouse suspicion.

Physical examination may reveal, in addition to neck stiffness, positive Kernig and Brudzinski signs. Cranial nerve palsies and papilledema are present in some cases. Hemiplegia may be noticed in a few cases who report late.

Lumbar puncture clinches the diagnosis.

Tuberculous meningitis manifests with neck stiffness and other features of raised intracranial pressure and meningeal irritation in its second stage. Child becomes progressively drowsy and even unconscious. Headache, vomiting, and feverishness become aggravated. Kernig sign is positive. Plantars are extensor. Ankle and patellar clonus may be elicitable, abdominal reflexes are absent. Hypotonia is usual. In small infants, anterior fontanel may be bulging. Cranial nerves involved are third, fourth, and seventh. Ocular paralysis, strabismus, nystagmus, and contracted pupils are common. Also, there may be papilledema. Choroid tubercles along the blood vessels of choroid plexus may be seen in a small proportion of the cases. This stage is followed in about a week or so by the third stage which is characterized by widespread paralysis and coma. Neck stiffness disappears in this terminal stage.

Lumbar puncture is a must to clinch the diagnosis.

Encephalitis may also manifest with meningeal irritation as a result of inflammatory reaction of meninges. Accompanying manifestations include change in sensorium, varying from lethargy to coma, fever, vomiting, and convulsions. Some children demonstrate peculiar behavior, hyperactivity, altered speech, and ataxia. Headache is common in older children whereas an infant may start with sheer gross irritability and feeding difficulty. What is remarkable about this condition is that the clinical picture shows rapid variation from hour to hour.

Diagnosis is essentially clinical. Lumbar puncture should always be done, not because encephalitis has any typical cerebrospinal fluid (CSF) picture but to rule out meningitis.

Cerebral malaria and brain abscess may manifest with meningeal signs in addition to other features characteristic of these conditions. A high index of suspicion helps in identifying them.

Retropharyngeal Abscess

Stiff neck may accompany retropharyngeal abscess complicating bacterial pharyngitis or resulting as an extension of a wound infection in the neighborhood or vertebral osteomyelitis.

Manifestations, occurring in a child who just has or is still having pharyngitis or nasopharyngitis, include abrupt onset of high fever, dysphagia, throat pain and distress, refusal of feed, noisy breathing, drooling, and hypertension of the neck.

Examination shows a distinct bulge in the posterior pharyngeal wall. Else, in a suspected case, a lateral film of the neck should be done to detect it as a retropharyngeal mass.

Retropharyngeal abscess may occur in caries spine as well (Fig. 56.1).

Cervical Lymphadenitis

Not infrequently, massive cervical lymphadenitis may produce a tender bulge in the posterior pharyngeal wall and cause skin manifestations to retropharyngeal abscess.

Viral Torticollis

Also called as rheumatic stiff neck, this condition is characterized by tender stiff neck, mainly on lateral or rotatory movements rather than on flexion, due to acute spasm of sternomastoid muscle, presumably as a result of a viral infection. It has nothing to do with rheumatic fever or rheumatoid arthritis.

Trauma

Stiff neck may result from trauma to the neck say a hard blow, leading to contusion and strain of the ligaments and muscles.

Congenital Anomalies

Congenital anomalies of the cervical vertebrae may be responsible for torticollis in some cases.

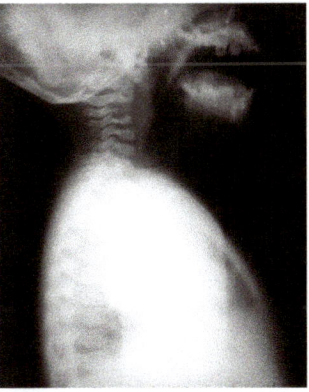

Fig. 56.1: *Retropharyngeal abscess*—Note the increase in the retropharyngeal space and erosion of body of C3 vertebra in the lateral view of cervical spine.

Congenital torticollis refers to a condition in which there is developmental shortening of the sternomastoid muscle of one side. Inability to turn the newborn's head 90° in both directions after 1 week of age should arouse suspicion of this diagnosis. You may feel a firm lump in the midportion of the affected muscle during the first 2–3 months. Left untreated, the muscle becomes fibrotic and shortened, resulting in permanent limitation of neck movements. The head and face also become asymmetrical.

This entity may well be the same as sternomastoid tumor.

Remaining Causes of Stiff Neck

Lumbar puncture, poliomyelitis, tetanus, intracranial hemorrhage or tumor, rheumatoid arthritis, meningeal leukemia, spastic cerebral palsy, myositis ossificans progressiva, etc.

FURTHER READING

1. Teichtahl AJ, McColl G. An approach to neck pain. *Rheumatology* 2013;42:774-777.

CHAPTER 57

Stridor

BACKGROUND

Stridor is defined as an audibly harsh, noisy inspiratory sound as a result of incomplete obstruction of the laryngeal area or trachea. Often it is accompanied by croupy cough, hoarseness, dyspnea, restlessness, and feeding difficulties.

HISTORY

In stridor manifesting at birth, always consider the possibility of trauma if intubation had been done, and obstruction caused by mucus, meconium or blood. This kind of stridor usually disappears within 24 hours.

Find out if the stridor is worsening? If the answer is affirmative, there is strong possibility of an anatomical obstruction or vocal cord paralysis.

Is the stridor accompanied by significant respiratory distress? Laryngeal atresia and tracheal atresia, both serious conditions, need to be considered in this situation.

Hoarseness accompanying stridor in a newborn suggests a laryngeal problem with the sole exception of laryngomalacia.

Stridor with brassy or barking cough in a newborn points to a tracheal problem.

Does the newborn tend to keep the neck in an hyperextended position? Does he have dysphagic symptoms? If yes, chances are of your dealing with a case of vascular rings.

PHYSICAL EXAMINATION

Physical examination should, in particular, ascertain if the newborn has severe dyspnea with cyanosis and chest retraction. Any glossoptosis, micrognathia, or choanal atresia?

In stridor manifesting during postneonatal period and later, find out if the child had been hale and hearty prior to the onset of this problem. Does he have fever, cough, hoarseness, sore throat or dyspnea? Is he in the habit of putting foreign body into his mouth?

While conducting clinical check-up, you must focus on certain vital points. Is the stridor purely inspiratory, expiratory or both? Is it intermittent, or persistent? Is there respiratory distress? Is there any extrinsic neck mass? Any evidence of injury? Is the throat congested?

INVESTIGATIONS

Mild stridor needs no investigations. In severe cases, tests are dictated by the likely impression arrived at through history and physical examination.

- Pulse oximetry may be useful to determine the extent and severity of the stridor and respiratory compromise.
- Arterial blood gas evaluation for moderate-to-severe cases.
- *Radiology*: Anteroposterior (AP) and lateral radiographs of the neck and chest are useful for evaluating the airway and lungs.
- Barium esophagography may be performed if vascular compression, tracheoesophageal fistula, gastroesophageal reflux (GER), or neurologic differential dysfunction is suspected.
- *Imaging*: Contrast-enhanced computed tomography (CT) can demonstrate mediastinal masses or aberrant vessels. Magnetic resonance imaging (MRI) may be helpful in delineating lesions of the upper airway and vascular anomalies.
- A pH probe or barium swallow in GER is suspected.

IMPORTANT DIFFERENTIALS

Stridor Manifesting in the Neonatal Period

Laryngomalacia

Also called as congenital laryngeal stridor, this condition is responsible for nearly 90% cases of stridor in the neonatal period. The cause is abnormal collapse of the supraglottic tissues (elongated or curved epiglottis, redundant aryeepiglottic folds) during inspiratory phase.

Manifestations occur usually after the first week or two of birth. Stridor is characteristically intermittent. It is mainly inspiratory though, at times, it may be partly expiratory. During sleep and rest, it disappears whereas crying or excitement aggravates it. It is much less in prone position but is increased in supine position. The voice, cry, feeding, and general health of the baby remain unaffected. Dyspnea with indrawing of the lower part of the chest during inspiration occurs in a large majority of the cases.

After the age of 6 months, the manifestations begin to regress. The condition disappears by the age of 18–24 months.

Atretic Obstructive Lesions in the Upper Airway

Congenital atretic lesions of the upper airway usually cause death soon after birth. In supraglottic web, the infant has inspiratory stridor in association with hoarseness, subdued cry, and chest indrawing. Laryngeal webs and cyst cause hoarse cry, dyspnea, and inspiratory stridor. Stridor as a result of subglottic pathology (congenital subglottic stenosis, hemangioma, angioma, papilloma, lymphangioma, polyps, etc.) is both inspiratory and expiratory. Hoarseness may be present. Cry is normal. Brassy or croupy cough may sometimes accompany the clinical picture.

Tracheomalacia, tracheal cyst or tracheal stenosis leads to expiratory stridor.

Laryngeal Edema/Obstruction

Laryngeal obstruction from presence of mucus, meconium or blood together with edema from trauma of intubation is an important cause of inspiratory stridor. It resolves well within 24 hours, particularly if aspiration of the obstructive stuff can be carried out under direct vision without loss of time.

Vocal cord paralysis is paralysis of the recurrent laryngeal nerve (usually right) which may occur in hydrocephalus-associated Arnold–Chiari malformation or in brainstem injury. Bilateral paralysis may occur.

Manifestations, more marked in bilateral involvement, include inspiratory stridor, hoarseness, weak cry, and choking during feeding.

Laryngoscopy shows lack of mobility of the vocal cords.

Vascular Rings

Stridor in vascular rings (double aorta or an abnormally placed subclavian artery) is, as a rule, intermittent and both inspiratory and expiratory though it may be purely inspiratory or expiratory. Accompanying features include intractable cough which may be brassy or bitonal, and opisthotonos. An attempt at flexing the neck worsens the stridor.

Diagnosis is by exclusion of other causes and by lateral X-ray of the airway.

Tumors

Outside compression from mediastinal or neck tumors (say lymphangioma, goiter, etc.) may produce stridor. There usually is some more evidence of compression, making the diagnosis easy.

Stridor Manifesting in Later Infancy and Childhood

Acute Laryngotracheobronchitis

This condition, caused usually by *Haemophilus influenzae* or parainfluenzae virus and also termed as croup, is the most common cause of acute inspiratory stridor. It occurs in children, usually under 3 years of age.

Following one or two days history of "cold", the child develops inspiratory stridor, usually at night. He begins to hyperventilate and is quite upset. As the stridor persists, cyanosis and lower chest retraction develops. With further progression of the disease, impairment of the consciousness occurs. Trachea and bronchi may become partially obstructed by thick secretions resulting in expiratory stridor and coarse rhonchi in the lung fields.

Acute Epiglottitis

This state of acute septicemia usually caused by *H. influenzae* type B, *Staphylococcus* or *Pneumococcus*, is characterized by rapid development of inspiratory stridor, dyspnea, muffling of the voice, dysphagia, and drooling. The child is febrile and flushed. With increasing respiratory effort, inspiratory stridor diminishes. Throat examination shows an intensely red and swollen epiglottis.

Foreign Body

Sudden development of inspiratory stridor in a child who was otherwise fine, particularly if he is left to eat unattended and is fond of taking small objects into the mouth, must arouse suspicion of a foreign body having got impacted in the larynx.

Diphtheria

Laryngeal diphtheria may be responsible for inspiratory stridor. Additional manifestations include hoarseness, aphonia, brassy or barking cough, dyspnea and cyanosis, restlessness, anxiety, and prostration. Neck shows lymphadenitis and brawny edema (bull-neck).

Diagnosis is by observing the characteristic membrane in the throat. In a vast majority of the cases, laryngeal involvement is secondary to faucial diphtheria. You may, however, readily see the membrane in the larynx by laryngoscopy.

In order to establish the diagnosis, you must take a throat or laryngeal swab and examine the smear for the organisms, which are seen as rods with bipolar bar.

Trauma

Any trauma to the larynx, resulting from instrumentation, corrosive agents or inhalation of smoke, may be responsible for laryngeal edema and acute stridor.

Laryngospasm

Laryngospasm, associated with tetany of whatsoever etiology, may manifest with inspiratory stridor, apneic episodes, and cyanosis. The attacks last over a few minutes and keep recurring.

Retropharyngeal Abscess

A retropharyngeal abscess manifests with inspiratory stridor only when pressure is put on the larynx. Clinical features include an abrupt onset of high fever, dysphagia, refusal of feeding, throat pain, hyperextension of the neck, and noisy respiration. A careful examination reveals a bulge in the posterior pharyngeal wall. This spectrum of manifestations is preceded by an acute nasopharyngitis or pharyngitis.

Retropharyngeal Lymphadenitis

A nonfluctuating lymphadenitis may produce a tender bulge in the retropharyngeal space and a clinical picture closely resembling retropharyngeal abscess.

FURTHER READING

1. Mancuso RF. Stridor in neonates. *Pediatr Clin North Am* 1996;43:1339-1356.
2. Griffiths AG. Chronic or recurrent respiratory symptoms. In: Kliegman RM, St Geme III JW, Blum NJ, et al (Eds). *Nelson Textbook of Pediatrics*, 21st edn. Philadelphia: Elsevier 2020:2161-2165.
3. Medscape. Stridor workup. Available at: http://emedicine.medscape.com/article/995267-workup#c5. Accessed on: 24 July 2019.

CHAPTER 58

Sudden Infant Death Syndrome

BACKGROUND

The term, *sudden infant death syndrome (SIDS)*, is applied to the sudden, unexpected death of an apparently healthy infant (typically 2–3-month-old) who was put to sleep without any suspicion of such an anticipation. A conventional autopsy fails to reveal the cause of death. When an apparently healthy infant suffers from an episode in which he stops breathing, develops cyanosis or pallor and becomes unresponsive but is successfully resuscitated, the term, apparent life-threatening event (ALTE) should be employed. This state has also been termed as near-miss or aborted SIDS. Such an infant runs significant risk of SIDS. In case of an infant with SIDS in a family, risk of the next or subsequent infant suffering from SIDS is five times the usual risk.

The crux of the pathologic findings points to occurrence of hypoxia preceding the tragic event. Paradoxically, autopsy shows no hyperplasia of the carotid bodies. This observation weighs against the presence of chronic hypoxia.

Etiology remains unclear. Allergy to cow's milk, enlargement of thymus, suffocation, deficiency of parathyroids or adrenals, hypernatremia and fulminant respiratory infection causing laryngeal obstruction, and/or spasm figure among the conditions that have been incriminated in its etiology. On top of all this, states such as prolonged sleep apnea associated with central nervous system (CNS) disorders, vascular rings, familial prolongation of QT interval (Romano Ward and Jervell and Lange-Nielsen syndromes), accidental suffocation, and child abuse and neglect (CAN) could camouflage as SIDS. A common etiology involving an abnormality of cardiorespiratory control, in which state of consciousness or CNS activity plays a modulating role, appears to be shared by all cases of true SIDS.

HISTORY

In case of infants at risk (low birth weight, near-miss, or ALTE, sibs of SIDS case, etc.), history should be obtained in relation to physiological handicaps before birth, e.g. low Apgar score, abnormality in control of respiration, heart rate, and temperature, and postnatal growth retardation. It is appropriate to question the parents about infant's feeding, medication, etc.

PHYSICAL EXAMINATION

Physical examination should obtain information on the infant's nutritional status, hydration, evidence of infection, CAN, and neurological handicap. Respiratory system must particularly be evaluated. He must also be observed while being given a feed.

With this clinical evaluation, it should be possible to rule out a known medical cause for the catastrophe.

INVESTIGATIONS

In suspected cases, investigations should include:
- Blood analysis for serum glucose, sodium, potassium, calcium, phosphorus, magnesium, blood urea nitrogen (BUN), pH, and blood gas analysis
- Urinalysis
- Microbiological tests as dictated by the merits of the case
- Electrocardiography (ECG) monitoring
- Electroencephalogram (EEG)
- Barium swallow
- Esophageal pH studies
- Chest X-ray
- Skeletal survey and 4–8-hour sleep studies.

DIFFERENTIALS

Apnea (Respiratory Pause)

Apnea of 20 seconds or more is significant. It may be of three types:
1. Central as a result of absent neurological output from the respiratory center.
2. Obstructive as a result of closure of the upper airway (even lower airway may be involved) so that the

infant fails to experience airflow despite considerable respiratory effort.
3. Mixed as a result of combination of an obstructive episode and central apnea. Though, apnea has been incriminated in the etiology of SIDS, the cause and effect relationship remains unclear.

Upper Airway Dysfunction

Anatomical and developmental anomalies of the upper airway may cause obstruction and, perhaps, SIDS or ALTE, e.g. posterior displacement of the tongue as in Pierre Robin syndrome, reduced airway diameter following neck flexion, cleft palate, laryngomalacia, tracheomalacia, bronchomalacia, laryngeal cleft or other anomalies, tracheoesophageal fistula of H-type, vascular rings, immature or abnormal neuromuscular control of oropharyngeal muscles, etc. In the presence of a viral respiratory infection, proneness to airway obstruction may be enhanced.

Hyperreactive Airway

Introduction of some fluids into the larynx may stimulate reflex apnea and reflux with aspiration, and cause SIDS.

Cardiac Anomalies (Arrhythmias)

The role of cardiac arrhythmias (R on T phenomenon, sick sinus syndrome, etc.) in the causation of SIDS remains debatable. No significant difference in cardiac rhythm is found between infants dying of SIDS and the normal controls. In ALTE, a proportion of the infants exhibit increased vagal tone. The resultant bradycardia is, perhaps, triggered by events such as a reflux.

Gastroesophageal Reflux

Reflux, a common finding in first 6 months of life, has been shown to produce apnea in some studies. How far it contributes to occurrence of SIDS remains unclear.

Abnormal Autonomic Nervous System and Chemical Mediators

Abnormality in autonomic nervous system in infants with ALTE is evidenced by increased heart rate, and decreased heart-rate viability, shorter QT index and, higher ventilatory response to CO_2. In SIDS, increased levels of dopamine in carotid bodies are found. In infants with abnormal autonomic nervous system, a relationship between SIDS and short-chain opioid peptides, e.g. B-casomorphin, has been postulated.

The role of chemical mediators such as catecholamines, endorphins, and serotonin in causation of SIDS has also been speculated.

Brainstem and Carotid Body Defects

Evidence suggests that brainstem and carotid body defects may be responsible for some cases of SIDS. The former circuit controls respiratory or cardiac stability. The integrity of the latter is important for oxygen responsiveness as also sheer survival.

Hyperthermia

Overwrapping leading to overheating of the preterm infants, who are susceptible to apnea when exposed to high environmental temperature, has been suggested as a factor in the etiology of SIDS. The concept, however, remains unproven.

FURTHER READING

1. Blair PS, Sidebotham P, Berry PJ, et al. Major epidemiologic changes in sudden infant death syndrome. A 20-year population-based study in UK. *Lancet* 2006;367:314-319.
2. Health Grove. Sudden infant death syndrome in India. Available at: http://global-disease-burden.healthgrove.com/l/91392/Sudden-Infant-Death-Syndrome-in-India. Accessed on: 24 July 2019.
3. Horn MH, Kinnamon DD, Ferraro N, et al. Smaller mandibular size in infants with history of an apparent life-threatening event. *J Pediatr* 2006;149:499-504.
4. Opdal SH, Rognum TO. New insight into sudden infant death syndrome gene: does it exist? *Pediatrics* 2004;114:e506-512.

CHAPTER 59

Tall Stature

BACKGROUND

By definition, *tall stature* is said to exist when an individual has the height that is above the 97th percentile for age. It is infrequent for the parents to seek advice for a child with tall stature. During the past 3 decades, only 18 adolescents and 3 toddlers were brought to the outpatient departments (OPDs) at Postgraduate Institute of Medical Education and Research, Chandigarh, Medical College, Shimla, Government Medical College, Jammu, and Narayana Medical College, Nellore, for this complaint. The incidence is, perhaps, not as low. It appears that tall stature is evidently socially more acceptable than short stature. Hence, parents do not care to seek advice for too tall children. Interestingly, the treatment given to this condition in the pediatric texts too varies from negligible to far too scant. Table 59.1 outlines the important causes of tall stature and Box 59.1 summarizes the clinical situations ending up with tallness.

TABLE 59.1: Etiology of tall stature.

System	Condition(s)
Genetic/chromosomal	Familial Marfan syndrome Klinefelter syndrome Primordial gigantism Beckwith–Wiedemann syndrome
Endocrinal	Congenital adrenal hyperplasia (in the early stage) Androgen-secreting adrenal tumors (in the early stage) Thyrotoxicosis True precocious puberty (in the early stage)
Pituitary gigantism Central nervous system (CNS) Metabolic	Hydrocephalus Homocystinuria

HISTORY

History should endeavor to obtain information about the abnormally tall parent(s) or close relative(s), as also about his intellectual performance. Is there any suggestion of precocious puberty or delayed puberty? Was the child very long right from the beginning or showed rapid linear growth in the subsequent few years? Did the height show sudden acceleration only recently?

BOX 59.1: Clinical situation ending up with tall stature.

Fetal overgrowth
- Maternal diabetes
- Cerebral gigantism
- Beckwith–Wiedemann syndrome
- Other insulin-like growth factor II (IGF-II) excess syndromes

Postnatal overgrowth
- Leading to tall stature in childhood
  – Familial
  – Cerebral gigantism
  – Beckwith–Wiedemann syndrome
  – Obesity of exogenous origin
  – Pituitary gigantism (excess growth hormone secretion)
  – McCune–Albright syndrome
  – Precocious puberty
  – Marfan syndrome
  – Klinefelter syndrome (XXY)
  – Short stature homeobox (SHOX) excess syndrome
  – Fragile excess syndrome
  – Homocystinuria
  – XYY syndrome
  – Hyperthyroidism
- Leading to tall stature in adulthood
  – Familial (constitutional)
  – Androgen/estrogen deficiency
  – Estrogen resistance (in males)
  – Testicular feminization
  – Adrenocorticotrophic hormone (ACTH) or cortisol deficiency
  – Adrenocorticotrophic hormone (ACTH) or cortisol resistance
  – Aromatase deficiency
  – Pituitary gigantism
  – Marfan syndrome
  – Klinefelter syndrome (XXY)
  – XYY syndrome.

PHYSICAL EXAMINATION

Physical examination, in the first instance, must record the accurate height and body proportions. Are there signs of raised intracranial pressure? Are there any other neurologic signs? Are there any abnormal features like arachnodactyly, antimongoloid slant of eyes, obesity, etc.?

INVESTIGATIONS

- X-ray for bone age
- Karyotyping
- Urine examination for homocystinuria
- Thyroid profile
- Growth hormone level.

Additional laboratory test(s) may be done bearing in mind the clinical impression.

DIFFERENTIALS

Familial Tall Stature

This kind of tallness can be recognized from the family history indicating that the child is taking after one or other parent or a close relative. The child is born with an above-average length. During all stages of growth, he shows a proportionate but above-average growth.

Marfan Syndrome

This autosomal dominant disease is characterized by tall stature with strikingly low upper segment–lower segment ratio, arm span more than height and long slender bones of forearm and long metacarpals together with multiple skeletal, cardiovascular, and ocular malformations (Figs. 59.1 and 59.2). Tallness and slimness are frequently seen right at birth and persist postnatally. Now two types of the conditions are recognized—infantile (congenital) and adult (Table 59.2).

Homocystinuria

This condition is characterized by clinical features that are similar to those seen in Marfan syndrome. The distinction can be established by urinary amino acid analysis.

Klinefelter Syndrome

This 47,XXY syndrome is characterized by, besides tallness, frank mental retardation or simply psychosocial, learning or school adjustment problems, slimness, long legs, poor weight, underdeveloped testes and phallus and delayed pubertal development. All tall boys, more so with mental

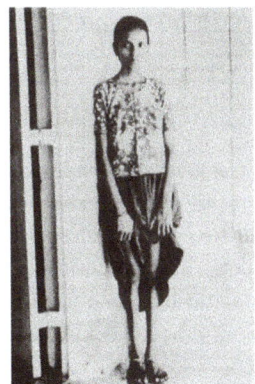

Fig. 59.1: *Marfan syndrome*—Note the striking arachnodactyly, tall statures (165 cm) with very low upper/lower segment ratio (0.8:1.0) and slimness in this 13-year-old girl. She had accompanying mitral valve prolapse.

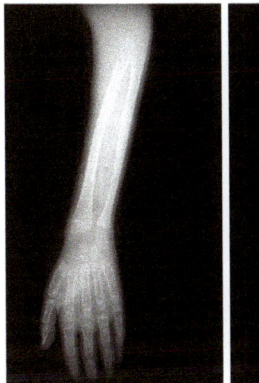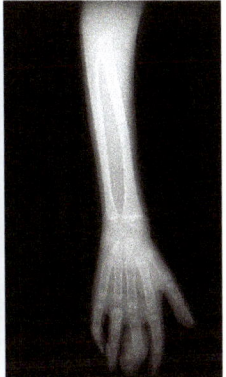

Fig. 59.2: *Marfan syndrome*—Note long slender bones of forearm and long metacarpals.

TABLE 59.2: Marfan syndrome vis-à-vis homocystinuria.

Feature	Marfan syndrome	Homocystinuria
Inheritance	Autosomal dominant	Autosomal recessive
Defect	Connective tissue disorder	Inborn error of metabolism
Cardiovascular component	Usually mitral incompetence, aortic root dilation	Rarely, risk of arterial thrombosis in dehydration
Diagnosis	Clinical	Urine examination
Treatment	Nothing specific	Responds favorably to dietary restriction of methionine plus pyridoxine
Risk to offsprings	1 in 2	Low
Prenatal diagnosis	Not yet available	Amniocentesis

retardation, must have karyotyping to exclude Klinefelter syndrome.

Cerebral Gigantism

Also termed as Sotos syndrome or primordial gigantism, in this condition rapid linear growth occurs during the first 4 years so that the child reaches 97th percentile from the birth length of over 90th percentile. Additional features include large hands and feet, a large head, antimongoloid slant (downslanting eyes), a high-arched palate, and mental retardation. A nonprogressive hypothalamic lesion is blamed for this disorder.

FURTHER READING

1. Gupte S, Abdullah SA, Singh UK. Tall stature. In: Gupte S (Ed). *Recent Advances in Pediatrics (Special Vol 13: Pediatric Endocrinology)*. New Delhi: Jaypee 2004:66-71.
2. Hindmarsh PC, Brook CGD. Tall stature. In: Brook CGD (Ed). *Clinical Pediatric Endocrinology*, 3rd edn. London: Blackwell 1995:195-209.
3. Tall Life. Tall stature: Disorders and syndromes. Available at: https://tall.life/tall-stature-disorders-and-syndromes. Accessed on: 24 July 2019.

CHAPTER 60

Vertigo

BACKGROUND

The term, *vertigo* (Latin, meaning "turning round"), denotes the sensation of moving around in space or having objects move about the person. The former is termed as subjective vertigo and the latter as objective vertigo.

It is often, though wrongly, employed for dizziness, lightheadedness or giddiness.

HISTORY

History should include time of onset of vertigo, presence or absence of preceding aura, relationship with meals, etc. Any preceding illness, especially in relation to the ears, trauma or drug intake. Any accompanying symptoms such as headache, hearing loss, tinnitus, nausea vomiting, nystagmus or visual complaint? Any psychosocial problem(s)? Any suggestion of hyperventilation?

PHYSICAL EXAMINATION

Physical examination, over and above general physical examination (GPE), should focus on ear, nose, and throat (ENT), central nervous system (CNS), and psychosocial evaluation. It is important to look for anemia in particular and record blood pressure.

INVESTIGATIONS

- Computed tomography (CT) scan of the petrous temporal bones
- Magnetic resonance imaging (MRI) of internal auditory meatus and brain
- Vestibular function tests
- Further tests in special circumstance, e.g.
  - Blood glucose monitoring and hemoglobin A1c (HbA1c) in suspected or coexisting diabetes mellitus
  - T3, T4, and thyroid-stimulating hormone (TSH) in suspected thyroid disease.

DIFFERENTIALS

Vasovagal Response (Syncope)

Severe shock or fright may set a neurogenic mechanism (vasovagal stimulation), causing syncope and vertigo.

Drugs

- *Analgesics*: Aspirin, indomethacin, antihistaminics, etc.
- *Antimicrobials*: Trimethoprim, gentamicin, nalidixic acid, kanamicin, isoniazid, sulfas, griseofulvin, minocycline, etc.
- *Tranquillizers*: Phenothiazines, diazepam, etc.
- *Anticonvulsants*: Carbamazepine, phenytoin, clonazepam, etc.
- *Diuretics*: Acetazolamide, thiazides, etc.

Anemia

Anemia leads to fall in cerebral perfusion and orthostatic hypotension. Upon arising from the supine position, the child may experience vertigo and even syncope.

Hypoglycemia

Symptoms, in addition to vertigo, include tachypnea, tachycardia, diaphoresis, generalized weakness, fainting, and seizures.

Epidemic Vertigo

The condition follows an upper respiratory infection (viral). It occurs in recurrences and subsides in a matter of a week or two.

Benign Paroxysmal Vertigo

Occurring at 1–3 years of age, a sudden attack of severe vertigo may be accompanied by vomiting and nystagmus.

The terrified child becomes pale, sweats profusely, cries, and clings to mother. The attack lasts for some seconds or minutes but recurrences may be seen over months and sometimes years. In contrast to epilepsy, sensorium is preserved. The condition may well be a migraine equivalent.

Remaining Causes of Vertigo

- Hyperventilation
- Seizure disorder
- Migraine
- Vestibular neuronitis
- Otitis media
- Raised intracranial pressure (RICP)
- Head injury
- Mumps
- Cerebellar tumor or abscess
- Allergy
- Heat stroke
- Ramsay Hunt syndrome.

FURTHER READING

1. Child Neurology Foundation. Vertigo. Available at: www.childneurologyfoundation.org/disorders/vertigo. Accessed on: 24 July 2019.
2. Illingworth RS. *Common Symptoms of Disease in Children.* Blackwell: Oxford 1983.

CHAPTER 61

Vomiting

BACKGROUND

Vomiting, a common symptom during infancy and childhood, is defined as forcible expulsion of contents of the stomach from the mouth. The strong contraction of the muscles of the abdominal wall and violent descent of diaphragm is the triggering factor that operates in its causation, irrespective of the actual cause.

The vomiting center lies in the cerebral medulla. Since it is under influence of chemoreceptors, disease affecting nearly any system—of course, brain is the most important—may cause vomiting. An obstructive lesion at pylorus or beyond, for instance, may cause vomiting by visceral afferents reaching the vomiting center.

HISTORY

History taking should pay special attention to the age of the child who vomits. Vomiting in the newborn infant may have altogether different implications than vomiting in later infancy and childhood. For instance, it is normal for a neonate to bring up small amounts of feed without being adversely affected as far as his health and well-being are concerned. Such vomiting, howsoever minor, in a young child should arouse suspicion of some organic problem.

It is of value to determine precisely its frequency and whether the problem is acute or it had been there in a recurrent form over quite a few months. What is the amount, color, and character of vomitus? Any relationship with feeding? Any abdominal discomfort or pain? Any accompanying drooling? Any suggestion of food poisoning? Does the child have associated diarrhea and dehydration? Any weight loss? Any convulsions, drowsiness or unconsciousness? Is there any history of trauma, especially to the head?

PHYSICAL EXAMINATION

Physical examination should ascertain the hydration and nutritional status of the child. Any evidence of infection? Any neurologic abnormality?

INVESTIGATIONS

- Serum electrolytes
- Urinalysis
- Ultrasound in pyloric stenosis
- Blood culture in sepsis
- Lumbar puncture (LP) in suspected meningitis.

DIFFERENTIALS

Vomiting in the Newborn

Benign

Swallowed amniotic fluid or blood may be responsible for vomiting in a few days after birth. Though the symptom causes much anxiety, it settles down in due course without any treatment.

Swallowed air due to erratic feeding, say far-too-rapid feeding or feeding a very large amount in a short time, is a common cause of vomiting or regurgitation in the newborn and early infancy. The vomitus is unchanged, contains no curd and is not malodorous. Vomiting in such cases occurs either soon after the feed or sometime within an hour's time. These babies with erratic feeding also suffer frequently from abdominal distention and colic. Accompanying these manifestations may be failure to thrive.

Organic

The common causes of organic vomiting in the newborn are septicemia and other infections such as meningitis, intrauterine infections causing encephalitis, otitis, gastroenteritis, and congenital obstructive defects of the gastrointestinal tract (GIT). The remaining causes include birth trauma, birth defects of central nervous system (CNS), hypoglycemia, and galactosemia.

The organic cause of vomiting should be considered in the presence of the following features:
- Persistent vomiting despite correction of feeding technique
- Accompanying abdominal distention

- Green vomitus which should be regarded as due to intestinal obstruction until and unless proved otherwise
- Poor feeding
- Dehydration, fever, septic umbilicus, bulging anterior fontanel, drowsiness, convulsions, etc.
- Failure to pass meconium in the first 24 hours
- Apparent peristalsis from right to left
- A palpable intra-abdominal mass
- Maternal hydramnios.

Septicemia: Vomiting may be the earliest symptom of this serious neonatal problem. Remaining manifestations include lethargy, refusal of feed, irritability, restlessness, loose motions, abdominal distention, fever or hypothermia, failure to gain weight, jaundice, respiratory distress, and skin eruptions. Umbilicus is often septic. Hepatosplenomegaly and pallor may accompany the clinical picture. Occurrence of seizures should arouse suspicion of meningitis.

Meningitis: Vomiting may well be the only manifestation of meningitis during neonatal period. Drowsiness, poor feeding, and convulsions may occur later. Bulging anterior fontanel may or may not occur. Neck stiffness is seldom present. In view of great emergency involved in the diagnosis and treatment of this condition, it is important that lumbar puncture is done immediately.

Hirschsprung's disease: Vomiting together with abdominal distention and failure to pass stools during the first week of life may suggest the diagnosis of this condition. Following rectal examination, the baby may have relief from these symptoms. Explosive discharge of feces and gas is characteristic. Episodes of constipation alternating with diarrhea, failure to gain weight and even weight loss, dehydration, hypoproteinemia, and edema are some of the other manifestations of this disorder.

A barium enema may show the following classical features of the disease:
- Abrupt change in caliber between the ganglionic and aganglionic segments
- Irregular contractions of the aganglionic segment, the so-called sawtooth contractions
- Parallel transverse folds in the dilated proximal portion of the colon
- Thickened, nodular, and edematous proximal colon which is reminiscent of protein-losing enteropathy
- Failure to pass out the barium.

However, the only conclusive evidence of congenital megacolon is absence of ganglion cells in the submucosa and intermuscular nerve plexus with or without increased number of nerve fibers in the rectal biopsy.

Esophageal atresia: In the most common type, esophageal atresia with distal tracheoesophageal fistula, the baby regurgitates and vomits all feeds and his mouth overflows with mucus and saliva. There is history of his having choked and vomited on his very first feed. Profuse chocking, coughing, cyanosis, excessive drooling, and abdominal distention are frequent.

Diagnosis is established by demonstrating air in the stomach and intestines in the plain X-ray of abdomen.

Alternatively, you may introduce a catheter down the infant's esophagus and take an X-ray film. In case of atresia, the catheter gets coiled in the blind upper pouch as seen in the plain X-ray film. You may introduce a small amount of diluted barium to confirm the diagnosis.

Since incidence of maternal hydramnios in such babies is high, it is a good practice to rule out the presence of esophageal atresia before giving feed to the baby, born to a mother with hydramnios.

Congenital hypertrophic pyloric stenosis: Vomiting, starting in the second half of the first month and progressively becoming forceful and projectile within 30 minutes of feeding, constant hunger, and failure to thrive are classical manifestations of this condition. Occasionally, greenish stools (starvation diarrhea), gastric hemorrhage or jaundice may be present. Dehydration, electrolyte imbalance—especially alkalosis, hypokalemia, hyponatremia, and tetany—may complicate the picture.

Barium meal study showing gross narrowing and elongation of pylorus, markedly distended stomach with retention of barium, and increased intensity of peristaltic waves confirm the diagnosis.

Chalasia of esophagus: Also called as gastroesophageal reflux; this condition results from incompetence of the lower esophageal sphincter. Manifestations (as a consequence of excessive reflux of the stomach contents into the esophagus) include vomiting, rumination, and failure to thrive. Vomiting characteristically occurs when the baby is returned to the cot (Figs. 61.1A and B).

Diagnosis may be confirmed by barium meal study, demonstrating reflux of contrast material from the stomach into the esophagus during respiration or by applying pressure over the abdomen and esophageal pH.

Hiatal hernia: In the most common form of hiatal hernia, cardiac end of stomach slides high up above the diaphragm and then back into the abdomen. It is frequently associated with reflux. Manifestations include regurgitation or vomiting (often projectile), failure to thrive, and anemia. Aspiration may cause pneumonia. Manifestations do not occur as long as the child is held upright. As soon as he is back to the cot, vomiting occurs.

Achalasia: This rare cause of vomiting in the neonate results from hypertonicity of the lower esophagus as a consequence of reduced ganglia in the mesenteric plexus.

Diagnosis is by radiologic demonstration of the obstruction at the cardiac end of the esophagus without organic stenosis.

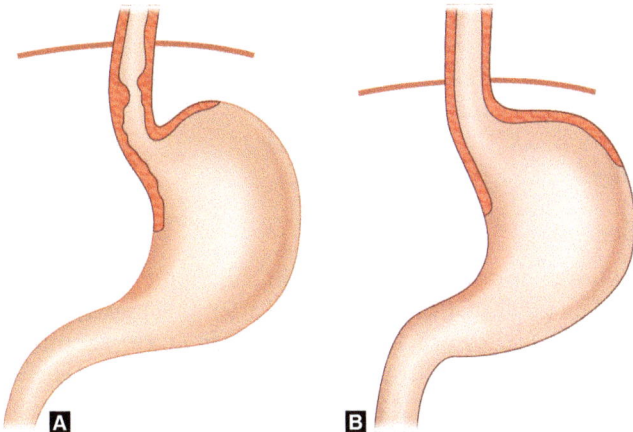

Figs. 61.1A and B: (A) Diagrammatic representation of the anatomy of the normal gastroesophageal junction, i.e. presence of intra-abdominal esophagus, well-developed lower esophageal sphincter (LES) and acute angle of Hiss, the factors that prevent gastroesophageal reflux (GER) in normal infants. (B) GE junction in GER, i.e. reduced length of intra-abdominal esophagus, poorly defined LES, and obtuse angle of Hiss, all favoring GER.

Obstruction of the small intestine: Vomiting from obstruction of the small intestine is frequent, persistent, bile-stained, copious, and nonprojectile. Accompanying features include abdominal distention, visible deep peristaltic waves, and diminished or, perhaps, absent bowel movements.

Upright X-rays of abdomen show the distribution of air in the intestine, thereby assisting in locating the site of obstruction.

Vomiting in Later Infancy

Benign

Faulty feeding: This is by far the most common cause of benign vomiting in infancy. This causes vomiting by introducing excessive "wind" into the stomach during the act of feeding.

The common type of faulty feeding in case of a breastfed baby is sucking an empty breast for quite a prolonged duration, resulting in air swallowing. Another type of defective feeding is "too rapid gulping" of milk because milk flows out of the distended breast very fast as is the case with the first morning feed.

In case of bottle-fed infant, the most common cause of faulty feeding and wind is the presence of an unduly small hole in the nipple. Also, anything that creates vacuum in the bottle (say the propped-up bottle) or obstructs the hole in the nipple (say, addition of cereals to the milk feed) is likely to cause swallowing of excess of air.

Overfeeding: Some mothers of low birth weight or preterm infants may develop an obsession to rather overfeed the infant whose capacity does not permit this overindulgence. Understandably, he begins to vomit. One wintry morning, a 2-month-old infant was referred to the author for vomiting quite a proportion of virtually every bottle feed. On detailed enquiry, it was learnt that the mother, in her overenthusiasm to make up for his low birth weight, was trying to push almost double the feed for the infant's needs down his throat. The infant showed dramatic response to the reduction in feed.

Too much crying: Not infrequently, the mother attempts to feed an excessively crying baby. As you would appreciate, such a baby (unless of course, he immediately stops crying as the nipple goes into his mouth) is likely to swallow considerable amount of air which may cause vomiting.

Erratic handling: If the infant is improperly handled after a feed, he may bring out some or the whole of it. In preterm infants, this is a common problem. The reason is that in such small babies, cardioesophageal sphincter is lax. A frequent mishandling observed is that the ignorant mother in the process of changing the nappy raises the lower part of the body after the feed. This facilitates bringing up of the feed.

Loneliness: Some infants react to loneliness and other indifferent attitudes of the mother by vomiting.

Too late or too early introduction of solids: If an infant is not offered solids by 6–7 months, the age at which he can chew well, he is likely to refuse them and to vomit them.

Foods dislike: The mother may push down the infant's throat a food that he dislikes or that he does not like in an amount that the mother wishes to feed to him. The result is that the baby vomits it.

Rumination: In this serious type of chronic regurgitation and vomiting, the infant, usually suffering from maternal or emotional deprivation, gags himself with the tongue or fingers, then pushes his abdomen in and out, arches his back and eventually succeeds in bringing the milk up. Thereafter, he virtually gargles with it, the milk alternately appearing and disappearing in the throat. On being observed, he may stop this activity. Else, he may vomit it and lie continuously in a small pool of regurgitated milk.

Organic causes of rumination, say hiatal hernia gastroesophageal reflux, esophageal stricture, achalasia or duodenal ulcer need to be excluded.

Travel sickness: Infrequently though, as young an infant as 5 or 6 months of age may begin experiencing motion sickness in an automobile, resulting in obscure vomiting.

Migraine: Occasionally, migraine may herald its onset in as young an infant as a 6-month-old with recurrent episodes of vomiting. Symptoms such as headache, abdominal pain, and fever manifest by 4–10 years.

Cow's milk allergy: Vomiting may be a symptom of allergy to cow's milk, usually to lactoglobulin, at times even to casein, bovine serum globulin, and bovine serum albumin.

Additional manifestations include diarrhea (usually watery), colic, skin rash (infantile eczema, urticaria, angioneurotic edema, etc.) anaphylaxis, unexplained crying, chronic cough with wheezing, otitis media, anemia, and failure to thrive.

Investigations may show eosinophilia, glucosuria, sucrosuria, lactosuria, aminoaciduria, renal tubular damage, acidosis, and pulmonary acidosis. Smear from rectal mucosa shows eosinophils.

Response to withdrawal of cow's milk is dramatic and challenge with this milk results in reappearance of the symptoms within 48 hours.

Organic

Infection: Occurrence of an infection should be suspected if a previously hale and hearty child suddenly begins to vomit, especially if he has accompanying fever and a sick look. Gastritis or gastroenteritis, upper respiratory infection, otitis media, urinary tract infection (UTI), whooping cough, viral hepatitis, meningitis, and encephalitis need to be considered in the differential diagnosis.

Obstructive GIT defects: Congenital obstructive lesions of the GIT responsible for vomiting in infancy include hypertrophic pyloric stenosis, chalasia, hiatal hernia, and tracheoesophageal fistula. The persistence of vomiting without any obvious cause, particularly if there had been imperforate anus or some other congenital anomaly of the GIT and/or congenital heart disease, should give a lead for this diagnosis. Positive history of hydramnios in the mother further supports this probability. X-ray of abdomen shows gas in the stomach. You may pass a Ryle's tube down the esophagus with the proximal end of the tube dipped in water. As you gradually withdraw it up the esophagus, occurrence of "bubbles" at the proximal end in water establishes the diagnosis of fistula.

Pylorospasm: It is a very, very rare disorder leading to recurrent vomiting in infancy.

Remaining organic causes of vomiting in later infancy: These include space-occupying lesions, peptic ulceration, gluten-induced enteropathy, appendicitis, Reye's syndrome, diabetes mellitus, uremia, ketotic hypoglycemia, galactosemia, and drugs and poisons, including salicylates, morphine, pethidine, anthelmintics, antibiotics, antihistaminics, antiepileptics, antidepressants, and anticancer agents.

Vomiting after Infancy

Benign

Nonorganic causes of vomiting in childhood include—(1) forcing the feed, (2) excitement of attending a party or the like, (3) anxiety or fear of going to school, (4) attention-seeking device in disturbed parent–child relationship, (5) imitation of another child having vomiting, (6) suggestion by overanxious parents, (7) finger insertion into the mouth, (8) migraine, and (9) travel or motion sickness.

Organic

Infection: Infections are a leading cause of organic vomiting in children beyond infancy as in infants. These include gastritis/otitis media, whooping cough, gastroenteritis, tonsillitis, UTI, viral hepatitis, Reye's syndrome, meningitis, encephalitis, appendicitis, pancreatitis, and mesenteric lymphadenitis.

Obstructive: GIT lesion intestinal obstruction of whatsoever etiology is an important cause of persistent vomiting in childhood.

Remaining cause of organic vomiting after infancy: Space-occupying lesions, torsion of undescended testis, uremia, diabetes mellitus, cholemia, hypercalcemia, and drugs.

FURTHER READING

1. Khan S, Di Lorenzo C. Chronic vomiting in children: new insights into diagnosis. *Curr Gastroenterol Rep* 2001;3:248-256.
2. Li BU, Misiewics L. Cyclic vomiting syndrome: A brain-gut disorder. *Gastroenterol Clin North Am* 2003;32:997-1019.
3. University of British Columbia. Approach to Vomiting. Available at: http://learn.pediatrics.ubc.ca/body-systems/gastrointestinal/approach-to-vomiting/vomiting. Accessed on: 24 July 19.

CHAPTER 62

Wheezing

BACKGROUND

The term, *wheezing*, is applied to the high-pitched rhonchi produced as a result of obstructive lower respiratory tract disease. The site of obstruction may be anywhere from the lower trachea to the small bronchi or large bronchioles.

Narrowing of the airway is not always due to bronchospasm. Factors such as mucosal edema and collection of large amounts of secretions too play a significant role in its causation. In infancy, wheeze occurs virtually exclusively due to mucosal edema and secretions. At this age, smooth muscles are yet to develop. Therefore, bronchospasm occurs not in infancy but later when the smooth muscles have developed.

Infants and children under 3 years of age are particularly prone to wheezing since their narrow airways are quite susceptible to the development of obstructive effect of bronchospasm, mucosal edema, and secretions.

Wheezing must be differentiated from "stridor". The latter is usually a medium- or low-pitched inspiratory sound resulting from narrowing of the upper airway, usually in the laryngeal area. It is frequently accompanied by hoarseness of voice and croupy cough.

Wheezing needs to be differentiated from "rattling" as well. The latter is secondary to air bubbling through fluid in the trachea or bronchi. It is heard without the aid of a stethoscope. Auscultatory finding is in the form of coarse crepitations (rales).

HISTORY

History must obtain information whether this is the first attack or the child had previous episodes of wheezing. Isolated attack of acute wheezing may accompany bronchiolitis or bronchopneumonia. Acute onset of severe wheezing in a healthy child who had been active and playing with crayons, peas, nuts, etc. a while ago should raise the suspicion of a foreign body aspirated into the lower respiratory tract. If recurrent or persistent wheezing dates back to birth, you must entertain the possibility of congenital structural defects of the lower respiratory tract.

Ascertain if the child appeared sick prior to the onset of wheezing. Does he suffer from any allergies? Any history of skin rash, eczema, etc.? Is he taking any medicines? Is the attack acute or insidious? Is it accompanied by fever, cough or respiratory distress?

In case of recurrent wheezing, find out if the child has a problem of recurrent or chronic diarrhea as well. In cystic fibrosis of pancreas, protracted diarrhea with stools highly steatorrheic and recurrent respiratory infection with wheezing are common manifestations. Is there any history of ascariasis or other worm infestations? Any history of recurrent abdominal pain, increase or decrease in appetite, pica or failure to thrive? In developing countries such as India, recurrent wheezing is often associated with tropical eosinophilia and hypereosinophilia accompanying ascariasis. Is there a family history of asthma?

PHYSICAL EXAMINATION

Physical examination must ascertain the magnitude of respiratory distress, if present. What is the state of hydration? Any respiratory acidosis? Is he febrile? Is he in congestive cardiac failure (CCF)? Any evidence of emphysema, bronchopneumonia or bronchiolitis? Presence of finger clubbing suggests a chronic lung infection. In uncomplicated bronchial asthma it is seen only rarely. Allergic rhinitis, eczema, urticaria, etc. point to the possibility of bronchial asthma or asthmatic bronchitis. Presence of nasal polyps suggests allergic conditions or cystic fibrosis. Mediastinal shift may mean a foreign body. You should make sure that CCF is not responsible for wheezing.

INVESTIGATIONS

- Chest X-ray
- Complete blood picture (CBP), including absolute eosinophil count in suspected tropical eosinophilia

- Pulmonary function testing [forced expiratory volume in one second (FEV1) and peak expiratory flow (PEF)]
- Sweat chloride in suspected cystic fibrosis.
- Bronchoscopy in suspected foreign body.
- Stool microscopy if absolute eosinophil count is quite high.

DIFFERENTIALS

Asthmatic Bronchitis

This, supposedly a mild form of bronchial asthma, occurs in first 5 or 6 years of life. The child develops typical "cold" which in another 1–3 days is followed by wheezing and dyspnea, often indistinguishable from bronchial asthma. This response to "cold" by wheezing and dyspnea is likely to stop once the child has crossed the age of 5 or 6 years. Remember that most remarkable feature of asthmatic bronchitis is that the child never wheezes in the absence of cold and in-between the attacks.

Bronchial Asthma

In this condition characterized by bouts of dyspnea, predominantly expiratory, as a result of temporary narrowing of the bronchi by bronchospasm, mucosal edema, and thick secretions, the child also wheezes when he is not having "cold". Though the onset of the disease in most instances is in the very first 2 years, the peak incidence is seen in 5–10 years age group. Boys suffer twice as much as girls. A strong family history of asthma is frequently available. There may be acute eczema and history suggestive of allergies to inhalants like pollen, dust and powder, foods like egg, meat, wheat and chocolate, and drugs like aspirin and morphine.

The onset of an asthmatic paroxysm is usually sudden and often occurs at night. Occasionally, it is preceded by the so-called asthmatic paroxysm in the form of tightness in the chest, restlessness, polyuria or itching.

A typical attack consists of marked dyspnea, bouts of cough and chiefly expiratory wheezing. Cyanosis, pallor, sweating, and restlessness are often present. Pulse is invariably rapid. The fulminant attack may subside in an hour or two, sometimes with vomiting or coughing up of viscid secretions. Some expiratory wheezing may, however, continue over several days though the child is otherwise comfortable.

In the event of a severe asthmatic paroxysm failing to respond to adequate doses of adrenaline and thereby persisting over hours or days, the condition is called status asthmaticus.

Generally, recurrent asthmatic attacks last over 2–7 or 10 days. Then, there is an interval of freedom which may vary from a few days to a few months.

Children with severe bronchial asthma over a prolonged period may develop a barrel-shaped chest deformity.

Diagnosis of bronchial asthma is usually clinical. All attempts should be made to detect the responsible allergen. X-ray of chest shows generalized emphysema (Fig. 62.1) and patchy atelectasis. Demonstration of eosinophilia in sputum or nasal secretions lends further support to the clinical impression.

Acute Bronchiolitis

This serious respiratory viral infection, occurring predominantly around the age of 6 months, is characterized by inflammation of the bronchioles, resulting in severe dyspnea.

Following a mild upper respiratory catarrh, the condition makes its appearance felt with dyspnea (rapid shallow breathing) and prostration. Cough is either absent or just slight. Mild-to-moderate fever is usually present. If dyspnea is marked (which usually is the case) air hunger, flaring of alae nasi, and cyanosis may occur. Also, dehydration and respiratory acidosis may develop.

Chest signs include intercostal, subcostal, and suprasternal retractions, hyper-resonant percussion note which is due to emphysema that may also push the liver and spleen downward, diminished breath sounds, widespread crepitations, and expiratory wheeze.

Diagnosis of bronchiolitis is generally obvious from the clinical picture. Chest X-ray shows emphysema, prominent bronchovascular markings and small areas of collapse. Screening reveals low-lying diaphragm with limited movements. Lungs are characteristically overinflated and intercostal spaces are wide.

Tropical Eosinophilia

This entity, a sort of allergic response to filarial infection, is an important cause of wheezy chest or bronchitis. Excepting infants under 1 year, it occurs at all ages.

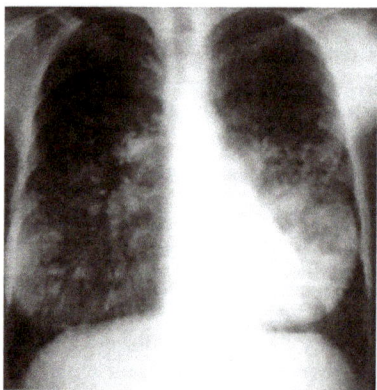

Fig. 62.1: *Chronic obstructive pulmonary disease*—Note the emphysematous changes with extensive parenchymal infiltration.

Chief manifestations have their onset insidiously. These include persistent cough (often simulating bronchial asthma), sometimes exertional dyspnea with wheezing, low-grade fever, anorexia, growth failure, and malaise. At times, vague abdominal manifestations may be present. Also, there may be enlargement of liver and lymph nodes. These manifestations tend to persist for months at a stretch without any significant systemic disturbance.

Investigations show that total leukocyte count (TLC) is increased, sometimes to as high as 100,000/cmm. Absolute eosinophil count varies from 4,000/cmm to 50,000/cmm, forming about 30–80% of all the cells.* Erythrocyte sedimentation rate (ESR) is usually high.

X-ray of chest is abnormal with increased reticular markings, coarse mottling (especially at the bases), and hilar prominence (eosinophilic lung, pulmonary eosinophilia, etc.) (Fig. 62.1). Peripheral lung fields are, as a rule, clear.

Foreign Body

Wheezing occurs when a foreign body lodges itself in the lower airway. There is history of choking followed by respiratory distress.

On physical examination, you may notice varying degree of dyspnea, asymmetrical chest expansion, decreased breath sounds, and unilateral wheezing.

X-ray of chest may show infiltration or consolidation confined to a specific segment or lobe of the lung.

Bronchoscopy has diagnostic as also therapeutic value.

Pneumonia

Unlike in adults, wheezing is a common accompaniment of the clinical picture of pneumonia in infancy and childhood, no matter whether the cause is viral, bacterial or fungal. Remaining manifestations include a mild upper respiratory infection followed by abrupt onset of fever, restlessness, apprehension, respiratory distress, air hunger, cyanosis, and cough.

Physical findings may show classical signs of consolidation or bronchopneumonia with exaggerated rhonchi.

X-ray of chest may or may not confirm the clinical impression since X-ray changes follow the actual lung changes by 2–4 days.

Tuberculosis

Wheezing as a result of enlarged mediastinal lymph nodes compressing the bronchi (as in tuberculosis) must seriously be investigated in areas where tuberculosis is rampant. High ESR, positive tuberculin (Mantoux) test/BCG diagnostic test, X-ray of chest revealing hilar prominence, and gastric lavage/sputum positive for acid-fast bacilli, especially in the presence of a positive family history of tuberculosis, all assist in confirming the diagnosis.

Cystic Fibrosis

Though relatively uncommon in India and other tropical and subtropical regions, cystic fibrosis is decidedly an important cause of wheezing.

This genetic disorder, involving not just the exocrine pancreas but also the sweat glands as also glands in the liver and exocrine glands elsewhere, starts manifesting early in infancy. Manifestations include chronic or recurrent diarrhea and recurrent respiratory infections, failure to thrive despite exceptionally good appetite, and multiple nutritional deficiencies. Stools are characteristically steatorrheic but may be loose. An obstinate catarrh or "frog in the throat" may be present ever since the first week of life. Abdominal distention, a palpable liver, clubbing and higher incidence of rectal prolapse, and nasal polyposis are some of the other manifestations. Complications include bronchiectasis, systemic amyloidosis, cor pulmonale, and cirrhosis. A typical picture of X-ray of chest is given in Figure 62.2.

When clinical picture arouses suspicion, fat balance studies to establish steatorrhea and D-xylose test to establish that steatorrhea is not exogenous in origin are indicated. Poor tryptic activity lends support to the clinical diagnosis. A high sweat chloride (60 mEq/L or more) is a "must" to confirm the diagnosis.

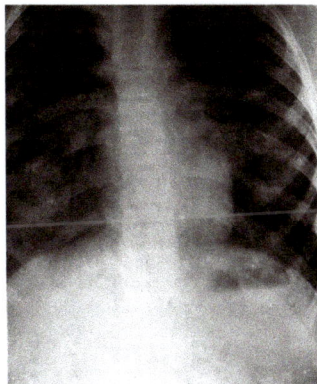

Fig. 62.2: X-ray of chest showing typical picture of cystic fibrosis in a child with wheezy chest and chronic diarrhea with failure to thrive since early infancy.

---

*Other causes of gross eosinophilia include parasitic infections (visceral larva migraines, ascariasis, ancylostomiasis, trichinosis, etc.), allergy (asthma, hay fever, etc.), malignancy (Hodgkin's lymphoma, leukemia, etc.), sarcoidosis, mycosis, drugs, and immune deficiency.

Drugs/Poisons

Aspirin, beta-blockers, penicillin, cephalosporin, erythromycin, ethionamide, neomycin, streptomycin, rifampicin, tetracyclines, lipiodol, vitamin K, indomethacin, ibuprofen, organophosphates, insecticide, tartrazine, etc.

Remaining Causes of Wheezing

Löffler syndrome, pulmonary hemosiderosis, CCF, congenital heart disease, vascular anomalies like pulmonary vascular rings, aspiration syndromes (prematurity, hiatal hernia, tracheoesophageal fistula, chalasia of esophagus, epilepsy, kerosene, paraffin, baby powder, etc.), bronchiectasis, post-pertussis, Kartagener's syndrome, anaphylaxis, bronchopulmonary dysplasia, immunodeficiency states, etc.

FURTHER READING

1. Irwin RS, Madison JM. The diagnosis and treatment of cough. *N Engl J Med* 2000;343:1715-1721.
2. Morice AH, Fontana GA, Sovijarvi AR, et al. The diagnosis and management of chronic cough. *Eur Respir J* 2004;24:481-492.
3. Morton RL, Sheikh S, Corbett ML, et al. Evaluation of the wheezy infants. *Ann Allergy Asthma Immunol* 2001;86:251-256.
4. Nethercott R, Mellis C. Investigating wheeze in children. *Med Today* 2003;4:20-26.

SECTION 3

Differential Diagnosis of Selected Clinical Signs

CHAPTER 63

Differential Diagnosis of Selected Clinical Signs

MICROGNATHIA (FIGS. 63.1 AND 63.2)

- Trisomy 13
- Progeria
- Treacher Collins syndrome
- Fetal alcohol syndrome
- Potter facies
- Pierre Robin syndrome.

STRIDOR IN FIRST FEW DAYS OF LIFE

- Laryngomalacia
- Vocal cords paralysis
- Laryngeal webs
- Vascular ring
- Congenital subglottic stenosis
- Hypocalcemia.

MACROCEPHALY

- Familial
- Hydrocephalus (Fig. 63.3)
- Subdural effusion
- Lipidosis
- Tuberous sclerosis
- Cerebral gigantism (Sotos syndrome)
- Megalencephaly
- Hydrancephaly
- Gangliosidosis.

MICROCEPHALY

- Familial
- Defects in brain development

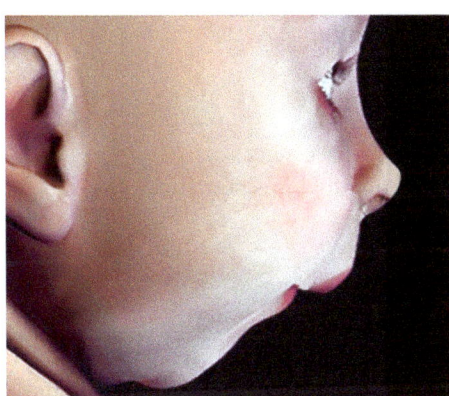

Fig. 63.1: *Micrognathia*—Note the very small mandible in relation to rest of the face.

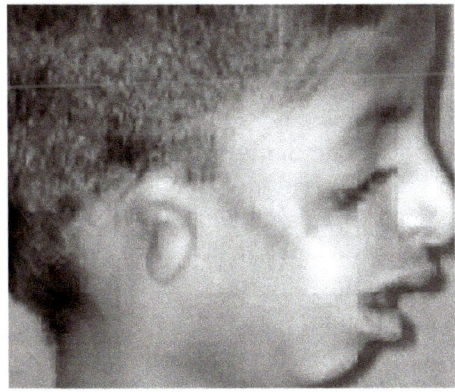

Fig. 63.2: *Micrognathia*—Note the very small mandible. Also present is malformed low-set ear.

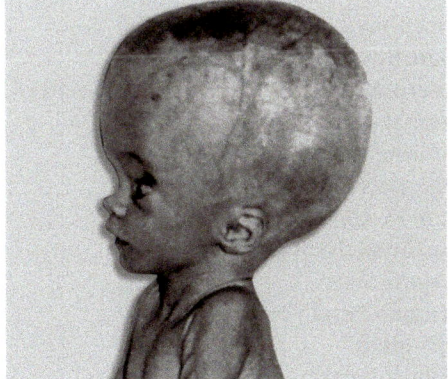

Fig. 63.3: *Large head secondary to congenital hydrocephalus*—Note the dilated scalp veins and "setting sun" sign as a result of downward deviation of eyes because of impingement of the dilated supraspinal recess on the tectum.

- Down syndrome
- Seckel dwarfism
- Intrauterine infections
- TORCH [toxoplasmosis, other (syphilis, varicella-zoster, parvovirus B19), rubella, cytomegalovirus, and herpes infections] or STORCH (Syphils, toxoplasmosis, varcella-zoster, rubella, cytomegalovirus, and herpes)
- Natal or postnatal disorders
- Anoxia
- Gross protein-energy malnutrition (PEM)
- Neonatal herpes virus infection
- Craniosynostosis (craniostenosis).

SPARSE AND LIGHT-COLORED SCALP HAIR

- Kwashiorkor
- Infantile tremor syndrome (ITS)
- Acrodynia
- Zinc deficiency
- Copper deficiency
- Acrodermatitis enteropathica.

FRONTAL/PARIETAL/OCCIPITAL BOSSING

- Vitamin D deficiency: rickets
- Thalassemia major
- Achondroplasia
- Congenital syphilis
- Ectodermal dysplasia
- Cleidocranial dysostosis
- Ehlers-Danlos syndrome
- Lowe syndrome
- Hallermann-Streiff syndrome
- Mucopolysaccharidosis.

LARGE ANTERIOR FONTANEL

- Vitamin D deficiency: rickets
- Protein-energy malnutrition
- Congenital hypothyroidism
- Hydrocephalus
- Prematurity
- Intrauterine growth restriction/retardation (IUGR)
- Congenital syphilis/rubella
- Achondroplasia
- Osteogenesis *imperfecta tarda*
- Trisomy 13, 18, and 21
- Cleidocranial dysostosis
- Apert syndrome
- Hallermann-Streiff syndrome
- Hydrocephaly
- Hypophosphatasia
- Pyknodysostosis

- Russell-Silver syndrome
- Thalassemia major
- Progeria.

CRANIOTABES

- Normal variant in first 3 months of life, especially in premature and low birth weight (LBW) infants
- Vitamin D deficiency: rickets
- Hydrocephalus
- Congenital syphilis
- Osteogenesis imperfecta tarda
- Treacher Collins syndrome
- Hypervitaminosis A
- Lacunar skull.

RICKETS WITH MENTAL RETARDATION

- Galactosemia
- Wilson disease
- Lowe syndrome
- Cystinosis
- Tyrosinemia
- Fructose intolerance.

BULGING ANTERIOR FONTANEL

- During excessive crying
- Raised intracranial pressure
  - Hydrocephalus
  - Meningitis
  - Encephalitis
  - Intracranial hemorrhage
  - Intracranial space-occupying lesion (ICSOL)
- Pseudotumor cerebri (otitic hydrocephalus)
  - Middle ear infection
  - Hypovitaminosis or hypervitaminosis A
  - Tetracycline toxicity
  - Nitrofurantoin toxicity
  - Nalidixic acid toxicity
  - Steroid therapy or sudden withdrawal
  - Lead poisoning
  - Iron-deficiency (chlorosis)
  - Diphtheria-pertussis-tetanus (DPT, triple) vaccine
  - Systemic lupus erythematosus (SLE)
  - Hypothyroidism
  - Hyperparathyroidism
  - Hypocalcemia
  - Congenital hypophosphatasia
  - Galactosemia
  - Addison's disease

- Obesity in prepubertal girls
- Overenthusiastic nutritional rehabilitation of grossly malnourished infants
- Mucopolysaccharidosis.

LOW-SET EARS

- Down syndrome
- Turner syndrome
- Trisomy 16 and 13
- Apert syndrome
- Carpenter syndrome
- *Cri-du-chat* (cat cry) syndrome
- Treacher Collins syndrome
- Idiopathic hypercalcemia
- Hurler syndrome.

SHORT NECK

- Down syndrome
- Congenital hypothyroidism
- Turner syndrome
- Noonan syndrome
- Mucopolysaccharidosis
  - Hurler syndrome, Morquio disease, etc.
- Klippel–Feil deformity
- Sprengel deformity.

DEPRESSED BRIDGE OF NOSE

- Racial
- Congenital hypothyroidism (cretinism)
- Down syndrome
- Thalassemia major
- Congenital syphilis
- Mucopolysaccharidosis (Hurler syndrome).

HYPERTELORISM

- Racial*
- Down syndrome*
- Congenital hypothyroidism (cretinism)*
- Trisomy 8
  - 4 p-
  - 5 p-
- Triploid syndrome
- Penta X, XXXX, XXXXX
- Aarskog syndrome
- Williams syndrome
- Noonan syndrome

- Fetal aminopterin syndrome
- Fetal warfarin syndrome
- Apert syndrome
- Pfeiffer syndrome
- Saethre–Chotzen syndrome
- Roberts syndrome
- Rubinstein–Taybi syndrome
- G syndrome
- Robinow syndrome
- Weaver syndrome
- Hypertelorism—hypospadias syndrome
- Sotos syndrome
- Larsen syndrome
- LEOPARD syndrome
- Sjögren–Larsson syndrome
- DiGeorge sequences
- Thalassemia major
- Ehlers–Danlos syndrome
- Waardenburg syndrome
- Chondrodystrophies
- Turner syndrome.

HYPOTELORISM

- Trisomy 13
- Holoprosencephaly
- Trigonocephaly
- Oculo-dental-digital syndrome.

PERIORBITAL EDEMA

- Excessive crying
- Acute conjunctivitis or blepharitis
- Kwashiorkor
- Acute nephritis or nephrotic syndrome
- Anemia
- Angioneurotic edema
- Congestive cardiac failure (CCF)
- Hypothyroidism
- Cavernous sinus thrombosis
- Dermatomyositis.

MONGOLOID (UPWARD AND LATERAL) SLANT OF EYES

- Racial
- Down syndrome
- Prader–Willi syndrome
- Ectodermal dysplasia

---

*These conditions are accompanied by only pseudohypertelorism, i.e. they give an impression of hypertelorism (increased distance between two eyes because of presence of flat nose). In true hypertelorism, the distance between two pupils (midpupillary distances) is actually increased and the eyes are set apart, because of congenital overdevelopment of the lesser wings and underdevelopment of the greater wings of the sphenoid.

- Laurence-Moon-Biedl syndrome.

EPICANTHAL FOLDS (FIG. 63.4)
- Skin folds covering medial canthi
- Normal trait in young children
- Down syndrome
- Other trisomies
- Single gene disorders.

ANTIMONGOLOID (DOWNWARD AND LATERAL) SLANT OF EYES (FIG. 63.5)
- Apert syndrome
- Treacher Collins syndrome
- Cerebral gigantism
- de Lange syndrome
- Whistling face syndrome
- *Cri-du-chat* (cat cry) syndrome
- Trisomy 16.

"SUNSET" SIGN
- Physiologic (2–4-month age)
- Hydrocephalus
- Kernicterus

- Asphyxia
- Pineal tumor.

PTOSIS (FIGS. 63.6 AND 63.7)
- Congenital
  - As an isolated anomaly
  - Marcus Gunn phenomenon (Marcus Gunn jaw winking syndrome)
  - Congenital fibrosis syndrome
- Acquired
  - Myasthenia gravis
  - Horner syndrome
  - Sturge-Weber syndrome
  - von Recklinghausen's syndrome
  - Fetal alcohol syndrome
  - Whistling face syndrome
  - Noonan syndrome
  - Moebius syndrome
  - Aarskog syndrome
  - Myotonic dystrophy
  - Botulism
  - Injury to upper lid or third nerve

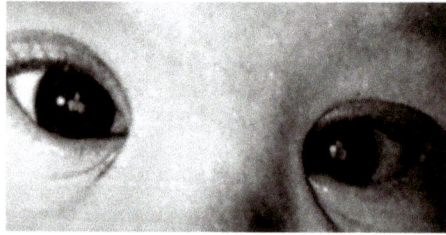

Fig. 63.4: *Epicanthal fold*—Note that the vertical (somewhat oblique) fold of skin, starting from upper lid, covers significant inner canthal area of left eye. As a result, the infant appears to have squint (pseudoesotropia).

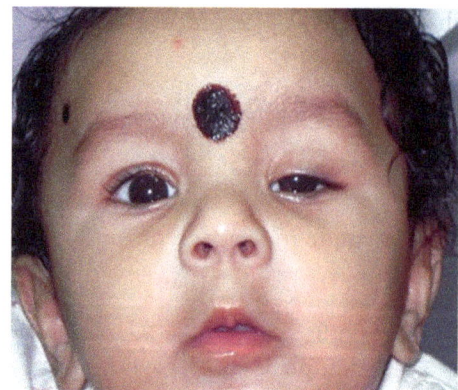

Fig. 63.6: Congenital ptosis in left eye.

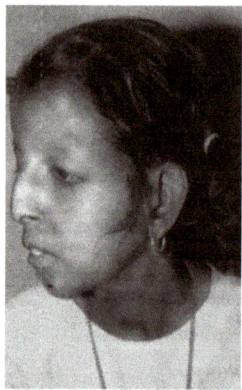

Fig. 63.5: *Antimongoloid slant*—Note the outward and downward inclination of the eyes (against upward and outward in case of mongoloid slant). Differential diagnosis includes Treacher Collins syndrome, Apert syndrome, and cerebral gigantism.

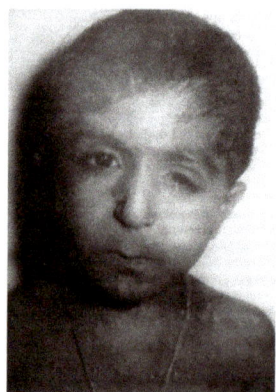

Fig. 63.7: *Unilateral congenital ptosis*—It usually occurs as an isolated finding and is the result of a localized dystrophy of the levator muscle with replacement of the striated fibers by fibrous tissue.

- Excessively sticky eyes
- *Drug-induced*: Mydriasis, vincristine, etc.

PROPTOSIS (EXOPHTHALMOS)

- Shallowness of the orbit
  - Craniosynostosis (craniostenosis)
  - Other craniofacial malformations
- Relatively increased tissue mass
  - Cavernous sinus thrombosis
  - Periorbital cellulitis
  - Orbital hemorrhage
  - Neoplasm (neuroblastoma, anterior meningocele, rhabdomyosarcoma, etc.)
  - Arteriovenous aneurysm
  - Chloroma
  - Neurofibromatosis
- Endocrinopathy
  - Thyrotoxicosis.

BLUE SCLERA

- Phenylketonuria (PKU)
- Osteogenesis imperfecta tarda.

SUBCONJUNCTIVAL HEMORRHAGE

- Whooping cough (pertussis)
- Severe cough
- Severe sneezing
- Leukemia
- Idiopathic thrombocytopenic purpura (ITP)
- Trauma (birth, mechanical injury, etc.)
- Inflammation (conjunctivitis).

WHITE REFLEX (CAT'S EYE)

- Cataract
- Retinoblastoma (Fig. 63.8)

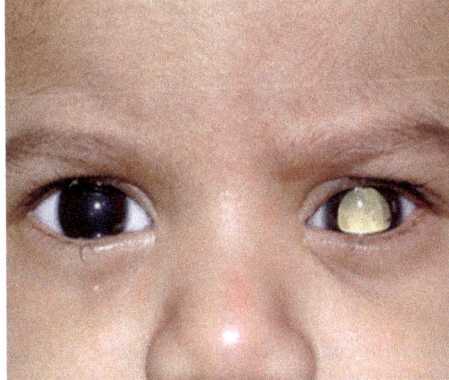

Fig. 63.8: Retinoblastoma—Note the white reflex in the left eye (leukocoria).

- Retrolental fibroplasia
- Pupillary membrane (persistent central hyaloid artery)
- Vitreous opacity
- Visceral larva migrans
- Retinal detachment.

CATARACT

- Developmental variant (Mittendorf dot)
- *Maternal infections*: TORCH, STORCH
- Metabolic disorders
  - Galactosemia
  - Diabetes mellitus (juvenile-onset)
  - Wilson disease (hepatolenticular degeneration)
  - Mucopolysaccharidosis
- Chromosomal disorders
  - Trisomy 13, 18, and 21
  - Turner syndrome
  - Deletion and duplication syndromes
- Drugs
  - Steroids
  - Vitamin D (both hypo and hyper)
  - Tetracyclines
  - Chlorpromazine
  - Radiation
- Trauma
  - CAN
  - Contusion
  - Penetrating injury
- Multisystem disorders
  - Kartagener syndrome
  - Marfan syndrome
  - Myopathies
  - Lowe syndrome
  - Progeria
  - Alport syndrome.

DISCOLORATION OF TEETH

- Poor orodental hygiene
- Caries
- Fluorosis
- Iron therapy
- Tetracycline therapy
- Neonatal hyperbilirubinemia
- Porphyria erythropetica
- Amelogenesis imperfecta.

MACROGLOSSIA

- Congenital hypothyroidism (cretinism)
- Glycogen storage disease
- Hurler syndrome

- Amyloidosis (primary)
- Pseudohypertrophic muscular dystrophy
- Beckwith syndrome (hypoglycemia with macroglossia).

GINGIVAL HYPERPLASIA

- Hydantoin sodium side effect
- Scurvy
- Bad orodental hygiene
- Epulis
- Hurler syndrome
- Xanthomatosis
- Diffuse fibromatosis
- Histiocytosis X.

BLINDNESS

- Congenital
  - *Cataract*: Developmental, rubella, galactosemia, etc.
  - Malformation
- Acquired
  - Vitamin A deficiency
  - Retinoblastoma
  - Optic atrophy
  - Retinal detachment
  - Retrolental fibroplasia
  - Trauma
  - Ophthalmia neonatorum
  - Acute exanthema.

PINPOINT PUPIL

- Structural lesions in pons
- Some metabolic disorders
- Mushroom or nutmeg poisoning
- Organophosphate poisoning
- *Drugs*: Morphine, heroin, barbiturates, clonidine, meprobamate, carbamate insecticide, pilocarpine eye drops.

IRIS COLOBOMA

- *Chromosomal syndromes*: Trisomy 13 4p, 13q, triploid, etc.
- CHARGE association
- Goltz syndrome
- Rieger syndrome.

ACUTE UVEITIS

- Inflammatory bowel disease (IBD)
- Kawasaki disease

- Enteropathic arthritis
- Pauciarticular juvenile rheumatoid arthritis (JRA) (type II)
- Ankylosing spondylitis.

DEAFNESS (HEARING LOSS)

- Congenital
  - *Genetic*: Isolated and complex—Pendred hypothyroidism, deafness syndrome, etc.
  - *Embryopathy*: Infections—TORCH/STORCH and drugs—thalidomide, streptomycin, etc.
  - *Idiopathic*: Nerve deafness and absent middle ear
- Acquired
  - *Infection*: Acute otitis media (AOM), chronic suppurative otitis media (CSOM), meningitis, mumps, etc.
  - *Perinatal*: Birth injury, asphyxia hyperbilirubinemia, prematurity, drugs like kanamycin and gentamicin, etc.
  - Head injury
  - Early otosclerosis.

PAROTID SWELLING (FIG. 63.9)

- Viral parotitis
  - Mumps
  - Parainfluenza 1 and 3
  - Coxsackie
  - Influenza A
  - Cytomegalovirus (CMV)
  - Epstein-Barr virus (EBV)
  - Enteroviruses
  - Lymphocytic choriomeningitis virus
  - Human immunodeficiency virus (HIV)

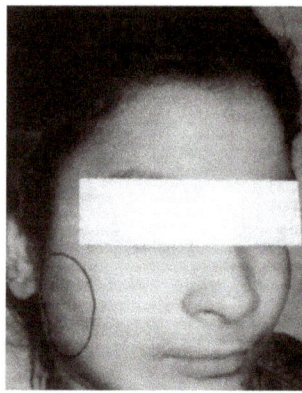

Fig. 63.9: *Recurrent parotid swelling*—It defined all diagnoses and therapies. Finally, it turned out to be human immunodeficiency virus (HIV) related.

- Pyogenic or purulent parotitis (usually *Staphylococcus aureus*)
- Sarcoidosis (often accompanied by uveitis)
- Sjögren syndrome
- Systemic lupus erythematosus
- Recurrent parotitis (autoimmune, allergy, infection, block of the Stensen's duct from calculus, injury or inspissated mucus)
- Mikulicz disease (bilateral painless parotid and lacrimal gland enlargement, dryness of mouth and eyes, etc.)
- Preauricular lymphadenopathy.

PREAURICULAR TAGS/PITS

- Goldenhar syndrome
- Treacher Collins syndrome
- Frontonasal dysplasia
- Wolf syndrome
- *Cri-du-chat* (cat cry) syndrome.

RETARDED (DELAYED) SPEECH

- Deafness
- Dumbness (elective mutism)
- Cerebral palsy
- Mental retardation
- Deprivation (emotional)
- Developmental delay
- Autism
- Sequel to serious central nervous system (CNS) infection in infancy (meningitis, encephalitis, cerebral malaria, etc.)
- Degenerative disorders.

PECTUS CARINATUM (PIGEON CHEST)

- Familial
- Rickets (Fig. 63.10)
- *Associations*: Scoliosis, mitral valve disease, coarctation of aorta, etc.

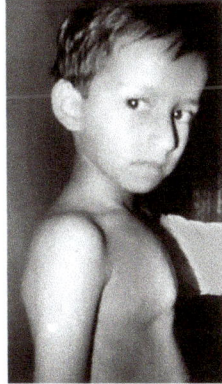

Fig. 63.10: Pectus carinatum (pigeon chest) in a child with nutritional rickets.

PECTUS EXCAVATUM (FUNNEL CHEST)

- Congenital deformity (Fig. 63.11)
- Marfan syndrome
- Ehler–Danlos syndrome
- Acquired
  - Chronic lung disease
  - Neuromuscular disease
  - Injury.

HARRISON SULCUS

- Vitamin D deficiency: rickets
- Asthma.

COSTOCHONDRAL BEADING

- Vitamin D deficiency: rickets (Fig. 63.12)
- Scurvy
- Achondroplasia.

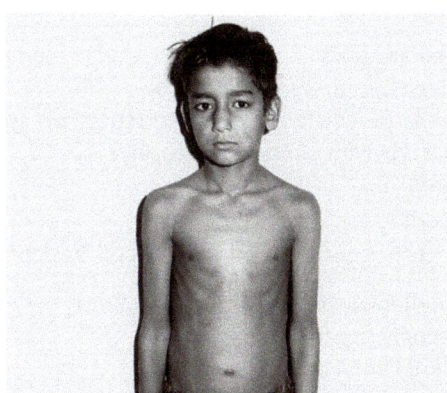

Fig. 63.11: Pectus excavatum (funnel chest) as a congenital deformity.

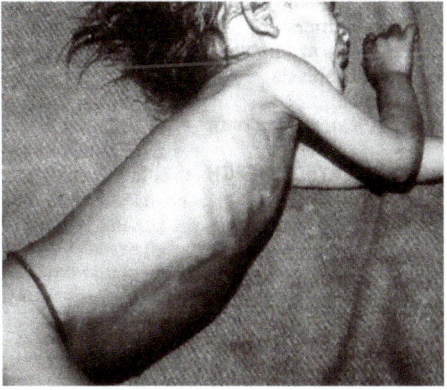

Fig. 63.12: *Costochondral prominence (beading)*—In nutritional rickets (rachitic rosary). It is smooth, rounded, and nontender. In scurvy (scorbutic rosary), it is sharp, angular, and tender.

SENILE APPEARANCE

- Progeria
- Cockayne syndrome
- Rothmund-Thomson syndrome
- Werner syndrome.

CONGENITAL LIMB HYPERTROPHY

- Neurofibromatosis
- Wilms tumor
- CHILD* syndrome
- Russell-Silver syndrome
- Beckwith-Wiedemann syndrome.

CLINODACTYLY

- Incurving, i.e. lateral curvature of little finger
- Isolated anomaly (Fig. 63.13)
- Down syndrome
- Russell-Silver syndrome
- Carpenter syndrome.

POLYDACTYLY

- Isolated anomaly
- Laurence-Moon-Biedl syndrome
- Majewski polydactyly syndrome (short-rib syndrome, polydactyly with chondrodystrophy)
- Trisomy 13.

KNOCK-KNEE DEFORMITY (GENU VALGUM)

- Intermalleolar distance more than 2 cm
- Physiologic (up to 4 years)
- Metabolic bone or skeletal disease
  - Rickets (vitamin D deficiency, nutritional, vitamin D resistant)
  - Renal osteodystrophy
  - Hypophosphatasia
- Bone or skeletal dysplasia
  - Metaphyseal dysplasia
  - Achondroplasia
- Asymmetrical growth arrest
  - Trauma
  - Infection
  - Tumors.

BOWLEG DEFORMITY (GENU VARUS)

- Physiologic (up to 2 years)
- Metabolic bone or skeletal disease
  - Rickets (vitamin D deficiency, nutritional, vitamin D resistant)
  - Renal osteodystrophy
  - Hypophosphatasia
- Bone or skeletal dysplasia
  - Metaphyseal dysplasia
  - Achondroplasia
- Asymmetrical growth arrest
  - Trauma
  - Infection
  - Tumors
  - Blount disease (tibia vara)
  - Congenital disorders
  - Neuromuscular disorders.

PAINFUL SWELLING OF THIGH

- Traumatic
- Subperiosteal hemorrhage of scurvy (Fig. 63.14)
- Hemophilia (usually in association with hemarthrosis of knee).

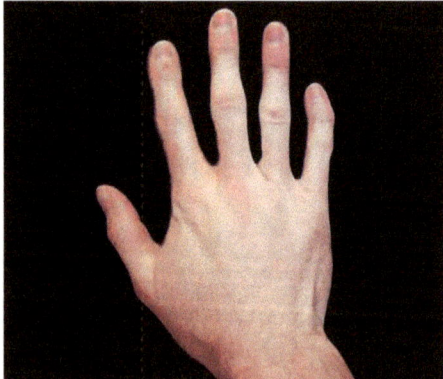

Fig. 63.13: *Clinodactyly*—Note the incurving of the little finger.

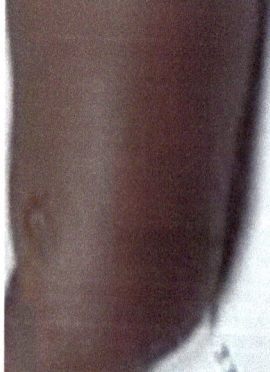

Fig. 63.14: *Subperiosteal hemorrhage*—Note the nontraumatic swelling of the thigh in an infant who also had bleeding gums and excessive irritability.

---

*Congenital hemidysplasia, ichthyosiform erythroderma, and limb defects.

Differential Diagnosis of Selected Clinical Signs

DRY, SCALY, HYPERKERATOTIC SKIN

- Vitamin A deficiency (Fig. 63.15)
- Linoleic acid deficiency
- Vitamin C deficiency
- Ichthyosis (Figs. 63.16 and 63.17).

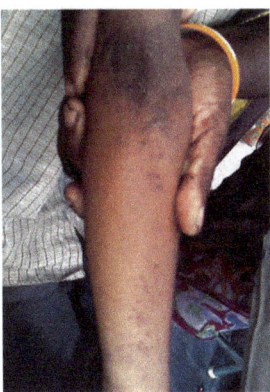

Fig. 63.15: Phrynoderma.

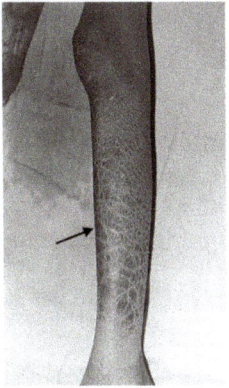

Fig. 63.16: *Ichthyosis vulgaris*—Note dry, hyperkeratotic scaly skin lesions primarily on the extensor surface of the legs. In this autosomal dominant disorder, lesions tend to worsen in winter and show some regression in summer.

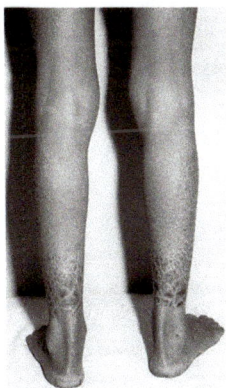

Fig. 63.17: *Ichthyosis vulgaris*—Note scanty lesions over back of legs.

SKIN TUBERCULOSIS

- Syphilitic chancre
- Leprosy
- Atypical mycobacterial infection
- Fungal infection
- Tularemia
- Cat-scratch disease
- Sporotrichosis
- Nocardiosis
- Leishmaniasis
- Foreign body reaction (e.g. nylon sutures)
- *Papular acne*: Rosacea.

SCROFULODERMA

- Skin involvement in tuberculous lymphadenitis
- Syphilitic gumma
- Deep fungal infection
- Actinomycosis
- Hidradenitis suppurativa.

SINUS BRADYCARDIA

- Physiologic variant
- Prematurity
- Hypoxemia
- Raised intracranial pressure (RICP)
- Hypothyroidism
- *Drugs*: Digoxin.

SINUS TACHYCARDIA

- Fever
- Anemia
- Congestive cardiac failure
- Hypovolemia
- Hyperthyroidism
- Drugs.

PAROXYSMAL SUPRAVENTRICULAR TACHYCARDIA

- Idiopathic
- Congenital heart disease [Ebstein's anomaly, transposition of the great arteries (TGA), single ventricle, atrial surgery]
- Endocardial fibroelastosis
- Sick sinus syndrome (SSS)
- Wolff–Parkinson–White syndrome (WPW syndrome)
- Hyperthyroidism
- *Drugs*: Theophylline, beta-agonists, decongestants (anticold agents).

INNOCENT CARDIAC MURMUR

- Classic vibratory systolic murmur (Still's murmur)
- Pulmonary ejection systolic murmur
- Pulmonary flow murmur of the newborn
- Venous hum (continuous)
- Carotid bruit (systolic).

CARDIOMEGALY WITHOUT MURMUR

- Congenital heart disease
  - Coarctation of aorta (in infants)
  - Ebstein's anomaly
- Myocardial disease
  - Endocardial fibroelastosis
  - Viral or idiopathic myocarditis
  - Glycogen storage disease (Pompe disease)
- Coronary artery disease
  - Kawasaki disease
  - Collagenosis (Periarteritis nodosa)
  - Anomalous origin of the left coronary artery from pulmonary artery
  - Calcification of coronary artery
  - Medial necrosis of coronary artery
- Miscellaneous
  - Pericardial effusion
  - Severe anemia
  - Beriberi
  - Protein-energy malnutrition
  - Respiratory disease leading to CCF
  - Peripheral arterial tone (PAT) with CCF
  - *Drug toxicity*: Adriamycin, radiation, etc.

ATRIAL FLUTTER OR FIBRILLATION

- *Congenital heart disease (CHD)*: Ebstein's anomaly
- Cardiomyopathy
- Wolff-Parkinson-White (WPW) syndrome
- Sick sinus syndrome
- Myocarditis
- Interatrial surgery
- Atrioventricular valve regurgitation.

UMBILICAL HERNIA

- Normal variant
- Prematurity
- Congenital hypothyroidism
- Down syndrome
- Mucopolysaccharidosis.

SCOLIOSIS

- Primary which may manifest in infancy or later
- Secondary
  - Rickets
  - Hemivertebrae
  - Marfan syndrome
  - Muscular dystrophy
  - Postpolio syndrome
  - Cerebral palsy
  - Spina bifida
  - Neurofibromatosis
  - Friedreich's ataxia.

FLAT FOOT

- Normal variation
- Congenital
  - Marfan syndrome
  - Ehlers-Danlos syndrome
  - Tarsal bone fusion
- Neurologic
  - Cerebral palsy
  - Spina bifida
  - Muscular dystrophy
- Nutritional
  - Rickets.

TALIPES EQUINOVARUS (CLUB FOOT)

- Familial
- Intrauterine posture
- Spina bifida
- Postpolio syndrome
- Arthrogryposis multiplex congenita (Fig. 63.18)
- Cerebral palsy
- Vertical talus.

CONGENITAL GOITER

- Iodine deficiency/excess
- Maternal goitrogen consumption
- Congenital hyperthyroidism
- Dyshomogenic defects.

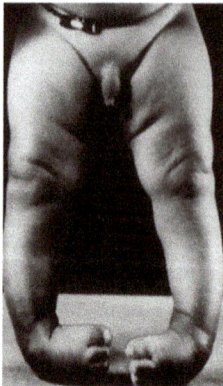

Fig. 63.18: Talipes equinovarus (club foot) in association with arthrogryposis multiplex congenita.

GYNECOMASTIA

- Normal pubertal development
- *Drugs*: Estrogens, phenothiazines, digoxin, meprobamate, reserpine, spironolactone, marijuana
- *Deficient androgen production*: Klinefelter syndrome, testicular failure, isolated luteinizing hormone (LH) deficiency (fertile eunuch)
- *Overproduction of estrogens*: Feminizing adrenal tumors
- *Local problems*: Carcinoma, lipoma, abscess, hemangioma, bruise, neurofibromatosis, etc.
- *Miscellaneous*: Pituitary/thyroid tumor, thyroid disease, etc.

SIMIAN CREASE

- Normal (4% neonates)
- Down syndrome (50% cases)
- Other trisomies.

CAFE-AU-LAIT SPOTS

- Normal variant
- Neurofibromatosis (von Recklinghausen's disease)
- Tuberous sclerosis
- Fanconi anemia
- Gaucher disease
- Ataxia telangiectasia
- Russell–Silver syndrome
- Pheochromocytoma
- Chronic myeloid leukemia
- McCune–Albright syndrome
- Multiple lentigines
- Ataxia telangiectasia
- Bloom syndrome
- Epidermal nevus syndrome
- Chédiak–Higashi syndrome.

DRUG-INDUCED LUPUS

- Hydralazine
- Isoniazid (INH)
- Procainamide
- Beta-blockers
- Anticonvulsants (probable)
- Quinidine
- Captopril
- D-penicillamine.

BUTTERFLY RASH

- Systemic lupus erythematosus
- Dermatomyositis
- Contact dermatitis
- Pemphigus erythematosus
- Mitral stenosis
- Hypothyroidism.

RECURRENCE OF FEVER IN MENINGITIS (ON TREATMENT)

- Phlebitis [intravenous (IV) puncture site]
- Drug fever
- *Superadded infection*: Viral, malaria, urinary tract infection (UTI)
- Drug resistance.

RECURRING MENINGITIS

- *Congenital defects*: Meningomyelocele, neurenteric cysts, midline or spinal dermal sinuses
- *Acquired defects*: Basal skull fracture
- Immunodeficiency
- Chronic relapsing encephalomyelitis
- *Inherently recurrent infections*: Mollaret's meningitis.

OPISTHOTONOS

- Tetanus
- Meningitis
- Kernicterus
- Dystonia or phenothiazine toxicity
- Strychnine poisoning
- Infantile Gaucher disease.

NECK RIGIDITY (STIFFNESS)

- Cervical lymphadenitis
- Retropharyngeal abscess
- Dystonia
- Meningitis
- Intracranial space-occupying lesion
- Subarachnoid hemorrhage
- Tetanus.

ACUTE ATAXIA

- Postinfection
- Chickenpox
- Echocardiography
- Coxsackie
- Drug-induced
- Antihistaminics
- Anticonvulsants
- Alcohol
- Intracranial space-occupying lesion
- Intracranial infections
- Hydrocephalus
- Miller–Fisher syndrome (ataxia, areflexia, ophthalmoplegia, etc.).

CHRONIC ATAXIA (STATIC)

- Postencephalitic
- Agenesis of cerebellar vermis
- Hydrocephalus.

CHRONIC ATAXIA (PROGRESSIVE)

Friedreich's ataxia.

CALF HYPERTROPHY

- Physiologic
- Duchenne muscular dystrophy (DMD)
- Hypothyroidism
- Becker muscular dystrophy
- Polymyositis
- Myotonia congenita
- Kugelberg-Welander syndrome.

PAINFUL/TENDER HEPATIC ENLARGEMENT

- Acute hepatitis
- Liver abscess
- Congestive cardiac failure
- Hepatoma.

DULL PERCUSSION NOTE (CHEST)

- Pleural effusion
- Consolidation
- Collapse
- Fibrosis
- Thickened pleura
- Bronchopneumonia
- Abscess.

PIGEON CHEST DEFORMITY

- Congenital
- Rickets
- Emphysema
- Skeletal dysplasia
- Mucopolysaccharidosis (MPS) (type 4)
- Marfan syndrome
- Noonan syndrome.

HEMIHYPERTROPHY

- Idiopathic
- Beckwith-Wiedemann syndrome
- Wilms tumor
- Neurofibromatosis
- Russell-Silver syndrome
- Adrenocortical carcinoma
- Cutis marmorata congenital.

MICROORCHIDISM

- Hypopituitarism
- Hypothyroidism
- Rudimentary tests syndrome
- Klinefelter syndrome
- Laurence-Moon-Biedl syndrome.

MACROORCHIDISM

- Sexual precocity
- Hypothyroidism
- Fragile-X syndrome
- Testicular tumor.

MICROPENIS

Less than 2 cm; normal 4-5 cm

- Hypopituitarism
- Down syndrome
- Klinefelter syndrome
- Laurence-Moon-Biedl syndrome
- CHARGE association
- Hypogonadotrophic hypogonadism
- Prader-Willi syndrome
- Kallmann syndrome
- Cornelia de Lange syndrome
- X-linked hypogammaglobulinemia
- Noonan syndrome
- Fanconi anemia
- William syndrome
- Rainbow syndrome
- Hallermann-Streiff syndrome
- Carpenter syndrome.

VAGINAL BLEEDING

- *Newborn*: Withdrawal bleeding in girls
- *Infancy and childhood*
  - *Before menarche*: Precocious puberty, exogenous estrogen vaginitis, foreign body, urethral prolapse, etc.
  - *After menarche*: Dysfunctional uterine bleeding (DUB), bleeding diathesis, gonorrhea, IUD, birth control pill, ectopic pregnancy, abortion, etc.

SYNDROME OF INAPPROPRIATE SECRETION OF ADH

- Central nervous system tumors
- Lung tumors
- Lymphoma
- Gastrointestinal carcinoma
- *Drugs*: Vincristine, cyclophosphamide.

ASCITES

- *Hypoproteinemia*: Kwashiorkor, nephrotic syndrome, protein-losing enteropathy

- Cirrhosis of liver
- Portal hypertension
- *Cardiac*: CCF
- *Infectious*: Tuberculosis, peritonitis, etc.
- Neoplasm
- *Iatrogenic*: Postdialysis, post-ventriculoperitoneal shunt, etc.
- Chylous.

GASTROENTERITIS WITH ARTHRITIS

- Infectious
- Salmonella
- Shigellosis
- Yersinia
- Adenovirus
- Tuberculosis
- Noninfectious
- Inflammatory bowel disease (ulcerative colitis, Crohn's disease, etc.)
- Anaphylactoid purpura.

GASTROINTESTINAL BLEEDING

- Upper
  - Bleeding from an oral or pharyngeal source
  - *Esophageal*: Varices, esophagitis, etc.
  - *Gastric*: Gastritis, ulcer, foreign body, vascular lesion, tear, etc.
- Lower
  - Dysentery (bacillary)
  - *Colitis*: Amebic, inflammatory bowel disease, pseudomembranous, radiation-induced, allergic, ischemic, etc.
  - *Vascular*: Hemangioma hemorrhoids, angiodysplasia, etc.
  - *Mass lesion*: Malignancy, polyposis, duplication, etc.
  - *Obstructive*: Intussusception, midgut volvulus, etc.
  - *Congenital*: Meckel's diverticulum (becoming "symptomatic" in a toddler).

ULCERATIVE COLITIS-LIKE MANIFESTATIONS

- Infectious colitis
  - Amebiasis
  - Giardiasis
  - *Clostridium difficile*
  - Cytomegalovirus
- Allergic colitis
- Crohn's disease
- Colitis of hemolytic uremic syndrome.

SOFT NEUROLOGIC SIGNS

- Occurring during normal development but not helpful in an individual child from clinical point of view; related to learning problems.
- Choreiform movements (upper limbs)
- Hyperactivity
- Short attention span
- Involuntary mirror movements of fingers on opposite hand (synkinesis)
- Poor motor incoordination
- Poorly performed alternating movements
- Inability to hop or tandem walk
- Failure to appreciate simultaneous touch to face and hands
- Mixed or confused laterality
- Inability to appreciate numbers drawn on the hand.

PREMATURE GRAYING OF HAIR

- Isolated dominant condition
- Autoimmune disorders
- Pernicious anemia
- Hyperthyroidism
- Hypothyroidism
- Progeria
- Werner syndrome.

POTTER FACIES AND SYNDROME (FIG. 63.19)

- Flat face
- Low-set ears
- Retrognathia
- Hypertelorism.

Mnemonic for Potter's syndrome

P: Pulmonary hypoplasia

O: Oligohydramnios

T: Twisted skin (wrinkly skin)

T: Twisted face (Potter's facies—low-set ears, retrognathia, hypertelorism)

E: Extremity deformities (limb deformities—club hands and feet, joint contractures, etc.)

R: Renal agenesis (bilateral).

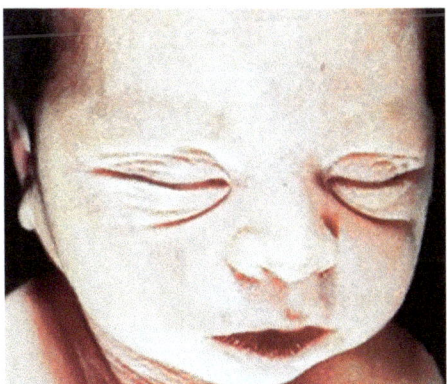

Fig. 63.19: *Potter facies*—Note the flat face, hypertelorism, and small mandible.

SECTION 4

Differential Diagnosis of Salient Laboratory Findings

CHAPTER 64

Differential Diagnosis of Salient Laboratory Findings

NORMOCYTIC ANEMIA

- Decreased production
- Hemolytic anemias
- Acute bleeding.

INCREASED MEAN CORPUSCULAR VOLUME (MACROCYTIC ANEMIA)

- Normal in the neonate
- Vitamin B_{12} or folic acid deficiency
- Hemolysis or hemorrhage (reticulocytes)
- Protein-energy malnutrition (PEM)
- Down syndrome
- Leukemia
- Congenital red blood cell (RBC) aplasia.

HYPOCHRONIC ANEMIA

- Iron deficiency
- Thalassemia
- Chronic infection or inflammation.

DECREASED MEAN CORPUSCULAR VOLUME (MICROCYTIC ANEMIA)

- Iron deficiency (RBC count decreased)
- Lead poisoning (RBC count decreased)
- Protein-energy malnutrition (RBC count decreased)
- Thalassemia major (RBC count remains normal)
- Chronic inflammation
- Sideroblastic anemia
- Copper deficiency.

INCREASED MEAN CORPUSCULAR HEMOGLOBIN CONCENTRATION

- ABO incompatibility
- Hereditary spherocytosis
- Autoimmune hemolytic anemia
- Hemolytic-uremic syndrome (HUS).

TARGET CELLS

- Red blood cell with an area of increased staining in the central pallor
- Thalassemia
- Sickle cell anemia
- Iron deficiency anemia (IDA) (Fig. 64.1)
- Lead poisoning
- Chronic liver disease
- Postsplenectomy.

BASOPHILIC STIPPLING

- Small basophilic inclusions throughout RBC cytoplasm
- Thalassemia
- Megaloblastic anemia (Fig. 64.2)
- Lead poisoning
- Dyserythropoiesis
- Liver disease
- Unstable hemoglobinopathies
- Pyrimidine 5'-nucleotidase deficiency.

HOWELL–JOLLY BODIES (FIG. 64.3)

- Small round cytoplasmic red cell inclusion with staining characteristics of nucleus

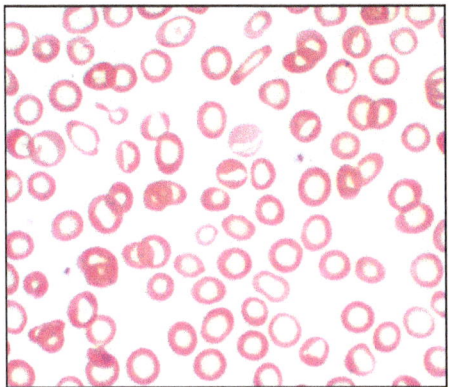

Fig. 64.1: *Iron deficiency anemia*—Note the microcytic–hypochromic red cells.

312 Section 4: Differential Diagnosis of Salient Laboratory Findings

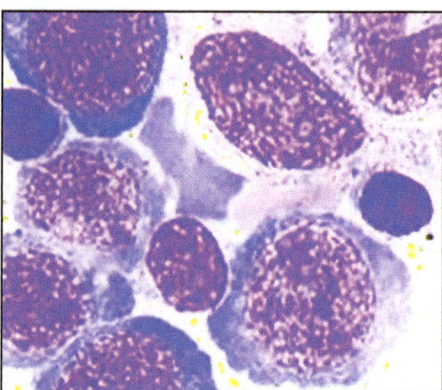

Fig. 64.2: *Megaloblastic anemia*—Note the large, nucleated immature, precursor of red blood cells (RBCs), seen in vitamin B_{12} or folic acid deficiency.

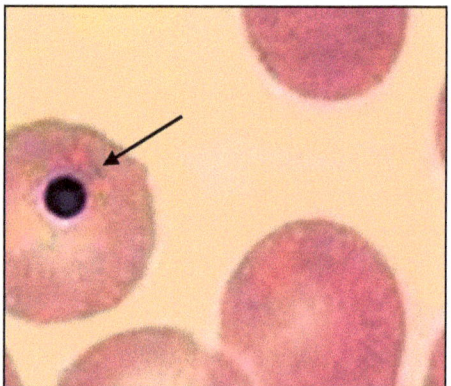

Fig. 64.3: *Howell–Jolly bodies*—Note the dot-like inclusion with staining characteristics of nucleus.

- Hemolytic anemia
- Megaloblastic anemia
- Postsplenectomy.

TEAR DROP CELLS (FIG. 64.4)

- Red blood cell resembling a tear drop
- Iron deficiency anemia
- Megaloblastic anemia
- Bone marrow fibrosis.

ELLIPTOCYTOSIS (FIG. 64.5)

- Elliptical or oval RBCs
- Hereditary elliptocytosis
- Iron deficiency anemia
- Thalassemia
- Myelofibrosis.

ACANTHOCYTOSIS (FIG. 64.6)

- Red blood cells with spicules of unequal length and uneven distribution over the surface
- Postsplenectomy

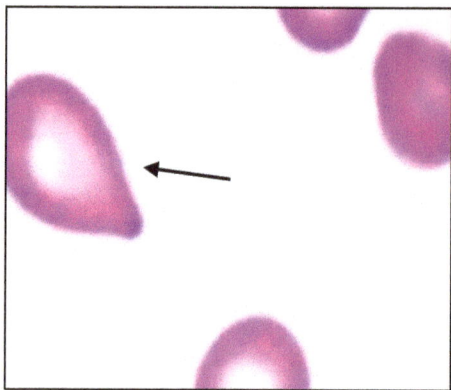

Fig. 64.4: *Tear drop cell*—Note the red cell resembling a tear drop.

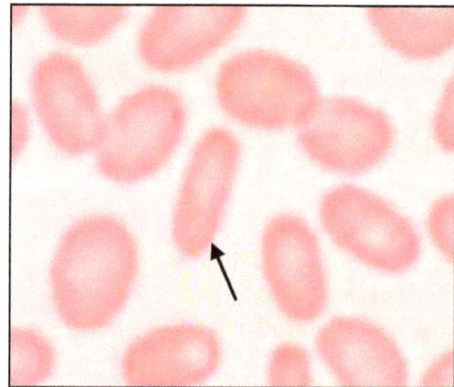

Fig. 64.5: *Elliptocyte*—Note the oval red cell.

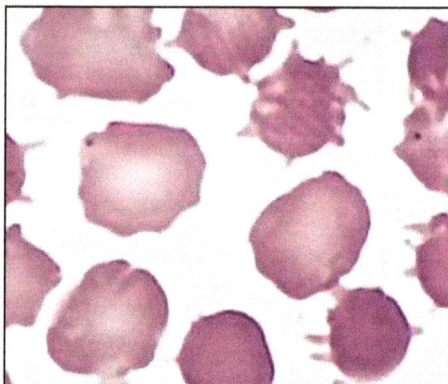

Fig. 64.6: *Acanthocytosis*—Note the red cells characterized by presence of unequal spicules.

- Liver disease
- Anorexia nervosa
- Starvation.

ROULEAUX FORMATION (FIG. 64.7)

- Red blood cells resembling stacks of coins
- Hyperfibrogenemia
- Hyperglobulinemia.

Differential Diagnosis of Salient Laboratory Findings

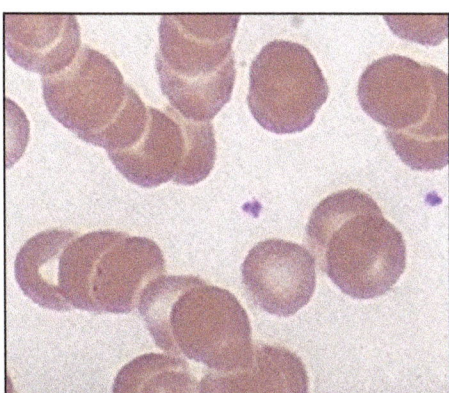

Fig. 64.7: *Rouleaux formation*—Note the aggregation of red cells.

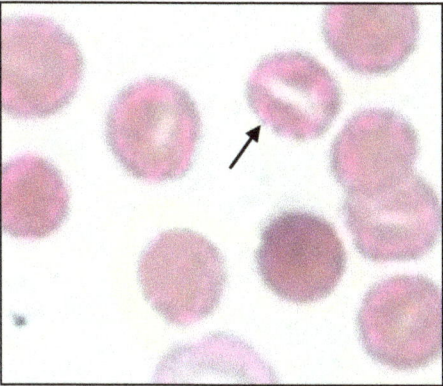

Fig. 64.8: *Stomatocyte*—Note the central slit in the red cell.

STOMATOCYTES (FIG. 64.8)

- Red blood cells having mouth-like form because of a central linear slit
- Hereditary stomatocytosis
- Hereditary spherocytosis
- Alcohol.

NEUTROPHILIA (NEUTROPHIL LEUKOCYTOSIS) (FIG. 64.9)

- Infection (usually bacterial)
- *Tissue destruction*: Trauma, burns, infarctions, gangrene neoplasm, etc.
- *Blood loss*: Hemorrhage, hemolysis, etc.
- *Drug therapy*: Steroids, poisons, etc.
- Myeloproliferative disease.

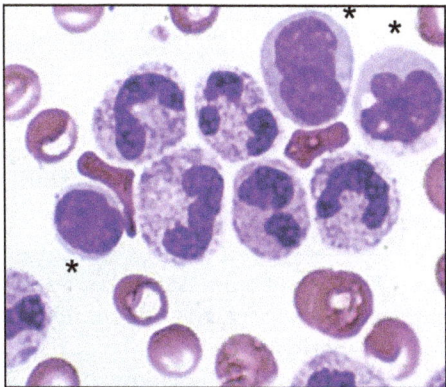

Fig. 64.9: Neutrophilia.

NEUTROPENIA (NEUTROPHIL LEUKOPENIA) (FIG. 64.10)

- *Infection*: Viral, overwhelming bacterial like typhoid brucellosis and malaria, etc.
- *Factor deficiency anemia*: Vitamin B_{12} and folic acid, infrequently iron
- Bone marrow depression
- Hypersplenism
- Systemic lupus erythematosus (SLE)
- Leukemia

EOSINOPHILIA (FIG. 64. 11)

- Allergy
- Asthma
- Hay fever
- Serum sickness
- Urticaria

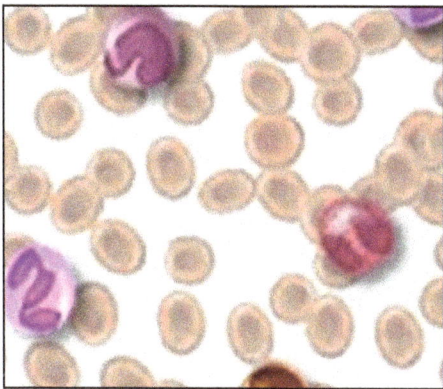

Fig. 64.10: *Neutropenia*—Note only very few neutrophils.

- Food sensitivity
- *Drugs*: Penicillins, nitrofurantoin, etc.
- *Parasitic infestation*: Ascariasis
- Tropical eosinophilia
- *Infections*: Convalescent phase
- Myeloproliferative disorders
- Reticulosis
- Leukemia
- Sarcoidosis.

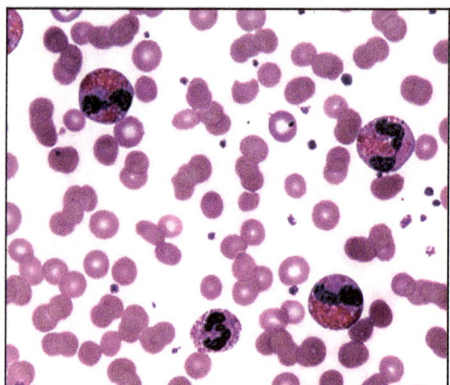

Fig. 64.11: Eosinophilia.

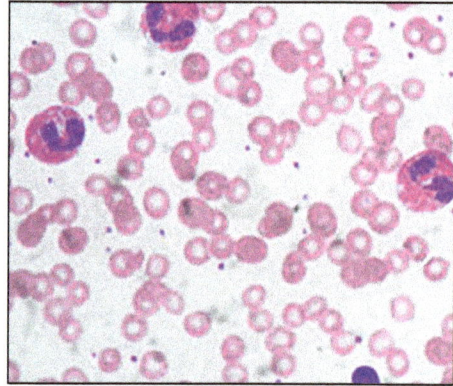

Fig. 64.12: Eosinopenia.

EOSINOPENIA (FIG. 64.12)

Cushing's disease
Steroid therapy
Pertussis
Acute illnesses.

LYMPHOCYTOSIS (FIG. 64.13)

- *Infections*: Infectious mononucleosis, exanthemata, influenza, hepatitis, pertussis, tuberculosis, syphilis, typhoid, brucellosis, etc.
- Convalescent phase of any infection
- Lymphocytic leukemia
- Reticulosis.

LYMPHOPENIA

- *Infections*: Acquired immunodeficiency syndrome (AIDS), tuberculosis, viral hepatitis, typhoid fever, etc.
- *Autoimmune disease*: Lupus
- *Malignancy*: Blood cancer, lymphomas
- Radiation
- Cancer chemotherapy
- Steroid therapy
- Cushing's disease
- Protein-energy malnutrition.

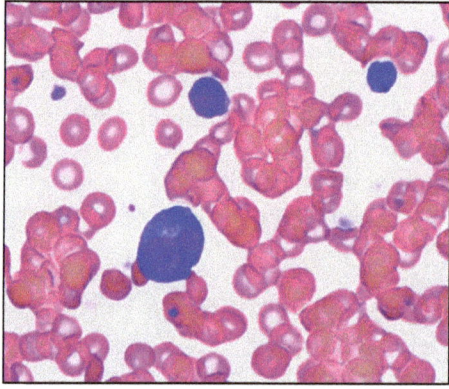

Fig. 64.13: Lymphocytosis.

MONOCYTOSIS (FIG. 64.14)

- Bacterial infections
  - Tuberculosis
  - Typhoid
  - Endocarditis
  - Brucellosis
  - Convalescence
- Protozoal infections
  - Malaria
  - Trypanosomiasis

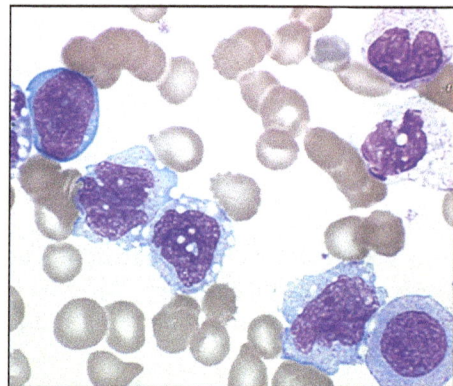

Fig. 64.14: Monocytosis.

- Chronic diseases
  - Ulcerative colitis
  - Crohn's disease
  - Connective tissue disease
- Malignancy
  - Myeloma
  - Monocytic leukemia
  - Lymphadenoma.

LEUKEMOID REACTION (FIG. 64.15)

- Markedly high total leukocyte count (TLC) with circulating immature cells but normal hemoglobin, platelets, and bone marrow
- Severe infections
- Tuberculosis
- Acute hemolysis.

THROMBOCYTOPENIA (FIGS. 64.16A AND B)

- Platelet count less than $150 \times 10^9/L$
- Poor megakaryocytosis
  - Bone marrow hypoplasia
  - Bone marrow infiltration.

POOR THROMBOCYTOPOIESIS

- Megaloblastic anemia
- Leukemia.

POOR PLATELET SURVIVAL

- Immune thrombocytopenic purpura (ITP)
- Drugs
- Acute infections, septicemia, malaria, etc.
- Thrombotic thrombocytopenia
- Hemolytic-uremic syndrome
- Disseminated intravascular coagulation (DIC).

SEQUESTRATION OF PLATELETS

Hypersplenism.

THROMBOCYTOSIS (FIG. 64.17)

- Platelet count more than $400 \times 10^9/L$
- Primary (essential)
  - Myeloproliferative disorders
- Secondary (reactive)
  - Acute infections or inflammations
  - Chronic infections or inflammatory disorders (tuberculosis, rheumatologic conditions, etc.)
  - Splenic hypofunction or asplenia
  - Acute hemorrhage
  - Iron deficiency anemia
  - Trauma
  - Leukemia [chronic myelogenous leukemia (CML), chronic lymphocytic leukemia (CLL), etc.].

HYPOCELLULAR BONE MARROW (FIG. 64.18)

- *Drug induced*: Carbamazepine, chloramphenicol
- *Chemical induced*: Benzene
- Virus induced

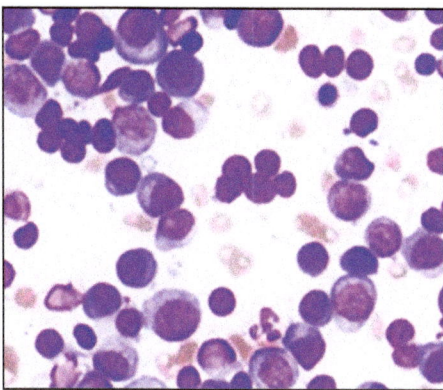

Fig. 64.15: *Leukemoid reaction*—Note the remarkably high total leukocyte count (TLC).

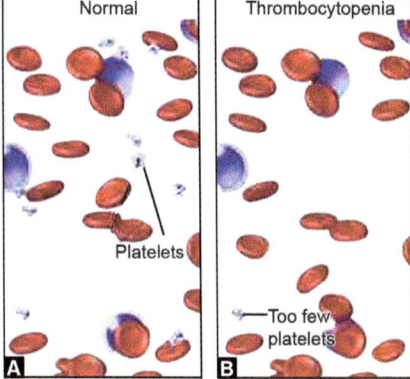

Figs. 64.16A and B: *Thrombocytopenia*—Note (A) several platelets in the normal and (B) only very few platelets representing thrombocytopenia.

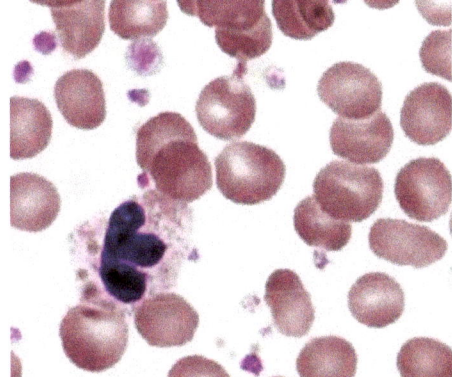

Fig. 64.17: *Thrombocytosis*—Note excess of platelets.

- Ionizing radiation
- Inherited bone marrow failure syndrome
- Aplastic anemia.

HYPERCELLULAR BONE MARROW (FIG. 64.19)

- Leukemias
- Myeloproliferative disorders

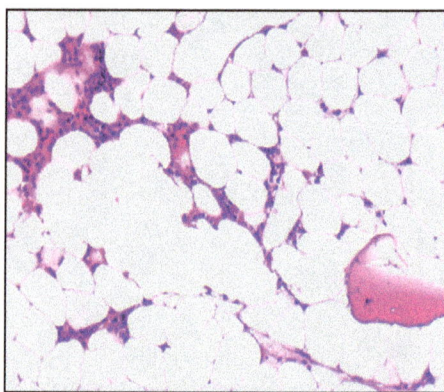

Fig. 64.18: Hypocellular bone marrow.

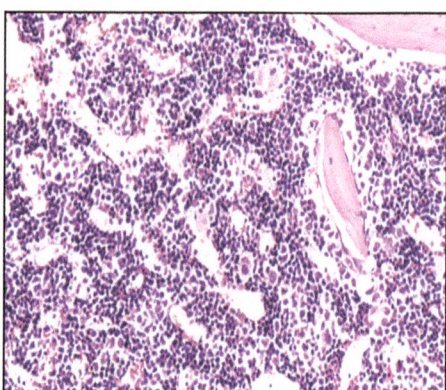

Fig. 64.19: Hypercellular bone marrow.

- Myelodysplasia
- Lymphomas
- Megaloblastic anemia
- Sideroblastic anemia
- Compensatory hyperplasia (following cell destruction).

MEGAKARYOCYTIC HYPERPLASIA

- Immune thrombocytopenic purpura
- *Reactive*: Chronic inflammatory disorders
- Essential thrombocythemia
- Myeloproliferative disorders.

MEGAKARYOCYTIC HYPOPLASIA (DEPRESSION)

- Aplastic anemia
- Viral infections
- Drug induced.

ERYTHROID HYPERPLASIA

- *Myeloid*: erythroid ratio less than 1:1; normal is equal to 2:1 to 4:1

- Hemolytic anemias
- Massive hemorrhage
- Polycythemia
- *Hemoglobin synthesis abnormalities*: Thalassemias, congenital sideroblastic anemia, etc.
- *Deoxyribonucleic acid (DNA) synthesis defects*: Folate or vitamin B_{12} deficiency, methotrexate, etc.

ERYTHROID HYPOPLASIA

- The M:E ratio more than 4:1 as a result of absence or suppression of RBC precursors
- Pure red cell aplasia
- Diamond–Blackfan syndrome
- Thymoma
- Parvovirus B19 infection.

LOW-SERUM PROTEINS (TOTAL)

- *Artefactual*: Blood drawn from an arm with intravenous (IV) drip running
- *Reduced synthesis*: Severe dietary deficiency, malabsorption, liver dysfunction, etc.
- *Increased loss*: Nephrotic syndrome, burns and exudates, protein-losing enteropathy.

HIGH-SERUM PROTEINS (TOTAL)

- *Artefactual*: Venipuncture stasis
- Fluid depletion
- *Hyperglobulinemia*: A paraprotein or polyclonal rise in gamma globulin.

LOW-SERUM ALBUMIN

See "Low-Serum Proteins (Total)".

HIGH-SERUM ALBUMIN

- *Artefactual*: Blood drawn from an arm with IV drip running
- Fluid depletion.

LOW ALPHA-1 GLOBULIN

- Nephrotic syndrome
- Alpha-1-antitrypsin deficiency.

HIGH ALPHA-1 GLOBULIN

- Tissue damage
- Inflammation.

LOW ALPHA-2 GLOBULIN

- Reduced albumin synthesis

- Protein-energy malnutrition
- Malabsorption syndrome
- Liver disease.

HIGH ALPHA-2 GLOBULIN

- Acute stress
- Nephrotic syndrome
- Diabetes mellitus
- Hyperthyroidism
- Adrenal insufficiency.

HIGH BETA GLOBULIN

- Biliary obstruction
- Nephrotic syndrome.

LOW GAMMA GLOBULIN

- *Protein loss*: Proteinuria as in nephrotic syndrome, burns, exudates, and protein-losing enteropathy
- Malabsorption syndrome
- Malnutrition.

HIGH GAMMA GLOBULIN

- Polyclonal
  - Chronic infections
  - Rheumatoid arthritis
  - Systemic lupus erythematosus
  - Liver disease
  - Sarcoidosis
- Monoclonal.

HIGH IMMUNOGLOBULIN G

- Infections
- Systemic lupus erythematosus
- Hashimoto's disease
- Liver disease.

LOW IMMUNOGLOBULIN G

- Nephrotic syndrome
- Congenital deficiency
- Malignancy.

LOW IMMUNOGLOBULIN A

- Congenital deficiency
- Protein-losing enteropathy
- *Drug therapy*: Gold, penicillamine, phenytoin, etc.

HIGH IMMUNOGLOBULIN A

- Cirrhosis (portal)
- Immunoglobulin A (IgA) nephropathy
- Autoimmune disorders.

LOW IMMUNOGLOBULIN M

Protein loss.

HIGH IMMUNOGLOBULIN M

- Chronic infections
- Biliary cirrhosis
- Connective tissue disorders (rheumatoid arthritis).

HIGH IMMUNOGLOBULIN E

- Asthma
- Allergic rhinitis
- Parasitic infestations
- Atopic dermatitis
- *Miscellaneous*: Cirrhosis, celiac disease, glomerulonephritis, paraproteinemia, etc.

LOW COMPLEMENT (C3, C4)

- Post-streptococcal acute glomerulonephritis
- Systemic lupus erythematosus nephritis
- Membranoproliferative glomerulonephritis
- Serum sickness
- Liver disease.

HIGH C-REACTIVE PROTEIN

- Rheumatic fever
- Rheumatoid arthritis
- Systemic vasculitis
- Septicemia (neonatal).

HIGH ALPHA-1-FETOPROTEIN

- Primary hepatoma
- Secondary hepatic carcinoma
- Tumors of alimentary tract
- Tumors of the gonads
- Cirrhosis
- Hepatitis
- Fetal death or neural tube defects in pregnancy.

HIGH CREATINE PHOSPHOKINASE

- *Muscle diseases*: Duchenne myopathy in which values are over 10 times the normal and precede the clinical

picture, viral myositis, toxoplasmosis, trichinosis, acute myoglobinuria, myotonias, neurogenic disease, severe exertion, seizures, intramuscular injection, etc.
- Hypothyroidism
- Hypoparathyroidism
- Rickets
- Chronic renal failure
- Shock
- Myocardial infarction
- *Drug therapy*: Alcohol, hypnotics, clofibrate, etc.

HIGH SERUM GLUTAMIC OXALOACETIC TRANSAMINASE OR ASPARTATE AMINOTRANSFERASE

- Liver disease
- Severe hemolysis
- Muscle damage
- Myocardial damage
- *Drugs*: Alcohol
- *Miscellaneous*: Trauma, shock, surgery, occult congestive cardiac failure (CCF), hypokalemia, severe exertion, etc.

HIGH SERUM GLUTAMIC-PYRUVIC TRANSAMINASE OR ALANINE AMINOTRANSFERASE

- Hepatic cirrhosis
- Hepatic metastasis.

HIGH ALKALINE PHOSPHATASE

- Rickets
- Paget's disease
- Bony metastasis
- Ankylosing spondylitis
- Liver disease.

LOW ALKALINE PHOSPHATASE

- Hypophosphatasia
- *Reduced bone growth*: Cretinism, vitamin C deficiency, achondroplasia, etc.
- Protein-energy malnutrition.

HIGH SERUM AMYLASE

- Acute pancreatitis
- Perforated peptic ulcer
- Mesenteric infarction
- Cholecystitis
- Ruptured aneurysm

- *Drug therapy*: Opiates, steroids, phenylbutazone, thiazides, etc.
- Following cholecystography
- Renal failure
- Salivary gland disease
- Macroamylasemia
- Metastatic tumors.

HIGH SERUM LACTATE DEHYDROGENASE

- Megaloblastic anemia
- Hemolysis
- Leukemia
- Acute liver congestion
- Acute intoxication
- Malignant disease, especially when accompanied by metastasis.

HIGH SERUM CALCIUM

- High intake of vitamin D, especially in renal failure, hypoparathyroidism, concomitant use of thiazide diuretics
- Primary hyperparathyroidism
- *Neoplasm*: Metastatic bone disease, pseudohyperparathyroidism
- Addison's disease
- Severe thyrotoxicosis
- Acromegaly
- Immobilization
- Paget's disease
- Dehydration
- Sarcoidosis
- Familial benign hypercalcemia.

LOW SERUM CALCIUM

- Vitamin D deficiency
- Hypoparathyroidism
- Renal failure
- Maternal diabetes, osteomalacia or hypoparathyroidism
- *Drug therapy*: Anticonvulsants, oral phosphates and calcitonin, anabolic, steroids estrogens, etc.

HIGH SERUM PHOSPHATE

- Vitamin D excess
- Hypoparathyroidism
- Diabetic ketosis
- Renal failure
- Healing fractures
- Hemolysis

- Acromegaly
- Neoplasm.

LOW SERUM PHOSPHATE

- Vitamin D deficiency
- Hyperparathyroidism
- Nutritional deficiency as during prolonged IV infusion or nasogastric suction, persistent vomiting, alcoholism, etc.
- Renal tubular disease
- *Acute infections*: Gram-negative septicemia.

HIGH SERUM MAGNESIUM

- High doses of magnesium as an antacid or cathartic
- Renal failure with hyperkalemia
- Hypercalcemia.

LOW SERUM MAGNESIUM

- Severe diarrhea
- Malabsorption
- Nasogastric aspiration
- Protein-energy malnutrition, especially in kwashiorkor
- Hypokalemia
- Hypocalcemia
- *Drug therapy*: Diuretics, gentamicin, cisplatin, etc.

HIGH SERUM UREA (AZOTEMIA)

- Reduced excretion
  - Reduced filtration
  - Increased reabsorption
- Catabolism of absorbed protein
  - High protein diet
  - Gastrointestinal bleed.

LOW SERUM UREA

- Anabolic states
- Low protein diet
- Liver failure
- Intravenous infusion.

HIGH SERUM UREA–CREATININE RATIO

- Protein catabolism
- Sodium and water depletion, e.g. diuretic therapy
- Congestive cardiac failure.

LOW SERUM UREA–CREATININE RATIO

- Reduced urea concentration

- High creatinine concentration
  - Dialysis
  - Drugs
  - Rhabdomyolysis.

AMINOACIDURIA

- *Nonspecific*: Fanconi syndrome
- *Congenital*: Cystinosis, Lowe syndrome, medullary cystic disease, idiopathic Fanconi syndrome, Wilson disease, galactosemia, glycogen, storage disease, etc.
- *Acquired*: Myelomatosis, amyloidosis, massive proteinuria, Sjögren's syndrome, heavy metal (lead mercury, cadmium, etc.) poisoning, phenols, outdated tetracyclines, etc.
- *Specific tubular defects*: Cystinuria
- Overflow aminoaciduria
- Phenylketonuria (PKU).

PHOSPHATURIA

- Renal tubular defects
  - Fanconi syndrome
  - Hereditary hypophosphatemic rickets
  - Renal tubular acidosis
- Primary hyperparathyroidism
- Secondary hyperparathyroidism.

SMELL AND TASTE AS CLUES TO DIAGNOSIS

- Acetone on breath diabetic ketoacidosis
- Mousy smell from urine PKU
- Smell of fresh maple sap from urine
- Maple syrup urine disease
- Fishy urine *Proteus* infection
- Excessively salty kiss (cystic fibrosis).

SIMPLE OBSERVATION ON URINE AS A CLUE TO DIAGNOSIS

- Color and concentration
- *Orange*: Jaundice, rifampicin
- *Red, dark tea or coke-colored*: Acute glomerulonephritis
- *Dilute watery*: Diabetes insipidus, polydipsia states, etc.

FROTHY: ALBUMINURIA

- Acute nephritis
- Alkaptonuria
- Melanotic sarcoma
- Casts
- *Granular or red cell*: Acute glomerulonephritis.

HYALINE: NORMAL

- Cloudiness
- *Dissolved urates*: Normal
- *Leukocytes*: Urinary tract infection (UTI).

PATHOGNOMONIC JEJUNAL BIOPSY FINDINGS

- Abetalipoproteinemia
- Lymphoma
- Amyloidosis
- Lymphangiectasia
  - *Giardia lamblia*.

HIGH SWEAT CHLORIDE

- Cystic fibrosis (>60 mEq/L)
- Insufficient sweat
  - Congenital hypothyroidism
  - Ectodermal dysplasia
  - Riley-Day syndrome
- Metabolic
  - Gb-6-PD deficiency
  - *Diabetes insipidus*: Nephrogenic
  - Mucopolysaccharidosis
- Protein-energy malnutrition
- Miscellaneous
  - Adrenal insufficiency (untreated)
  - Fucosidosis
  - Celiac disease
  - Familial cholestasis.

FALSE NEGATIVE SWEAT CHLORIDE

- Peripheral edema
- Cloxacillin
- Hypoparathyroidism
- Klinefelter syndrome (XXY)
- Hypogammaglobulinemia
- Hypohidrosis
- Atopic dermatitis
- Glycogen storage disease (type I).

FALSE NEGATIVE TUBERCULIN (MANTOUX) TEST

- Immunosuppression
- Severe PEM
- Immunosuppressant therapy (steroids)
- Diseases
  - Human immunodeficiency virus (HIV) malignancy
  - Tuberculous meningitis (TBM), miliary tuberculosis
- Exanthemata
  - Measles
  - Mumps
  - Chickenpox
- Young infants
- Stress of surgery, burns, etc.
- During incubation period.

XANTHOCHROMIC CEREBROSPINAL FLUID

- Froin's syndrome
- Guillain-Barré syndrome (GBS)
- Deep icterus
- Old subarachnoid hemorrhage.

ALBUMINOCYTOLOGICAL DISSOCIATION

- Guillain-Barré syndrome
  - *Cerebrospinal fluid (CSF)*: Cells nearly normal, proteins quite high
- Froin's loculation syndrome or spinal subarachnoid block [CSF—cells within normal range, proteins high (more than twice upper limit of normal) xanthochromia, clot on standing].

SECTION 5

Differential Diagnosis of Selected Radiologic Signs

CHAPTER 65

Differential Diagnosis of Selected Radiologic Signs

MEDIASTINAL SHIFT

- Conditions pushing the mediastinum
  - Empyema or massive pleural effusion
  - Pneumomediastinum
  - Large mass (tumor)
- Conditions pulling the mediastinum
  - Atelectasis (collapse)
  - Fibrosis
  - Agenesis
  - Surgical resection.

HILAR ENLARGEMENT (FIG. 65.1)

- Nonspecific bronchopneumonia (secondary to viral infections like measles, chickenpox, influenza, etc., mycoplasma, or rickettsia). Usually, hilar enlargement is bilateral. The hilar borders are indistinct, the perihilar markings are exaggerated with streaky densities extending outward, and there are peribronchial and interstitial infiltrates.
- *Tuberculosis:* The hilar enlargement is usually unilateral
  - Pulmonary arterial or venous hypertension
- *Lymphoma:* The hilar enlargement may be unilateral initially but soon it becomes bilateral with widening of the mediastinum and has remarkably sharp borders.
- *Sarcoidosis:* The hilar enlargement is bilateral, lobulated, and well defined with calcification at times.
- *Lymphoblastic leukemia:* The hilar enlargement is bilateral and resembles sarcoidosis.

ENLARGEMENT OF ANTERIOR MEDIASTINUM

- Thymic enlargement (Figs. 65.2A and B)
- Thymoma
- Dermoid cyst

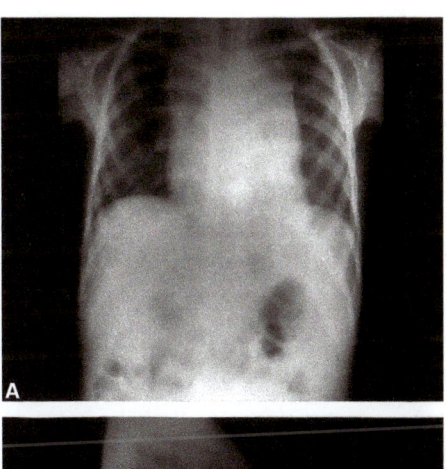
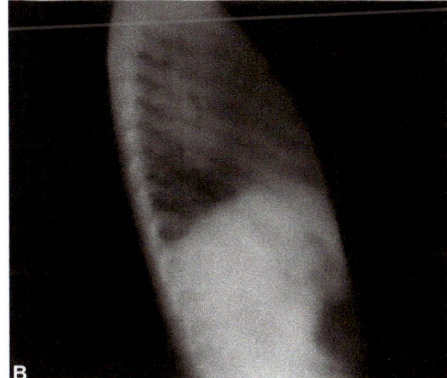

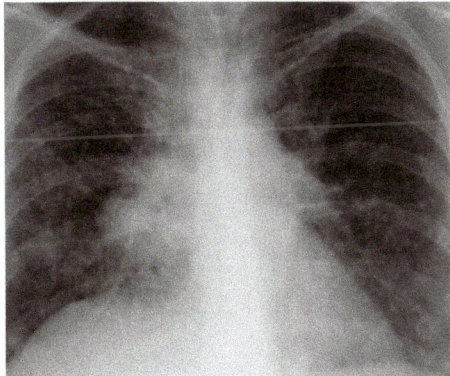

Fig. 65.1: *Bilateral hilar enlargement*—Differentials include infections (viral, tuberculous, mycoplasma or rickettsial infections, sarcoidosis, etc.), lymphoma, metastasis, leukemia, and pulmonary arteriovenous hypertension.

Figs. 65.2A and B: Widened anterior mediastinum (thymus).

- Teratoma
- Substernal goiter.

ENLARGEMENT OF THE SUPERIOR MEDIASTINUM

- Thymus (Fig. 65.3)
- Lymphoma.

ENLARGEMENT OF THE MIDDLE MEDIASTINUM

- Atypical location of the thymus
- Persistence of left superior vena cava
- Widening of right superior vena cava
- Bronchogenic cyst
- Pericardial cyst
- Lymphoma
- Neuroblastoma
- Testicular tumor
- Pericardial cyst
- Cardiac myxoma
- Angiomatous lymphoid hamartoma.

ENLARGEMENT OF THE POSTERIOR MEDIASTINUM (FIG. 65.4)

- Atypical location of the thymus
- Neurogenic tumors like neurofibroma, neurofibrosarcoma, and neuroblastoma
- Hemangioma
- Meningocele.

MULTIPLE FINELY GRANULAR SHADOWS (MILIARY MOTTLING) IN THE LUNGS

- *Miliary tuberculosis (Figs. 65.5A and B):* Miliary lesions are very small but equal in size. The number of the lesions decreases in craniocaudal direction. There is invariably an enlargement of the hilar or paratracheal lymph nodes.
- *Miliary bronchopneumonia (Fig. 65.6):* The lesions are of varying size and not well defined. They decrease from hilum to periphery. The involvement of the hilum with streaky densities is usual. This kind of bronchopneumonia is frequent in measles and pertussis.
- Staphylococcal pneumonia (Fig. 65.7)

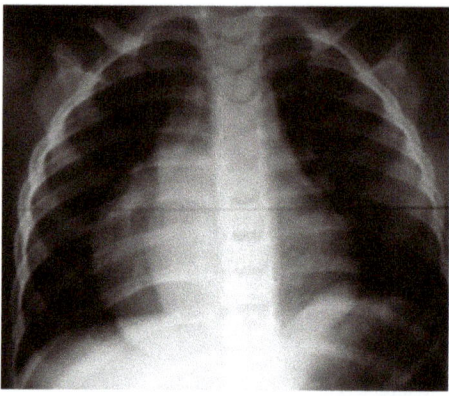

Fig. 65.4: Posterior medastinum widening (neuroblastoma)—Note the shadow behind the cardiac shadow on right side.

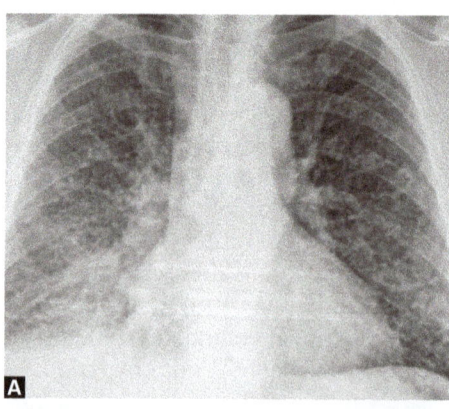

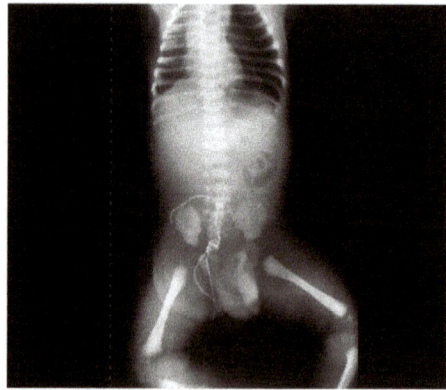

Fig. 65.3: Superior mediastinal widening (thymus shadow).

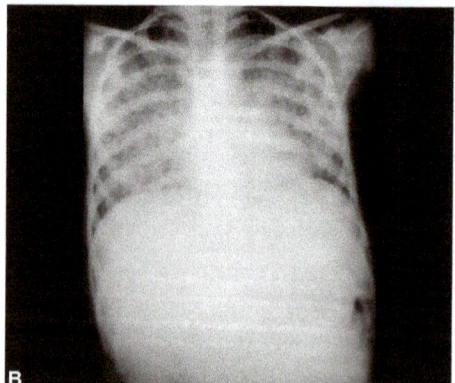

Figs. 65.5A and B: *Miliary mottling* in disseminated pulmonary tuberculosis. It needs to be differentiated from conditions such as tropical eosinophilia, miliary bronchopneumonia seen in measles or pertussis, pulmonary hemosiderosis, pulmonary edema, etc.

- Tropical eosinophilia (Fig. 65.8)
- Fungal infections
- Aspiration pneumonia
- Pneumocystis carinii (jiroveci) pneumonia
- Sarcoidosis
- Lymphoma
- Leukemia
- Methotrexate lung
- Thyroid malignancy
- Idiopathic pulmonary hemosiderosis
- Pulmonary alveolar proteinosis
- Pulmonary alveolar microlithiasis
- Pulmonary edema
- Uremic lung.

SOLITARY LUNG DENSITIES

- Congenital cysts
- Acquired cysts
- Pneumonic infiltrates
- Localized effusions
- Eosinophilic infiltrate
- Tuberculoma
- Echinococcosis
- Abscesses
- Aspergillosis.

MULTIPLE LUNG DENSITIES

- Bronchopneumonia (Fig. 65.9)
- Bronchogenic dissemination in tuberculosis

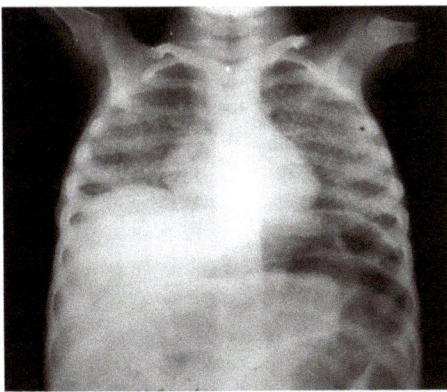

Fig. 65.6: Miliary bronchopneumonia (expiratory/film).

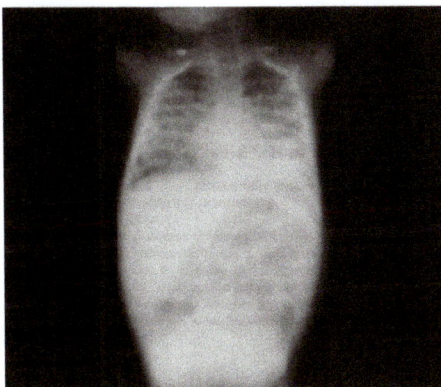

Fig. 65.7: *Staphylococcal pneumonia*—Note the pneumatoceles of different sizes in contrast to the diffuse bronchopneumonia of pneumococcal etiology. Here the lung involvement is patchy. A fast progression from bronchopneumonia to effusion or pneumothorax is strongly suggestive of staphylococcal pneumonia.

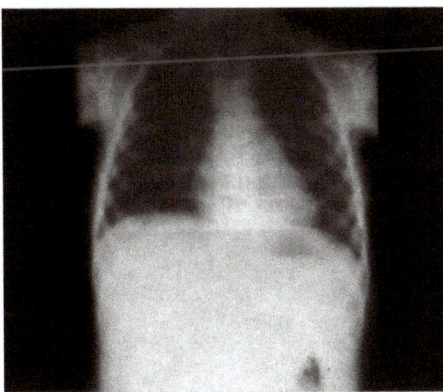

Fig. 65.8: Tropical eosinophilia.

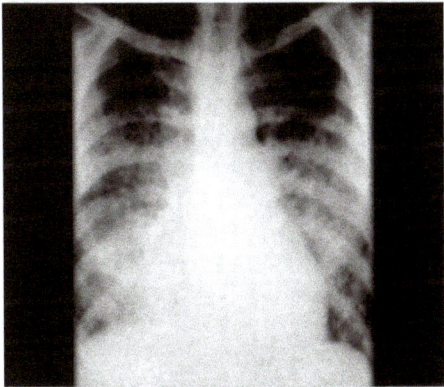

Fig. 65.9: Viral bronchopneumonia in chickenpox.

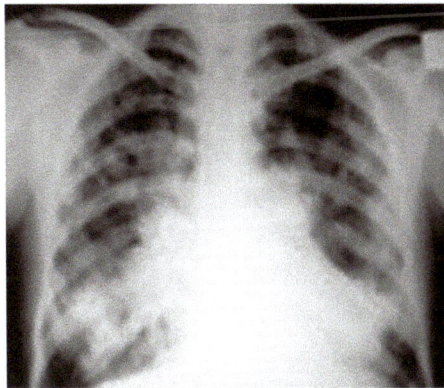

Fig. 65.10: Multiple hydatid cysts.

- Septic pulmonary infarction
- Multiple hydatid cysts (*see* Fig. 65.10).

LARGE LUNG DENSITY

- Lobar pneumonia or consolidation (Fig. 65.11)
- Atelectasis
- Abscess
- Tuberculosis
- Pulmonary sequestration
- Pulmonary agenesis
- Pleural effusion or empyema (Figs. 65.12 and 65.13)
- Hydropneumothorax (Fig. 65.14).

OVERWHELMING INTERSTITIAL CHANGES IN LUNG FIELD

- Pertussis
- Cystic fibrosis
- Pneumocystis carinii pneumonia
- Sinobronchitis
- Congenital pulmonary lymphangiectasia
- Congenital lesions of the heart with pulmonary edema or congestion due to enhanced pulmonary blood flow
- Wilson-Mikity syndrome
- Interstitial pulmonary fibrosis (Hamman-Rich syndrome)
- Collagenosis
- Scleroderma
- Histiocytosis.

UNILATERAL INCREASE IN LUNG RADIOLUCENCY

- Rotation into the oblique position of the subject
- Congenital lobar emphysema (infantile lobar emphysema)
- Emphysema secondary to a foreign body in the main stem bronchus
- Macleod's syndrome (unilateral or partial bronchial obstruction).

PULMONARY EDEMA (UNILATERAL)

- Pulmonary edema if the child's position is decubitus

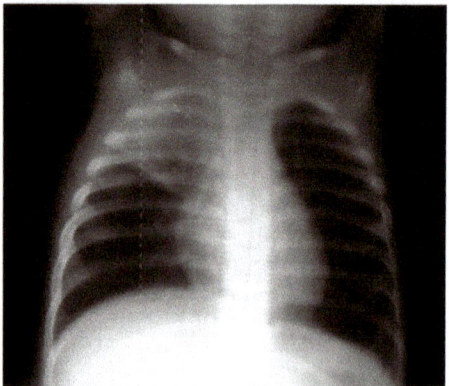

Fig. 65.11: Consolidation (right upper lobe).

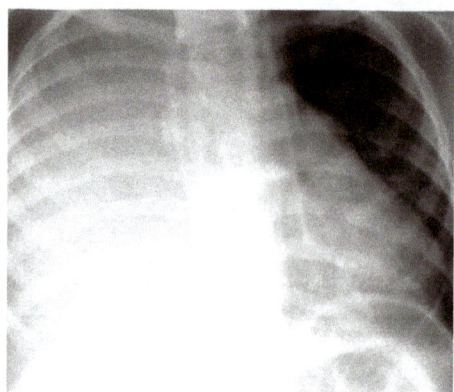

Fig. 65.13: Empyema.

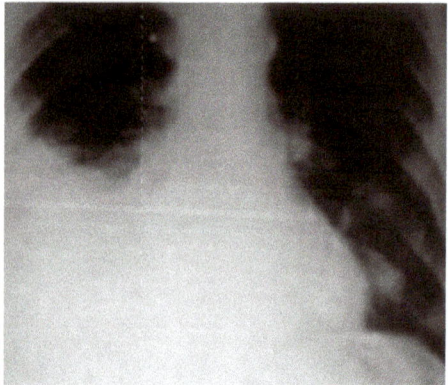

Fig. 65.12: *Pleural effusion (right)*—Note the curved line.

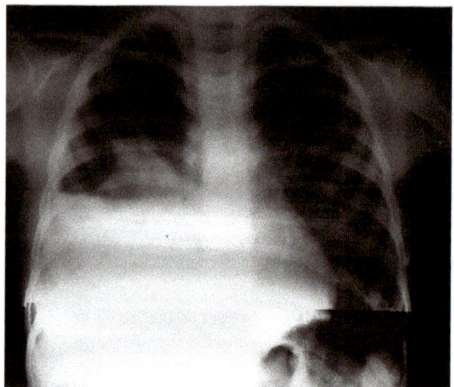

Fig. 65.14: Hydropneumothorax.

Differential Diagnosis of Selected Radiologic Signs

- Rapid removal of fluid or air from pleural space on one side only
- Pulmonary lymphangiectasia.

PULMONARY METASTASES

- Wilms tumor
- Ewing sarcoma
- Rhabdomyosarcoma
- Fibrosarcoma
- Synovial sarcoma
- Hodgkin lymphoma.

MIDDLE LOBE CONSOLIDATION (FIG. 65.15)

- Asthma
- Tuberculosis
- Acute infection
  - *Pseudomonas aeruginosa*
  - *Klebsiella*.

ENLARGED CARDIAC SHADOW

- Congestive cardiac failure (CCF)
- Pericardial effusion (Fig. 65.16)
- Myocarditis (Fig. 65.17)
- Ventricular septal defect (VSD)
- Cardiomyopathy (Fig. 65.18).

AIR BRONCHOGRAM

- Hyaline membrane disease (HMD)
- Pulmonary edema
- Pneumatic consolidation
- Adult respiratory distress syndrome (ARDS)
- Sarcoidosis.

OPAQUE HEMITHORAX

- Massive pleural effusion
- Atelectasis/collapse/fibrosis, consolidation
- Thickened pleura (tuberculous)
- Pulmonary agenesis.

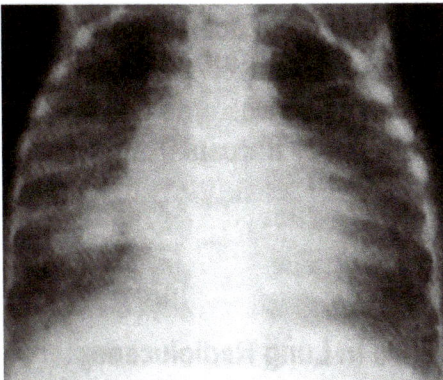

Fig. 65.15: Right middle lobe consolidation—Differential diagnosis includes pseudomonas or Klebsiella infection, asthma, and tuberculosis.

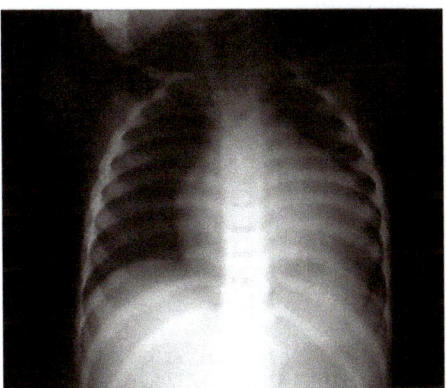

Fig. 65.17: Myocarditis.

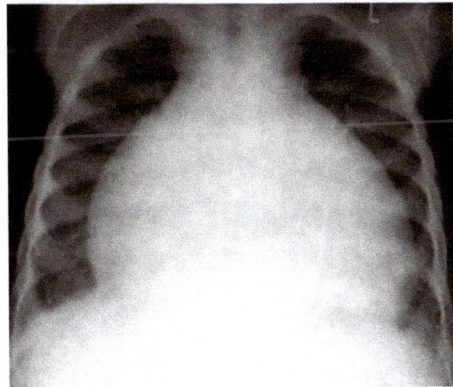

Fig. 65.16: *Pericardial effusion*—Note the symmetrically enlarged (flask-shaped) heart with sharp, well-defined, Stenciled borders, and wide base with acute angle between right border and right hemidiaphragm. Cardiothoracic (CT) ratio is 0.8 against the normal 0.5.

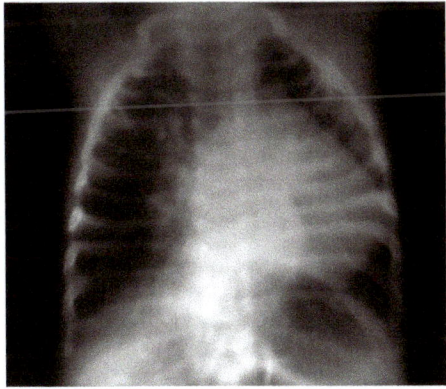

Fig. 65.18: Cardiomyopathy.

KERLEY LINES IN CHEST X-RAY

- A sign of interstitial pulmonary edema
- Left ventricular failure (LVF)
- Mitral stenosis
- Sarcoidosis
- Pneumoconiosis
- Lymphangiectasia.

NODULAR OPACITIES IN CHEST X-RAY

- Tuberculomas
- Pyogenic abscesses
- Fungal messes
- Secondaries (Cannon-ball metastases)
- Hyd C
- Hamartomes.

CALCIFICATION IN CHEST X-RAY

- Tuberculosis
- Hemosiderosis
- Fungal infection.

RETICULAR GRANULAR PATTERN IN CHEST X-RAY

- Hyaline membrane disease
- Meconium aspiration syndrome (MAS)
- Congenital pneumonia
- Pulmonary edema
- Pulmonary hemorrhage.

SOAP BUBBLE APPEARANCE IN ABDOMEN FILM OF NEONATES

- Meconium ileus
- Meconium plug
- Necrotizing enterocolitis
- Atresia or severe stenosis
- Hirschsprung's disease
- Fecolith
- Pulmonary stenosis
- Pulmonary hypertension
- As a part of cardiomyopathy with global enlargement.

LEFT VENTRICULAR ENLARGEMENT

- Ventricular septal defect
- Aortic regurgitation
- Mitral valve disease
- Cardiomyopathy.

LEFT ATRIAL ENLARGEMENT

- Ventricular septal defect
- Patent ductus arteriosus (PDA)
- Mitral valve disease.

RIGHT-SIDED HEART

- Cardiomyopathy (Fig. 65.18)
- Dextrocardia (Fig. 65.19)
- Large pleural effusion or empyema (left lung)
- Space-occupying lesion, say large hydatid cyst, tumor, etc. (left lung)
- Collapse (right lung).

ABNORMAL INTRA-ABDOMINAL AIR COLLECTION

- Abnormally located bowel segment
  - Inguinal hernia
- Pneumoperitoneum
- Retropneumoperitoneum
  - Perforation
- Gas in bowel wall
  - Gastric pneumatosis
  - Rupture of a lung bulla
- Gas within abscess
  - Subphrenic
  - Hepatic
  - Renal or perirenal
- Gas in biliary system
  - Stone
  - Cholecystitis
  - Tumor with hepatobiliary fistula
  - Surgery.

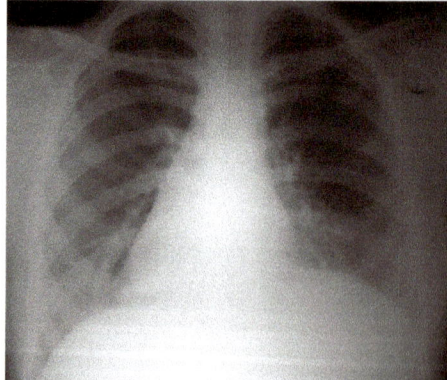

Fig. 65.19: *Dextrocardia with situs inversus and bronchiectasis*—Note the apex of the heart on the right side and left dome of diaphragm at higher level.

BOWEL SHOWING OPAQUE MATERIAL (CALCIFICATION/OPACITIES) IN ABDOMINAL FILM

- Iron
- Salicylates
- Phenothiazine
- Chloral hydrate.

INTRA-ABDOMINAL CYST

- Omental cyst
- Mesenteric cyst
- Choledochal cyst
- Ovarian
- Intestinal duplication
- Pancreatic pseudocyst
- Abscess
- Meckel's diverticulum
- Lymphangioma
- Mesenteric lymphoma
- Intramural tumor
- Absent kidney
  - Congenital
  - Nephrectomy
- Small kidney
  - Renal hypoplasia
  - Renal atrophy
- Ectopic kidney
  - Pelvic
  - Intrathoracic
  - Crossed fused ectopia
- Obliteration of perirenal fat
  - Perirenal abscess
  - Perirenal hematoma
  - Renal tumor.

UNILATERAL SMALL KIDNEY

- Congenital hypoplasia
- Infarction
- Atrophy
  - Postinflammatory
  - Postradiation
  - Postobstruction
  - Reflux
  - Ischemia (renal artery stenosis).

BILATERAL SMALL KIDNEY

- Chronic glomerulonephritis
- Hypotension
- Alport syndrome

- Nephrosclerosis
- Embolic disease.

UNILATERAL LARGE KIDNEY

- Acute pyelonephritis
- Renal vein thrombosis
- Obstructive uropathy
- Arterial obstruction
  - Infarct
- Hypertrophy
- Duplication.

BILATERAL LARGE KIDNEY

- Glomerular disease
  - Acute glomerulonephritis
  - Systemic lupus erythematosus (SLE)
  - Diabetes insipidus
- Amyloidosis
- Edema of kidney
- Acromegaly
- Sickle-cell anemia
- Bilateral duplication
- Acute urate nephropathy
- Leukemia.

DOUBLE BUBBLE APPEARANCE

- Duodenal atresia (Figs. 65.20 and 65.21)
- Annular pancreas
- Malrotation of midgut with volvulus
- Ladd's bands
- Meconium ileus (Fluid levels + bubbles)
- Ileal atresia
- Meconium plug syndrome
- Atresia of colon
- Small left colon syndrome
- Hirschsprung's disease.

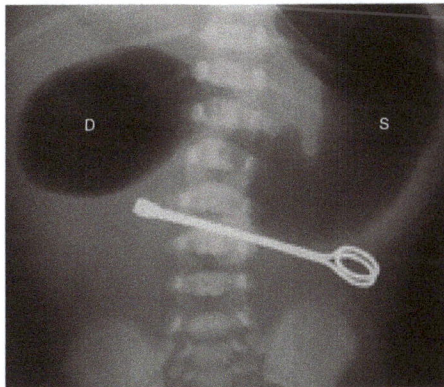

Fig. 65.20: Double bubble sign in duodenal atresia.

MULTIPLE AIR-FLUID LEVELS

- Intussusception (Fig. 65.22)
- Worms
- Tuberculosis
- Calculi
- Tuberculous peritonitis
- Tuberculous lymph nodes
- Addison disease
- Wolman disease
- Calcification following neonatal shock
- Calculi
- Foreign body
- Schistosomiasis
- Amebic cyst
- Hydatid cyst
- Tuberculosis
- Hemangioma
- Hepatoma
- *Calculi*: Intrahepatic biliary, gallbladder, etc.
- Cysticercosis
- Myositis
- Radio-opaque tumors (abdominal)
- Nephroblastoma (Wilms tumor)
- Neuroblastoma
- Teratoma
- Dermoid.

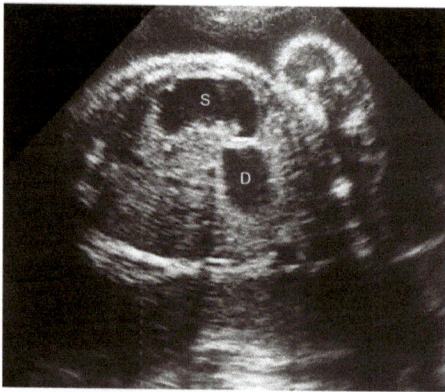

Fig. 65.21: *Duodenal atresia*—Note the double bubble sign on ultrasonography.

ABSENT RADII

- Fanconi anemia
- VATER [vertebrae, anus, trachea, esophagus, renal (kidneys)] syndrome
- Thrombocytopenia with absent radius (TAR) syndrome
- Holt–Oram syndrome
- Aase syndrome.

WORMIAN BONES (FIG. 65.23)

Intrasutural ossicles in lambdoid, posterior sagittal, and temporal squamosal sutures
- *Normal:* Up to 6 months
- Hypothyroidism
- Hypophosphatasia
- Down syndrome
- Cleidocranial dysostosis
- Rickets (during healing)
- Progeria
- Menkes kinky hair disease
- Osteogenesis imperfecta
- Pyknodysostosis.

HAIR-ON-END APPEARANCE (SKULL)

Widening of diploic space and thinning of outer table with coarse trabeculae, giving rise to "hair-on-end appearance
- Thalassemia (Fig. 65.24)
- Sickle-cell anemia
- Spherocytosis
- G-6-PD deficiency
- Chronic iron deficiency anemia (IDA) (Fig. 65.25)

ABNORMAL SKULL SHAPE

- Normal variant
- Craniosynostosis (Fig. 65.26)
- Rickets
- Chondrodystrophy.

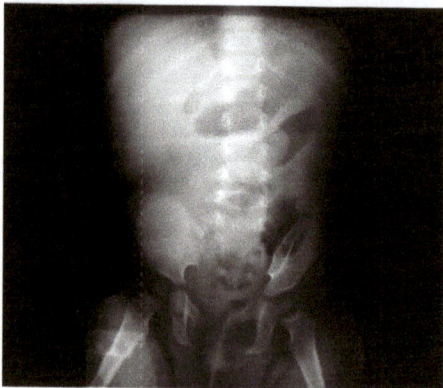

Fig. 65.22: Intussusception.

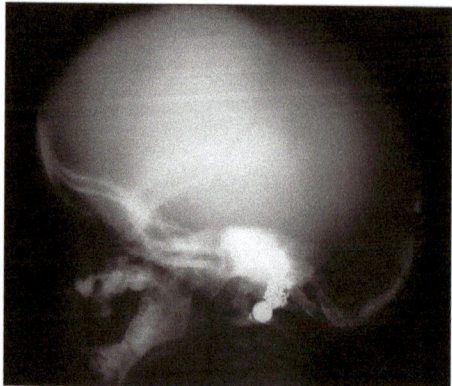

Fig. 65.23: Wormian bones in lambdoid sutures.

CRANIOSYNOSTOSIS

- Premature closure of skull sutures
- Primary
- Secondary
  - Microcephaly
  - *In association with syndromal states*: Down, Apert, Carpenter, Treacher Collins, Hurler, achondroplasia, etc.
  - *Metabolic*: Rickets, hypercalcemia, hyperthyroidism, hypervitaminosis D
  - *Hematologic*: Sickle-cell anemia, thalassemia
  - *Iatrogenic*: After shunt operation.

J-SHAPED SELLA TURCICA

- Normal variant
- Osteogenesis imperfecta
- Neurofibromatosis
- Achondroplasia
- Mucopolysaccharidosis
- Chronic hydrocephalus
- Optic glioma.

INTRACRANIAL CALCIFICATION

- *Cytomegalovirus (CMV)*: Seen as a calcified mold of the ventricles
- *Toxoplasmosis*: Seen as diffuse intracranial calcifications spread in both cerebral hemispheres
- *Rubella*: Infrequent
- Herpes simplex
- Fahr syndrome (Fig. 65.27)
- Down syndrome
- Hyperparathyroidism
- Sturge-Weber syndrome (tram-track appearance)
- Craniopharyngioma (suprasellar calcification) (Fig. 65.28)
- Tuberculosis (basal calcification).

SUTURAL DIASTASIS

- Hydrocephalus (Figs. 65.29 and 65.30)
- Traumatic (after the closure of sutures).

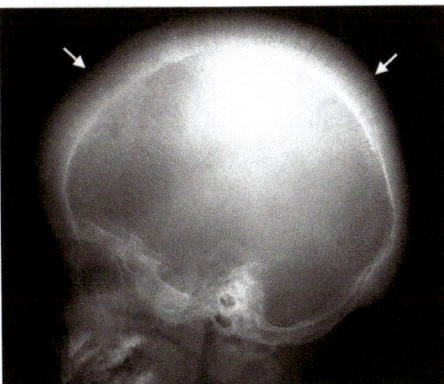

Fig. 65.24: Hair-on-end appearance in thalassemia major.

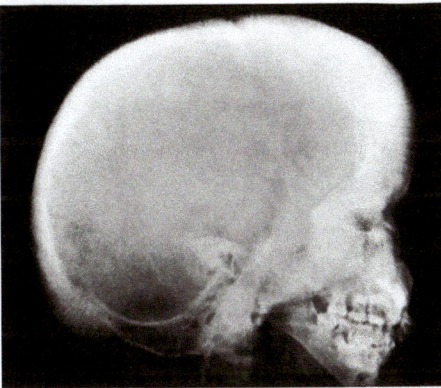

Fig. 65.25: Hair-on-end appearance in chronic iron deficiency anemia.

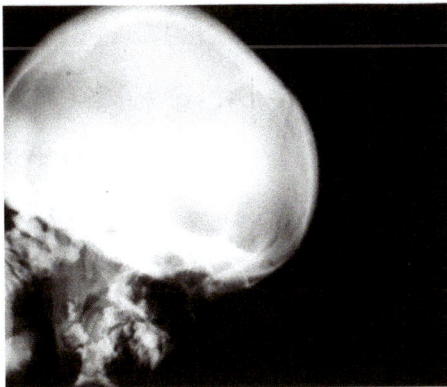

Fig. 65.26: Scaphocephaly with shoe-like sella in Hurler syndrome.

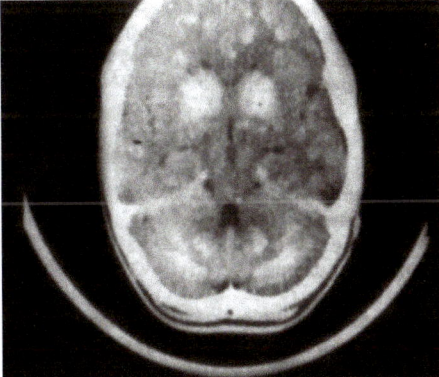

Fig. 65.27: *Fahr syndrome*—Computed tomography (CT) scan showing calcification in the basal ganglia in a patient who presented with hyperkinetic syndrome comprising of agitation, restlessness, rigidity, and tremor. There was no overt parathyroid disease. Some evidence suggested "familial" occurrence of the symptom complex. Note that calcification of basal ganglia can also occur in hyperparathyroidism and, occasionally, in Down syndrome.

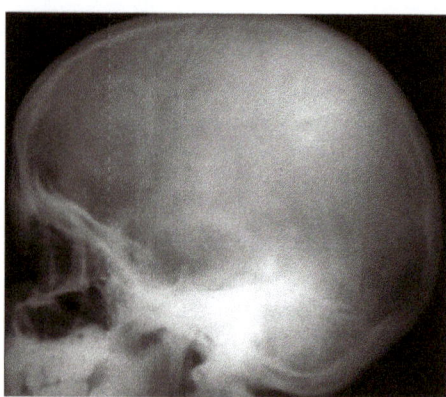

Fig. 65.28: *Craniopharyngioma*—Note the enlarged sella turcica.

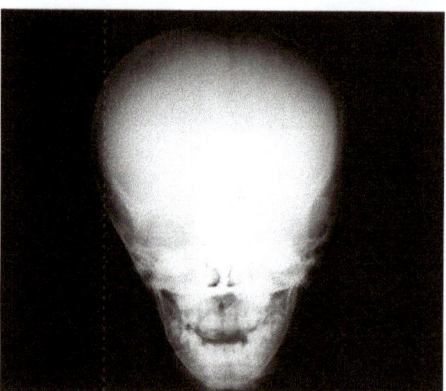

Fig. 65.29: *Hydrocephalus*—Note the enlarged skull with sutural diastasis.

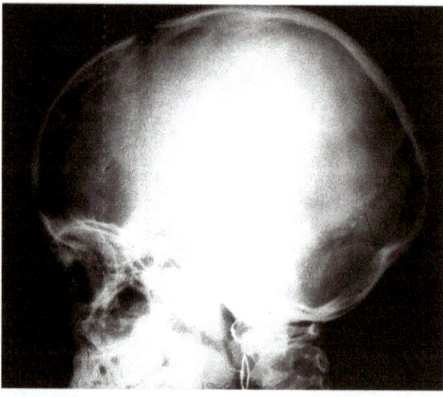

Fig. 65.30: *Hydrocephalus*—Note the enlarged skull with sutural diastasis in the lateral view.

SILVER/COPPER-BEATEN APPEARANCE (FIGS. 65.31 AND 65.32)

- Raised intracranial pressure (RICP)
- Meningomyelocele.

INCREASED BONE DENSITY

- Osteopetrosis
- Fluorosis
- Pyknodysostosis.

ENHANCING LESIONS (NEUROIMAGING)

- Tuberculosis
- Neurocysticercosis (Figs. 65.33A to D)
- Abscess
- Early glioma
- Metastases
- Toxoplasmosis
- Arteriovenous malformations.

NONENHANCING LESIONS (NEUROIMAGING)

- Neurocysticercosis
- Hydatid disease
- Cystic astrocytoma
- Porencephaly
- Colloid cyst of third ventricle
- Neurocysticercosis
- Multiple myeloma
- Hydatid cyst.

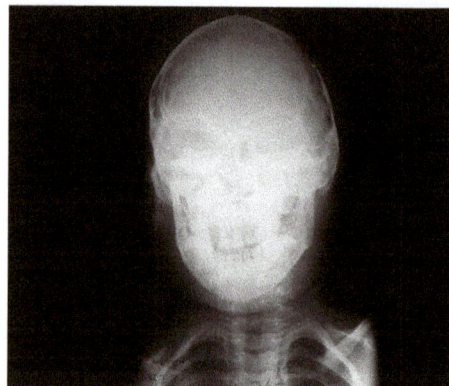

Fig. 65.31: *Intracranial space-occupying lesion (ICSOL)*—Note the lacunar skull with silver-beaten appearance.

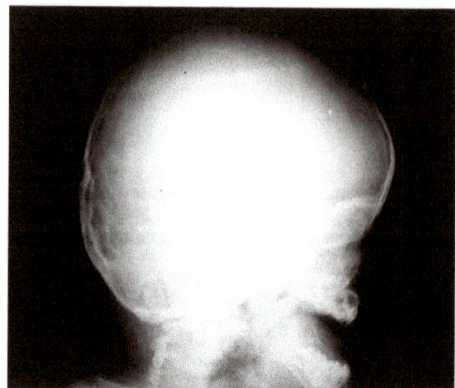

Fig. 65.32: *Intracranial space-occupying lesion (ICSOL)*—Note the lacunar skull with silver-beaten appearance (lateral view).

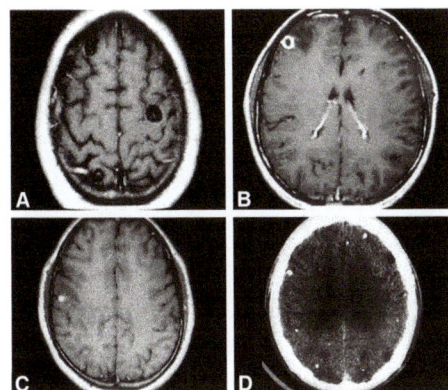

Figs. 65.33A to D: Four stages of neurocysticercosis.

CALCIFICATION (NEUROIMAGING)

- Tuberculosis
- Neurocysticercosis
- Tuberous sclerosis
- Toxoplasmosis
- Cytomegalovirus infection.

METACARPAL SIGN

- Shortening of metacarpals, usually fourth and fifth. A line drawn along the heads of the fourth and fifth metacarpals intersects the head of the third metacarpal.
- A normal variant in 10% individuals.
- Pseudohypoparathyroidism (Albright's hereditary osteodystrophy)
- Turner syndrome.

PATHOLOGIC FRACTURES

- Osteogenesis imperfecta (Fig. 65.34)
- Nutritional rickets (Fig. 65.35) or osteomalacia
- Scurvy (Fig. 65.36)
- Bone tumors—both primary and secondary (Fig. 65.37).
- Severe osteoporosis from any cause.

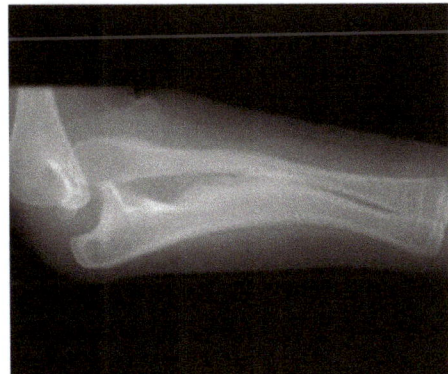

Fig. 65.34: Pathologic fractures with deformities in osteogenesis imperfecta.

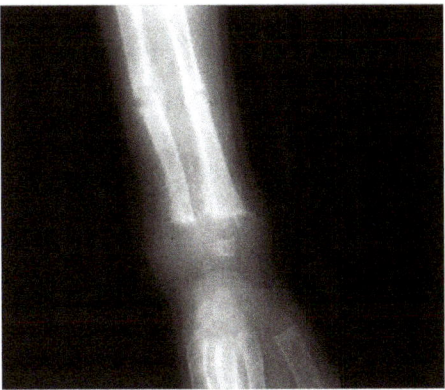

Fig. 65.35: *Nutritional rickets*—Note the classical radiologic changes at the wrist: cupping, fraying (blurring like bristles of toothbrush) and flaring (splaying) of the metaphysis. Also seen are pathologic fractures of radius and ulna, poor bone density (because of osteoporosis) and increased distance between epiphysis and metathesis (due to loss of zone of provisional calcification).

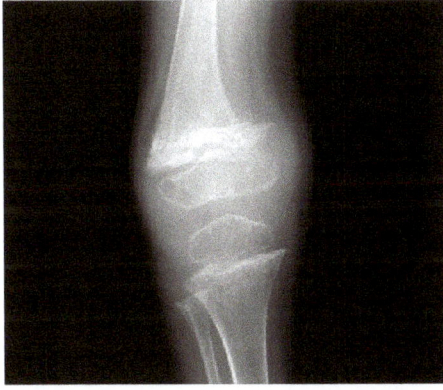

Fig. 65.36: *Scurvy*—Note the small pathologic fractures at upper end of fibula and lower end of femur. Also seen are thinning of the cortex, signet ring, white line of Hilton, Pelken spur, corner sign, etc.

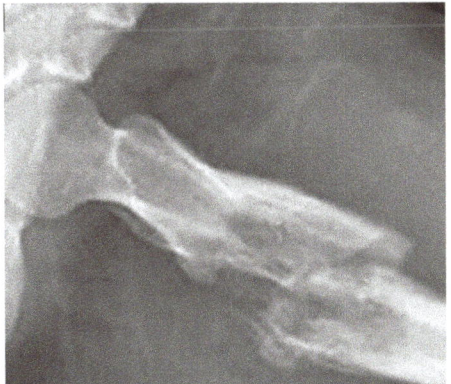

Fig. 65.37: Pathologic fracture from secondaries.

Index

Page numbers followed by *b* refer to box, *f* refer to figure, *fc* refer to flowchart, and *t* refer to table

A

Abdomen, anatomical topography of 225*f*
Abdominal discomfort 34*f*
Abdominal distension 11*f*, 55, 56
   etiology of 55, 55*t*
   history 55
   investigations 56
   massive 40*f*
   physical examination 55
Abdominal mass 225
   history 225
   investigations 226
   parietal lump 226
   physical examination 225
Abdominal pain 58, 59*t*
   causes of 60*b*, 64
   chronic 59*b*, 62
   history 60
   investigations 60
   physical examination 60
   recurrent 24*f*, 58
   types of recurrent 58
Abetalipoproteinemia 73
Abscess 7*f*
   appendiceal 249
   fecal brown 16*f*
   iliopsoas 232*f*
   large 35*f*
   liver 62
   lumbodorsal 16*f*
   lung 83, 101, 161, 248
   pelvic 249
   retropharyngeal 273, 273*f*, 277
   subperiosteal 43*f*
   subphrenic 62
Acanthocytosis 312, 312*f*
Acetazolamide 129, 175, 164, 194, 283
Achalasia 286
Achondroplasia 24*f*, 260*f*
Aciduria, organic 10*f*
Acquired immunodeficiency syndrome 116, 183, 183*b*, 223, 250
Acrocyanosis 103*f*
Acrodermatitis enteropathica 39*f*, 10*f*, 116
Acrodynia 10*f*
Acute abdominal pain 60
   causes of 59*b*
Acute diarrhea
   causes of 111*b*, 115
   etiology of 111
Acute respiratory distress syndrome 119
Adenoid facies 49*f*
Adenoidectomy 171

Adenoma sebaceum 25*f*
Aerophagy 56
Air bronchogram 327
Air-fluid levels, multiple 330
Alanine aminotransferase 318
Albinism 236
Albright's hereditary osteodystrophy 20*f*, 238
Albright's syndrome 238
Albumin, high serum 316
Albuminocytological dissociation 320
Albuminuria 319
Alkaline phosphatase, low 318
Alkalosis 230
Alkylating agents 43*f*
Allergy
   food 63*f*
   history of 100
Alopecia 10*f*
   acquired diffuse 43*f*
Alpha-1-antitrypsin deficiency 13*f*, 126
Alpha-thalassemia 134
Alveolar capillary dysplasia 122
Ambiguous genitalia 16*f*, 29*f*, 44*f*, 65
   classification of 65*b*
   diagnosis of 66*fc*
   history 65
   investigations 65
   physical examination 65
Amebiasis, chronic 151
Amelia 35*f*
Aminoaciduria 319
Aminophylline 129, 194
Amitriptyline 164
Amphetamine 192, 194
Amylase, high serum 318
Anagen effluvium 43*f*
Anal fissure 45*f*, 75, 91
Anal orifice, placement of 90
Anaphylactoid purpura 62, 132, 258
Anasarca 132
Ancylostoma duodenale 58
Ancylostomiasis 151
Androgen action defect 65
Anemia 68, 69, 69*b*, 71
   acquired hypoplastic 71
   aplastic 52*f*, 69, 71
   autoimmune hemolytic 71, 201
   clinical grading of 68*t*
   congenital
      hemolytic 70
      hypoplastic 71
   drug-induced hemolytic 200
   hemolytic 70
   history 68

   hypochronic 311
   investigations 68
   macrocytic 311
   physical examination 68
   severe 28*f*
   types of 49*f*
   unexplained 70
   WHO grading of 68*t*
Angioma 276
Anhidrotic ectodermal dysplasia 37*f*, 252
Anisocytosis 70, 184
Anorectal defect, level of 28*f*
Anorectal stenosis 90
Anorexia 34*f*, 69, 183, 222
Anotia 17*f*
Anterior mediastinum, enlargement of 323
Antibody
   antinuclear 251
   blocking 197
Anticonvulsants 10*f*
Antidiarrheal drug 112
Antihistamines 154, 194
Antimalarials 71
Antimetabolites 43*f*, 71
Antimongoloid slant 39*f*, 298, 298*f*
Aorta syndrome, coarctation of 128
Aortic stenosis 128, 167
Apert syndrome 39*f*, 48*f*, 266, 298*f*
Aphasia 163
Apnea 278
Appendicitis
   acute 60
   chronic 249
   diagnosis of 60
Apt's test 170
Arachnodactyly 15*f*, 39*f*
Arachnoid villi 210
Argemone mexicana 137
Arnold-Chiari malformation 36*f*, 210*f*
Arrhythmias 279
Arthralgia 203, 205, 206, 222, 223
Arthritis 203, 223, 307
   juvenile idiopathic 205
   pauciarticular juvenile idiopathic 17*f*
Arthrogryposis multiplex congenita 304*f*
Arthropathy, hemophiliac 13*f*
Ascariasis 151, 182
Ascaris lumbricoides 58, 125, 231
Ascites 55, 57, 306
   massive 13*f*
Ascitic fluid collects 57
Ash-leaf spot 6*f*
Aspiration, massive 118
Aspirin 60, 175, 283

Asthma 5f, 327f
   bronchial 101, 122
   history of 100
   severe 103
Astrocytoma 73
Ataxia 72
   acute 305
   causes of 73
   history 72
   investigations 72
   physical examination 72
   progressive 73f
   telangiectasia 6f, 73
Atelectasis 125
Athetosis 192
Atopy 5f
Atresia
   biliary 199t
   extrahepatic biliary 14f, 180f, 199
Atretic obstructive lesions 276
Atrial enlargement, left 328
Atrial flutter 304
Atrial septal defect 29f, 127, 166, 168, 264
Atrial tachycardia, paroxysmal 127
Attention-seeking device 64, 164
Auerbach's plexuses 91
Aura 163
Auspitz sign 8f
Autonomic nervous system, abnormal 279
Autosomal dominant
   disorder 303f
   syndrome 23f
Autosomal recessive disorder 33f
Autosplenectomy 64
Azathioprine 61
Azotemia 319

B

Babinski's sign 73
Bacteremia, severe 268
Bacterial infections
   generalized 249
   localized 248
Bad breath 161
Bad oro-dental hygiene 161
Barium enema 61
Basilar impression syndrome 165
Basophilic stippling 311
Bassen-Kornzweig syndrome 73
B-casomorphin 279
BCG diagnostic test 249
Beckwith syndrome 175
Beef tapeworm 151
Beeturia 173
Behcet disease 247
Belladonna poisoning, sign of 87
Bile syndrome 200
Bitot spot 32f
Blastomyces dermatitidis 251
Blastomycosis 251
Bleeding diathesis 13f
Blepharitis 10f
Blindness 300

Blood
   count, complete 133
   dyscrasias 75
   in stools 74
      causes of 76
      history 74
      physical examination 74
   loss 69
      acute 43f
   picture, complete 68, 254
   pressure, systolic 128
   urea nitrogen 278
Blue sclera 299
Bluish purple gums 81
Body mass index 237
Bone
   age
      interpretation of 262b
      through radiology 261t
   density, increased 332
Bordet-Gengou medium 178
Boric acid 43f
Bornholm's disease 62, 78
Bottle baby disease 25f, 157
Bowleg deformity 26f, 302
Brain
   damage 108
   development 265
   tumor 36f, 73, 252
Brainstem 279
Brandt's syndrome 116
Breastfeeding 39f
Bronchial foreign body 188
Bronchiectasis 83, 101, 328f
Bronchiolitis, acute 123, 123f
Bronchitis
   acute 100
   asthmatic 124
Bronchomalacia 279
Bronchopneumonia 34f, 123f
   hospital-acquired 30f
Brucellosis 249
   acute 221
   chronic 222
Brudzinski signs 218, 273
Bruises, aging of 242t
Brushfield spots 5f
Buffalo hump 3f
Bulging anterior fontanel 296
Bull-neck appearance 21f
Bullous dermatosis, chronic 9f
Burkitt lymphoma 51f
Butterfly rash 305

C

Café-au-lait spots 6f, 305
Caffey disease 81, 253
Calcium, high serum 318
Calf hypertrophy 306
Campomelic syndrome 66
Campylobacter 114
   jejuni 111
Cancer chemotherapy 43f

Cancrum oris 159
Candida albicans 114
Candidiasis 5f
Canker sores 160
Caput succedaneum 136
Carbamazepine 154, 164, 283
Carbohydrate malabsorption 115
Cardiac disease origin, cyanosis of 104
Cardiac failure, congestive 30f, 57, 101, 103,
      125, 127, 128f, 132, 134, 174, 238, 289
Cardiac murmur, innocent 304
Cardiomyopathy 128, 327f
   hypertrophic 129f
Cardiorespiratory distress, severe 126
Cardiovascular disorders 83, 135
Cardiovascular system 73
Carotid body defects 279
Carpal bones 261
Carpenter syndrome 31f, 266
Cataract 299
   congenital 236
Cavernous sinus thrombosis 43f
Celecoxib 60
Celiac disease 18f, 30f, 39f, 57, 57f, 109, 113,
      115, 151, 194
Cellulitis 7f
Central nervous system 93, 106, 147, 171,
      190, 193, 209, 268, 272, 278, 283, 285
   congenital malformation of 95
   diagnosis of 249
Cephalhematoma 197
   large 199
Cephaloridine 71
Cephalosporins 71
Cerebellar
   ataxia
      acute 72
      congenital 146
   disease 236
Cerebral
   abscess 95
   diplegia 269
   gigantism 21f, 298f
   hemorrhage 119
   malaria 95, 273
   palsy 26f, 49f, 146
   perfusion pressure 248
Cerebrospinal fluid 94, 164, 185, 193, 194f,
      245, 249, 273
Cervical
   lymphadenitis 35f, 272
      tumor-bearing 24f
   lymphadenopathy 222, 272
Chancre 222
Chassaignac's paralysis 203
Cheilosis 159
Chest
   deformity 126
   dull percussion note 306
   pain 77, 77b
      benign 77
      causes of 78
      history 77
      investigations 77

organic 78
   physical examination 77
  wall compliance 30*f*
  X-ray 328
   findings, grading of 118*t*
Chickenpox 256, 325*f*
  rash 257*f*
Child abuse 41*f*
  and neglect 79, 79*f*, 80*f*
   history 79
   investigations 80
   nonorganic failure to thrive 80
   physical abuse 80
   physical examination 79
   sexual abuse 80
  physical indicators of 80*b*
Childhood disability, causes of 35*f*
Chlamydia 207
  trachomatis 223, 251
Chlamydial infection 251
Chloramphenicol 71
Chlorpromazine 164, 272
Choanal atresia 121
Cholecystitis 62
Chondroitin sulfate 185
Choreoathetosis 192
Chromosomal syndromes 300
Chronic ataxia
  progressive 306
  static 306
Chronic obstructive pulmonary disease 290*f*
Cirrhosis 37*f*
  biliary 13*f*, 57*f*
  childhood 186*f*
  clinical diagnosis of 13*f*
Cleft
  lip 12*f*
  palate 12*f*, 29*f*, 279
Clinodactyly 302, 302*f*
Clitoris, hypertrophied 44*f*
Clonazepam 194, 237
Clostridium difficile 75, 114
Club foot 304
Clubbing 42*f*, 82
  causes of 84
  history 82
  physical examination 82
Coarctation of aorta 29*f*, 168
Cobbler-stone 231
Cold
  agglutinin disease 202
  injury 134
Collodion baby 7*f*
Coloboma 14*f*
Color blindness, total 236
Coma 85
  central nervous system infections 88
  dehydration and electrolyte imbalance 88
  diabetic ketoacidosis 87
  drugs and poisons 87
  head injury 87
  hepatic 181
  history 85
  hypoglycemic shock 87
  hysteria 88
  liver disease 88
  nonketotic hyperosmolar 87
  physical examination 86
   fever 86
   fundoscopy 86
   head and body 86
   limbs 86
   neck rigidity 86
   reflexes 86
  remaining causes of 88
  seizure disorder 87
  syncopal attacks 88
  uremic 88
Conjunctiva, palpebral 24*f*
Conjunctivitis 13*f*
Consciousness, stages of depressed 85
Conservative hydrostatic reduction 61, 75
Constipation 63, 89, 157
  childhood 91
  chronic 18*f*, 138
  history 89
  investigations 90
  later infancy 91
   benign 91
   organic 91
  neonatal 90
   and early infancy 90
   benign 90
   early infancy 90
   organic 90
  physical examination 90
  severe chronic 138
Cooley anemia 70
Coombs' test 71
Copper-beaten appearance 332
Cor pulmonale 126
Corpora cavernosa 38*f*
Cortical hyperostosis, infantile 81
Corticosteroids 61
Costochondral beading 301
Costochondral prominence 301*f*
Costochondritis 78
Cough 100
  causes of 102
  chronic 100
  history 100
  investigations 100
  physical examination 100
  severe 22*f*, 62
  uninterrupted 23*f*
Coumarins 43*f*
Cow's milk 69
  allergy 60, 63, 69, 76, 134
  protein intolerance 156
Coxa vara, congenital 214
Coxsackie stomatitis 159
Craniofacial dysmorphism 33*f*
Craniopharyngioma 154, 332*f*
Craniosynostosis 20*f*, 42*f*, 265, 331
  microcephaly secondary to 266*f*
Craniotabes 296
C-reactive protein 248
  high 317
Crohn's disease 63, 76, 116, 231, 253
Croupy cough 275
Crouzon's syndrome 48*f*
Cryptophthalmos, bilateral 15*f*
Cryptosporidiosis 116
Cubitus valgus 33*f*
Curling's ulcer 171
Curth's modified profile sign 83
Cushing's syndrome 3*f*, 241, 263
Cushing's ulcer 171
Cyanosis 42*f*, 45*f*, 103, 105, 177
  central 103, 104*f*
  congenital heart
   disease 104
   failure 105
  defect 104
  history 103
  investigations 103
  peripheral 103
  physical examination 103
  upper airway obstruction 104
Cyclopentolate 194
Cyclophosphamide 71, 129, 175
Cycloserine 194
Cystic fibrosis 10*f*, 18*f*, 42*f*, 57, 82, 83, 103, 109, 115, 152, 289, 291*f*
Cysticercosis 93
Cysts
  congenital 187
  intra-abdominal 329
Cytomegalic inclusion disease 250
Cytomegalovirus 14*f*, 107, 247
  infection 221, 243

D

Da Costa syndrome 77
Dandy-Walker
  anomaly 210
  cyst 210*f*
de Lange syndrome 39*f*
Deafness 106, 300
  congenital 107
   genetic 107
   nongenetic 107
  history 107
  physical examination 107
  postnatal 108
   genetic 108
   nongenetic 108
  special tests 107
Defective feeding, types of 287
Degenerative diseases 138
Dehydration 56
  fever 156
  severe 35*f*
Demeclocycline 154
Dengue
  fever 253
  hemorrhagic fever 245
   grading of 245*b*
  shock syndrome 245
Dental
  caries 15*f*
  eruption 37*f*

Depression 316
Dermatitis
    atopic 5f
    herpetiformis 257, 257f
Dermatomyositis 251
Dermatophytosis 5f
Dermoid cyst 227
Devil's grip 78
Dextrocardia 328f
Diabetes
    insipidus 153, 253
    maternal 134
    mellitus 153, 159, 263, 288
Diamond sign 82
Diaper rash 11f
Diaphragm, paralysis of 121
Diarrhea 60, 69, 111, 157
    acute 111, 112
    chronic 10f, 18f, 42f, 57f, 109, 112, 112b, 113, 115, 194
        anemia 115
        intestinal parasitic infestations 115
        iron-deficiency 115
        protein-energy malnutrition 115
    cow's milk allergy 116
    history 112
    infective 114
    noninfective 114
    persistent 111, 113
    physical examination 113
        acute 113
        chronic 113
        persistent 113
    relevant investigations 113
        acute 113
        chronic 113
        persistent 113
Diarrheal disease 111f
Diastolic murmur 166, 168
    aortic incompetence 168
    mitral stenosis 169
    pulmonary incompetence 168
    tricuspid stenosis 169
Diazepam 137, 164, 283
Diclofenac 60
Dietary intake, poor 91
DiGeorge syndrome 39f
Digestive function, altered 112
Digital clubbing 82f
Diphenhydramine 71
Diphenoxylate HCl 57
Diphenylhydantoin sodium 160
Diphtheria 276
Disseminated intravascular coagulation 46f, 47f
Diverticulitis 232
Doll's eye phenomenon 86
Doll's head maneuver 86
Dorsal meningocele 16f
Double bubble appearance 329
Down's syndrome 3f-5f, 26f, 39f, 56, 146, 146f, 166, 331f
Dropsy, treatment of 137

Drowsiness, progressive 22f, 35f
Drug toxicity 72
Duchenne muscular dystrophy 216f
Duodenal atresia 330f
    double bubble sign in 329f
Duodenal ulcer disease 63
D-xylose malabsorption 194
Dysentery 75
Dysmorphic facial features 12f
Dysphagia 272
Dysplasia 216f
    developmental 213
Dyspnea 117, 118, 122, 190, 275, 290
    history 117
    investigations 117
    physical examination 117
Dystonia 36f
Dysuria 60, 130
    acute glomerulonephritis 130
    drugs 131
    history 130
    investigations 130
    physical examination 130
    physiologic 130
    urinary
        lithiasis 130
        tract infection 130

E

Ebstein-Barr syndrome 219
Ectopic anus 90
Eczema 5f
    infantile 288
Edema 132
    after neonatal period, localized 136
    angioneurotic 136, 288
    cardiac cause 133
    etiology of 132b
    generalized 134
    history 132
    in newborn, localized 136
        abdominal wall 136
        face 136
        genitalia 136
        head 136
        limbs 136
    non-pitting 136
    nutritional 134
    physical examination 132
    pitting 136
    renal 134
Edwards' syndrome 48f
Effort syndrome 77
Ehler-Danlos syndrome 18f, 245
Eisenmenger complex 105
Ejection systolic murmur 167, 168
Elbow 261
Electrolyte imbalance 134
Elliptocyte 312f
Elliptocytosis 312
Ellis-Van-Creveld syndrome 29f, 31f
Embryonic testicular regression syndrome 66

Emotional disturbance 138
Emphysema 125, 179
Empyema 83, 124, 326f
Encephalitis 72, 95, 273
Encephalocele, cranial 16f
Encephalopathy, hypoxic ischemic 119
Encopresis 45f, 138
    history 138
    investigations 138
    local defects 139
    physical examination 138
    types of 138
Endemic tropical sprue 152
Endocarditis, infective 83, 249
Endogenous obesity 238
    Cushing's syndrome 238
    genetic syndromes 238
    hypothalamic dysfunction 238
    hypothyroidism 238
    polycystic ovaries 238
    Prader-Willi syndrome 238
Entamoeba histolytica 62, 112, 114, 115, 182, 231
Enteric bacteria, gram-negative 204
Enteric infections 111
Enterobius vermicularis 130, 131
Enterocolitis, necrotizing 61, 75
Enteroteratoma 227
Enuresis 140
    anatomical defects 141
    emotional deprivation 141
    enuresis 140
    familial 141
    history 140
    investigations 140
    mental retardation 141
    neurogenic bladder 141
    physical examination 140
    primary 140
        poor toilet training 140
    regressive 140
    secondary 140, 141
        metabolic disorders 141
        psychological 141
        worm infestation 141
    types of 140
    urinary tract infection 141
Enzyme 198
Eosinopenia 314, 314f
Eosinophilia 313, 314f
    tropical 124, 325f
Ephedrine 164, 194
Epicanthal fold 298, 298f
Epidemic dropsy 136
Epidermolysis bullosa simplex 9f
Epigastrium 226
Epiglottitis, acute 189, 276
Epilepsy 97, 284
    abdominal 63
    classification of 97, 97b
    evidence of 63
    focal 98
    grand mal 97

idiopathic 97
organic 97
simulating states 98
Epistaxis 142, 171
    allergy 143
    bleeding disorders 143
    causes of 143
    congenital vascular defect 143
    foreign body 143
    history 142
    investigations 142
    nasal polyposis 143
    physical
        and emotional stress and strain 143
        examination 142
    recurrent 143
    remaining causes of 143
    solar radiation 143
    systemic diseases 143
    trauma 143
    upper respiratory infection 143
Epstein-Barr virus 221, 256
Erysipelas 7f
Erythema
    infectiosum 256
    multiforme 10f
    toxicum 255f
Erythrocyte sedimentation rate 248, 291
Erythroid
    hyperplasia 316
    hypoplasia 316
Escherichia coli 61, 75, 111, 198, 269
Esophageal atresia 286
Esophageal sphincter, lower 286
Esophageal varices 171f
Esophagus 286
    chalasia of 286
    foreign body in 171
Ethambutol 164
Ethionamide 194
Ethosuximide 164
Eunuchoid stature 109
Evening colic 63
Exomphalos major 227f
Exomphalos minor 227f
Exophthalmos 299
Extracorporeal membrane oxygenation 122
Extremity, lower 35f
Eyebrows, absence of 37f
Eyelid, left upper 14f
Eyes
    antimongoloid slant of 298
    bulge 23f
    downslanting 282
    mongoloid slant of 297
    movements 43f
        limitation of 24f

F

Face edema 136
Facial palsy 31f
Facies, hemolytic 42f

Fahr syndrome 331f
Failure to thrive 148
    environmental deprivation 150
    history 148
    investigations 149
    maternal 150
    nutritional deprivation 149
    physical examination 149
    remaining causes of 152
    social 150
    tuberculosis 152
False penile urethra, development of 67
Fanconi anemia 6f
Fatty acid deficiency 10f
Febrile seizures 95
Fecal pellets 90f
Fecal soiling 138
Fecolith 45f, 55, 90, 91f
Feeding problems 155
    bottle addiction 157
    change in bowel habit 157
    choking 157
    colic 156
    dehydration fever 156
    excessive crying 156
    history 155
    investigations 155
    overfeeding 157
    physical examination 155
    poor mothering 157
    regurgitation 155
    sucking difficulties 156
    swallowing difficulties 156
    underfeeding 157
    vomiting 156
Femoral epiphysis, slipped capital 214
Fenfluramine 154, 194
Fertile eunuch 109
Fetal
    alcohol syndrome 46f, 166, 191
        part of 14f
    hemoglobin level 68
    transfusion syndrome 28f
Fetoprotein, high alpha-1 317
Fetor hepaticus 88
Fetor oris 161
Fever
    blisters 248
    enteric 249, 268f
    glandular 221
    high 223
    recurrence of 305
Fever of unknown origin 246
    collagen disorders 251
    dehydration fever 252
    drug fever 252
    factitious fever 252
    history 246
    infections 248
    investigations 248
    malignancies 251
    malingering 252
    miscellaneous causes of 253

normal high temperature 253
    physical examination 247
Fibrillation 304
Fibrin-split products 243
Fibrocystic disease 152
Fibrous tissue 298f
Finger-nose test 191
Flaccid paralysis, acute 21f
Flaky-paint dermatosis 35f
Flat foot 304
Flexible flat feet 20f
Floppy baby syndrome 144, 144f
    causes of 144b
    central etiology 145
    drugs 147
    investigations 144
    peripheral etiology 145
    physical examination 144
    remaining causes of 147
Fluctuation sign 83
Follicle stimulating hormone 262
Francisella tularensis 222
Friedreich ataxia 73
Frohlich's syndrome 238
Fructose intolerance 95
Full-blown disease 221
Fungal infection 143, 251
Funnel chest 41f, 301, 301f
Furazolidone 71

G

Galactorrhea 240
Galactosemia 95, 185, 200
Gallop rhythm 167
Gamma globulin
    high 317
    low 317
Gastric aspirate cytology 120
Gastritis 75
    acute 61
    chronic 63
Gastroenteritis 35f, 156, 307
Gastroesophageal junction, anatomy of
        normal 287f
Gastroesophageal reflux 156, 279, 286
Gastrointestinal bleeding 307
Gastrointestinal disorders 84
    Crohn's disease 84
    multiple polyposis 84
    regional ileitis 84
    steatorrhea 84
    ulcerative colitis 84
Gastrointestinal tract 122, 171, 285
Gastroschisis 227f
Gaucher's cells 51f, 185
Gaucher's disease 6f, 57, 71, 185
Genetic disorders 5f
Genitalia
    external 173
    female 66
    infantile 109
    normal 109

Gentamicin 283
Genu valgum 30f, 211, 302
Genu valgus 15f
Genu varum 15f, 211
Genu varus 302
German measles 221
Giardia lamblia 58, 75, 112, 115
Giardiasis, chronic 151
Gingival hyperplasia 300
Gingivostomatitis
    aphthous ulcers 160
    avitaminosis 159
    chronic mouth breathing 160
    dental defects 160
    drugs 160
    fibromatosis gingivae 160
    history 159
    hypovitaminosis 159
    infections 159
    investigations 159
    physical examination 159
Glasgow coma scale, modified 85t
Glaucoma, primary congenital 43f
Globulin
    high alpha-1 316
    high alpha-2 317
    low alpha-1 316
    low alpha-2 316
Glomerulonephritis, acute 27f, 57, 62
Glucose-6-phosphate dehydrogenase 71
    deficiency 197
Glucuronyl transferase 198
Glutamic-pyruvic transaminase,
    high serum 318
Gluten
    hypersensitivity 134
    sensitivity 194
Glycogen storage disease 21f, 34f, 37f
Goiter 41f
    congenital 304
Goldenhar syndrome 39f
Gonadal failure, primary 110
Gonadal intersex, true 65
Gonadotropin-releasing hormone 109
Gower's sign 216
Granuloma, eosinophilic 252
Granulomatous disease, chronic 16f, 223
Graves' disease 190
Great arteries, transposition of 30f, 103
Great vessels, transposition of 29f, 128
Griseofulvin 283
Group B streptococcal infection 120
Growth
    chart 148f, 149f
    constitutional delay of 109
    hormone deficiency 263
Guillain-Barré syndrome 21f, 26f
Gut-brain intersection 58f
Gynecomastia 36f, 305

H

Haemophilus influenzae 204, 258, 276

Hair
    light-colored 10f
    on-end appearance 331f
    premature graying of 307
Hairy cell leukemia 50f
Hairy pinna 36f
Halitosis 161
    bronchiectasis 162
    chronic rhinitis 161
    foreign body in nose 161
    history 161
    infections 162
    investigations 161
    lung abscess 162
    physical examination 161
    remaining causes of 162
Hallermann-Stroff syndrome 29f
Haloperidol 87
Halstrea's antibody-dependent immune 245
Hamartoma, pathologically 23f
Hamman-Rich syndrome 126
Hand-Schuller-Christian disease 252
Harrison sulcus 211, 301
Hay fever 5f
Head injury, severe 36f
Headache 163
    causes of 165
    drugs 164
    history 163
    investigations 163
    physical examination 163
    related to
        epilepsy 164
        eye problems 164
        psychiatric disease 164
        psychological problems 164
        sinusitis 164
    severe 22f
    tension 164
    vascular 163
Hearing
    loss 300
    phases of 106b
Heart
    disease 103
        congenital 82, 103, 127
        cyanotic congenital 83
        history of 100
    failure 121
    murmurs 166
        history 166
        investigations 167
        physical examination 167
    rate viability 279
    right-sided 328
Heat rash 256
Helicobacter pylori infection 57, 63
Hemangioma 179, 187, 276
    capillary 9f
Hematemesis 170, 267
    causes of 172
        pediatric 170, 170b
    drugs 171

hemorrhagic disease 171
history 170
in later infancy
    and childhood 171
    blood dyscrasias 172
    chalasia 171
    corrosive esophagitis 172
    drugs 172
    esophageal varices 171
    hiatal hernia 171
    peptic ulceration 171
    swallowed blood 171
    violent retching 172
in newborn 170
investigations 170
physical examination 170
remaining causes of 171
swallowed maternal blood 170
Hematogenous diseases 183, 231
    anemias 270
    hypersplenism 270
    thrombocytopenic purpura 270
Hematoma 27f, 242f
Hematuria 11f, 69, 173, 174, 229, 230
    bleeding diathesis 175
    drugs 175
    factitious hematuria 175
    foreign body 175
    hemolytic uremic syndrome 174
    hemorrhagic cystitis 175
    Henoch-Schönlein purpura 174
    history 173
    investigations 173
    meatal ulceration 175
    nephropathy 173
    nephrotic syndrome 174
    physical examination 173
    remaining causes of 176
    renal
        calculus 175
        tuberculosis 175
        vein thrombosis 175
    trauma to perineum 175
    urethral carbuncle 175
    urethritis 175
    urinary tract infection 174
    Wilms' tumor 175
Hemichorea 191
Hemicrania 163
Hemihypertrophy 215, 215f, 306
Hemiparesis 163
Hemiplegia 215
Hemoglobin
    abnormal 103, 105
    physiologic reduction of 69
Hemoglobinuria 173
Hemolysis 201
Hemolytic disease 70, 132, 134, 197
Hemolytic uremic syndrome 71, 244
Hemophilia 18f
    diagnosis of 206
Hemoptysis 177
    bronchiectasis 177

foreign body 177
history 177
investigations 177
physical examination 177
remaining causes of 178
whooping cough 178
Hemorrhage
adrenal 57
gastric 230
subarachnoid 36*f*
subconjunctival 13*f*, 299
subperiosteal 302*f*
Hemorrhagic disease 74
Hemosiderosis 185
Henoch-Schönlein purpura 62, 69, 174, 203, 244, 258*f*
Heparin 43*f*
Hepatic disorders 84
Hepatitis
A 181*t*
B 13*f*, 181*t*
Hepatitis
amebic 182
chronic
active 182, 182*f*
persistent 182
idiopathic neonatal 199
neonatal 199, 199*t*
Hepatoblastoma 11*f*, 186*f*
Hepatoma 11*f*
Hepatomegaly 179
in later infancy 181
and childhood 181
congestive hepatomegaly 184
infections 181
inflammations 181
malignant diseases 186
nutritional problems 184
storage diseases 184
in newborn 179
alpha-1-antitrypsin deficiency 180
cholesterol storage disease 181
congestive cardiac failure 179
erythroblastosis fetalis 180
extrahepatic biliary atresia 180
galactosemia 180
gangliosidoses 181
intrauterine infections 180
neonatal hepatitis 180
septicemia 180
Wolman disease 181
investigations 179
physical examination 179
Hepatotoxic drugs 187
Hereditary hemorrhagic telangiectasia 245
Hermaphroditism 65
female 65
male 65
true 66
Hernia
congenital inguinal 26*f*
diaphragmatic 121, 121*f*, 125
hiatal 62, 286
Herpes gingivostomatitis 159

Herpes labialis 10*f*
Herpes simplex 257*f*
virus 14*f*
Herpes zoster 10*f*, 78, 257*f*
High alkaline phosphatase 318
High arched palate 37*f*
High sweat chloride 320
Hilar enlargement 323
bilateral 323*f*
Hip
and knee 261
congenital dislocation of 213, 216*f*
developmental dysplasia of 213
tuberculosis of 214
Hirschsprung's disease 89, 90, 91, 286
Histiocytosis 252
Histoplasmin skin test 270
Histoplasmosis 251
Hoarseness 144, 188, 275
acute laryngitis 189
congenital laryngeal anomalies 189
foreign body 188
history 188
investigations 188
physical examination 188
remaining causes of 189
trauma to larynx 188
weakness of laryngeal muscles 189
Hodgkin's lymphoma 22*f*, 57, 84, 223, 231, 251, 271
Homocystinuria 281*t*
Hookworm 112
infestation 69
Horseshoe kidney 175
Howell-Jolly bodies 311, 312*f*
Human chorionic gonadotropin 109
Human immunodeficiency virus 16*f*, 107, 183, 250, 300*f*
Human placental lactogen 19*f*
Huntington's chorea 191
Hurler's disease 26*f*
Hurler's syndrome 38*f*, 211, 331*f*
Hyaline membrane disease 118, 119
Hydatid
cysts, multiple 325*f*
disease 182
Hydrocephalus 209*b*, 211*f*, 332*f*
acquired 25*f*
congenital 22*f*, 34*f*, 44*f*, 210, 210*f*, 295*f*
Hydrochloric acid 172
Hydropneumothorax 125*f*, 326*f*
Hydrops fetalis 26*f*
Hydrops gallbladder 232
Hygroma, cystic 35*f*, 42*f*
Hymenolepis nana 75, 114, 151
Hyoscine 194
Hyperbilirubinemia
severe neonatal 108
unconjugated 197*b*
Hypercellular bone marrow 315, 316*f*
Hyperesthesia 10*f*
Hyperkinetic syndrome 331*f*
Hyperlipemia 21*f*
Hyperlipidemia 34*f*

Hyperplasia, congenital adrenal 19*f*, 44*f*, 67
Hyperprolactinemia 110
Hyperreactive airway 279
Hypertelorism 3*f*, 17*f*, 297
Hypertension 27*f*, 163
benign intracranial 164
extrahepatic portal 13*f*
portal 57
Hyperthermia 279
Hyperthyroidism 41*f*
Hypertrophic pyloric stenosis, congenital 286
Hyperuricemia 21*f*
Hyperventilation 126
Hypervitaminosis
A 43*f*, 81
D 154
Hypoalbuminemia 57
Hypocalcemic tetany 94
Hypocellular bone marrow 315, 316*f*
Hypochondria
left 226
right 226
Hypochondrium
left 231
gallbladder 232
gut 231
hypogastrium 232
iliopsoas sheath 232
kidney 232
lymph nodes 231
right and left lumbar regions 231
right iliac fossa 231
testis 232
umbilical region 231
urinary bladder 232
right 228
adrenals 230
aorta 231
epigastrium 230
gallbladder 229
gut 229
kidney 229, 230
liver 228
lymph nodes 231
pancreas 230
subphrenic abscess 229
Hypogastrium 228
Hypoglycemia 21*f*, 29*f*, 34*f*, 72, 94, 96, 197
Hypogonadism
hypergonadotropic 110
hypogonadotropic 109
Hypokalemia 91, 230
Hypomagnesemia tetany 96
Hyponatremia 230
Hypoparathyroidism, idiopathic 96
Hypopharynx, posterior 21*f*
Hypospadias 25*f*
Hypotelorism 297
Hypothalamic-pituitary region 110
Hypothermia 197, 218
Hypothyroidism 45*f*, 56, 107*f*
congenital 19*f*, 24*f*, 146, 146*f*, 200
goitrogenous 21*f*

Hypotonia 146
    benign congenital 26f, 145
    severe 91
Hypoxia, high altitude 127
Hypsarrhythmia 98
Hysteria 129
Hysterical fits 98

I

Ibuprofen 60
Ichthyosis
    congenital 7f
    vulgaris 8f, 303f
Icterus 195
    gravis 197
Iliac fossa
    left 228
    right 61, 227
Imipramine 129, 194
Immersion burns 80f
Immune
    function, altered 112
    thrombocytopenic purpura 46f, 244, 258f
Immunoglobulin A nephropathy 174
Immunologic disorders 35f
Imperforate anus 28f
Impetigo 5f, 257f
Indian Childhood Cirrhosis 57, 186, 253
Indomethacin 60, 283
Infant's muscles 145
Infantile tremor syndrome 10f, 191, 191f
Infections
    bacterial 248
    chronic 263
    congenital 269
Infectious diseases 5f
Infestations 5f
Inflammation 13f
Inflammatory bowel disease 246
Inflammatory skin diseases 5f
Inguinal canal 65
Inguinal hernia 227f
Inguinal lymphadenitis 223
Intensive investigational workup 262b
International League against Epilepsy 97b
Interphalangeal joints, proximal 17f, 205
Interstitial pneumonia 183
Intestinal intraluminal causes 112
Intestinal mucosal causes 112
Intestinal obstruction 23f
Intestinal parasitosis 91, 112, 148, 150
Intestinal tuberculosis 229, 230
Intestinal worm infestation 63, 68
Intra-abdominal air collection,
    abnormal 328
Intracranial calcification 331
Intracranial pressure 265
Intracranial space-occupying lesion 332f
Intracranial tumors 235
Intrauterine growth retardation 30f, 259
Intrauterine infections 14f, 197, 199, 265
Intravenous substance abuse 129

Intraventricular hemorrhage 122
Intussusception 61, 75, 330f
Involuntary movements 190
    athetosis 192
    choreiform movements 191
    drug-induced 192
    history 190
    myoclonus 192
    physical examination 190
    psychogenic 192
    seizure 192
    tics 192
    tremors 190
Iodine deficiency 21f
Iris
    coloboma 300
    periphery of 5f
Iron
    absorption, inadequate 69
    deficiency anemia 311f
        causes of 69b
        chronic 24f, 331f
    supply, inadequate 69
Irritability 193
    acrodynia 194
    colic 194
    drugs 194
    food intolerance 194
    history 193
    hypoglycemia 194
    insecurity 194
    investigations 193
    narcotic withdrawal syndrome 193
    physical examination 193
    pink disease 194
    serious infections 193
    teething 194
Irritable bowel syndrome 116
Isonex 129
Isoniazid 283

J

Japanese encephalitis 34f
Jaundice 195
    acholuric 70
    breast-milk 198
    congenital acholuric 70, 201
    familial nonhemolytic 198
    in later infancy and childhood 200
    in newborn 196
        after first week 200
        first day 196
        fourth to seventh day 198
        second or third day 198
    persistent 200
    physical examination 195
    physiologic 198
Jejunal biopsy 18f
Jitteriness tremors 191
Jittery tremors 191
Joint
    ankles 215

    distal interphalangeal 17f
    feet 215
    fixed 206
    hips 213
    knees 214
    spine 215
Joint pain 203
    acute leukemia 207
    ankylosing spondylitis 207
    drugs 207
    gut arthropathy 207
    hemarthrosis 206
    Henoch-Schönlein purpura 206
    history 203
    investigations 203
    physical examination 203
    psoriasis 207
    reactive arthritis 207
    Reiter disease 207
    remaining causes of 208
    rheumatic fever 205
    septic arthritis 204
    serum sickness 206
    sickle cell anemia 206
    systemic lupus erythematosus 206
    trauma 203
    tuberculous arthritis 204
    viral arthritis 204
Jugular venous pressure 105, 127, 133, 134
Juxta-articular cysts 206

K

Kala-azar 269f
Kallmann syndrome 109
Kanamicin 147, 283
Kaposi sarcoma 183
Kartagener's syndrome 292
Kasabach-Merritt syndrome 244
Kawasaki disease 33f, 44f, 223, 247, 256, 256f
Kayser-Fleischer ring 33f, 190
Keck's classification 166t
Keratomalacia 39f
Kernig signs 218, 273
Ketoacidosis, diabetic 87f
Ketotic hypoglycemia 288
Kidneys 57
    bilateral
        large 329
        small 329
    unilateral
        large 329
        small 329
Kiesselbach's area 143
Kiesselbach's plexus 142
Klebsiella 114, 198
    aeruginosa 198
    infection 327f
Klinefelter syndrome 110
Knock-knee deformity 30f, 302
Krammer's guidelines 196t
Kwashiorkor 10f, 28f, 35f, 135f
    type 57

L

Labyrinthitis, acute 72
Lactate dehydrogenase 185, 244
   high serum 318
Lactic acidosis 21f, 34f
Lactose 63
Lange-Nielsen syndromes 278
Large head 209
   causes of 209b
   cerebral gigantism 211
   gangliosidosis 212
   history 209
   hydrancephaly 212
   hydrocephalus 210
   investigations 210
   megalencephaly 211
   physical examination 209
   vitamin D deficiency 211
Laryngeal cleft 279
Laryngeal disease 100
Laryngitis
   acute infectious 189
   acute spasmodic 189
Laryngomalacia 279
Laryngospasm 277
Laryngotracheobronchitis, acute 189, 276
Laurence-Moon-Biedl syndrome 33f, 238
Lead encephalopathy 96
Lead poisoning 91
Legg-Calve-Perthes disease 214
Leishmania donovani 182, 269
Leprosy 143
Lethargy 144, 218
   anemia 218
   chronic fatigue syndrome 219
   history 218
   infections 218
   investigations 218
   low-grade infection 218
   physical examination 218
   postictal stage 218
   remaining causes of 219
Letterer-Siwe disease 252
Leukemia 13f, 16f, 57, 69, 252, 267, 323f
   acute
      lymphoblastic 38f, 207
      lymphocytic 50f, 223
      myeloid 50f
   chronic
      lymphocytic 50f
      myeloid 50f
Leukemoid reaction 315, 315f
Leukocoria 299f
Leukocytosis 178
Leydig cell 109
   tumors 239
Limb hypertrophy, congenital 302
Limping 213
   bones 213
   history 213
   investigations 213
   joints 213
   neuromuscular frame 215

   physical examination 213
   remaining causes of 217
Lips, mucosal pigmentation of 23f
Listeria monocytogenes 198
Liver
   abscess, amebic 182
   biopsy 13f, 199
   cirrhosis of 152, 200
   disease, chronic 14f, 37f, 134, 199
   disorder 135, 142
   function test 133, 170
Lobar emphysema, congenital 122
Lobe consolidation, middle 327
Löffler's syndrome 124
Lovibond profile sign 82, 83f
Low serum
   albumin 316
   calcium 318
   magnesium 319
   phosphate 319
   proteins 316
   urea 319
Lower lobe pneumonia 62
Lumbar regions
   left 226
   right 226
Lump, intra-abdominal 225, 228
Lung
   cysts 122
      congenital 122
   density
      large 326
      multiple 325
   disease 120
      chronic 82
   fields, peripheral 124
   radiolucency 326
Luteinizing hormone 239, 262
Lymph glands, groups of 220f
Lymphadenitis
   acute 221
   chronic 222
      septic 222
   filarial 223
Lymphadenopathy 220, 223
   bilateral inguinal 35f
   chronic 183
   drugs 224
   history 220
   immunologic disorders 223
   infections 221
   inflammations 221
   investigations 221
   malignant diseases 223
   neoplastic diseases 223
   physical examination 221
Lymphangiectasia, congenital pulmonary 122
Lymphangioma 276
Lymphedema precox 137f
Lymphocytosis 314, 314f
Lymphogranuloma venereum 251
Lymphoma 323f
Lymphopenia 314

Lymphoreticulosis, benign 223
Lysergic acid diethylamide 87

M

Macrocephaly 295
   causes of 209, 209b
Macroglossia 118, 299
Macroorchidism 306
Maculopapular rash 255
Magnesium, high serum 319
Malabsorption states 151
Malabsorptive disorders, major 111
Malaria 250, 267, 268f
   chronic 16f, 182f
Malignant diseases 231
Mallory-Weiss syndrome 172
Malnutrition 134
   acute 22f, 150f
   chronic 22f, 149, 150f
Malodorous breath 161
Mantoux test 249, 291, 320
Maple syrup urine disease 10f, 95
Marble bone disease 31f, 71
Marfan's syndrome 15f, 39f, 147, 281f, 281t
Mass, palpable hard 90
Mastoiditis 249
Maternal blood, swallowed 74, 170
Maternal drug addiction 191
McCune-Albright syndrome 6f
Meadow's syndrome 175
Mean corpuscular volume 311
   increased 311
Measles 40f, 255, 255f
   encephalitis 22f
Meatal stenosis 131
Meckel's diverticulum 61, 69, 75
Meckel-Gruber syndrome 16f, 31f
Meconium aspiration syndrome 119, 119f, 122
Meconium ileus 61, 90, 90f
Meconium plug syndrome 90
Medastinum widening, posterior 324f
Mediastinal shift 323
Mediastinal widening, superior 324f
Mediastinum
   enlargement
      of middle 324
      of posterior 324
      of superior 324
   widened anterior 323f
Medulloblastoma 73
Mefenamic acid 60, 71
Megakaryocytic hyperplasia 316
Megaloblastic anemia 312f
Meningitis 16f, 36f, 286, 305
   recurring 305
Meningocele 18f
   anterior 57
   cranial 17f
Meningococcemia 245, 257, 258f
Meningomyelocele 22f, 210f
Mental development index 69

Mental retardation 138, 296
   microcephaly with 19f
Mesenteric lymphadenitis 61
Metabolic acidosis 185
Metabolic diseases 26f
Metabolism, inborn errors of 197, 231
Metacarpal bones 261
Metacarpal sign 333
Metacarpophalangeal joints 17f
Metachromatic leukodystrophy 211
Metastasis 323f
Methemoglobinemia 103
Methicillin 175
Methotrexate 129
Methylphenidate 192
Microangiopathic hemolytic anemia 52f
Microcephaly 295
   microphthalmia 16f
Microcytic anemia 311
Microcytic-hypochromic anemia, severe 184
Micrognathia 37f, 46f, 295, 295f
Microorchidism 306
Micropenis 306
Microphthalmia 14f
Micturition, frequency of 153
   attention-seeking device 154
   cystitis 153
   diabetes
      insipidus 154
      mellitus 154
   drugs 154
   history 153
   investigations 153
   physical examination 153
   posterior urethral valves 154
   remaining causes of 154
Migraine 163
   partial 163
Miliaria rubra 256
Miliary bronchopneumonia 325f
Milkmaid sign 191
Milroy's disease 37f, 132, 136f
Minocycline 283
Mitotic inhibitors 43f
Mitral incompetence 168
Molloscum contagiosum 258f
Monday morning pain 64
Moniliasis 159
Monocytosis 314, 314f
Mononucleosis, infectious 183, 250, 256, 256f
Monozygotic twins 28f
Moon-Biedl syndrome 110
Mouth breathing 101, 233
   adenoids 233
   choanal atresia 233
   deviated nasal septum 234
   foreign body 234
   habit 234
   history 233
   investigations 233
   maternal medication 233
   nasal
      allergy 233
      polyp 234
   physical examination 233

Mucoviscidosis 152
Mumps 42f, 136
Murmur 304
   continuous 169
   innocent 166
   soft mid-diastolic 168
Muscle 147
   flabby abdominal 56
   pains 272
   power, grading of 213b
   traumatic avulsion of 214
Muscular dystrophy 216
Musculoskeletal disorder 213
Myalgia 222
   epidemic 62, 78
Myasthenia
   gravis 145, 189
   neonatal 26f
Myocarditis 127, 327f
Myoclonic epilepsy, infantile 98
Myoglobinuria 173
Myopathy 217
Myotonic muscular dystrophy 216f, 217

N

Nail-patella syndrome 176
Nalidixic acid 283
Nappy rash 11f
Nasal discharge, unilateral 161
Natal teeth 29f
Nausea 34f
Neck
   lymph glands of 220f
   rigidity 305
   short 297
Neonatal jaundice 196f, 197, 198f
   causes of 196b
Neoplastic disease 35f
Nephritic syndrome 134
Nephritis 174
   acute 135, 173
      poststreptococcal 173
Nephroblastoma 11f, 230
Nephrotic syndrome 11f, 57, 133, 135f
Nerves, peripheral 147
Neuroblastoma 11f, 57, 186, 229, 252, 324f
Neurocysticercosis 97f
   stages of 333f
Neurofibromatosis 6f
Neurologic signs, soft 307
Neurological defects 138
Neuromuscular
   disorder 213
   junction 147
Neuropathic state 101
Neutropenia 313, 313f
Neutrophil
   leukocytosis 313
   leukopenia 313
Neutrophilia 313, 313f
Niacin deficiency 160
Nicotinamide adenine dinucleotide,
   deficiency of 105

Niemann-Pick
   cell 185
   disease 71, 185, 199
Nikolsky sign 7f
Nitric acid test 137
Nitroblue tetrazolium test 223
Nitrofurantoin 71
   rifampicin 129
Noncardiac pulmonary edema 119
Nondigestive tract 60b
Nonenhancing lesions 332
Non-Hodgkin's lymphoma 11f, 224, 252, 271
Nonsteroidal anti-inflammatory drugs 60
Nontyphoidal salmonellosis 96
Noonan's syndrome 37f, 110, 264
Normocytic anemia 311
Nose
   depressed bridge of 297
   picking 143
Nursemaid's elbow 203
Nutritional anemia 69
Nutritional deficiencies 109
Nutritional disorders 134
Nutritional marasmus 27f
Nutritional rickets 26f, 211, 301f, 333f
Nystagmus 235
   congenital 236
      jerky 236
      pendular 236
   history 235
   investigations 235
   labyrinthine 236
   optokinetic 235
   organic 235
   physical examination 235
   physiologic 235
   simulating eye movements 236

O

Obesity 56, 126, 157, 237
   causes of 238
   endogenous 238
   exogenous 237
   history 237
   hypoventilation 238
   investigations 237
   physical examination 237
Ocular motor dysmetria 236
Oliguria 35f
Omphalocele, congenital 226
Opaque hemithorax 327
Ophthalmoplegia 43f
Opisthotonos 36f, 305
   causes of 36f
Optic atrophy, congenital 236
Oral malodor 161
Oral thrush 159
Organic vomiting, causes of 285
Oropharynx, posterior 21f
Orthopnea 117
Osgood-Schlatter disease 215
Osler-Weber-Rendu disease 245
Osmotic diarrhea 111, 114
Osteitis 78

Osteochondritis 214
Osteogenesis imperfect
    congenital 27f
        deformities in 333f
    tarda 81
Osteomyelitis 16f, 204, 249
Osteopetrosis 31f
Ototoxic drugs, administration of 107
Oxycephaly 265
Oxyuriasis 151

P

Pain, colicky abdominal 62
Palpation, abdominal 60
Palpitations 190
P-aminosalicylic acid 244
Pancreas 57
Pancreatic cyst 57
Pancreatitis
    acute 61
    chronic 57
Pancreatogenous steatorrhea 149
Pansystolic murmur 168
Paper chromatography 137
Papilloma 276
Para-aminosalicylate sodium 129
Para-aminosalicylic acid 62
Paranasal sinusitis 24f
Parasitic infections 250
Parathyroid disease 331f
Paronychia 10f
    congenital 29f
Parotid gland, swelling of 61
Parotid swelling 300
    recurrent 300f
Parthenium 132
Pasqualini syndrome 109
Patau syndrome 14f, 47f
Patent ductus arteriosus 127, 166, 269
Pathologic fracture 333, 333f
Pectus carinatum 301, 301f
Pectus excavatum 41f, 301, 301f
Pel-Ebstein fever 251
Pemphigus vulgaris 9f
Penicillin 10f, 71, 129
Peptic ulcer 61
Periappendicitis 249
Pericardial effusion 327f
Pericarditis 78
    constrictive 57
Pericardium 26f, 57
Perinatal hypoxia 107
Perinephric abscess manifests 230
Periodic acid-Schiff 180
Periodic fever 253
Periodic syndrome 64
Periorbital cellulitis 24f, 43f
Periorbital edema 173, 297
Peritoneum 26f
Peritonitis
    acute 61
        primary 61
        secondary 61
    sign of 56, 60

Perleche 159
Persistent fetal circulation 122
Perthes disease 214
Pertussis 13f, 23f, 101
Peter's anomaly 12f
Peter's plus syndrome 12f
Peutz-Jeghers syndrome 23f
Pharyngitis, bacterial 273
Phenacetin 71
Phenothiazines 283
Phenylbutazone 71
Phenylketonuria 194, 265
Phenytoin 159, 283
Philtrum, smooth 43f
Phocomelia 43f
Phosphate, high serum 318
Phosphaturia 319
Phosphokinase, high creatine 317
Photophobia 195
Phrynoderma 303f
Pickwick papers 126
Pierre-Robin syndrome 29f, 37f, 46f, 118
Pigeon chest 301, 301f
    deformity 306
Pinpoint pupil 300
Pituitary dwarf 24f, 32f
Plasmodium falciparum infection 95
Platelet
    sequestration of 315
    survival, poor 315
Platypnea 117
Plethoric chubby appearance 36f
Pleura 26f
Pleural effusion 121, 124, 326f
    massive 124f
Pleurisy 78
Pleuritis 101
Pleurodynia 62, 78
Pneumatocele 124f
    multiple 124f
Pneumatosis intestinalis 75
Pneumococcus 204, 276
Pneumonia 78, 100, 120, 123
    eosinophilic 124
    postnatal 120
Pneumonic consolidation 123f
Pneumonitis 134
Pneumoperitoneum 55
Pneumothorax 120, 121f, 125
    neonatal 121f
Poikilocytosis 70, 184
Polio 213
Poliomyelitis 21f, 215
Polyarteritis nodosa 251
Polyarticular arthritis, juvenile idiopathic 17f
Polychromasia 202
Polycystic kidney 229
Polydactyly 16f, 20f, 31f, 45f, 302
Polydypsia 141
Polymerase chain reaction 254
Polyp 69, 75
    internal 75
Polyphagia 141
Polysyndactyly 31f

Polyuria 91, 141
Pontine glioma 73
Popliteal cysts 214
Porphyria 62
Postmeasles
    encephalomyelitis 22f
    pigmentation 41f
Postpolio residual paresis 35f, 215f
Pott's spine 27f, 204
Potter's facies 15f, 122, 307, 307f
Potter's syndrome 122, 307
Prader-Willi syndrome 144, 147
Precocious pseudopuberty 240
    adrenogenital syndrome 240
    feminizing adrenal tumors 241
    tumors of testes 241
    virilizing adrenocortical tumors 241
Precocious puberty 36f, 239
    boys 239
    central 239
    girls 239
    history 239
    investigations 240
    physical examination 239
Priapism 38f
Prickly heat 256
Prickly poppy 137
Primaquine 71
Primidone 194
Prochlorperazine 272
Progeria 16f
Proglottids 151
Proptosis 299
Prostatitis 131
Protein
    bound iodine, low 146
    energy malnutrition 26f, 56, 133, 144
    high serum 316
Provocative stimulus 47f
Pseudoesotropia 298f
Pseudohermaphroditism
    female 67
    male 66, 66f
Pseudo-Hirschsprung's disease 91
Pseudohypertelorism 3f, 147
Pseudohypertrophy 216
    muscular dystrophy 216f
Pseudohypoparathyroidism 20f
Pseudomembranous
    colitis, antibiotic-associated 75
    enterocolitis 61
Pseudomonas 198, 327f
    aeruginosa 114
Psittacosis 251
Psoriasis 8f
    besides 5f
Psychiatric stress 43f
Psychogenic epilepsy 98
Psychogenic involuntary movements 192b
Psychogenic pain abdomen 64
Psychomotor epilepsy 98
Ptosis 298
    congenital 298f
    familial 25f
    unilateral congenital 298f

Pubertal stages
 in boys 260t
 in girls 260t
Puberty
 constitutional delay of 109
 delayed 109, 110f
 signs of 240, 241
Pulmonary agenesis 122
Pulmonary alveolar
 microlithiasis 126
 proteinosis 126
Pulmonary arteriovenous hypertension 323f
Pulmonary disorders 83
 chronic suppuration 83
Pulmonary edema 324f, 326
Pulmonary embolism 78, 127
Pulmonary hemorrhage 119
 massive 120
Pulmonary hemosiderosis 126, 324f
Pulmonary hyperplasia 122
Pulmonary hypertension, persistent 119, 122
Pulmonary infarction 78, 127
Pulmonary metastases 327
Pulmonary stenosis 168
Pulmonary tuberculosis 83, 221
Pulmonary veno-occlusive disease 126
Pupillary reaction, pattern of 86
Purpura 242
 complicating 9f
 episodes of 242
 fulminans 245
 history 242
 in later infancy and childhood 244
 nonthrombocytopenic 244
 physical examination 242
 thrombocytopathic 244
 thrombocytopenic 244
Purpura in newborn 243
 causes of 243
 disseminated intravascular
  coagulation 243
 hemolytic disease 243
 immune neonatal thrombocytopenia 243
 intrauterine infections 243
 maternal medication during pregnancy 243
 septicemia 243
Pyelonephritis 62
Pyemic abscesses, part of multiple 16f
Pyogenic meningitis 94, 95, 272, 273
Pyrexia 37f, 222
 of unknown origin, etiology of 246b
Pyridoxine deficiency 160

Q

Q fever 251
Quinidine 71

R

Rachitic rosary 301f
Radioactive iodine, low 146

Rash 254
 appearance of 22f
 causes of neonatal 255
 history 254
 investigations 254
 physical examination 254
Rash in infancy 255
 and childhood 255
 Henoch-Schönlein purpura 258
 herpes simplex-type i 257
 herpes zoster 257
 immune thrombocytopenic purpura 258
 impetigo 257
 leukemia 258
 molluscum contagiosum 257
 petechial 257
 purpuric 257
 vesicular 256
Rash in newborn 254
 erythema toxicum 254
 herpes simplex 255
 impetigo neonatorum 255
 neonatal
  miliaria 255
  varicella 255
 staphylococcal skin infection 254
Rectal prolapse 18f, 49f
Red blood cells 68, 173, 244
 normal 49f
Red cell production, inadequate 71
Redman syndrome 45f
Refsum's syndrome 73, 73f
Reifenstein syndrome 67
Renal disorders 135
Renal function test 133
Renal tuberculosis 229
Renal tubular acidosis 26f
Rendu-Osler-Weber disease 143
Respiratory distress 46f, 118b, 223
 syndrome 29f, 118f, 118t, 119t
  idiopathic 118
Respiratory infection 42f
Respiratory insufficiency 27f
Respiratory origin, cyanosis of 104
Respiratory stability 279
Respiratory tract infections
 lower 100
 upper 100
Restlessness 275
Reticular granular pattern 328
Retinoblastoma 299f
Retrolental fibroplasia 236
Retropharyngeal lymphadenitis 277
Reye's syndrome 126, 184, 288
Rhesus isoimmunization 23f
Rheumatic chorea 191
Rheumatic fever 205f
Rheumatic heart disease 129
Rheumatic pericarditis 129
Rheumatic stiff neck 273
Rheumatoid arthritis 246
 juvenile 205f, 223, 251
Rheumatoid rash 223

Rhizomelia 33f
Rhizomelic chondrodysplasia 33f
Rib
 crack of 78
 fracture of 78
Riboflavin deficiency 159
Rickets 26f, 57f, 211, 296
 advanced refractory 30f
Rickettsial diseases 251
Rickettsial infection 251
Rifampicin 71
Ritter's disease 7f
Rose-Bengal test 199
Roseola infantum 255, 255f
Rose-Thorn arthritis 208
Rotavirus 114
Rotor's syndrome 199
Rouleaux formation 312, 313f
Roundworm 112
Rubella 14f, 243, 256
 syndrome, congenital 11f
Russell-Silver syndrome 4f
Ryle's tube trauma 75

S

Sacral lipoma 16f
Sacrococcygeal teratoma 47f
Salicylates 71, 129
Salmonella 16f, 61, 75, 114, 204
 typhi 183, 268
Sarcoidosis 253
Scabies 8f
Scalp hair, light-colored 296
Scalp veins, prominent 210
Scaphocephalic skull 266f
Scaphocephaly 266f
Scarlet fever 44f, 256
 rash 256f
Schamroth sign 82, 82f
Schistosoma mansoni infection 16f
Schizocytes 243
Sclerema 134
Scoliosis 30f, 304
Scorbutic rosary 32f
Scrofuloderma 222f, 303
Scrotal edema, idiopathic 136
Scrotal tongue 147
Scrotum 65
Scurvy 13f, 160, 333f
Seborrhea, infantile 5f
Seborrheic dermatitis 11f
 infantile 5f
Secretory function, altered 112
Seizure 36f, 93
 accidental injection of anesthesia 94
 atypical febrile 22f
 disorders
  acute 95
  chronic 97
  recurrent 97
 drug 95
  withdrawal syndrome 94

electrolyte imbalance 94
history 93
hypocalcemia 94
hypoglycemia 94
hypomagnesemia 94
in later infancy 95
infections 94
investigations 93
metabolic disorders 95
perinatal problems 94
physical examination 93
pyridoxine dependency 94
Seizures in newborn 93
   accidental injection of anesthesia 94
   drug 95
      withdrawal syndrome 94
   electrolyte imbalance 94
   hypocalcemia 94
   hypoglycemia 94
   hypomagnesemia 94
   infections 94
   metabolic disorders 95
   perinatal problems 94
   pyridoxine dependency 94
Sella turcica, J-shaped 331
Senile appearance 302
Sensorium 272, 284
Sepsis, neonatal 21f, 38f
Septic arthritis 214
Septicemia 183, 198, 200, 249, 286
   advanced fulminant 243
   neonatal 180
Serotonin 279
Serum
   ascites albumin gradient 13f
   glutamic
      oxaloacetic transaminase 180, 250
      pyruvic transaminase 180, 250
   hepatitis 181
   sickness 253
Sex maturation 240
Sex maturity stages
   in boys 260t
   in girls 260t
Sexually transmitted disease 223
Shagreen patch 6f
Shigella 61, 111, 114, 207
   infection 75
Shigellosis 96
Shoe-like sella 331f
Short stature 259, 263f
   causes of 259b
   chromosomal disorders 264
   chronic visceral diseases 263
   constitutional 262
   disproportionate 12f, 259
   emotional deprivation 263
   endocrinopathy 263
   familial 262
   genetic 262
   history 259
   investigations 261
   nutritional stunting 263
   physical examination 259

   primordial dwarfism 263
   proportionate 259
   skeletal disorders 263
   sophisticated tests 262
Shoulder 261
Sibling's development 239
Sick sinus syndrome 279
Sickle cell 50f, 69
   anemia 38f, 64, 68, 70, 184, 203, 253
   disease 16f, 143, 165, 267
Silk glove sign 228
Silver-beaten appearance 332, 332f
Silverman-Russell syndrome 45f
Silver-Russell syndrome 263
Simian crease 305
Sinus
   bradycardia 303
   tachycardia 303
Sinusitis 163, 164, 249
Situs inversus 328f
Skeletal dysplasia 66
Skin 24f
   dry 303
   hyperkeratotic 303
   rash 254b
   scaly 303
   tuberculosis 303
Skull roentgenogram 265
Skull shape, abnormal 330
Skull sutures, premature union of 265
Small head 265
   craniostenosis 265
   craniosynostosis 265
   familial 266
   history 265
   investigations 265
   microcephaly 265
   normal variation 266
   physical examination 265
   small infant 266
Small intestine, obstruction of 287
Snakebite 12f, 40f, 49f
Soap bubble appearance 328
Sodium excretion 57
Soft palate 21f
Soft tissue edema 21f
Solitary lung densities 325
Sore throat 272
Sotos syndrome 19f, 21f, 211
Sparse 10f, 296
Spasmus nutans 236
Spastic cerebral palsy 17f
Speech
   delayed 301
   phases of 106b
   retarded 301
Spherocyte 50f, 69
Spherocytic cell 70
Spherocytosis 68, 202
   congenital 200, 201
   hereditary 70, 200, 201
Sphincter
   external 139
   internal 139

Spider leg deformity 230
Spinal cord 147
Spinal muscular atrophy 145, 145f
   hereditary 26f
Splenic cysts, suspicion of 271
Splenic enlargement 267
Splenohepatomegaly 270f
Splenomegaly 267
   abscess 271
   congestive 231, 271
   extrahepatic biliary atresia 271
   hemangioma 271
   hematogenous diseases 270
   inborn errors of metabolism 271
   infections 268
      brucellosis 269
      common viral 270
      enteric fever 268
      histoplasmosis 270
      hydatid disease 270
      infectious mononucleosis 270
      infective endocarditis 269
      intrauterine 269
      kala-azar 269
      malaria 268
      neonatal hepatitis 270
      septicemia 268
      tuberculosis 268
   investigations 268
   malignant diseases 271
   nutritional recovery syndrome 271
   physical examination 267
   splenic cysts 271
   Still's disease 271
   systemic lupus erythematosus 271
   tropical 14f
Squint 298f
Staphylococcal
   gingivitis 159
   pneumonia 124f, 325f
Staphylococcus 5f, 114, 276
   albus 269
   aureus 182, 198
Starvation diarrhea 230, 286
Steatorrhea 82
Stein-Leventhal syndrome 238
Stenosis, congenital subglottic 276
Sternomastoid
   muscle 273
   tumor 23f
Steroid 132, 237
   therapy 43f
Stevens-Johnson syndrome 8f, 160
Stiff neck 272
   cervical lymphadenitis 273
   congenital anomalies 273
   history 272
   investigations 272
   meningitis 272
   phenothiazine toxicity 272
   remaining causes of 274
   retropharyngeal abscess 273
   trauma 273
   viral torticollis 273

Still's disease 231
Stomach, foreign body in 171
Stomatitis, aphthous 18f
Stomatocyte 313, 313f
Strawberry tongue 44f
Streptococcal gingivitis 159
Streptococcus 5f, 204
    viridans 269
Streptomycin 129
Stridor 275
    congenital laryngeal 275
    history 275
    investigations 275
    laryngeal edema 276
    laryngomalacia 275
    obstruction 276
    physical examination 275
    tumors 276
    vascular rings 276
Strongyloides stercoralis 63, 75, 112
Strongyloidiasis 151
Strychnine poisoning 36f
Sturge-Weber syndrome 93, 165
Sudamina 256
Sudden infant death syndrome 156, 278
    investigations 278
    physical examination 278
Sudden severe weight loss 43f
Sulfas 10f, 71, 129, 283
Sunken eyes 35f
Sunset sign 34f, 298
Superior vena cava 133
Sutural diastasis 331
Sweat chloride, false negative 320
Sweating 222
    absence of 248
Swyer syndrome 66
Syphilis 81, 93, 143, 222
    congenital 269
Systemic bacterial infections 174
Systemic disease 132
Systemic lupus erythematosus 19f, 187, 191, 246, 251
    nephropathy 174
Systolic murmurs 166, 167
    six grades of 166t

T

Tachycardia, paroxysmal supraventricular 303
Taenia
    saginata 151
    solium 115
Talipes equinovarus 304, 304f
    congenital 30f
Tall stature 280, 280b
    cerebral gigantism 282
    etiology of 280t
    familial 281
    history 280
    homocystinuria 281
    investigations 281
    Klinefelter syndrome 281
    Marfan syndrome 281
    physical examination 281
Tanner's pubertal staging 109
Tapeworms 58, 63, 112, 151
Target cells 50f, 184, 311
Taste 319
Tay-Sachs disease 211
Tear drop cell 312, 312f
Teeth, discoloration of 299
Temporal lobe epilepsy 98
Tender hepatic enlargement 306
Testes, absence of 65
Testicular hormone deficiency 65
Tetanus 36f, 47f, 94
    neonatal 34f
Tetracyclines 165
Tetralogy of Fallot 104, 128, 167f
Thalassemia 68
    major 70, 70f, 270f, 331f
Thalidomide baby 43f
Thallium 43f
Thiabendazole 165
Thiazides 61, 283
Thigh, painful swelling of 302
Thiouracil 43f
Thorazine 175
Threadworms 130
Thrombocytopenia 245, 315, 315f
Thrombocytopenic purpura
    drug-induced 244
    idiopathic 13f, 51f, 52f, 75
Thrombocytopoiesis, poor 315
Thrombocytosis 52f, 315, 315f
Thrombophlebitis 19f
Thrombopoietin deficiency 244
Thrombosis 57
Thyroid
    enlarged 190
    stimulating hormone 21f, 189, 263, 283
Thyrotoxicosis 19f
Thyroxine 194
Tics 101, 192
    types of 192
Tietze syndrome 78
Tiredness 69
Todd's paralysis 93
Toddler's diarrhea 116
Toilet training, poor 91, 140
Tongue protrudes 23f
Tonic-clonic movements 93
Tonsillar diphtheria 21f
Tonsillectomy 171
Tonsillitis 272
    acute 62, 171
Torticollis, congenital 274
Total leukocyte count 249, 291
Toxic
    alopecia 43f
    hepatitis 201
    shock syndrome 44f
    synovitis 214
Toxocara canis 246
Toxoplasma gondii 246
Toxoplasmosis 93, 243, 246, 250
    acquired 222
    congenital 269
Tracheoesophageal fistula 122
Tracheomalacia 279
Transient synovitis 214
Transient tachypnea 120, 120f
Trauma, abdominal 74
Treacher-Collins syndrome 39f, 298f
Trendelenburg limping 213, 215f
Trepopnea 117
Trichinosis 250
Trichobezoar 230
Trichuriasis 151
Trichuris trichiura 63, 112
Tricuspid atresia 29f, 104
Tricyclic antidepressants 147
Triflupromazine 272
Trigonocephaly 44f
Trimethoprim 164, 283
Trisomy 13 47f
Trisomy 18 48f
Troxidone 164, 194
True precocious puberty 240
    constitutional precocity 240
    hypothyroidism 240
    Mccune-Albright syndrome 240
    organic brain lesions 240
    rare causes of 240
Truncus 105
Tuberculin test 249, 291
    false negative 320
Tuberculosis 82, 143, 149, 249, 327
    diagnosis of 40f
    disseminated 36f
    generalized 268f
    history of 100
Tuberculous
    cervical lymphadenopathy 24f
    lymphadenitis 222f
    meningitis 3f, 24f, 273
    spondylitis 27f
Tuberous sclerosis 6f, 25f
Tularemia 249
Turner's syndrome 4f, 24f, 33f, 36f, 39f, 110, 199, 238, 264
    male 37f
Twin-twin transfusion 28f
Typhoid 267
Typhus 256
Tyrosinosis 57

U

Ulcerative colitis 61, 64, 69, 76, 116, 307
Ulcers 18f
    aphthous 160
Umbilical granuloma 20f, 226, 227f
Umbilical hernia 304
    large 226f
Umbilical region 226
Upper airway 276
    dysfunction 279

Upper extremity 35f
Upper lobe, right 123f, 326f
Urea, high serum 319
Urea-creatinine ratio, high serum 319
Uremia 230, 288
Urethra, local factors involving 131
Urinary tract infection 64, 246, 249, 288
Urine
    dipstick 133
    color of 60
Uterine hernia syndrome 66
Uveitis, acute 300

V

Vaginal bleeding 306
Valproate 237
Valvular pulmonic stenosis 128
Vanishing testes syndrome 110
Vasculitis 247
Vena cava, inferior 57
Veno-occlusive disease 200
Ventricular enlargement, left 328
Ventricular septal defect 29f, 127f, 166
    large 127
Versinia enterocolitica 114
Vertebral column, diseases of 78
Vertebral osteomyelitis 273
Vertigo 283
    anemia 283
    benign paroxysmal 283
    drugs 283
    epidemic 283
    history 283
    hypoglycemia 283
    investigations 283
    physical examination 283
    remaining causes of 284
    vasovagal response 283
Vesicular rash 256
Vibrio cholerae 114
Vincent's angina 159, 162
Vincristine 129, 164
Violent sneezing 13f
Viral bronchopneumonia 325f
Viral exanthema 254
Viral hepatitis 34f, 62, 200, 250
Viral infections 250
Viral myalgia 78, 272
Virilized clitoris 66f
Visceral larva migrans 246, 250
Visual defects 163
Vitamin
    A deficiency 39f
    D 30f
    D deficiency 57f
        rickets 26f, 151f
    deficiency 199
        diseases 150
    K 71
        deficiency 143, 271
Vitiligo 6f
Vocal cord paralysis 276
Vomiting 22f, 34f, 285
    history 285
    in later infancy 287
    investigations 285
    physical examination 285
    projectile 156
    severe 91
Vomiting after infancy 288
    benign 288
    infection 288
    obstructive 288
    organic 288
Vomiting in newborn 285
    benign 285
    organic 285
von Gierke disease 21f, 34f, 185
von Recklinghausen's disease 165
von Willebrand disease 143, 245
Vulvitis 154

W

Waardenburg syndrome 107f
Weight gain, excessive 157
Weil's disease 183
Werdnig-Hoffmann disease 144, 145, 189
Wheezing 289
    acute bronchiolitis 290
    asthmatic bronchitis 290
    bronchial asthma 290
    cystic fibrosis 291
    drugs 292
    foreign body 291
    history 289
    investigations 289
    physical examination 289
    pneumonia 291
    poisons 292
    remaining causes of 292
    tropical eosinophilia 290
    tuberculosis 291
White reflex 299
Whooping cough 18f, 101
    diagnosis of 178
Widal's test 221
Wilm's tumor 11f, 57, 175, 229, 230, 252
Wilson's disease 185, 190
Wilson-Mikity syndrome 120
Wing-beating 190
Wiskott-Aldrich syndrome 244
Wormian bones 330, 330f
Worms sign, bag of 191
Worsening sensorium 22f

X

Xanthochromic cerebrospinal fluid 320
Xerophthalmia 32f
XXY syndrome 281

Y

Yersinia 204
    enterocolitica 61, 114, 207, 250
    infection 250

Z

Zinc deficiency 10f
Zoonotic infection 246

EU GSPR Authorised Reprsentative
Logos Europe, 9 rue Nicolas Poussin
1700, La Rochelle, France
Phone: +33 (0) 6 67 93 73 78
E-mail: contact@logoseurope.eu

www.ingramcontent.com/pod-product-compliance
Ingram Content Group UK Ltd.
Pitfield, Milton Keynes, MK11 3LW, UK
UKHW050430150426
5217IPUK00019B/1329